CARDIOVASCULAR DISEASE

DISEASE

Epidemiology, Prevention, and Rehabilitation

A Guide to the Literature
Volume I: 1960 - 1973

CARDIOVASCULAR

DISEASE

Epidemiology, Prevention, and Rehabilitation

A Guide to the Literature
Volume I: 1960 - 1973

Senta S. Rogers, Ph.D.

Scientific and Coordinating Editor
Senior Staff Scientist

Irvin C. Mohler, M.A.

Administrative Editor
Research Instructor in Medical and Public Affairs and in Medicine

Division of Rehabilitation Medicine of the Department of Medicine and
Science Communication Division of the Department of Medical and Public Affairs
of the George Washington University Medical Center, Washington, D.C.

IFI/PLENUM • NEW YORK - WASHINGTON - LONDON

Library of Congress Cataloging in Publication Data

Rogers, Senta S
    Cardiovascular disease: epidemiology, prevention, and rehabilitation.

    CONTENTS: v. 1. 1960-1973.
    1. Cardiovascular system—Diseases—Bibliography.   1. Mohler, Irvin C., joint
author. II. Title. [DNLM: 1. Cardiovascular diseases—Bibliography. ZWG100
R729c]
Z6664.H3R63   016.6161   74-17250
ISBN 0-306-67191-3 (v. 1.)

The preparation of this volume was supported in part by
SRS Grant No. 16-P-57538/3-02.

Published in 1974 by IFI/Plenum Data Company
A Division of Plenum Publishing Corporation
227 West 17th Street, New York, N.Y. 10011

United Kingdom edition published by Plenum Press, London
A Division of Plenum Publishing Company, Ltd.
4a Lower John Street, London W1R 3PD, England

Printed in the United States of America

Foreword

Coronary heart disease (CHD) is a term used to define a constellation of manifestations which result from or are associated with atherosclerosis of the coronary arteries. These manifestations include angina pectoris, myocardial infarction, congestive heart failure, dysrhythmias and sudden death. The disease is ubiquitous throughout the Western world and its incidence is of near-epidemic proportions. In the years following World War II a great proportion of the available research resources had been devoted to understanding CHD. It is now well established that the disease process begins in early life, is insidious in its development, and its occurrence can be predicted by the establishment of a "risk profile". The latter refers to the presence or absence of risk factors. Hypertension, hypercholesterolemia and heavy cigarette smoking are clearly established risk factors, as are sex and age. Other conditions thought to predispose one to CHD even though the "risk" is not clearly established include diabetes mellitus, obesity, personality traits, sedentary living habits, and emotional stress. It is estimated that 1.33 million Americans succumb to a cardiac event annually. Of these, 600,000 die either acutely or during the first year of survival. Of the survivors, approximately half can look forward to returning to a reasonably normal life while the remainder may require additional medical or surgical interventions. Thus, the profile of the potential CHD has been identified, a great deal is known about the manifestations of angina pectoris and myocardial infarction, and progress has been made in developing rehabilitation programs for patients with angina pectoris and/or myocardial infarction.

This bibliography was conceived as a mechanism for synthesizing the available reference material dealing with the epidemiology, prevention and rehabilitation of CHD. While the volume may be found to have many deficiencies it is the hope of Dr. Rogers, Irv Mohler and myself that it will form a contribution to help those investigators who will pursue the study of this disease process. We are grateful to the Social and Rehabilitation Service of the Department of Health, Education, and Welfare for the support they provided to this project, and to those many members associated with the National Exercise and Heart Disease Study whose stimulation helped make this volume a reality.

John Naughton, M.D., Professor of Medicine
Director, Rehabilitation Research
& Training Center 9
Washington, D.C. 20037

Introduction

The idea of a bibliography on cardiovascular diseases and rehabilitation was germinating for a long time in Dr. Naughton's mind until one day in 1972 he suggested that a guide to the literature be compiled. The present collection of 5,005 citations is the response to that suggestion. It is designed to further research efforts in rehabilitation and prevention of coronary heart disease.

The literature citations compiled herein cover a wide area such as: anticoagulants, antiarrhythmic drugs, effects of diet, refined carbohydrates, saturated fats, smoking, hemodynamics, hypertension, hyperlipidemia, hyperglycemia, biochemical tests, artificial pacemakers, economic and psychosocial factors, and heart response to exercise.

The principal and pivotal emphasis is on physical activity/exercise in the rehabilitation of heart disease patients. The 1960-1973 period is covered extensively and earlier articles have been included because of chronological or historical interest. Citations are arranged alphabetically by last name and numbered for easy reference in the accompanying author and subject indexes. The author index uses the exact name as given in the citation, hence in the case of several initials, there are several entries depending on the initials used. With Slavic and Japanese names, there is often a transliteration problem and several versions of the same name might also be encountered in the author index.

The List of Publications Cited is arranged alphabetically. There are 756 journals cited. The journals most widely used are: Circulation, American Journal of Cardiology, American Heart Journal, Annals of Internal Medicine, Archives of Internal Medicine, British Heart Journal, Journal American Medical Association, Journal of Chronic Diseases, Lancet, and New England Journal of Medicine.

It is sincerely hoped that this bibliography will become a useful tool to those engaged in cardiovascular research and that it will lead to cross-fertilization of ideas in searches for precursors and predisposing factors of coronary heart diseases and eventually in the eradication of heart disease as a scourge of our times. Many people have been involved in bringing this bibliography to fruition and warm thanks are hereby rendered to: Theresa K. West, Manager of the project where the idea of this work was generated and Dr. Elzberry Waters, Jr. Acting Director, Science Communication Division where the idea became a reality; Irvin C. Mohler who administered the overall effort; Britta Demello who is responsible for the Author Index and typed many entries; April Commodore, Mildred Harrell, Linda Pleasant, and Marcy Nadel for typing pàrt of the manuscript; Helen Selvig and James Karesh who both ably checked literature references; Patricia Soo Chan Sing, Debbie Michaelson, and Stephen Peter Zisk who worked on the Subject Index; Shelley

Bader, Jane Ferguson, Martha Laredu, and Jackie Schulman of the Paul Himmelfarb Medical Library who generously helped with all "hard searches"; Howard E. Foster who Xeroxed thousands of cards and pages, and lastly but not least Helmuth Scherer and Gerda Carroll of Domonetics, Inc. for a job well done with computer typesetting. To Robert N. Ubell and Plenum Press a hearty thank you.

Senta S. Rogers, Ph.D.

Contents

"The heart is the beginning of life . . . . . . it is the heart by whose virtue and pulse the blood is moved, perfected, made apt to nourish, and is preserved from corruption and coagulation; it is the household divinity which, discharging its function, nourishes, cherishes, quickens the whole body, and is indeed the foundation of life, the source of all action"

William Harvey. An Address
"On the motion of the heart and blood." 1628

"Diseases of the heart and blood vessels are the most serious threat to the health of the American people; they cause one out of every two deaths in the nation—taking more than 900,000 lives a year"

"The Heart Future",
American Heart Association, New York, 1962 p. 1.

"—Medical experience has shown that work appropriate to the cardiac status results in the long run in less harm than inactivity itself, of which the psychological and socioeconomic consequences may be disastrous for the family and the community as a whole"

WHO, Technical Report Series.
Rehabilitation of Patients with Cardiovascular Diseases.
Geneva, 1966.

0001
ABARQUEZ, R.F., JR., C. DAYRIT, AND E.V. VALDEZ.
Comparative sensitivities of the dynamic exercise ECG, postexercise ECG and combined ECG method tests among Filipino coronary patients.
Journal Philippine Medical Association 42(9):539-560, 1966.

0002
ABARQUEZ, R.F., A.H. FREIMAN, F. REICHEL, AND J.S. LADUE.
The precordial electrocardiogram during exercise.
Circulation 22:1060, 1960.

0003
ABBASI, A.S., R.N. MACALPIN, L.M. EBER, AND M.L. PEARCE.
Echocardiographic diagnosis of idiopathic hypertrophic cardiomyopathy without outflow obstruction.
Circulation 46(5):897-904, 1972.

0004
ABBASI, A.S., R.N. MACALPIN, L.M. EBER, AND M.L. PEARCE.
Left ventricular hypertrophy diagnosed by echocardiography.
New England Journal Medicine 289:118, 1973.

0005
ABBOTT, J.A.
The fidelity of the externally recorded human pulse.
American Journal Medical Sciences 258:40-51, 1969.

0006
ABBOTT, J.A., AND M.M. SCHEINMAN.
Nondiagnostic electrocardiogram in patients with acute myocardial infarction. Clinical and anatomic correlations.
American Journal Medicine 55:608, 1973.

0007
ABERG, H., AND L. NORDGREN.
Maintenance of sinus rhythm after conversion of atrial fibrillation and fibrillatory wave rate.
Upsala Journal Medical Sciences 78(1):38-40, 1973.

0008
ABERG, H., AND L. NORDGREN.
On the association between failure in converting atrial fibrillation and fibrillatory wave rate.
Upsala Journal Medical Sciences 78(1):41-42, 1973.

0009
ABERG, H., G. STRÖM, AND I. WERNER.
Heart rate during exercise in patients with atrial fibrillation.
Acta Medica Scandinavica 191(4):315-320, 1972.

0010
ABERG, H., G. STRÖM, AND I. WERNER.
The effect of digitalis on the heart rate during exercise in patients with atrial fibrillation.
Acta Medica Scandinavica 191(5):441-445, 1972.

0011
ABRAHAMS, J.P. AND J.E. BIRREN.
  Reaction time as a function of age and behavioral predisposition to coronary heart disease.
  Journal Gerontology 28(4):471, 1973.

0012
ABRAHAMSEN, A.M., AND F. KIIL.
  Exercise performance and electrocardiographic changes as indices of effort of long-acting nitrates in angina pectoris.
  British Medical Journal 1:456-458, 1966.

0013
ABREZOL, R.
  Psychological assistance to exercising Alpine climbers.
  Minerva Medica 63:2956-2962, 1972.

0014
ABUZEID, H.A.H., AND J.M. CHAPMAN.
  Relationship between hemoglobin level and some risk factors in ischemic heart disease—Los Angeles heart study.
  Circulation 48(4):8, 1973.

0015
ACKER, D., F. BOEHM, D.E. ASKEW, AND H. ROTHMAN.
  Electrocardiogram changes with intrauterine contraceptive device insertion.
  American Journal Obstetrics Gynecology 115(4):458-461, 1973.

0016
ACKER, J.E., JR.
  Factors affecting the employment of patients treated in coronary care units for myocardial infarction.
  Journal Tennessee Medical Association 61:1200-1201, 1968.

0017
ACKER, J.E., JR.
  Role of the nurse in rehabilitation of the myocardial infarction patient.
  Journal South Carolina Medical Association 65(Suppl. 1):65, 1969.

0018
ACKER, J.E.
  Factors affecting the employment of coronary care treated patients after myocardial infarction.
  Malattie Cardiovascolari 10:453-456, 1969.

0019
ACKER, J.E.
  Exercise programs aiding in primary prevention or rehabilitation of heart disease.
  Malattie Cardiovascolari 10:457-459, 1969.

0020
ACREE, P.W.
  Pacemaker in the management of complete heart block.
  Journal Louisiana State Medical Society 116(7):244-248, 1964.

0021
ACTIS DATO, A., G. BALDRIGHI, F. PASSONI, ET AL.
  Coronarographic patterns and surgical management in nine cases of Prinzmetal's angina.
  Minerva Medica 63(89):4901-4913, 1972.

0022
ADAMS, C.W.
  Introduction (Symposium on Exercise and the Heart).
  American Journal Cardiology 30(7):713, 1972.

0023
ADDARII, F.
  Vectocardiographic investigations in sportsmen.
  Münchener Medizinische Wochenschrift 114(45):1966-1968, 1972.

0024
ADELMAN, A.G., E.D. WIGLE, N. RANGANATHAN, ET AL.
  The clinical course in muscular subaortic stenosis. A retrospective and prospective study of 60
  hemodynamically proved cases.
  Annals Internal Medicine 77(4):515-525, 1972.

0025
ADGEY, A.A.J., J.S. GEDDES, H.C. MULHOLLAND, D.A.J. KEEGAN, AND J.F. PANTRIDGE.
  Incidence, significance, and management of early bradyarrhythmia complicating acute myocardial
  infarction.
  Lancet 2:1097, 1968.

0026
ADOLFSSON, L., N.H. ARESKOG, AND T. RASMUSON.
  Effects of alprenolol and sorbidnitrate during exercise in patients with coronary insufficiency.
  European Journal Clinical Pharmacology 3(2):68-73, 1971.

0027
ADOLPH, R.J.
  Diagnosis and medical management of complete atrioventricular block.
  Heart Bulletin 17(1):16-20, 1968.

0028
ADSETT, C.A., AND J.G. BRUHN.
  Short-term group psychotherapy for post-myocardial infarction patients and their wives.
  Canadian Medical Association Journal 99(12):577-584, 1968.

0029
AGLE, D.P., O.D. RATNOFF, AND G.K. SPRING.
  The anticoagulant malingerer. Psychiatric studies of three patients.
  Annals Internal Medicine 73(1):67-72, 1970.

0030
AGRESS, C.M., AND M.J. BINDER.
  Cardiogenic shock.
  American Heart Journal 54:458, 1957.

0031
AGRESS, C.M., AND S. WEGNER.
  The vibrocardiographic exercise test for coronary insufficiency.
  American Journal Cardiology 9:541-546, 1962.

0032
AGRUSS, N.S., E.Y. ROSIN, R.J. ADOLPH, AND N.O. FOWLER.
  Significance of chronic sinus bradycardia in elderly people.
  Circulation 46(5):924-930, 1972.

0033
AHLBORG, B.
  Capacity for prolonged exercise in man.
  Försvarsmedicin 3(Suppl.1):1, 1967.

0034
AHLQUIST, R.P.
  Isoproterenol in cardiology.
  Amercian Heart Journal 86:149, 1973.

0035
AHMED, S.H., M.T. El-Rakhawy, A.ABDALLA, AND R.G. HARRISON.
  A new conception of coronary artery preponderance.
  Acta Anatomica (Basel) 83(1):87-94, 1972.

0036
AHMED, S.S., G.E. LEVINSON, C.J. SCHWARTZ, AND P.O. ETTINGER.
  Systolic time intervals as measures of the contractile state of the left ventricular myocardium in man.
  Circulation 46(3):559-571, 1972.

0037
AHRENS, E.H.
  Hardening of the arteries: Can it be prevented by appropriate diet?
  Journal Rehabilitation 32:93, 1966.

0038
AHUJA, M.M.S., V. GOSSAIN, C.K. BHAN, AND V. KUMAR.
  Vascular disease in north Indian diabetics in relation to diet and blood lipids.
  In: Shafrier, P., Ed. Impact of insulin on metabolic pathways, p. 423.
  New York, Academic Press, 1972.

0039
AISENBERG, R.B., P.H. WOLFF, A. ROSENTHAL, AND A.S. NADAS.
  Psychological impact of cardiac catheterization.
  Pediatrics 51:1051, 1973.

0040
AKHMEDZHANOV, M. IU., ET AL.
  Sanatorium—Health resort treatment and problems of rehabilitation of patients with myocardial infarct.
  Sovetskaya Meditsina 32:55-57, 1969.

0041
AKHREM-AKHREMOVICH, R.M., D.M. ARONOV, Y.T. PUSHKAR, V.A. SOBOLEVA, Z.V.
KRUKOVSKAYA, L.K. PAVELCHUK, V.M. STARK, A.A. MODOROVA, AND E.I. NIKITINA.
Stage-by-stage treatment and methods in the rehabilitation of patients with myocardial infarction
and chronic coronary insufficiency.
Kardiologiya 11(1):91-98, 1971.

0042
AKHREM-AKHREMOVICH, R.M., D.M. ARONOV, N.A. BELAYA, S.G. VORONINA, M.G. SHARF-
NADEL, Y.T. PUSHKAR, A.A. KRAMER, A.Z. EVENTOV, AND P.A. ALEKSEEV.
Significance of intensive training in the compensation of cardiovascular disorders in patients after
myocardial infarction.
Kardiologiya 12:26-31, 1972.

0043
ALARCÓN-FALCÓN, H.
Comparative electrocardiographic and ballistocardiographic tests after exercise.
Anales de la Facultad de Medicina, Universidad Naional Mayor de San Marcos de Lima
48(2):277-296, 1965.

0044
AL-BAZZAZ, F.J. AND H. KAZEMI.
Arterial hypoxemia and distribution of pulmonary perfusion after uncomplicated myocardial
infarction.
American Review Respiratory Diseases 106(5):721-728, 1972.

0045
ALBRINK, M.J., ET AL.
Serum lipids, hypertension and coronary artery disease.
American Journal Medicine 31:4, 1961.

0046
ALDERMAN, E.L., A. BRANZI, W. SANDERS, ET AL.
Evaluation of the pulse contour method of determining stroke volume in man.
Circulation 46(3):546-558, 1972.

0047
ALDERMAN, E.L., H.J. MATLOF, N.E. SHUMWAY, AND D.C. HARRISON.
Evaluation of enzyme testing for the detection of myocardial infarction following direct coronary
surgery.
Circulation 48:135-140, 1973.

0048
ALDES, J.H., ET AL.
A program to effect vocational restoration of "unemployable" cardiac cases.
Diseases Chest 54:518-522, 1968.

0049
ALDES, J.H., S. GRABIN, AND S.P. STEIN.
A comprehensive cardiac rehabilitation programme.
Medical Journal Australia 2:511-513, 1968.

0050
ALEKSANDROV, A.A., A.A. KRAMER, S.M. ZHDANOVA, AND V.I. METELITSA.
Epidemiological study of the spread of hypertension and association of some risk factors with the level of arterial pressure.
Terapevticheskii Arkhiv 44:81-84, 1972.

0051
ALEKSANDROW, D., S. CZAPLICKI, AND A. MICHJLIK.
Distribution of coronary risk factors in a sample population of men aged 40 years.
Kardiologia Polska 15:121, 1972.

0052
ALEXANDER, C.S.
Cobalt beer cardiomyography. A clinical and pathologic study of twenty-eight cases.
American Journal Medicine 53(4):395-417, 1972.

0053
ALEXANDER, J.T.
Exercise and coronary heart disease.
Cardiovascular Research Center Bulletin 8:2-7, 1969.

0054
ALGARRA VIDAL, F.J.
The electrocardiogram and phonocardiogram in essential arterial hypertension.
Revista Española de Cardiologia 21:60-80, 1968.

0055
ALIMURUNG, M.M.
Modern living and heart disease.
Journal Philippine Federation Private Medical Practitioners 13:655, 1964.

0056
ALLEN, J.
The use of isometric exercises in a geriatric treatment program.
Geriatrics 20:346-347, 1965.

0057
ALLESSIE, M.A., F.I.M. BONKE, AND F.J. SCHOPMAN.
Circus movement in atrial muscle as a mechanism of supraventricular tachycardia.
Journal Physiologie 65(2):324A, 1972.

0058
ALLISON, S.P., M.J. CHAMBERLAIN, AND P. HINTON.
Intravenous glucose tolerance, insulin, glucose, and free fatty acid levels after myocardial infarction.
British Medical Journal 4:776-778, 1969.

0059
ALMAJAN, E., ET AL.
Psychological aspects of the coronary patient.
Revue de Médecine Psychosomatique (Paris) 12:65-71, 1970.

0060
ALPERT, J., O.A. LARSEN, AND N.A. LASSEN.
Blood flow in the calf muscles during walking: effect of daily muscular exercise in patients with occlusive arterial disease.
Scandinavian Journal Clinical Laboratory Investigation (Suppl.) 19(100):90, 1967.

0061
ALTLAND, N.R.
Personality correlates of acute myocardial infarction.
Dissertation Abstracts 26(2):1157-1158, 1965.

0062
ALTLAND, N.R., ET AL.
Personality differentiation of patients with coronary artery disease.
Maryland State Medical Journal 15:63-65, 1966.

0063
AMIEL, M., AND F. PINET.
70 mm intensifier fluorography in vascular examinations, particularly selective coronarography.
Medica Mundi 17(2):84-92, 1972.

0064
AMSTERDAM, E.A., R. GORLIN, AND S. WOLFSON.
Evaluation of long-term use of propranolol in angina pectoris.
Journal American Medical Association 210(1):103-106, 1969.

0065
ANBE, D.T., AND G. FINE.
Cardiac lymphangioma and lipoma. Report of a case of simultaneous occurrence in association with lipomatous infiltration of the myocardium and cardiac arrhythmia.
American Heart Journal 86:227, 1973.

0066
ANDER, S., ET AL.
Psychological factors in myocardial infarction.
Lakartidningen 68:3695-3699, 1971.

0067
ANDERSEN, J.A., AND B. FISCHER-HANSEN.
Arrhythmias and symptoms during treadmill testing three weeks after myocardial infarction in 100 patients.
British Heart Journal 35(8):781, 1973.

0068
ANDERSEN, K.L.
Ethnic group differences in fitness for sustained and strenuous muscular exercise.
Canadian Medical Association Journal 96:832-833, 1967.

0069
ANDERSEN, K.L., R.J. SHEPHARD, H. DENOLIN, E. VARNAUSKAS, AND R. MASIRONI.
Fundamentals of exercise testing.
Geneva, World Health Organization, 1971.

0070
ANDERSON, D.E.
   Vocational rehabilitation of cardiac patients.
   Medical Journal Australia 55(10);74-75, 1968.

0071
ANDERSON, D.E.
   A modern cardiac aphorism.
   Medical Journal Australia 57-1(15):769-771, 1970.

0072
ANDERSON, E.W., R.J. ANDELMAN, J.M. STRAUCH, N.J. FORTUIN, AND J.H. KNELSON.
   Effect of low-level carbon monoxide exposure on onset and duration of angina pectoris.
   Annals Internal Medicine 79:46, 1973.

0073
ANDERSON, F.I., T.J. TSAGARIS, G. TIKOFF, J.L. THORNE, A.M. SCHMIDT, AND H. KUIDA.
   Hemodynamic effects of exercise in patients with aortic stenosis.
   American Journal Medicine 46(6):872-885, 1969.

0074
ANDERSON, M.T., G.B. LEE, B.C. CAMPION, K. AMPLATZ, AND N. TUNA.
   Cardiac dysrhythmias associated with exercise stress testing.
   Circulation 44(Suppl. II):135, 1971.

0075
ANDERSON, M.T., G.B. LEE, B.C. CAMPION, K. AMPLATZ, AND N. TUNA.
   Cardiac dysrhythmias associated with exercise stress testing.
   American Journal Cardiology 30(7):763, 1972.

0076
ANDERSON, T.W.
   The changing pattern of ischemic heart disease.
   Canadian Medical Association Journal 108:1500, 1973.

0077
ANDERSON, T.W.
   Nutritional muscular dystrophy and human myocardial infarction.
   Lancet II:298, 1973.

0078
ANDERSON, T.W., D. HEWITT, L.C. NERI, G. SCHREIBER, AND F. TALBOT.
   Water hardness and magnesium in heart muscle.
   Lancet II:1391, 1973.

0079
ANDRADE, Z.A., AND A.R.L. TEIXEIRA.
   Changes in the coronary vasculature in endomyocardial fibrosis and their possible significance.
   American Heart Journal 86:152, 1973.

0080
ANDRESS, M.R., AND M.L. THOMAS.
   Renal arteriovenous fistula resulting in death from cardiac failure: Report of a case.
   Australasian Radiology 16:137, 1972.

0081
ANDRIANGE, M., G. CALAY, J. GACH, AND N. LISIN.
   Shock in myocardial infarction. Treatment of cardiogenic shock with dopamine.
   Acta Clinica Belgica 26(5):249-261, 1971.

0082
ANFOSSI, F., P.L. ROSSI, AND G. SATTA.
   On the rehabilitation of subjects with prior myocardial infarct. Personal observations and consider-
   ations.
   Annali della Sanita Pubblica 28:147-163, 1967.

0083
ANGELINI, P., R. LUFSCHANOWSKI, A. BRUSCA, AND R.D. LEACHMAN.
   Electrocardiogram and coronary angiography. A study of 215 patients with clinical diagnosis of
   ischaemic heart disease.
   Gazzetta Italiana di Cardiologia 2(4):471-483, 1972.

0084
ANGELINO, P.F., B. SEVERGNINI, N. DE BENEDICTIS, AND C. BELLI.
   Electrocardiographic telemetry in the rehabilitation of acute myocardial infarction and severe
   coronary insufficiency.
   Bollettino della Società Italiana di Cardiologia 16(9):559-569, 1971.

0085
ANJILVEL, L.
   Familial hyperlipoproteinemia in an isolated part of Newfoundland.
   Canadian Medical Association Journal 109:894, 1973.

0086
ANTONI, H.
   Physiological principles of the induction and interruption of auricular and ventricular fibrillation
   by electrical currents.
   Herz Kreislauf 4:324, 1972.

0087
ANTONINI, F.M., C. FUMAGALLI, E. PETRUZZI, G. BERTINI, S. MORI, AND P. TINTI.
   Prognostic significance of hyperglycemia in acute myocardial infarction.
   Acta Diabetologica 10(3):645-55, 1973.

0088
ANTONIOLI, G., G. BAGGIONI, AND P. ALBONI.
   Reciprocal rhythm induced by ventricular pacing.
   Gazzetta Italiana di Cardiologia 2(5):702-709, 1972.

0089
ANTONIOTTI, F.
   Medical and social aspects of the invalid citizen in Italian society.
   Rivista degli Infortoni e delle Malattie Professionali 58(4):653-668, 1971.

0090
ANTONIS, A., AND I. BERSOHN.
   Serum-triglyceride levels in South African Europeans and Bantu in ischaemic heart-disease.
   Lancet 1:998-1002, 1960.

0091
ANTONOVSKY, A.
   Social class and the major cardiovascular diseases.
   Journal Chronic Diseases 21:65-106, 1968.

0092
ARCHER, M., S. RINZLER, AND G. CHRISTAKIS.
   Social factors affecting participation in a study of diet and coronary heart disease.
   Journal Health Social Behavior 8:22-31, 1967.

0093
ARCHIBALD, K.C., ET AL.
   Rehabilitation of the elderly cardiac patient.
   Geriatrics 25:133-141, 1970.

0094
ARESKOG, N.H.
   Exercise test standardization with special regard to diagnosis of coronary insufficiency.
   Scandinavian Journal of Clinical Laboratory Investigation (Suppl.)24(110):113, 1969.

0095
ARESKOG, N.H.
   ECG and pain reaction to work test, physical work capacity, and coronary angiogram in coronary heart disease.
   Malattie Cardiovascolari 10(1/2):35-39, 1969.

0096
ARESKOG, N.H.
   Effects of propranolol on coronary insufficiency at work test.
   Malattie Cardiovascolari 10(1/2):41-45, 1969.

0097
ARESKOG, N.H., AND L. ADOLFSSON.
   Effects of a cardio-selective beta-adrenergic blocker (ICL 50172) at exercise in angina pectoris.
   British Medical Journal 3:601-603, 1969.

0098
ARESKOG, N.H., L. ADOLFSSON, AND T. RASMUSON.
   Effects of alprenolol and sorbidnitrate at exercise in patients with coronary insufficiency.
   Scandinavian Journal Clinical Laboratory Investigation (Suppl.) 24(110):114, 1969.

0099
ARESKOG, N.H., L. BJÖRK, V.O. BJÖRK, I. CULLHED, A. HALLEN, and G. STRÖM.
   Diagnosis of coronary insufficiency by graded submaximal exercise test.
   Scandinavian Journal Clinical Laboratory Investigation (Suppl.) 19(100):54, 1967.

0100
ARESKOG, N.H., L. BJÖRK, V.O. BJÖRK, I. CULLHED, A. HALLEN, AND G. STRÖM.
   Heart-rate reaction to graded submaximal exercise test and work tolerance in coronary heart disease in relation to heart volume and degree of coronary angiographic changes.
   Scandinavian Journal Clincial Laboratory Investigation (Suppl.)19(100):71, 1967.

0101
ARESKOG, N.H., L. BJÖRK, V.O. BJÖRK, A. HALLEN, AND G. STRÖM.
Physical work capacity, ECG reaction to work test, and coronary angiogram in coronary artery disease.
Acta Medica Scandinavica (Suppl.) 472:9-35, 1967.

0102
ARESKOG, N.H., AND A. HALLEN.
Relations between ECG and anginal pain response to exercise.
Scandinavian Journal Clinical Laboratory Investigation (Suppl.) 19(100):69, 1967.

0103
ARGUELLE, A.E., C. HOFFMAN, M. CHEKHERD, AND A. CERVETTO.
Corticoadrenal and adrenergic overactivity in male patients with chronic myocardial infarction.
Journal Steroid Biochemistry 4(4):427-432, 1973.

0104
ARIMA, T., S. YAMASAKI, K. YAMADA, J. GINNOUCH, S. ISHIDA, F. OOSHIMA, K. TAKAYAMA, H. TOSHIMA, AND N. KIMURA.
Clinical studies of serum gamma-glutamyl transpeptidase activity in myocardial infarction.
Japanese Circulation Journal 37(8):906, 1973.

0105
ARMSTRONG, A. B. DUNCAN, M.F. OLIVER, D.G. JULIAN, K.W. DONALD, M. FULTON, W. LUTZ, AND S.L. MORRISON.
Natural history of acute coronary heart attacks: Community Study.
British Heart Journal 34:67, 1972.

0106
ARMSTRONG, T.G., B.S. LEWIS, AND M.S. GOTSMAN.
Systolic time intervals in constrictive pericarditis and severe primary myocardial disease.
American Heart Journal 85(1):6-12, 1973.

0107
ARMSTRONG, W., S. ELLIOTT, AND J. OSBORN.
Oxygen debt and ventilatory "R" during exercise in patients with heart disease.
Clinical Research 16(3):161, 1968.

0108
ARNOLD, G., AND C. HARTUNG.
Histomechanical properties of the chordae tendineae of the human heart.
Biomedizinische Technik 17(5):169-173, 1972.

0109
ARNULF, G., AND Y. GRAND
Ventricular fibrillation after release of a coronary artery occlusion.
Archives des Sciences Physiologiques 25(3):343-351, 1971.

0110
ARONOV, D.M.
The tolerance of patients with coronary insufficiency to physical exertion.
Kardiologiya 10(4):51-58, 1970.

0111
ARONOV, D.M., AND I.P. ILYUSHINA.
The dynamics of some indices of the blood coagulation and anticoagulation systems under the effect of physical exertion in young persons suffering from coronary insufficiency.
Kardiologiya 11(3):69-75, 1971.

0112
ARONOV, D.M., AND Z.M. KISELEVA.
Activity of blood monoamine oxidase and catecholamine excretion in coronary insufficiency in young persons.
Kardiologiya 11(8):34-38, 1971.

0113
ARONOW, W.S.
Medical treatment of angina pectoris. III. Pharmacology of sublingual nitrites as antianginal drugs.
American Heart Journal 84(2):273-275, 1972.

0114
ARONOW, W.S.
The medical treatment of angina pectoris. V. Long acting nitrites as antianginal drugs.
American Heart Journal 84(4):567-569, 1972.

0115
ARONOW, W.S.
The medical treatment of angina pectoris. VI. Propranolol as an antianginal drug.
American Heart Journal 84(5):706-709, 1972.

0116
ARONOW, W.S.
The medical treatment of angina pectoris. VII. Newer beta-adrenergic blockers as antianginal drugs.
American Heart Journal 84(6):834, 1972.

0117
ARONOW, W.S.
Thirty-month follow-up of maximal treadmill stress test and double Master's test in normal subjects.
Circulation 47:287-290, 1973.

0118
ARONOW, W.S.
Thirty-month follow-up of resting and postexercise apexcardiogram in asymptomatic subjects.
Circulation 47:807-812, 1973.

0119
ARONOW, W.S., A.F. BOWYER, AND M.A. KAPLAN.
External isovolumic contraction times and left ventricular ejection time/external isovolumic contraction time ratios at rest and after exercise in coronary heart disease.
Circulation 43(1):59-65, 1971.

0120
ARONOW, W.S., AND H.M. CHESLUK.
Evaluation of nitroglycerin in angina in patients on isosorbide dinitrate.
Circulation 42:61, 1970.

0121
ARONOW, W.S., AND H.M. CHESLUK.
Sublingual isosorbide dinitrate therapy versus sublingual placebo in angina pectoris.
Circulation 41:869, 1970.

0122
ARONOW, W.S., ET AL.
Resting and postexercise apexcardiogram correlated with maximal treadmill stress test in normal subjects.
Circulation 44:397-402, 1971.

0123
ARONOW, W.S., ET AL.
Effect of halofenate on exercise performance in coronary heart disease.
Clinical Pharmacology Therapeutics 14(3):366, 1973.

0124
ARONOW, W.S., P.R. HARDING, W.H. NELSON, ET AL.
Treatment of arrhythmias with tolamidol.
Clinical Pharmacology Therapeutics 13(6):856-860, 1972.

0125
ARONOW, W.S., C.N. HARRIS, M.W. ISBELL, ET AL.
Effect of freeway travel on angina pectoris.
Annals Internal Medicine 77(5):669-676, 1972.

0126
ARONOW, W.S., M.A. KAPLAN, AND D. JACOB.
Tobacco: A precipitating factor in angina pectoris.
Annals Internal Medicine 69(3):529-536, 1968.

0127
ARONOW, W.S., N.P. PAPAGEORGE'S, R.R. UYEYAMA, AND J. CASSIDY.
Maximal treadmill stress test correlated with postexercise phonocardiogram in normal subjects.
Circulation 43:884, 1971.

0128
ARONOW, W.S., R.R. UYEYAMA, J. CASSIDY, AND J. NEBOLON.
Resting and postexercise phonocardiogram and electrocardiogram in patients with angina pectoris and in normal subjects.
Circulation 43(2):273-277, 1971.

0129
ARSTILA, M.
Pulse-conducted triangular exercise-ECG test. A feed-back system regulating work during exercise.
Acta Medica Scandinavica (Suppl.) 529:3-109, 1972.

0130
ARSTILA, M., V. KALLIO, AND H. WENDELIN.
Propranolol and LB 46 (Prinodolol) in angina pectoris.
Annals Clinical Research 5:91, 1973.

0131
ARSTILA, M., P. VIHERAE, AND I. VAELIMAEKI.
Semiautomatic controller of linear heart rate acceleration in ergometric exercise test.
Proceedings of the National Meeting Biophysics Biotechnology, Finland 1:159-161, 1973.

0132
ARTAMONOV, V.N.
Determination of permitted loads of physical exercises for elderly persons.
Fizicheskaya kul'tura istochnik dolgoletiya (Physical culture as a source of longevity), pp. 234-244. Moscow, Fizkul't. Sport., 1965.

0133
ARTHUR, R.J.
Stoic coronary personality.
New England Journal Medicine 280:333-334, 1969.

0134
ARVEDSON, O.
A method to display the results of computer discrimination between normal ECG's and ECG's in patients with coronary insufficiency.
Scandinavian Journal Clinical Laboratory Investigation 17:199-200, 1965.

0135
ASCOOP, C.A., M.L. SIMOONS, W.G. EGMOND, AND A.V.G. BRUSCHKE.
Exercise test, history, and serum lipid levels in patients with chest pain and normal electrocardiogram at rest: Comparison to findings of coronary arteriography.
American Heart Journal 82(5):609-617, 1971.

0136
ASKANAS, Z.
Materials on the influence of the rehabilitation and treatment on readaptation of patients with recent myocardial infarction.
In: Plavšić, C. and M.M. Gertler, Eds. The first international biennial conference on cardiac rehabilitation, Dubrovnik, Yugoslavia, 1969.

0137
ASKANAS, Z.
Rehabilitation of patients with newly diagnosed myocardial infarction.
Kardiologiya 12:28-36, 1972.

0138
ASKANAS, Z.
Rehabilitation of patients with new myocardial infarction. Part 1.
Kardiologiya 12:24-32, 1973.

0139
ASKANAS, Z., ET AL.
The role of the psychologist in the rehabilitation of patients with recent myocardial infarction.
Polski Tygodnik Lekarski 21:1308-1311, 1966.

0140
ASKANAS, Z., ET AL.
Evaluation of the effectiveness of hospital physical rehabilitation in patients with recent myocardial infarct.
Kardiologia Polska 13:17-22, 1970.

0141
ASKANAS, Z., Z. KRASZEWSKA, S. RUDNICKI, K. SLIDZIEWSKI, R.J. ZOCHOWSKI, AND J. BARYLAK.
Radioelectrocardiographic control during rehabilitation.
Malattie Cardiovascolari 10(1-2):79-89, 1969.

0142
ASKANAS, Z., D. LISZEWSKA, AND J. TYLKA.
Interaction between psychic and somatic risk factors of myocardial infarction.
Scandinavian Journal Rehabilitation Medicine 2-3:85-86, 1970.

0143
ASKANAS, Z., H. OSTROWSKA, AND S. SIEK.
Personality of the patients with myocardial infarction.
Polski Tygodnik Lekarski 20(35):1327-1329, 1965.

0144
ASKANAS, Z., J. TYLKA, S. RUDNICKI, H. OSTROWSKA, J. BARYLAK, AND K. TYMINSKA.
Assessment of the effectiveness of the hospital method of psychological rehabilitation of patients with recent myocardial infarct.
Kardiologia Polskă 13:293-300, 1970.

0145
ASLAN, A., AND A. VRABIESCU.
Changes with age in cardiac dynamics appraised by study on the electrocardiogram on effort, of the Rv — Tv interval referring to the heart rate.
Fiziologia Normală Patologică 16(6):509-522, 1970.

0146
ASOKAN, S.K., T.L. CREWS, P.E. CUNDEY, JR., AND M.J. FRANK.
Effects of lidocaine on potassium, sodium, and water in ischaemic myocardium.
Cardiovascular Research 6(5):482-489, 1972.

0147
ASPLUND, J., O. EDHAG, L. MOGENSEN, O. NYQUIST, E. ORINIUS, AND A. SJOGREN.
Four cases of massive digitalis poisoning.
Acta Medica Scandinavica 189(4):293-297, 1971.

0148
ÅSTRAND, I.
Aerobic work capacity in men and women with special reference to age.
Acta Physiologica Scandinavica 49(Suppl.169):1, 1960.

0149
ÅSTRAND, I.
Exercise electrocardiograms in a 5-year follow-up study.
Acta Medica Scandinavica 173(3):257-268, 1963.

0150
ÅSTRAND, I.
Exercise electrocardiograms recorded twice with an 8-year interval in a group of 204 women and men 48-63 years old.
Acta Medica Scandinavica 178:27, 1965.

0151
ÅSTRAND, I.
Prognostic value of exercise electrocardiogram in older men.
Scandinavian Journal Clinical Laboratory Investigation 23(3):271-276, 1969.

0152
ÅSTRAND, I.
Exercise electrocardiogram, its prognostic significance.
In: Halonen, P. and A. Louhija, Eds. Advances in Cardiology vol 8. Early diagnosis of coronary heart disease, pp. 142-147. Basel, Switzerland. S. Karger, 1973.

0153
ÅSTRAND, I., T.E. CUDDY, J. LANDEGREN, R.O. MALMBORG, AND B. SALTIN.
Hemodynamic response to exercise during atrial flutter and sinus rhythm.
Acta Medica Scandinavica 173(1):121-127, 1963.

0154
ÅSTRAND, I., B. KYLIN, AND I.M. LIDSTROM.
Electrocardiograms and exercise test in health check. A study on forest workers.
Scandinavian Journal Clinical Laboratory Investigation 23(1):31-41, 1969.

0155
ÅSTRAND, I., AND T. LUNDMAN.
The exercise electrocardiogram in coronary heart disease. Its prognostic value.
Scandinavian Journal Clinical Laboratory Investigation 22(4):301-306, 1968.

0156
ÅSTRAND, P.-O.
Experimental studies of physical working capacity in relation to sex and age.
Copenhagen, Munksgaard, 1952.

0157
ÅSTRAND, P.-O.
Measurement of maximal aerobic capacity.
Canadian Medical Association Journal 96:732-734, 1967.

0158
ÅSTRAND, P.-O., ET AL.
Cardiac output during submaximal and maximal work.
Journal Applied Physiology 19:268-274, 1964.

0159
ÅSTRAND, P.-O., AND K. RODAHL.
Textbook of work physiology.
New York, McGraw-Hill, 1970.

0160
ASTROM, H.
Effect of posture on circulation and respiration at rest and during exercise in heart disease.
Acta Physiologica Scandinavica (Suppl.) 347:5-86, 1970.

0161
ASTRUP, T. AND P. BRAKMAN.
Responders and non-responders in exercise-induced blood fibrinolysis.
In: Larsen, O.A., and R.O. Malmborg, Eds. Coronary heart disease and physical fitness. Copenhagen, Munksgaard, 1971.

0162
ATLAS, P., AND S. CLEJAN.
Hyperlipoproteinemia—major predisposing factor in myocardial infarction in young adults.
Israel Journal Medical Sciences 9(4):560, 1973.

0163
ATTINGER, E.O.
Biomechanics, patient care and rehabilitation.
In: Kenedi, R.M., Ed. Biomechanics and related bioengineering topics, pp. 29-60. London, Pergamon, 1965.

0164
AUCHINCLOSS, J.H., JR.
Transient response of oxygen transfer to exercise.
Federation Proceedings 27(2):231, 1968.

0165
AUCHINCLOSS, J.H., JR., AND R. GILBERT.
Estimation of maximum oxygen uptake with a brief progressive stress-test.
Journal Applied Physiology 34:525-26, 1973.

0166
AVEZOU, F., J.M. MALLION, B. DENIS, B. ROSSIGNOL, AND P. MARTIN-NOEL.
Results of research into coronary reserves after exertion in 80 patients with myocardial infarction.
Annales de Cardiologie et d'Angéiologie (Paris) 21:269-277, 1972.

0167
AZUMA, K., K. HAGINO, K. AKABOSHI, K. SHIMIZU, K. SHINMURA, H. SHINMURA, T. KASATANI, Y. KASAHARA, O. NAKANO, K. MUROTA, S. YASUI, T. TAKKAKI, AND K. INAMORI.
A studies on the management of essential hypertension. IV. On the relationship between salt metabolism and effectiveness of diuretics.
Japanese Circulation Journal 31(1):191-192, 1967.

0168
AZUMA, K., K. HAGINO, K. SHIMIZU, K. TAKETO, AND N. TAKEMOTO.
Effects of benzoctamine hydrochloride on psychosomatic diseases of the circulatory organs.
Journal Japanese Psychomatic Society 12:298, 1972.

0169
BABKA, J.C., AND C.J. PEPINE.
Hyperkinetic cardiovascular state in polymyositis.
Chest 64:243, 1973.

0170

BACANU, G., L. ANGHELESCU, AND L. POPA.
Diagnosis of diabetes mellitus in patients with myocardial infarction.
Medicina Internă 17:413-416, 1965.

0171

BACHE, R.J., Y. WANG, AND J.C. GREENFIELD, JR.
Left ventricular ejection time in valvular aortic stenosis.
Circulation 47(3):527-533, 1973.

0172

BACHMANN, K.
Acute and chronic coronary insufficiency. Angina pectoris: diagnosis and indications.
Langenbecks Archiv für Chirurgie 332(Kongr.B):267-272, 1972.

0173

BACOS, J.M., AND T.W. MATTINGLY.
The critical period of heart attack.
Journal Rehabilitation 32:29, 1966.

0174

BADARAU, G., L. FITERMAN, G. BLINDU, AND B. ABABEI.
The problem of recovery of cardiovascular patients.
Revista Medico-Chirurgicală a Societații de Medici și Naturalisti din Iași 71:496-506, 1967.

0175

BADGER, G.F., ET AL.
Myocardial infarction in the practices of a group of private physicians. IV. Factors related to the longevity of patients with mycardial infarction during the first five years.
Journal Chronic Diseases 21:473-482, 1968.

0176

BAGLEY, R.N.
Massive corticosteroid therapy of myocardial infarction.
Clinician 36(10):421-422, 1972.

0177

BAHL, A.L., T.K. BASU, AND R.N. CHUGH.
Precocious ischemic heart disease evaluation of different risk factors.
Indian Journal Medical Science 24(11):722-728, 1970.

0178

BAHLER, R.C., AND C.A. MacLEOD.
Atrial pacing and exercise in the evaluation of patients with angina pectoris.
Circulation 43(3):407-419, 1971.

0179

BAHNSON, C.B., AND W.I. WARDELL.
Parent constellation and psychosexual identification in male patients with myocardial infarction.
American Psychologist 16:349, 1961.

0180
BAIRD, J.R.C. AND J. LINNELL.
   The assessment of beta-adrenoreceptor blocking potency and cardioselectivity in vitro and in vivo.
   Journal Pharmacy Pharmacology 24(11):880-885, 1972.

0181
BAJPAI, P.C., M. HASAN, A.K. GUPTA, AND K.B. KUNWAR.
   Electrocardiographic changes in hypomagnesemia.
   Indian Heart Journal 24(3):271-276, 1972.

0182
BAKER, B.B., J.A. WAGNER, AND W.G. HEMENWAY.
   Succinylcholine induced hyperkalemia and cardiac arrest.
   Archives Otolaryngology 96(5):464-465, 1972.

0183
BAKER, L.D., S.J. LESHIN, G.V.R.K. SHARMA, AND J.V. MESSER.
   The relative effects of exercise and isoproterenol in eliciting regional metabolic abnormalities in
   cineangiographically quantitated human coronary artery disease.
   American Journal Cardiology 23:104, 1969.

0184
BAKKER, C.B., M. BOGDONOFF, H.K. HELLERSTEIN, W.L. KRAUS, J.P. NAUGHTON, M.F.
   REISER, R.H. ROSENMAN, J.J. SCHWAB, AND N.K. WENGER'
   Heart disease and sex: Response to questions.
   Medical Aspects Human Sexuality 5(6):24-35, 1971.

0185
BALCON, R., J. HOY, W. MALLOY, AND E. SOWTON.
   Haemodynamic comparison of atrial pacing and exercise in patients with angina pectoris.
   British Heart Journal 31(2):168-171, 1969.

0186
BALKE, B., ED.
   Physiological aspects of sports and physical fitness.
   The Athletic Institute, 1968.

0187
BALKE, B., J. NAUGHTON, AND J. BRUCH.
   The role of physical activity in the treatment of coronary heart disease.
   In: Hanekopf, G., Ed. XVI Weltkongress für Sportmedizin. Kiln-Berlin, Deutscher Ärzte Verlag,
   1966.

0188
BALKE, B., J. NAUGHTON, AND G. SEVELIUS.
   Cardiac output and stroke volume within man's potential range of energy expenditure.
   Excerpta Medica, International Congress Series no. 742, 1962.

0189
BALKE, B., AND R.W. WARE.
   An experimental study of "physical fitness" of Air Force personnel.
   U.S. Armed Forces Medical Journal 10:675-688, 1959.

0190
BALL, K.
The unimportance of diet in the treatment of coronary heart disease.
Modern Geriatrics 2(7):402-405, 1972.

0191
BALL, K.P., ET AL.
Low-fat diet in myocardial infarction. A controlled trial.
Lancet 2:501-504, 1965.

0192
BALOGH, Z., M. BLAZEK, AND J. TARJAN.
Selection of cardiac and articular patients requiring balneotherapy on the basis of the Master test and balneo tolerance test.
Rheumatologia Balneologia Allergologia 13(2):106-110, 1972.

0193
BANERJEA, J.C.
Rehabilitation of cardiac patients.
Indian Heart Journal 16(1):1-4, 1964.

0194
BANTEA, C., P. KALMÁR, AND C. JAKOBS.
A simple method for intracardial EKG registration in patients with intracardial catheter (two modifications).
Thoraxchirurgie Vaskuläre Chirurgie 21:239, 1973.

0195
BARANOV, V.A.
Changes of the terminal part of the ECG ventricular complex under the effect of physical exercises in patients with myocardial infarction.
Kardiologiya 7(12):89-94, 1967.

0196
BARANOV, V.A.
Effect of exercise therapy on the contractile function of the myocardium during ischemic heart diseases. (Clinical and ballistocardiographic studies.)
Kardiologiya 8(5):30-37, 1968.

0197
BARATS, S.S., AND V.S. VOLKOV.
Incidence and outcome of myocardial infarction among laborers and office personnel engaged in industry.
Sovetskaya Meditsina 33(10):127-129, 1970.

0198
BARBOSA, J., A.S. LOPES, J.S. LOPES, ET AL.
The action of oxyfedrine on ventricular dynamics in ischemic heart disease.
Arquivos Brasileiros de Cardiologia 25(3):231-239, 1972.

0199
BARCKOW, D., H. HEIDRICH, AND H. FRISIUS.
Cardiovascular changes during artificial ventilation in patients in an intensive care unit.
Deutsche Medizinische Wochenschrift 97(28):1059-1063, 1972.

0200
BARNARD, R.J., G.W. GARDNER, N.V. DIACO, R.N. MACALPIN, AND A.A. KATTUS.
Cardiovascular responses to sudden strenuous exercise—heart rate, blood pressure, and ECG.
Journal Applied Physiology 34(6):833-837, 1973.

0201
BARNARD, R.J., R. MACALPIN, A.A. KATTUS, AND G.D. BUCKBERG.
Ischemic response to sudden strenuous exercise in healthy men.
Circulation 48:936, 1973.

0202
BARNES, R.J.
Associated factors in coronary artery disease in the Chinese.
Asian Journal Medicine 8(10):419-424, 1972.

0203
BARNETT, G.O., S.M. FOX, III, A.J. MALLOS, J.C. GREENFIELD, JR., AND D.L. FRY.
The significance of the instantaneous aortic blood ejection velocity.
Journal Clinical Investigation 39:971, 1960.

0204
BARRY, A.J., J.W. DALY, E.D.R. PRUETT, J.R. STEINMETZ, N.C. BIRKHEAD, AND K.
RODAHL.
Effects of physical training in patients who have had myocardial infarction.
American Journal Cardiology 17(1):1-8, 1966.

0205
BARRY, A.J., J.R. STEINMETZ, H.F. PAGE, AND K. RODAHL.
The effects of physical conditioning on older individuals. II. Motor performance and cognitive
function.
Journal Gerontology 21:192-199, 1966.

0206
BARRY, H.J.
Physical activity and psychic stress/strain.
Canadian Medical Association Journal 96:848-851, 1967.

0207
BARRY, W.H., E.L. ALDERMAN, P.O. DAILY, AND D.C. HARRISON.
Diagnosis and treatment of a case of recurrent ventricular tachycardia.
American Heart Journal 84(2):235-241, 1972.

0208
BARTEL, A.G., V.S. BEHAR, R.H. PETER, E.S. ORGAIN, AND Y. KONG.
Exercise stress testing in evaluation of aortocoronary bypass surgery. Report of 123 patients.
Circulation 48:141-148, 1973.

0209
BARTELSTONE, H.J., N. KAHN, AND I.D. MANDEL.
Salivary potassium concentration as an indicator of digitalis toxicity.
IADR Program and Abstracts, p. 169, 1969.

0210
BARTH, P.
 Smoking and vascular diseases.
 Diagnostik 5(8):355, 1972.

0211
BASSETT, D.R., AND W.G. SCHROFFNER.
 Coronary heart disease in Chinese men in Hawaii. Serum lipids, plasma glucose, and cardio-
 vascular, anthropometric, and related findings. Comparisons and findings with Japanese men.
 Archives Internal Medicine 125(3):478-487, 1970.

0212
BASSLER, T.J.
 Cardiac rehabilitation.
 Journal American Medical Association 226:790, 1973.

0213
BASTIAANS, J.
 Psychoanalytic investigations on the psychic aspects of acute myocardial infarction.
 Psychotherapy Psychosomatics 16:202-209, 1968.

0214
BASU, S.K.
 Rehabilitation in cardiovascular and pulmonary diseases.
 Indian Medical Journal 61(6):151, 1967.

0215
BATSEVICH, A.A.
 Clinico phonocardiographic analysis of the opening click of the mitral valve.
 Vrachebnoe Delo 10:24-27, 1972.

0216
BATTOCK, D.J., H. ALVAREZ, AND C.A. CHIDSEY.
 Effects of propranolol and isosorbide dinitrate on exercise performance and adrenergic activity in
 patients with angina pectoris.
 Circulation 39:157-170, 1969.

0217
BATTOCK, D.J., H. ALVAREZ, AND C.A. CHIDSEY.
 Effects of propranolol and isosorbide dinitrate on exercise performance and adrenergic activity in
 patients with angina.
 American Journal Cardiology 23(1):105, 1969.

0218
BAUBINENE, A.V., AND R.A. YATSKUNAITE.
 The method of assessing ECG changes in epidemiological investigations of ischemic heart disease.
 Kardiologiya 11:130-132, 1971.

0219
BAUM, O.V., AND E.D. DUBROVIN.
 Physicomathematical model of genesis of electrocardiograms.
 Biophysics 16(5):934-941, 1971.

0220
BAUMAN, D.J., AND T.J. TSAGARIS.
   Continuous heart murmur following aortocoronary bypass surgery.
   Chest 64:269, 1973.

0221
BAUMANN, P.C.
   The prehospital phase in acute myocardial infarction.
   Schweizerische Medizinische Wochenschrift 102(5):1810-1815, 1972.

0222
BEARD, E.F., E. GARCIA, G.E. BURKE, AND W.E. DEAR.
   Postexercise electrocardiogram in screening for latent ischemic heart disease. A study with clinical
   follow-up observation.
   Diseases Chest 56(5):405-408, 1969.

0223
BECK, D.
   Psychosomatic aspects of functional heart diseases.
   Schweizerische Medizinische Wochenschrift 95:395-399, 1965.

0224
BECK, D.
   Psychodynamic factors in brief therapy represented by the example of functional cardiac dis-
   orders.
   Folia Clinica Internacional (Barcelona) 16:28-33, 1966.

0225
BECK, R.H.
   Electrocardiographic results after maximum exercise in the detection of early coronary disease.
   Journal American Osteopathic Association 67:537-543, 1968.

0226
BECK, R.H., G. BURCHETT, S.J. CALISE, ET AL.
   Physical activity in maintaining and developing total body and cardiovascular health.
   Journal American Osteopathic Association 70(10):1047-1056, 1971.

0227
BECK, W.
   Problems of geriatric surgery. II.
   Heilberufe 24(4):104-109, 1972.

0228
BECK, W., AND V. SCHRIRE.
   Endomyocardial fibrosis in Caucasians previously resident in tropical Africa.
   British Heart Journal 34(9):915-918, 1972.

0229
BECKER, A.E., M.J. BECKER, D.G. CLAUDON, AND J.E. EDWARDS.
   Surface thrombosis and fibrous encapsulation of intravenous pacemaker catheter electrode.
   Circulation 46(2):409-412, 1972.

0230
BECKER, M.C., ET AL.
   Rehabilitation of the patient with a permanent pacemaker.
   Geriatrics 22:106-111, 1967.

0231
BECKURTH, J.R., ET AL.
   Recent trends in the medical treatment of hypertension.
   Virginia Medical Monthly 91:435-442, 1964.

0232
BEDFORD, E.
   Cardiology in the days of Laennec. The story of auscultation of the heart.
   British Heart Journal 34(12):1193-1198, 1972.

0233
BEDNARZEWSKI, J., AND P.B. KOLBER.
   Conduction disturbances in myocardial infarction in the light of observation of 1000 cases.
   Polski Tygodnik Lekarski 27(32):1686-1689, 1972.

0234
BEDRAK, E., G. BEER, AND K.I. FURMAN.
   Fibrinolytic activity and muscular exercise in heat.
   Journal Applied Physiology 19:469-71, 1964.

0235
BEFELER, B., F.J. HILDNER, R.P. JAVIER, L.S. COHEN, AND P. SAMET.
   Cardiovascular dynamics during coronary sinus, right atrial, and right ventricular pacing.
   American Heart Journal 81:372-380, 1971.

0236
BEISER, G.D., S.E. EPSTEIN, M. STAMPFER, AND E. BRAUNWALD.
   The comparative hemodynamic effects of treadmill and supine bicycle exercise in patients with
   cardiac impairment.
   Physiologist 10(3):122, 1967.

0237
BEISER, G.D., S.E. EPSTEIN, M. STAMPFER, B. ROBINSON, AND E. BRAUNWALD.
   Studies on digitalis. XVII. Effects of ouabain on the hemodynamic response to exercise in
   patients with mitral stenosis in normal sinus rhythm.
   New England Journal Medicine 278(3):131-137, 1968.

0238
BELLER, G.A., T.W. SMITH, W.H. ABELMANN, E. HABER, AND W.B. HOOD, JR.
   Digitalis intoxication: A prospective clinical study with serum level correlations.
   New England Journal Medicine 284-989, 1971.

0239
BELLET, S.
   Clinical disorders of the heart beat, (3 ed.).
   Philadelphia, Lea and Febiger, 1971.

0240
BELLET, S., S. DELIYIANNIS, AND M. ELIAKIM.
The electrocardiogram during exercise as recorded by radioelectrocardiography. Comparison with the postexercise electrocardiogram (Master two-step test).
American Journal Cardiology 8:385-400, 1961.

0241
BELLET, S., M. ELIAKIM, S. DELIYIANNIS, AND D. LA VAN.
Radioelectrocardiography during exercise in patients with angina pectoris. Comparison with the postexercise electrocardiogram.
Circulation 25 (1 Part 1):5-14, 1962.

0242
BELLET, S., O.F. MULLER, A.B. HERRING, AND H. MOUALLEM.
Effect of vasodilator drugs on the exercise electrocardiogram in anginal patients studied by radioelectrocardiography.
Circulation 26(4 Part 2):686-687, 1962.

0243
BELLET, S., O.F. MULLER, A.B. HERRING, AND D.W. LA VAN.
Effect of erythrityl tetranitrate on the electrocardiogram as recorded during exercise by radioelectrocardiography.
American Journal Cardiology 11(5):600-608, 1963.

0244
BELLET, S., O.F. MULLER, D.W. LA VAN, G.J. NICHOLS, AND A.B. HERRING.
Radioelectrocardiography during exercise in patients with the anginal syndrome. Use of multiple leads.
Circulation 29(3):366-375, 1964.

0245
BELLET, S., L.R. ROMAN, J.B. KOSTIS, AND A. SLATER.
The stress effect of automobile driving in normal subjects and patients with coronary disease.
American Journal Cardiology 23:106, 1969.

0246
BELLET, S., L.R. ROMAN, G.J. NICHOLS, AND O.F. MULLER.
Detection of coronary prone subjects in a normal population by radioelectrocardiographic exercise test. Follow-up studies.
American Journal Cardiology 19(6):783-787, 1967.

0247
BELLONE, M., L. COSCARELLI, AND A. ZAGAMI.
Anesthesia and the electrocardiogram in coronary patients.
Acta Anesthesiologica (Padova) 23(1):55-71, 1972.

0248
BEMILLER, C.R., C.J. PEPINE, AND A.K. ROGERS.
Long term observations in patients with angina and normal coronary arteriograms.
Circulation 47(1):36-43, 1973.

0249
BENAIM, R., M. CHAPELLE, AND P. CHICHE.
  Action of phenytoin on atrioventricular and intraventricular conduction in humans.
  Annales de Cardiologie et d'Angéiologie 21(4):379-388, 1972.

0250
BENAK, R.T.
  Congestive heart failure, the patient and the community.
  American Journal Public Health 54:1706-1710, 1964.

0251
BENCHIMOL, A., K.B. DESSER, AND J.L. GARTLAN, JR.
  Left ventricular blood flow velocity in man studied with the Doppler ultrasonic flowmeter.
  American Heart Journal 85(3):294-301, 1973.

0252
BENCHIMOL, A., AND E.G. DIMOND.
  Apexcardiogram in ischemic heart disease; effect of exercise and nitroglycerin on the atrial
  contraction.
  Circulation 24(4 Part 2):884-885, 1961.

0253
BENCHIMOL, A., AND E.G. DIMOND.
  The apexcardiogram in normal older subjects and in patients with arteriosclerotic heart disease:
  Effect of exercise on the "a" wave.
  American Heart Journal 65:789, 1963.

0254
BENCHIMOL, A., E.G. DIMOND, AND Y-B. LI.
  The effect of heart rate, exercise and nitroglycerin on the cardiovascular dynamics in patients
  with complete heart block.
  American Journal Cardiology 13(1):96, 1964.

0255
BENCHIMOL, A., J.G. ELLIS, AND E.G. DIMOND.
  Hemodynamic consequences of atrial and ventricular pacing in patients with normal and abnormal
  hearts: Effect of exercise at a fixed atrial and ventricular rate.
  American Journal Medicine 39(6):911-922, 1965.

0256
BENCHIMOL, A., ET AL.
  Left ventricular end-diastolic pressure and cardiac output at rest and during exercise in patients
  with angina pectoris.
  Cardiologia 53:261-279, 1968.

0257
BENCHIMOL, A., H. FLEMING, AND K.B. DESSER.
  Abnormal apexcardiogram associated with rheumatic left ventricular dysfunction.
  Chest 64:225, 1973.

0258
BENCHIMOL, A., H.M. LOWE, AND P.R. AKRE.
  Cardiovascular response to exercise during atrial fibrillation and after conversion to sinus rhythm.
  American Journal Cardiology 16:31-41, 1965.

0259
BENCHIMOL, A., S. MATSUO, K.B. DESSER, ET AL.
Coronary artery blood flow velocity during ventricular tachycardia in man.
American Journal Medical Sciences 264(4):277-282, 1972.

0260
BENCHIMOL, A., R.B. VOTH, M.D. SINGH, H.A. PALMERO, and E.G. DIMOND.
Cardiac function in heart block at a variable heart rate: Effect of exercise at various fixed rates (man).
Circulation 304(4 Suppl. 3):45-46, 1964.

0261
BENCHIMOL, A., T.F. WANG, K.B. DESSER, AND J.L. GARTLAN, JR.
The Valsalva maneuver and coronary arterial blood flow velocity. Studies in man.
Annals Internal Medicine 77(3):357-360, 1972.

0262
BENESTAD, A.M.
Determination of physical work capacity and exercise tolerance in cardiac patients.
Acta Medica Scandinavica 183:521-529, 1968.

0263
BENESTAD, A.M.
Assessment of physical work capacity in cardiac patients.
Tidsskrift for den Norske Laegeforening 89:1189-1191, 1969.

0264
BENESTAD, A.M.
The deteriorative effect of myocardial infarction upon physiological indices of work capacity.
Acta Medica Scandinavica 191(1/2):67-75, 1972.

0265
BENISCH, B.M., A. FAYEMI, M.A. GERBER, AND J. AXELROD.
Mycoplasmal pneumonia in a patient with rheumatic heart disease.
American Journal Clinical Pathology 58(3):343-348, 1972.

0266
BENJAMIN, B.
Bereavement and heart disease.
Journal Biosocial Science 3(1):61-67, 1971.

0267
BENNETT, M.A., AND B.L. PENTECOST.
Suppression of ventricular tachyarrhythmias by transvenous intracardiac pacing after acute myocardial infarction.
British Medical Journal 4:468-470, 1970.

0268
BENNETT, M.A., AND B.L. PENTECOST.
Warning of cardiac arrest due to ventricular fibrillation and tachycardia.
Lancet (North American Edition) 1:1351-1352, 1972.

0269

BENNETT, N.B., C.M. OGSTON, AND D. OGSTON.
The effect of prolonged exercise on the components of the blood fibrinolytic enzyme system.
Journal Physiology (London) 198:479, 1968.

0270

BENTON, J.G., H. BROWN, AND H.A. RUSK.
Energy expended by patients on the bedpan and bedside commode.
Journal American Medical Association 144:1443-1447, 1950.

0271

BENZING, G., III, J. HELMSWORTH, J. STOCKERT, AND S. KAPLAN.
Human myocardial performance during surgical treatment of cardiac defects.
Journal Thoracic Cardiovascular Surgery 59(6):800-809, 1970.

0272

BERG-LARSEN, R.
A psychodynamic evaluation of patients with myocardial infarction with regard to their future occupational and social adjustment.
Psychotherapy Psychosomatics 18:294-298, 1970.

0273

BERGLUND, G., AND L. HANSSON.
A within-patient comparison of alprenolol and propranolol in hypertension.
Acta Medica Scandinavica 193:547, 1973.

0274

BERGMAN, H., AND E. VARNAUSKAS.
The hemodynamic effects of physical training in coronary patients.
Medicine Sport 4:138-147, 1970.

0275

BERGMAN, H., AND E. VARNAUSKAS.
Placebo effect in physical training of coronary heart disease patients.
In: Larsen, O.A. and R.O. Malmborg, Eds. Coronary heart disease and physical fitness, pp. 48-51.
Baltimore, University Park Press, 1971.

0276

BERGSTRÖM K., AND U. SÄWE.
Improved diagnosis of acute myocardial infarction by frequent serum enzyme determinations.
Acta Medica Scandinavica 193:515-523, 1973.

0277

BERGSTRÖM, G., AND A. SVANBORG.
Dietary treatment of acute myocardial infarction.
Acta Medica Scandinavica 181(6):717-721, 1967.

0278

BERGY, G.G., AND D.R. SPARKMAN.
Analysis of experience in workmen's compensation for heart cases. Factors influencing the decision re compensability in heart attacks occurring among industrial workers.
Circulation 33:461-473, 1966.

0279
BERKARDA, B., G. AKOKAN, AND U. DERMAN.
Fibrinolytic response to physical exercise in males.
Atherosclerosis 13(1):85-91, 1971.

0280
BERKOWITZ, W.D., A.L. WIT, C. STEINER, S.H. LAU, AND A.N. DAMATO.
The effects of propranolol on atrioventricular and intraventricular conduction.
American Journal Cardiology 23:106, 1969.

0281
BERNARD, R., H. LEWINSON, A. CORNIL, AND J.P. THYS.
Electrical pacing in myocardial infarction (90 observations).
Acta Cardiologica 27(6):665-679, 1972.

0282
BERNATECK, F.
Problems and objectives of physical-dietetic follow-up treatment after heart surgery.
Archiv für Physikalische Therapie (Leipzig) 16:123-128, 1964.

0283
BERNATECK, F.
Rehabilitation of patients with heart and circulatory diseases in the spa.
Zeitschrift für Aerztliche Fortbildung (Jena) 59:835-836, 1965.

0284
BERNI, A.J., M.W. LUTTGES, AND D.E. DICK.
Electrocardiogram monitoring: Computerized detection of ventricular changes induced by drugs.
Science 179:1338-1340, 1973.

0285
BERNREITER, M.
The use of additional leads in the early diagnosis of posterior myocardial infarction.
Angiology 16:452-459, 1965.

0286
BERNSTEIN, D., D.R. RICHMOND, D. COLES, AND R. HAWKER.
Exercise and right atrial pacing in the evaluation of patients with ischemic heart disease.
Australian New Zealand Journal Medicine 1(3):323, 1971.

0287
BERSAY, C.
Myocardial infarction and psychosomatic factors.
Coeur et Médecine Interne 9(3):323-326, 1970.

0288
BERSCH, W.
On the moderation band of the left heart chamber.
Basic Research Cardiology 68:225, 1973.

0289
BERTINI, G., L. GIGLIOGI, C. FUMAGALLI, AND S. MORI.
Auriculoventricular block in the acute phase of myocardial infarction.
Cardiologia Pratica 23(2):151-156, 1972.

0290
BESSE, P., H. BRICAUD, AND P. BROUSTET.
Changes in heart contraction in the course of angina pectoris.
Revue du Praticien 22(34):4805-4812, 1972.

0291
BETELMAN, R.A.
Extrasystolic arrhythmia in ostensibly healthy persons older than 50 years, on the basis of many years of clinical and electrocardiographic observation.
Terapevticheskii Arkhiv 44(8):86-89, 1972.

0292
BETHELL, H.J.N., AND P.G.F. NIXON.
P wave of electrocardiogram in early ischaemic heart disease.
British Heart Journal 34(11):1170-1175, 1972.

0293
BETTICA-GIOVANNINI, R.
The cardiopathies, a medical, psychological and social problem, in the studies of Prof. Franco De Matteis.
Giornale di Batteriologia, Virologia ed Immunologia 60:516-519, 1967.

0294
BEZZUBIK, V.G, AND S.A. KOZYREVA.
Myocardial infarction in persons over 70 years old.
Kardiologiya 10(3):142-144, 1970.

0295
BEZZUBIK, V.G, N.P. VOSHCHANOVA, AND S.A. KOZYREVA.
Life span and immediate causes of death in persons who had myocardial infarctions when over 70 years of age.
Kardiologiya 12:37, 1972.

0296
BIALKOWSKA, M., B. CYBULSKA, AND W.B. SZOSTAK.
Some metabolic indices in coronary artery disease.
Polski Tygodnik Lekarski 27(40):1550-1553, 1972.

0297
BIASCO, G., A. MICCOLI, AND P. RIZZON.
Hemodynamic changes caused by amiodarone in patients with ischemic heart disease.
Bolletino della Società Italiana di Cardiologia 17(7):401-406, 1972.

0298
BIASE, M., Di, S. CESARIO, G. BRINDICCI, AND P. RIZZON.
Incidence of the atrioventricular block with acute myocardial infarction associated with intraventricular conduction disorders of bi- and trifascicular type.
Bollettino della Società Italiana di Cardiologia 17(8):587-594, 1972.

0299
BICKELMANN, A.G., ET AL.
The response of the normal and abnormal heart to exercise: A functional evaluation.
Circulation 28:238-250, 1963.

0300
BIERENBAUM, M.L., A.B. CALDWELL, P. WATSON, AND V. MOLLEK.
Fats and fatty acids in excess.
Journal American Dietetic Association 50(5):368-371, 1967.

0301
BIERENBAUM, M.L., ET AL.
Modified-fat dietary management of the young male with coronary disease. A five-year report.
Journal American Medical Association 202(13):1119-1123, 1967.

0302
BIERENBAUM, M.L., D.P. GREEN, A.B. CALDWELL, AND E.H. KELLY.
Blood cholesterol and coronary heart disease. Preliminary report.
Journal Medical Society New Jersey 58(4):134-138, 1961.

0303
BIERENBAUM, M.L., D.P. GREEN, A. FLORIN, A.I. FLEISCHMAN, AND A.B. CALDWELL.
Modified fat dietary management of the young coronary male. A five-year controlled study.
Circulation 31(Suppl. 2):3, 1965.

0304
BIERENBAUM, M.L., R.I. RAICHELSON, T. HAYTON, AND D. GREEN.
Decreased catecholamine excretion and angina pectoris with diazepam in stressed arteriosclerotic heart disease patients.
Federation Proceedings 31(2):289, 1972.

0305
BIERENBAUM, M.L., H. YACOWITZ, AND A.I. FLEISCHMAN.
Studies on the mechanism of the hypolipemic action of dietary calcium in man.
Circulation 31(Suppl. 2):3, 1965.

0306
BIERSNER, R.J., E.K.E. GUNDERSON, AND R.H. RAHE.
Relationship of sports interests and smoking to physical fitness.
Journal Sport Medicine 12:124, 1972.

0307
BIGGER, J.T., JR., AND B.N. GOLDREYER.
The mechanism of supraventricular tachycardia.
Circulation 42:673-688, 1970.

0308
BILINSKII, E.A., AND A.A. POPOV.
Vectorcardiographic analysis of electrocardiograms under physical loading.
Vrachebnoe Delo 1:134-135, 1968.

0309
BILLIMORIA, J.D., J. DRYSDALE, D.C. JAMES, AND N.F. MacLAGAN.
Determination of fibrinolytic activity of whole blood. With special reference to the effect of exercise and fat feeding.
Lancet 2:471-5, 1959.

0310
BILODEAU, C.B., AND T.P. HACKETT.
  Issues raised in a group setting by patients recovering from myocardial infarction.
  American Journal Psychiatry 128(1):73-78, 1971.

0311
BINAGHI, G., ET AL.
  Evaluation with the exercise test of the significance of the post-extrasystolic beat in the diagnosis
  of coronary insufficiency.
  Folia Cardiologica (Milano) 26:239-247, 1967.

0312
BINAGHI, G., L. BRUNO, P. GIANI, G. MORTARINO, L. BANDERA, AND G. FOLLI.
  Relation between cardiac work and coronary insufficiency caused through effort in angina
  patients.
  Bollettino della Società Italiana di Cardiologia 15(2):55-61, 1970.

0313
BING, G.T.
  Cardiovascular disease in Djakarta, Indonesia, in private and in municipal outpatient practice.
  Tropical Geographical Medicine 22:289-296, 1970.

0314
BING, O.H.L., W.W. BROOKS, AND J.V. MESSER.
  Effects of isoproterenol on heart muscle performance during myocardial hypoxia.
  Journal Molecular Cellular Cardiology 4(4):319-328, 1972.

0315
BING, R.J.
  Rehabilitation in heart disease.
  Archives Environmental Health 3(3):304-307, 1961.

0316
BING, R.J., AND K. HELLBERG.
  Coronary blood flow in relation to angina pectoris.
  Circulation 46(6):1146-1154, 1972.

0317
BIÖRCK, G., AND E.M. WEDELIN.
  The return to work of patients with myocardial infarction.
  Acta Medica Scandinavica 175:215, 1964.

0318
BIRKETT, D.A., AND D.A. CHAMBERLAIN.
  Beta-adrenergic blockage in angina pectoris: A method of treadmill assessment.
  British Medical Journal 2:500-502, 1966.

0319
BISHOP, J.M., AND N. SEGEL.
  The circulatory effects of intravenous pronethalol in man at rest and during exercise in the supine
  and upright positions.
  Journal Physiology (London) 169:112P-114P, 1963.

0320
BISHOP, L.F., AND P. REICHERT.
   The interrelationship between anxiety and arrhythmias.
   Psychosomatics 11(4):330-334, 1970.

0321
BISHOP, L.F., AND P. REICHERT.
   Emotion and heart failure.
   Psychosomatics 12(6):412-415, 1971.

0322
BISSONNETTE, G.
   The rehabilitation of the employee with heart disease. A challenging responsibility of the occupational health nurse.
   American Association Industrial Nurses Journal 14:6-9, 1966.

0323
BITTAR, N., J.A. SOSA, AND R.F.P. CRONIN.
   Abnormal lactate-pyruvate extraction ratios during exercise in patients with coronary artery disease.
   Canadian Medical Association Journal 96:341, 1967.

0324
BJERKELUND, C.
   Therapeutic level in long-term anticoagulant therapy after myocardial infarction.
   American Journal Cardialogy 11(2):158-163, 1963.

0325
BJERKELUND, C.
   Work capacity after myocardial infarct.
   Tidsskrift for den Norske Laegeforening 86:548-550, 1966.

0326
BJÖRNTORP, P., M. FAHLÉN, J. HOLM, T. SCHERSTÉN, AND J. STENBERG.
   Changes in the activity of skeletal muscle succinic oxidase after training.
   In: Larsen, O.A. and R.O. Malmborg, Eds. Coronary heart disease and physical fitness, pp. 138-142, Baltimore, University Park Press, 1971.

0327
BJURÖ, T., H. SANNE, J. STENBERG, AND E. VARNAUSKAS.
   Mobilization after acute coronary infarction.
   In: Larsen, O., and R.O. Malmborg, Eds. Coronary heart disease and physical fitness, pp. 180-182. Baltimore, University Park Press, 1971.

0328
BLACHLY, P.H., ET AL.
   Vocational and emotional status of 263 patients after heart surgery.
   Circulation 38:524-532, 1968.

0329
BLACK, A., M.M. BLACK, G.G. GENSINI, AND S. DI GIORGI.
   Exertion and acute coronary artery injury.
   Circulation 31(Suppl. 2):3, 1965.

0330
BLACK, D.P.
Management of myocardial infarction in a rural area.
Canadian Medical Association Journal 109:863, 1973.

0331
BLACKBURN, H.W.
Developments in exercise electrocardiography.
Proceedings Medical Section American Life Convention 57:145-170, 1969.

0332
BLACKBURN, H.W.
Measurement in exercise electrocardiography: The Ernst Simonson Conference. Springfield, Ill.
Thomas, 1969.

0333
BLACKBURN, H.W., ET AL.
The exercise electrocardiogram: Differences in interpretation. Report of a technical group on
exercise electrocardiography.
American Journal Cardiology 21(6):871-880, 1968.

0334
BLACKBURN, H., H.L. TAYLOR, AND A. KEYS.
The electrocardiogram in prediction of five-year coronary heart disease incidence among men aged
forty through fifty-nine.
Circulation 41(Suppl. I):154, 1970.

0335
BLACKBURN, H.W., H.L. TAYLOR, AND A. KEYS.
Prognostic significance of the post-exercise electrocardiogram: Risk factors held constant.
American Journal Cardiology 25:85, 1970.

0336
BLACKBURN, H.W., H.L. TAYLOR, N. OKAMOTO, P. RAUTAHARJU, P.L. MITCHELL, AND A.C.
KERKHOF.
Standardization of the exercise electrocardiogram. A systematic comparison of chest lead con-
figurations employed for monitoring during exercise.
In: Karvonen, M.J., and A.J. Barry, Eds. Physical activity and the heart, pp. 101-133. Springfield,
Ill. Thomas, 1967.

0337
BLACKBURN, H.W., H.L. TAYLOR, T.C. PUCHNER, AND A. KEYS.
Relationship of resting and postexercise electrocardiographic abnormalities to obesity, hyper-
tension, and hypercholesteremia in working men.
Circulation 24(4 Part 2):887-888, 1961.

0338
BLACKBURN, H. W., G. WINCKLER, J. VILANDRÉ, J. HODGSON, AND H.L. TAYLOR.
Exercise Tests.
Medicine Sport 4:78, 1970.

0339
BLACKET, R.B., J. WOODHILL, AND M.A. MISHKEL.
Diet, hypercholesterolaemia and coronary heart disease.
Medical Journal Australia 52-1:59, 1965.

0340

BLACKET, R.B.
   Diet in the prevention of heart disease.
   Medical Journal Australia 60-1:969, 1973.

0341

BLACKMON, J.R., L.B. ROWELL, J.W. KENNEDY AND R.D. TWISS.
   Normal adaptations to moderate through maximal upright exercise in patients with mitral stenosis.
   Clinical Research 14(1):122, 1966.

0342

BLAKE, T.M., P.H. LEHAN, K.R. BENNETT, AND J.R. GALYEAN, III.
   Exercise tests and coronary artery disease.
   Southern Medical Journal 65:769-770, 1972.

0343

BLANKENHORN, D.H., H.P. CHIN, AND F.Y.K. LAU.
   Ischemic heart disease in young adults: metabolic and angiographic diagnosis and prevalence of
   type IV hyperlipoproteinemia.
   Annals Internal Medicine 69:21, 1968.

0344

BLANTON, J.H., M. RODRÍGUEZ, R. COSTAS, JR., A.A. COLÓN, M. FELIBERTI, H. BENSON, R.
   AIXALÁ, AND M.R. GARCÍA-PALMIERI.
   A dietary study of men residing in urban and rural areas of Puerto Rico.
   American Journal Clinical Nutrition 18:169-175, 1966.

0345

BLEIFELD, W., P. HANRATH, W. MERX, ET AL.
   Acute myocardial infarction. I. Hemodynamics of the left ventricle.
   Deutsche Medizinishe Wochenschrift 97(47):1807-1815, 1972.

0346

BLEIFER, D.J., S.B. BLEIFER, AND R. OKUN.
   Perhexiline maleate in angina pectoris. A controlled, double blind clinical trial.
   Geriatrics 27(9):109-115, 1972.

0347

BLISS, B.P., C.J.C. KIRK, AND R.G. NEWALL.
   Abnormalities in glucose tolerance, lipid and lipiprotein levels in patients with atherosclerotic
   peripheral arterial disease.
   Angiology 23(2):69-75, 1972.

0348

BLOCK, M.B., M. GAMBETTA, L. RESNEKOV, AND A.H. RUBENSTEIN.
   Spontaneous hypoglycaemia in congestive heart failure.
   Lancet 2:736-738, 1972.

0349

BLOEHS, V.
   Is there an old heart?
   Zeitschrift für Alternsforschung 25(2):163-168, 1971.

0350
BLOHMKE, M., ET AL.
Results of a medical and social survey of coronary disease.
Revista Clinica Expañola 112:621-628, 1969.

0351
BLOHMKE, M., ET AL.
Results of a medical and social investigation of coronary diseases.
Minerva Medica 60:1184-1192, 1969.

0352
BLOMQVIST, C.G.
Use of exercise testing for diagnostic and functional evaluation of patients with arteriosclerotic heart disease.
Circulation 44(6):1120-1136, 1971.

0353
BLOMQVIST, G.
The Frank lead exercise electrocardiogram. A quantitative study based on averaging technic and digital computer analysis.
Acta Medica Scandinavica 178(Suppl. 440):5, 1965.

0354
BLOMQVIST, G.
Exercise and performance evaluation. Why evaluate performance?
Journal South Carolina Medical Association (Suppl.) 65(12):1-4, 1969.

0355
BLOMQVIST, G., I. ÅSTRAND, B. EKBLOM, AND P. HALL.
Computer analysis of vectorcardiographic changes during and after exercise in patients with coronary disease and in normal subjects.
In:Karvonen, M.J., and A.J. Barry. Eds. Physical activity and the heart, pp. 134-143. Springfield, Ill. Thomas, 1967.

0356
BLOMQVIST, G., AND J. M. ATKINS.
Repeated exercise testing in patients with angina pectoris: Reproducibility and follow-up results.
Circulation 44(Suppl. II):76, 1971.

0357
BLOMQVIST, G., B. SALTIN, AND J.H. MITCHELL.
Acute effects of ethanol ingestion on the response to submaximal and maximal exercise in man.
Circulation 42(3):463-470, 1970.

0358
BLOOMER, W.E., M.H. ELLESTAD, A.J. BELAND, J.A. COPE, AND E.R. PALAREA.
Evaluation of myocardial revascularization with arterial implants. An objective study using electrocardiography and maximal stress testing.
Annals Internal Medicine 73(6):913-919, 1970.

0359
BLOOR, C.M., AND A.S. LEON.
   Interaction of age and exercise on the heart and its blood supply.
   Laboratory Investigation 22:160, 1970.

0360
BLOUIN, S., L. AUBIN, AND G.R. DAGENAIS.
   Functional evaluation of patients with ischemic heart disease.
   Union Médicale du Canada 101:2650, 1972.

0361
BLÜMCHEN, G., H. KIEFER, H. ROSKAMM, D. WALDMANN, D. BÜCHNER, AND H. REINDELL.
   Comparison of the coronary angiographic findings of 127 patients with anamnesis, risk factors for
   coronary disease, resting and stress EKG.
   Zeitschrift für Kreislaufforschung 58(2):149-167, 1969.

0362
BOBBA, P., J.A. SALERNO, AND A. CASARI.
   Transient left posterior hemiblock. Report of four cases induced by exercise test.
   Circulation 46(5):931-938, 1972.

0363
BOCK, H., AND E.O. KRASEMANN
   Primary functions in rehabilitation. Social and medical responsibility. Based on the example of re-
   habilitation of heart-attack patients.
   Das Öffentliche Gesundheitswesen 35:445, 1973.

0364
BOGDANIK, T., M. WARMUS, Z. BOWSZYCOWA, ET AL.
   The mathematical model of the electrical heart position in healthy patients and in heart
   hypertrophy.
   Materia Medica Polona 4:60, 1972.

0365
BOISSIER, J.R., C. ADVENIER, AND J.F. GIUDICELLI.
   Cardiovascular effects of 2,5-dimethoxy-4-methylamphetamine (STP or DOM).
   Therapie 27(6):989-999, 1972.

0366
BOLOOKI, H., A. GHAHRAMA, S. MALLON, L. SOMMER, G. KAISER, AND A. VARGAS.
   Long-term follow-up of patients with impending and early myocardial infarction treated by emer-
   gency myocardial revascularization.
   Circulation 48(4):147, 1973.

0367
BOLOOKI, H., AND J.R. JUDE.
   Current trends towards management of patients with cardiac arrest.
   Pahlavi Medical Journal 1(2):50-65, 1970.

0368
BOLOOKI, H., J.R. JUDE, L.S. SOMMER, AND L. LEMBERG.
   Cardiac and systemic hemodynamic findings and surgery in patients with cardiogenic shock and
   low perfusion state due to acute myocardial infarction.
   Bulletin de la Société Internationale de Chirurgie 31(5):411-417, 1972.

0369
BONAMI, M., ET AL.
  Experimental approach to the personality and occupational rehabilitation of the coronary patient.
  Acta Psychiatrica Belgica 70:579-590, 1970.

0370
BONAMI, M., ET AL.
  Psychologic reaction and attitudes following myocardial infarction.
  Acta Psychiatrica Belgica 72:80-95, 1972. (French)

0371
BONNER, D.C.
  Rehabilitation instead of bed rest?
  Geriatrics 24:109-118, 1969.

0372
BOOTSMA, B.K., J. STRACKEE, J.J. DENIER VON DEN GON, AND F.L. MEIJLER.
  Random behavior of RR intervals in patients with atrial fibrillation (AF) at rest and during exercise.
  Circulation 40 (Suppl. 3):48, 1969.

0373
BOOYENS, J., AND W.R. KEATINGE.
  The expenditure of energy by men and women walking.
  Journal Physiology 138:165, 1957.

0374
BOPP, P., P.C. FOURNET, B. HAENNI, AND R. VALLET.
  Risks and complications of catheterization and angiocardiography.
  Schweizerische Medizinische Wochenschrift 102(42):1497-1502, 1972.

0375
BORCHGREVINK, C.F., C. BJERKELUND, A.M. ABRAHAMSEN, G. BAY, P. BORGEN, B. GRANDE, I. HELLE, J. KJORSTAD, A.M. PETERSEN, T. RORVIK, T. THORSEN, AND A. ODEGAARD.
  Long-term anticoagulant therapy after myocardial infarction in women.
  British Medical Journal 3:571-574, 1968.

0376
BORDIA, A., S.K. SHARMA, A. MATHUR, AND L.M. SANGHVI.
  Serum magnesium, serum cholesterol and serum lipoproteins in cases of coronary artery disease.
  Indian Heart Journal 24(3):277-281, 1973.

0377
BORG, G.
  Perceived exertion as an indicator of somatic stress.
  Scandinavian Journal Rehabilitation Medicine 2(2/3):92-98, 1970.

0378
BORG, G., AND H. LINDERHOLM.
  Exercise performance and perceived exertion in patients with coronary insufficiency, arterial hypertension and vasoregulatory asthenia.
  Acta Medica Scandinavica 187(1/2):17-26, 1970.

0379
BORGES, S., J. FELDMAN, E.J.S. CARMO, JR., ET AL.
Multiple aneurysms of the coronary arteries. Presentation of one case with diagnosis in life.
Arquivos Brasileiros de Cardiologia 24(6):63-67, 1971.

0380
BORNEMISZA, P.
Glucosetoleranz bei Arteriosklerotikern, Fettsüchtigen und Gesunden. (Glucose tolerance in athero-sclerotics, obese, and normal people.)
Medizinische Klinik 67:258-261, 1972.
0381
BORNHOFEN, E.
Heart and circulation of the aging human.
Fortschritte der Medizin 90(33):1209-1212, 1972.

0382
BORTNER, R.W.
A short rating scale as a potential measure of Pattern A behavior.
Journal Chronic Diseases 22(2):87-91, 1969.

0383
BORTNER, R.W., R.H. ROSENMAN, and M. FRIEDMAN.
Familial similarity in Pattern A behavior: Fathers and sons.
Journal Chronic Diseases 23(1):39-43, 1970.

0384
BORUN, E.R., J.M. CHAPMAN, AND F.J. MASSEY, JR.
Computer analysis of Frank lead electrocardiographic data recorded in an epidemiologic study.
American Journal Cardiology 18:664, 1966.

0385
BOSNJAKOVIC, V.B., L.R. BENNETT, L.D. GREENFIELD, and W.R. VINCENT.
Dual-isotope method for diagnosis of intracardiac shunts.
Journal Nuclear Medicine 14:514, 1973.

0386
BOTTIGER, L.E., L.A. CARLSON, L. ENGSTEDT, AND L. ORO.
The effect of long-term heparin treatment in ischaemic heart disease.
Journal Atherosclerosis Research 5:253, 1965.

0387
BOUHEY, J., C. KLEPPING, C. PORTIER, AND B. CHALON.
Syncopal attacks due to cardiac dysrhythmia in a female with chronic potassium depletion.
Revue Médicale de Dijon 7(9):509-515, 1972.

0388
BOUJJA, H.
Resumption of work following myocardial infarction.
Revue de Médecine de Tours 5(6):495-496, 1971.
0389
BOUJOFF, G.V.
The postcoronary patient: psychological management.
Applied Therapeutics 10:655-657, 1968.

0390
BOURASSA, M.G., L. CAMPEAU, M.A. BOIS, AND O. RICO.
Myocardial lactate metabolism at rest and during exercise in ischemic heart disease.
American Journal Cardiology 23:771-777, 1969.

0391
BOUVRAIN, Y., P.F. BOUCHET, G. MOTTE, AND P. ROCHE.
Bundle branch block in the acute phase of myocardial infarction.
Archives des Maladies du Coeur et des Vaisseaux 65(6):649-657, 1972.

0392
BOYER, J.L.
Adult fitness starter program for individuals considered to be at high risk for coronary heart disease.
Journal South Carolina Medical Association (Suppl.) 65(12):99-100, 1969.

0393
BOYER, J.L., AND F.W. KASCH.
Exercise therapy in hypertensive men.
Journal American Medical Association 211:1668-1671, 1970.

0394
BOYER, J.M.
Effects of chronic exercise on cardiovascular function.
Physical Fitness Research Digest 2:1, 1972.

0395
BOYLE, D.M., M.J. WALSH, J.M. BARBER, ET AL.
Early mobilisation and discharge of patients with acute myocardial infarction.
Lancet, II:57-60, 1972.

0396
BOYLE, E., JR.
Types of elevated serum lipid levels in man, and their management.
Journal American Geriatric Society 10(10):822-830, 1962.

0397
BOYLE, E., JR.
Biological patterns in hypertension by race, sex, body weight, and skin color.
Journal American Medical Association 213(1):1637-1643, 1970.

0398
BOYLE, J.A., AND A.R. LORIMER.
Early mobilization after uncomplicated myocardial infarction. Prospective study of 538 patients.
Lancet (North American Edition) 2:346-349, 1973.

0399
BOYLES, P.W.
Improved long-term survival following myocardial infarction with fibrinolytic therapy.
Angiology 16(6):346-350, 1965.

0400
BOYLES, P.W.
Fibrinolytic activity and thromboembolism.
Clinical Pharmacology Therapeutics 13:534-538, 1972.

0401
BOZYK, Z.
Invalid pensions after myocardial infarction received by men in the Mokotow quarter of the city of Warsaw in the years 1955-1964.
Przeglad Epidemiologiczny 22:435-438, 1968.

0402
BRACELAND, F.J.
Psychiatric aspects.
Journal Rehabilitation 32:53, 1966.

0403
BRADFORD, H.A.
Anticoagulants in the management of various thromboembolic diseases.
Angiology 15:35-41, 1964.

0404
BRAMMEL, H.L.
Coronary heart disease rehabilitation.
Cardiac Rehabilitation Unit. University of Colorado Medical Center, July 1971.

0405
BRANDALEONE, H.
Driving and the coronary patient.
Journal Rehabilitation 32:97, 1966.

0406
BRANN, I.
The significance of the electrocardiographic pattern for assessment of the degree and type of left ventricular hypertrophy. Correlation of haemodynamic state to electrocardiogram at rest and during work.
Cardiologia 46(1):3-24, 1965.

0407
BRAUNWALD, E.
Control of myocardial oxygen consumption. Physiologic and clinical considerations.
American Journal Cardiology 27(4):416-432, 1971.

0408
BRAUNWALD, E., AND L.S. COHEN.
Amelioration of exercise-induced angina pectoris in idiopathic hypertrophic subaortic stenosis with beta-adrenergic blockage.
Circulation 33(Suppl. III):64, 1966.

0409
BRAUNWALD, E., ET AL.
Studies on cardiac dimensions in intact, unanesthetized man. III. Effects of muscular exercise.
Circulation Research 13:460, 1963.

0410
BRAUNWALD, E., AND E.R. KELLY.
The effects of exercise on central blood volume in man.
Journal Clinical Investigation 39:413, 1960.

0411
BRAUNWALD, E., J. ROSS, JR., AND E.H. SONNENBLICK.
Mechanisms of contraction of the normal and failing heart.
New England Journal Medicine 277:794, 853, 910, 962, 1012, 1967.

0412
BRAUNWALD, E., J. ROSS, JR., J.H. GAULT, D.T. MASON, C. MILLS, I.T. GABE, AND S.E. EP-
STEIN.
Assessment of cardiac function.
Annals Internal Medicine 70(2):369-399, 1969.

0413
BRECKENRIDGE, C.G., AND W.A. SPENCER.
Rehabilitation medicine—Research and methods.
Southern Medical Bulletin 55(1):24-28, 1967.

0414
BRENNAN, R.E.
Frequency of use of diet in the treatment of coronary heart disease in four Pittsburgh hospitals,
and some factors related to adherence to diet in the population studied.
Dissertation Abstracts 27:3162-B, 1967.

0415
BRESLOW, L., AND P. BUELL.
Mortality from coronary heart disease and physical activity of work in California.
Journal Chronic Diseases 11:421-444, 1960.

0416
BRICAUD, H., J.P. BROUSTET, AND P. BROUSTET.
Rehabilitation of cardiac patients.
Nouvelle Presse Médicale 1(18):1199-1202, 1972.

0417
BRICKNER, P.W., AND A. KAUFMAN.
Case finding of heart disease in homeless men.
Bulletin New York Academy Medicine 49(6):475-484, 1973.

0418
BRIGGS, M.H., ET AL.
Androgens and exercise.
British Medical Journal 3:49, 1973.

0419
BROWN, D.F., J.T. DOYLE, AND S.H. KINCH.
Serum triglycerides in health and in ischemic heart disease.
New England Journal Medicine 273:947, 1965.

0420
BRISSE, B., AND F. BENDER.
Catecholamines and 11-hydroxycorticoids in the serum of patients with cardiac insufficiency under stress.
Medizinische Welt 22:1067, 1971.

0421
BRISTOW, J.D., R.L. CRISLIP, C. FARREHI, W.E. HARRIS, R.P. LEWIS, D.W. SUTHERLAND, AND H.E. GRISWOLD.
Left ventricular volume measurements in man by thermodilution.
Journal Clinical Investigation 43(6):1015-1024, 1964.

0422
BRISTOW, J.D., ET AL.
The effects of supine exercise on left ventricular volume in heart disease.
American Heart Journal 71(3):319-329, 1966.

0423
BRISTOW, J.D., F.E. KLOSTER, M.H. LEES, V.D. MENASHE, H.E. GRISWOLD, AND A. STARR.
Serial cardiac catheterizations and exercise hemodynamics after correction of tetralogy of Fallot: Average follow-up 13 months and 7 years after operation.
Circulation 41(6):1057-1066, 1970.

0424
BROCHIER, M., AND PH. MORAND.
Readaptation of cardiac patients after myocardial infarction.
Revue de Médecine de Tours 5(8):647-652, 1971.

0425
BRODER, G., AND K. AMBE.
Exercise recovery systolic time interval test for coronary artery disease.
Clinical Research 20(3):365, 1972.

0426
BRODY, A.J.
Master two-step exercise test in clinically unselected patients.
Journal American Medical Association 171:1195, 1959.

0427
BRODY, D.A., G.D. COPELAND, J.W. COX, JR., ET AL.
Experimental and clinical aspects of total electrocardiographic alternation.
American Journal Cardiology 31(2):254-259, 1973.

0428
BROUSTET, J.P., A. CHOUSSAT, H. BRICAUD, ET AL.
Rehabilitation of coronary patients.
Annales de Cardiologie et d'Angéiologie 21(2):111-127, 1972.

0429
BROUSTET, J.P., M. DUBECQ, J. BOULOUMIE, P. BARON, AND A. BEAUFFIGEAU.
The rehabilitation of cardiac cases.
Bordeaux Médical 5(9):1009-1020, 1972.

0430
BROWE, J.H., D.M. MORLLEY, M.C. McCARTHY, AND R.M. GOFSTEIN.
  Diet and heart disease study in the cardiovascular health center.
  Journal American Dietetic Association 48:101-108, 1966.

0431
BROWN, D.F., AND J.T. DOYLE.
  Pre-beta lipoproteinemia. Its bearing on the dietary management of serum lipid disorders as related to ischemic heart disease.
  American Journal Clinical Nutrition 20(4):324-332, 1967.

0432
BROWN, H.B.
  The national diet-heart study: Implications for dietitians and nutritionists.
  Journal American Dietetic Association 52:279-287, 1968.

0433
BROWN, H.B.
  Food patterns that lower blood lipids in man.
  Journal American Dietetic Association 58:303-311, 1971.

0434
BROWN, K.W.G., R.L. MacMILLAN, N. FORBATH, F. MEL'GRANO, AND J.W. SCOTT.
  Coronary unit: An intensive-care centre for acute myocardial infarction.
  Lancet 2:349-352, 1963.

0435
BROWN, L.B., ET AL.
  Social effects of myocardial infarction in men under the age of 50 years: A review after one to eight years.
  Medical Journal Australia 2:125-128, 1969.

0436
BROWN, R.G., L.A.G. DAVIDSON, T. McKEOWN, AND A.G.W. WHITFIELD.
  Coronary-artery disease. Invluences affecting its incidence in males in the seventh decade.
  Lancet 2:1073, 1957.

0437
BROWN, R.W., AND A.J. GOBLE.
  Effect of propranolol on exercise tolerance of patients with atrial fibrillation.
  British Medical Journal 2:279-280, 1969.

0438
BROWNE, I.W., AND T.P. HACKETT.
  Emotional reactions to the threat of impending death. A study of patients on the monitor cardiac pacemaker.
  Irish Journal Medical Science 6:177-187, 1967.

0439
BROŽEK, J., A. KEYS, AND H. BLACKBURN.
  Personality differences between potential coronary and noncoronary subjects.
  Annals New York Academy Sciences 134:1057-1064, 1966.

0440
BROŻEK, J., ET AL.
   Skinfold distributions in middle-aged American men: A contribution to norms of leanness — fatness.
   Annals New York Academy Science 110:492-502, 1963.

0441
BRUCE, R.A.
   Evaluation of functional capacity and exercise tolerance of cardiac patients.
   Modern Concepts of Cardiovascular Disease 25:321-326, 1956.

0442
BRUCE, R.A.
   Exercise testing of patients with coronary heart disease: Principles and normal standards for evaluation.
   Annals Clinical Research 3(6):323-332, 1971.

0443
BRUCE, R.A., J.R. BLACKMON, J.W. JONES, AND G. STRAIT.
   Exercise testing in adult normal subjects and cardiac patients.
   Pediatrics, 32(Part II):742-756, 1963.

0444
BRUCE, R.A., L.A. COBB, J.H. MORLEDGE, AND S. KATSURA.
   Effects of posture, upright exercise, and myocardial stimulation on cardiac output in patients with diseases affecting diastolic filling and effective systolic ejection of the left ventricle.
   American Heart Journal 61:476-487, 1961.

0445
BRUCE, R.A., M. COOPER, G. GEY, AND R. EARLY.
   Earlier detection of coronary heart disease.
   Clinical Research 20(2):161, 1972.

0446
BRUCE, R.A., ET AL.
   The effects of digoxin on fatiguing static and dynamic exercise in man.
   Clinical Science 34:29, 1968.

0447
BRUCE, R.A., ET AL.
   Coronary disease and exercise.
   Texas Medicine 65:73-77, 1969.

0448
BRUCE, R.A., ET AL.
   Introductory report on ST responses to maximal exercise, quantitative measurements, time course and relationships.
   Malattie Cardiovascolari 10:15-34, 1969.

0449
BRUCE, R.A., AND T.R. HORNSTEN.
   Exercise stress testing in evaluation of patients with ischemic heart disease.
   Progress Cardiovascular Diseases 11:371-390, 1969.

0450
BRUCE, R.A., T.R. HORNSTEN, AND J.R. BLACKMON.
Myocardial infarction after normal responses to maximal exercise.
Circulation 38:552, 1968.

0451
BRUCE, R.A., J.W. JONES, AND G.A. STRAIT.
Anaerobic metabolic responses to acute maximal exercise in male athletes.
American Heart Journal 67:643-650, 1964.

0452
BRUCE, R.A., AND W. KLUGE.
Defibrillatory treatment of exertional cardiac arrest in coronary disease.
Journal American Medical Association 216(4):653-658, 1971.

0453
BRUCE, R.A., F. KUSUMI, AND D. HOSMER.
Maximal oxygen intake and nomographic assessment of functional aerobic impairment in cardio-vascular disease.
American Heart Journal 85:546, 1973.

0454
BRUCE, R.A., Y-B. LI, G.E. DOWER, AND K. NILSON.
Polar cardiographic responses to maximal exercise and to changes in posture in healthy middle-aged men.
Journal Electrocardiology 6:91, 1973.

0455
BRUCE, R.A., AND J.R. McDONOUGH.
Stress testing in screening for cardiovascular disease.
Bulletin New York Academy Medicine 45:1288-1305, 1969.

0456
BRUCE, A., B. ROWELL, S. KASSER, AND A. MURRAY.
Variations and disparities in blood pressure responses to upright exercise in health and disease.
Malattie Cardiovascolari 10(1-2):275-288, 1969.

0457
BRUCE, R.A., AND S. R. YARNALL.
Computer-aided diagnosis of cardiovascular disorders.
Journal Chronic Diseases 19:473-484, 1966.

0458
BRUCE, T.A., C.B. CHAPMAN, O. BAKER, AND J.N. FISHER.
The role of autonomic and myocardial factors in cardiac control.
Journal Clinical Investigation 42:721-726, 1963.

0459
BRUHN, J.G., B. CHANDLER, AND S. WOLF.
A psychological study of survivors and nonsurvivors of myocardial infarction.
Psychosomatic Medicine 31(1):8-19, 1969.

0460
BRUHN, J.G., ET AL.
   Social aspects of coronary heart disease in two adjacent, ethnically different communities.
   American Journal Public Health 56:1493-1506, 1966.

0461
BRUHN, J.G., ET AL.
   Social characteristics of patients with coronary heart disease.
   American Journal Medical Sciences 251:629-637, 1966.

0462
BRUHN, J.G., K.E. McCRADY, AND A. DUPLESSIS.
   Evidence of "Emotional Drain" preceding death from myocardial infarction.
   Psychiatry Digest 29:34-40, 1968.

0463
BRUHN, J.G., A.E. THURMAN, JR., B.C. CHANDLER, AND T.A. BRUCE.
   Patients' reactions to death in a coronary care unit.
   Journal Psychosomatic Research 14:65-70, 1970.

0464
BRUHN, J.G., AND S. WOLF.
   Studies reporting "low rates" of ischemic heart disease: A critical review.
   American Journal Public Health 60(8):1477-1495, 1970.

0465
BRUHN, J.G., S. WOLF, AND B.V. PHILIPS.
   A psycho-social study of surviving male coronary patients and controls followed over nine years.
   Journal Psychosomatic Research 15:305-313, 1971.

0466
BRUMMER, P., E. LINKO, AND V. KALLIO.
   Myocardial infarction treated by early ambulation. Effect of prolonged anticoagulant therapy on the immediate prognosis after discharge from hospital.
   American Heart Journal 62:478-480, 1961.

0467
BRUNDAGE, B.H., AND M.D. CHEITLIN.
   Left ventricular angiography as a function test.
   Chest 64:70-74, 1973.

0468
BRUNNER, D.
   The influence of physical activity on incidence and prognosis of ischemic heart disease.
   In: Raab, W., Ed. Prevention of ischemic heart disease: Principles and practices, pp. 236-243. Springfield, Ill. Thomas, 1966.

0469
BRUNNER, D.
   Active exercise for coronary patients.
   Rehabilitation Record 9:29-31, 1968.

0470
BRUNNER, D., S. ALTMAN, N. MESHULAM, AND K. LOEBL.
Coronary risk factors in Yemenites living different time spans in Israel.
In: Plavšić, C. and M.M. Gertler, Eds. The first international biennial conference on cardiac rehabilitation. Dubrovnik, Yugoslavia, 1969.

0471
BRUNNER, D., AND G. MANELIS.
Myocardial infarction among members of communal settlements in Israel.
Lancet 2:1049, 1960.

0472
BRUNNER, D., AND G. MANELIS.
Physical activity at work and ischemic heart disease.
In: Larsen, O., and R.O. Malmborg, Eds. Coronary heart disease and physical fitness, pp. 244-250. Baltimore, University Park Press, 1971.

0473
BRUNNER, D., G. MANELIS, AND K. LOEBL.
Influence of manual labor and occupation on the five-year mortality of middle-aged patients with initial myocardial infarction.
Circulation 26(4 Part 2):693, 1962.

0474
BRUNNER, D., AND N. MESHULAM.
Prevention of recurrent myocardial infarction by physical exercises in coronary patients.
Israel Journal Medical Sciences 4(5):1090, 1968.

0475
BRUNNER, D., AND N. MESHULAM.
Prevention of recurrent myocardial infarction by physical exercise.
Israel Journal Medical Sciences 5:783-785, 1969.

0476
BRUNNER, D., AND N. MESHULAM.
Active rehabilitation of coronary patients, a step in preventive cardiology.
Proceedings International Congress Gerontology 8(2):103, 1969.

0477
BRUNNER, D., N. MESHULAM, AND F. ZERYKIER.
Active rehabilitation in coronary patients.
In: Plavšić, C. and M.M. Gertler, Eds. The first international biennial conference on cardiac rehabilitation. Dubrovnik, Yugoslavia, 1969.

0478
BRUNZELL, J.D., W.R. HAZZARD, D. PORTE, JR., AND E.L. BIERMAN.
Evidence for a common saturable, triglyceride removal-mechanism for chylomicrons and very low density lipoproteins in man.
Journal Clinical Investigation 52:1578, 1973.

0479
BRUSCHKE, A.V.G., A.W. HANSSEN, AND F. VON HERPEN.
  Comparison of coronary angiogram with other parameters (history, electrocardiogram, vector-cardiogram, two-step test, serum lipids) in patients with anginal complaints.
  British Heart Journal 33(1): 150, 1971.

0480
BRUSIS, O.A.
  Rehabilitating coronary patients through exercise.
  Postgraduate Medicine 44:131-135, 1968.

0481
BUCHBINDER, N.A., AND W.C. ROBERTS.
  Active infective endocarditis confined to mural endocardium. A study of six necropsy patients.
  Archives Pathology 93(5):435-440, 1972.

0482
BUCKLIN, R.
  Heart disease and the law.
  Medical Trial Technique Quarterly 17:294-301, 1971.

0483
BÜDINGEN, F., AND H.C. MOELLER.
  On the therapy of coronary insufficiency.
  Therapie der Gegenwart 103:436-454, 1964.

0484
BUELL, P., AND L. BRESLOW.
  Mortality from coronary heart disease in California men who work long hours.
  Journal Chronic Diseases 11:615-626, 1960.

0485
BULEY, L.E.
  Incidence, causes and results of airline pilot incapacitation while on duty.
  Aerospace Medicine 40:64, 1969.

0486
BUNDE, C.A., I.L. GRUPP, AND G. GRUPP.
  Effects of the antianginal agent perhexilene maleate on exercise induced tachycardia in human volunteers.
  Federation Proceedings 28(2):672, 1968.

0487
BURCH, G.E.
  Cardiac causalgia and hoarseness.
  American Heart Journal 84(3):420, 1972.

0488
BURCH, G.E.
  The etiology of arteriosclerosis. A thought.
  American Heart Journal 83(3):434-436, 1972.

0489
BURCH, G.E.
   A primer of venous pressure.
   Springfield, Ill., Thomas, 1972.

0490
BURCH, G.E.
   On exercising the heart.
   American Heart Journal 85:835, 1973.

0491
BURCH, G.E.
   The practice of cardiology today.
   American Heart Journal 85(3):291-293, 1973.

0492
BURCH, G.E.
   Ischemic cardiomyopathy.
   American Heart Journal 86:276, 1973.

0493
BURCH, G.E.
   A sign of cardiac arrest.
   American Heart Journal 86:138, 1973.

0494
BURCH, G.E., ET AL.
   Selected problems in electrocardiography.
   Annals Internal Medicine 52:587, 1960.

0495
BURCH, G.E., ET AL.
   Potentials and limitations of patients after myocardial infarction.
   American Heart Journal 71:830-837, 1966.

0496
BURCH, G.E., AND T. GILES.
   Aspects of the influence of psychic stress on angina pectoris.
   American Journal Cardiology 31(1):108-110, 1973.

0497
BURGALASSI, S.
   The sociological problem of aging people.
   Giornale di Gerontologia 21:349, 1973.

0498
BURGGRAF, G.W., AND J.O. PARKER.
   Hemodynamic effects of amyl nitrite in coronary artery disease.
   American Journal Cardiology 32:772, 1973.

0499
BURKART, F., S. BAROLD, AND E. SOWTON.
  Hemodynamic effects of repeated exercise.
  American Journal Cardiology 20(4):509-515, 1967.

0500
BURKHARDT, H., G. ROLL, AND D. LOEW.
  Study of platelet function in myocardial infarction and the possibility of modifying it by means
  of acetysalicylic acid.
  Medizinische Welt 23:1074, 1972.

0501
BURRMANN, H., H. SCHNEIDER, H-W. WACHE, AND H. BARTELS.
  Studies on the correlations of decreased postprandial glucose tolerance with age, body weight,
  blood pressure, cholesterol, as well as asymptomatic and established Diabetes Melitus in a closed
  country population in the second half of life.
  Zeitschrift für Innere Medizin 26:690-694, 1971.

0502
BURRY, H.C.
  Athletic fitness: its role in prevention of accidents and injuries.
  Practitioner 206:227-233, 1971.

0503
BURTON, A.C.
  The importance of the shape and size of the heart.
  American Heart Journal 54:801-810, 1957.

0504
BUSKIRK, E.R.
  Problems related to conduct of athletics in hot environments.
  In: Balke, B., Ed., Physiological aspects of sports and physical fitness, p. 33. The Athletic Insti-
  tute, 1968.

0505
BUSKIRK, E.R.
  An introduction to exercise and performance evaluation.
  Journal South Carolina Medical Association (Suppl.) 65(12):4-7, 1969.

0506
BUSKIRK, E.R., D. HARRIS, J. MENDEZ, AND J. SKINNER.
  Comparison of two assessments of physical activity and a survey method for calorie intake.
  American Journal Clinical Nutrition 24:1119-1125, 1971.

0507
BUSKIRK, E., AND H.L. TAYLOR.
  Maximal oxygen intake and its relation to body composition, with special reference to chronic
  physical activity and obesity.
  Journal Applied Physiology 11:72, 1957.

0508
BUSLENKO, N.S., AND B.A. KUZNETSOVA.
Serotonin content in the blood and 5-oxyindolacetic acid titer in the urine of patients with ischaemic disease of the heart.
Kardiologiya 12(9):39-43, 1972.

0509
BUSNENGO, E.
The Macruz index and clinical evaluation in electrocardiography in the selection and control of air crews.
Rivista di Medicina Aeronautica 35:62-72, 1972.

0510
BUSNENGO, E., AND P. ROTA.
Changes in duration of the QT interval in the electrocardiogram during muscular exercise. I. Duration of the QT interval in the constant muscular exercise test.
Rivista di Medicina Aeronautica e Spaziale 29:398-406, 1966.

0511
BUSNENGO, E., AND P. ROTA.
Changes in the QT interval in the electrocardiogram during muscular work. II. Duration of the QT interval in the strenuous exercise test.
Rivista di Medicina Aeronautica e Spaziale 30:425-436, 1967.

0512
BUTLER, V.P., JR.
Digoxin: Immunological approaches to measurement and reversal of toxicity.
New England Journal Medicine 283:1150, 1970.

0513
BUTTRAM, W.R., JR.
The diagnosis and treatment of heat reactions.
In: Balke, B. Ed., Physiological aspects of sports and physical fitness, pp. 45-46. The Athletic Institute, 1968.

0514
BUXMAN, J., R.E. DRICKEY, AND D. WERDEGAR.
Employment practices as deterrents to rehabilitation of patients with cardiovascular illness.
Clinical Research 17(2):409, 1969.

0515
BUYUKOZTURK, K., B. KINGSLEY, AND N.L. SEGAL.
The influences of heart rate, age and sex on the movements of mitral valve.
Acta Cardiologica 27(4):427-444, 1972.

0516
BUZINA, R., AND A. KEYS.
Blood coagulation after a fat meal.
Circulation 14:854, 1956.

0517
BUZZI, A., AND B. CARBAJAL.
Tratamiento anticoagulante prolongado. (Long term anticoagulant therapy.)
Revista de la Asociacion Médica Argentina 74(1):30-35, 1960.

0518
CADY, L.D., JR., ET AL.
   Computed cardiographic pattern diagnosis.
   Methods Information Medicine 4:92-96, 1965.

0519
CADY, L.D., JR., M.M. GERTLER, AND L.A. NOWITZ.
   Coronary disease factors.
   Behavioral Science 9:30-32, 1964.

0520
CAFFREY, B.
   Social stress and cardiovascular disease. Factors involving interpersonal and psychological character-
   istics. A review of empirical findings.
   Milbank Memorial Fund Quarterly 45(Suppl.):119-139, 1967.

0521
CAFFREY, B.
   Reliability and validity of personality and behavioral measures in a study of coronary heart
   disease.
   Journal Chronic Diseases 21:191-204, 1968.

0522
CAFFREY, B.
   Behavior patterns and personality characteristics related to prevalence rates of coronary heart
   disease in American monks.
   Journal Chronic Diseases 22:93-103, 1969.

0523
CAHEN, P., J. DEPOUILL, S. QARD, AND P. CHAZAUD.
   Myocardial ischemia during exercise electrocardiographic criteria—data recorded in 553 patients
   with selective coronarography.
   Lyon Médical 229:969-80, 1973.

0524
CAIN, H.D., AND A.J. BURLANDO.
   Cardiac response during rehabilitation therapy.
   Clinical Research 15(3):105, 1967.

0525
CAIN, H.D., W.G. FRASHER, JR., AND R. STIVELMAN.
   Graded activity program for safe return to self-care myocardial infarction.
   Journal American Medical Association 177:111, 1961.

0526
CALDWELL, J.R., AND O.A. CARRETERO.
   Plasma renin and blood pressure after sympathetic stimulation in normotensive and hypertensive
   patients.
   American Journal Cardiology 29(4):466-469, 1972.

0527
CALDWELL, J.R., S. COBB, M.D. DOWLING, AND D. DE JONGH.
   The dropout problem in antihypertensive treatment: A pilot study of social and emotional factors influencing a patient's ability to follow antihypertensive treatment.
   Journal Chronic Diseases 22(8/9):579-592, 1970.

0528
CALESNICK, B.
   Medical management of coronary artery disease, a résumé of its pharmacology.
   Angiology 14(1):17-22, 1963.

0529
CALIFANO, J.E., AND H.A. RUGGIERO.
   Electrovectorcardiography in the differential diagnosis of myocardial infarction.
   Prensa Médica Argentina 59(35):1313-1318, 1972.

0530
CALL, R.W., B. CLYMAN, J.W. COPEMAN, AND D.R. KASERMAN.
   The use of posterior lead in cardiovascular stress testing.
   Journal Occupational Medicine 12:241-5, 1970.

0531
CALL, R.W., C. CLYMAN, AND D.R. KASERMAN.
   Practical use of stress testing in industry.
   Journal Occupational Medicine 10(11):649-654, 1968.

0532
CALLEJA, H.B., AND M.X. GUERRERO.
   Prolonged PR interval and coronary artery disease.
   British Heart Journal 35(4):372-376, 1973.

0533
CALVIN, J.R., AND P.W. ACREE.
   Current management of complete heart block.
   Journal Louisiana State Medical Society 120:297-303, 1968.

0534
CALVY, G.L., L.D. CADY, M.A. MUFSON, J. NIERMAN, AND M.M. GERTLER.
   Serum lipids and enzymes. Their levels after high-caloric, high-fat intake and vigorous exercise regimen in Marine Corps recruit personnel.
   Journal American Medical Association 183:1, 1963.

0535
CALVY, G.L., L.H. COFFIN, JR., M.M. GERTLER, AND L.D. CADY.
   The effect of strenuous exercise on serum lipids and enzymes.
   Military Medicine 129:1012-6, 1964.

0536
CAMPBELL, D.A.
   A study of the preventive health behavior of a group of men with increased risk for the development of coronary heart disease.
   Dissertation Abstracts, International Section B Science and Engineering 32(3):1678-B, 1971.

0537
CANDIOLO, B.
A new beta-adrenergic blocking agent in the treatment of angina pectoris.
Prensa Medica Argentina 59(34):1283-1286, 1972.

0538
CAÑIZARES, C., C. DE LEON, F. CAÑIZARES, AND A. MARTINEZ.
Correlation of the levels of coagulability, fibrinolysis, and lipids with physical activity, hormonal and nutritional states.
Sangre 16(4):377-386, 1971.

0539
CANTONE, A.
Physical effort and its effects in reducing alimentary hyperlipaemia.
Journal Sports Medicine Physical Fitness 4:32, 1964.

0540
CANTWELL, J.D.
Postinfarction cardiac rehabilitation.
American Family Physician 8:137, 1973.

0541
CANTWELL, J.D., J.E. DAWSON, AND G.F. FLETCHER.
Supraventricular tachyarrhythmias. Treatment with edrophonium.
Archives Internal Medicine 130(2):221-224, 1972.

0542
CANTWELL, J.D., AND G.F. FLETCHER.
Cardiac complications while jogging.
Journal American Medical Association 210:130-132, 1969.

0543
CAQUET, R., AND S. DESCHE LABARTHE.
Endocarditis caused by drugs of addiction.
Gazette Médicale de France 79(31):5269-5270, 1972.

0544
CARDILLO, T.E.
A two-year study of myocardial infarction in industry.
Journal Occupational Medicine 9:175-182, 1967.

0545
CARDUS, D.
Effects of 10 days recumbency on the response to the bicycle ergometer test.
Aerospace Medicine 37:993-999, 1966.

0546
CARDUS, D.
Computer processing of data generated by a bicycle ergometer test.
Journal Sports Medicine Physical Fitness 7:155-161, 1967.

0547
CARDUS, D.
O$_2$ alveolar-arterial tension difference after 10 days recumbency in man.
Journal Applied Physiology 23:934-937, 1967.

0548
CARDUS, D., AND R.K. ZEIGLER.
Heart beat frequency curves. A mathematical model.
Computers Biomedical Research 1:508-526, 1968.

0549
CARLSON, L.A.
Viewpoints of a diet experiment.
Nordisk Medicin 77(21):669, 1967.

0550
CARLSON, L.A., AND L.E. BÖTTIGER.
Ischaemic heart disease in relation to fasting values of plasma triglycerides and cholesterol.
Lancet 1:865-868, 1972.

0551
CARLSON, R.B., S. KLINE, C. APSTEIN, ET AL.
Lactate metabolism after aortocoronary artery vein bypass grafts.
Annals Surgery 176(5):680-685, 1972.

0552
CARNES, G.D.
Understanding the cardiac patient's behavior
American Journal Nursing 71:1187-1188, 1971.

0553
CARROLL, D.G.
Cardiac rehabilitation. Part III. Follow-up after myocardial infarction.
Maryland State Medical Journal 17(1):78-79, 1968.

0554
CARRUTHERS, M.O., AND P. TAGGART.
Study of plasma catecholamine and lipids responses to emotional stress.
Quarterly Journal Medicine 40:578-579, 1971.

0555
CARSON, P., M. NEOPHYTO, H. TUCKER, AND T. SIMPSON.
Exercise program after myocardial infarction.
British Medical Journal 4:213-216, 1973.

0556
CASAR, F.P.
Psychogenesis and psychological problems of coronary disease.
Revista Española de Cardiologia 19:239-244, 1966.

0557
CASH, J.D.
Effect of moderate exercise on the fibrinolytic system in normal young men and women.
British Medical Journal 2:502, 1966.

0558
CASH, J.D., AND D.G. WOODFIELD.
  Fibrinolytic response to moderate, exhaustive and prolonged exercise in normal subjects.
  Nature 215:628, 1967.

0559
CASSEL, J.
  Social stress and cardiovascular disease. Factors involving sociocultural incongruity and change.
  Appraisal and implications for theoretical development.
  Milbank Memorial Fund Quarterly 45(Suppl.):41-45, 1967.

0560
CASSEL, J.C.
  Review of 1960 through 1962 cardiovascular disease prevalence study.
  Archives Internal Medicine 128:890-895, 1971.

0561
CASSEL, J., S. HEYDEN, A.G. BARTEL, B.H. KAPLAN, H.A. TYROLER, J.C. CORNONI, AND
  C.G. HAMES.
  Occupation and physical activity and coronary heart disease.
  Archives Internal Medicine 128:920-928, 1971.

0562
CASSEM, N.H., ET AL.
  How coronary patients respond to last rites.
  Postgraduate Medicine 45:147-152, 1969.

0563
CASSEM, N.H., AND T.P. HACKETT.
  Psychiatric consultation in a coronary care unit.
  Annals Internal Medicine 75(1):9-14, 1971.

0564
CASTELLANOS, A., A.S. AGHA, C.S. CASTILLO, AND M.P. TESSLER.
  Functional properties of the human atrioventricular and intraventricular conduction system during
  premature atrial stimulation.
  Cardiovascular Research 6(6):716-724, 1972.

0565
CASTELLANOS, A., JR., L. LEMBERG, AND A.G. ARCEBAL.
  Mechanisms of slow ventricular tachycardias in acute myocardial infarction.
  Diseases Chest 56(6):470-476, 1969.

0566
CASTLE, L.W., W. SIEGEL, W.L. PROUDFIT, AND F.A. HEUPLER.
  Ventricular fibrillation and coronary atherosclerosis with normal maximal exercise test, report of a
  case.
  Cleveland Clinic Quarterly 39:163-66, 1972.

0567
CASTON, J., L. COOPER, AND H.W. PALEY.
  Psychological comparison of patients with cardiac neurotic chest pain and angina pectoris.
  Psychosomatics 11(6):543-550, 1970.

0568
CATHEY, C., H.B. JONES, J. NAUGHTON, J.F. HAMMARSTEN, AND S. WOLF.
The relation of life stress to the concentration of serum lipids in patients with coronary artery disease.
American Journal Medical Sciences 244(4):421-441, 1962.

0569
CAULFIELD, J.B., W.B. DUNKMAN, AND R.C. LEINBACH.
Cardiogenic shock. Myocardial morphology with and without artificial left ventricular counter-pulsation.
Archives Pathology 93(6):532-536, 1972.

0570
CAY, E.L., N.J. VETTER, A.E. PHILIP, AND P. DUGARD.
Psychological reactions to a coronary care unit.
Scandinavian Journal Rehabilitation Medicine 2-3:78-84, 1970.

0571
CAY, E.L., N. VETTER, A.E. PHILIP, AND P. DUGARD.
Psychological influences determining return to work after a coronary thrombosis.
Rehabilitation 81:27-35, 1972.

0572
CAY, E.L., N. VETTER, A. PHILIP, AND P. DUGARD.
Psychological status during recovery from an acute heart attack.
Journal Psychosomatic Research 16:425-35, 1972.

0573
CAY, E.L., N. VETTER, A.E. PHILIP, AND P. DUGARD.
Psychological reactions to a coronary care unit.
Journal Psychosomatic Research 16(6):437-447, 1972.

0574
CAY, E.L., N. VETTER, A. PHILIP, AND P. DUGARD.
Return to work after a heart attack.
Journal Psychosomatic Research 17:231-43, 1973.

0575
CEBOLLA, R.R., M.V. PALACIOS, F.J. ALGARRA VIDAL, AND A. TALENS HERNANDIS.
Significance of auricular gallop rhythm in acute myocardial infarction. Study of phonomechan-ography.
Revista Española de Cardiologia 25:443-450, 1972.

0576
CEJKA, V., A.J. BLEIJENB, N. BELTVAND, A.E. MEINDERS, AND A.J. DUNNING.
Glucose tolerance, plasma IRI response and stress in acute phase of myocardial infarction.
Acta Endocrinologica S177:127, 1973.

0577
CENTER, S., AND P. TARJAN.
The clinical application of low output pacemakers.
Journal Thoracic Cardiovascular Surgery 64:935, 1972.

0578
CERNOHORSKÝ, J.
  The role of ECG after exercise in the determination of precordial pain.
  Sbornik Vĕdeckých Praci Lékařské Fakulty Karlovy University 12(5):523-528, 1969.

0579
CHACCUR, E., J.C. LINARES, AND A. BISTENI.
  Value of diazepam in the treatment of ventricular arrhythmias.
  Archivos del Instituto de Cardiologia de Mexico 42:391, 1972.

0580
CHAKRABARTI, R., E.D. HOCKING, and G.R. FEARNLEY.
  Reaction pattern to three stresses-electroplexy, surgery, and myocardial infarction—of fibrinolysis and plasma fibrinogen.
  Journal Clinical Pathology 22:659, 1969.

0581
CHALANT, C.H., C. HAHN, B. FAIDUTTI, ET AL.
  Surgical management of fresh infarctions.
  Archives des Maladies du Coeur et des Vaisseaux 65(6):685-690, 1972.

0582
CHAMBERLAIN, J.
  Evaluation of screening for chest and heart diseases. Preventive Techniques for the Modern Community.
  The Chest and Heart Association, pp. 1-7. London, England, 1971.

0583
CHANDRARAINA, P.A.N., N.D. NANDA, P.M. SHAH, M. HODGES, AND R. GRAMINK.
  Echocardiographic study of left atrial size in acute myocardial infarction.
  Circulation 46 (Suppl. 2):138, 1972.

0584
CHANEY, D.S. AND L. ANDREASEN.
  Relaxation and neuromuscular tension control and changes in mental performance under induced tension.
  Perceptual Motor Skills 34:677-678, 1972.

0585
CHAPMAN, B.L.
  Correlation of mortality rate and serum enzymes in myocardial infarction. Test of efficiency of coronary care.
  British Heart Journal 33(5):643-646, 1971.

0586
CHAPMAN, B.L.
  Relation of cardiac complications to SGOT level in acute myocardial infarction.
  British Heart Journal 34(9):890-896, 1972.

0587
CHAPMAN, C.B., ED.
  Physiology of muscular exercise.
  American Heart Association Monograph No. 15. New York, The American Heart Association, 1967.

0588
CHAPMAN, J.M., A.H. COULSON, V.A. CLARK, AND E.R. BORUN.
The differential effect of serum cholesterol, blood pressure and weight on the incidence of myocardial infarction and angina pectoris.
Journal Chronic Diseases 23:631-645, 1971.

0589
CHAPMAN, J.M., L.S. GOERKE, W. DIXON, D.B. LOVELAND, AND E. PHILLIPS.
Measuring the risk of coronary heart disease in adult population groups. The clinical status of a population group in Los Angeles under observation 2-3 years.
American Journal Public Health 47:33, 1957.

0590
CHAPMAN, J.M., AND F.J. MASSEY, JR.
The interrelationship of serum cholesterol, hypertension, body weight, and risk in coronary heart disease.
Journal Chronic Diseases 17:933, 1964.

0591
CHATTERJEE, K., W.J. MANDEL, J.K. VYDEN, ET AL.
Cardiovascular effects of bretylium tosylate in acute myocardial infarction.
Journal American Medical Association 223(7):757-760, 1973.

0592
CHAUBEY, B.S., AND H.C. ATTAL.
Treatment of digitalis induced arrhythmias with LB 46 (Visken).
Indian Heart Journal 24(Suppl. 1):215-223, 1972.

0593
CHAVERO, E.P., L.H. PÉREZ, J.A. LORENZO, L.C. LÓPEZ, J. MARTÍNEZ, AND J. BENÍTEZ.
Two years of experience in the coronary care unit.
Archivos del Instituto de Cardiologia de Mexico 40(6):785-796, 1970.

0594 CHAZOV, E.I.
Problems of myocardial infarction therapy.
Sovetskaya Meditsina 34(4):3-9, 1971.

0595
CHERASKIN, E., AND W.M. RINGSDORF, JR.
Carbohydrate-fat consumption and cardiovascular complaints.
Journal Oral Medicine 24(3/4):124-130, 1969.

0596
CHENEY, H.L.
The long-term management of patients with coronary heart disease.
Journal Medical Association Georgia 54:162, 1965.

0597
CHENG, T.O.
Atrial Pacing: its diagnostic and therapeutic applications.
Progress Cardiovascular Diseases 14:230-247, 1971.

0598
CHENG, T.O.
   Cardiac Pacing: the state of the art.
   Journal American Geriatric Society 20(10):473-484, 1972.

0599
CHENG, T.O., T. BASHOUR, AND G.A. KELSER, Jr.
   Complete heart block occurring during right heart catheterization in a patient with left bundle
   branch block and prolonged P-R interval studied by bundle of His recording atrial pacing.
   Medical Annals District of Columbia 41(12):742-5, 1972.

0600
CHENG, T.O., T. BASHOUR, B.K. SINGH, AND G.A. KELSER.
   Myocardial infarction in the absence of coronary arteriosclerosis. Result of coronary spasm?
   American Journal Cardiology 30(6):680-682, 1972.

0601
CHENG, T.O., G. ERTEM, AND Z. VERA.
   Heart sounds in patients with cardiac pacemakers.
   Chest 62(1):66-70, 1972.

0602
CHERCHI, A.
   Electrocardiogram and metabolism during physical exercise in normal and cardiac patients.
   Malattie Cardiovascolari 10(1/2):109-128, 1969.

0603
CHERCHI, A.
   Electrocardiographic diagnosis of coronary insufficiency during exertion.
   Malattie Cardiovascolari 10:47-59, 1969.

0604
CHERCHI, A., ET AL.
   Quantitative evaluation of the electrocardiographic changes in the RS-T segment during muscular
   exercise.
   Bollettino della Società Italiana di Cardiologia 14:363-385, 1969.

0605
CHERCHI, A., M. LIXI, G. PORRAZZO, M.P. ESU, P. SASSU, AND P. MONTALDO.
   The metabolic and hemodynamic response in patients with mitral stenosis upon progressive
   orthostatic muscular exercise: I. Cardiac output.
   Bollettino della Società Italiana di Cardiologia 14(4):459-479, 1969.

0606
CHEREVATOV, B.G.
   The reaction of a healthy and affected heart to physical exertion according to radioelectro-
   cardiographic data.
   Klinicheskaya Meditsina 49(1):36-41, 1971.

0607

CHERRIER, F., J. ROBERT, M. CUILLIERE, AND H. MABILLE.
Measurement of coronary blood flow with the aid of Xenon[133] during selective coronary arteriography. Preliminary study.
Archives des Maladies du Coeur et des Vaisseaux, 65(12):1473-1481, 1972.

0608

CHETKOWSKA, E., M. EDELMAN, AND J. ZUCHOWSKA.
Postinfarction scars manifesting themselves as paroxysmal arrhythmia.
Wiadomosci Lekarskie 25(15):1329-1331, 1972.

0609

CHEVROLLE, J., ET AL.
Problems raised by return to work of myocardial infarct convalescents at the Régie Nationale des Usines Renault.
Gazette Médicale de France 72:2997-3003, 1965.

0610

CHEVROLLE, J.
Problems connected with the resumption of work by convalescents from a myocardial infarction. Review of 110 cases.
Presse Médicale 74:746, 1966.

0611

CHIANG, B.N., E.R. ALEXANDER, R.A. BRUCE, D.J. THOMPSON, AND NONG TING.
Factors related to ST-segment depression after exercise in middle-aged Chinese men.
Circulation 40(3):315, 1969.

0612

CHIANG, B.N., L.V. PERLMAN, AND L.D. OSTRANDER, JR.
Relationship of premature systoles to coronary heart disease and sudden death in the Tecumseh epidemiologic study.
Annals Internal Medicine 70:1159-1166, 1969.

0613

CHIANG, B.N., L.V. PERLMAN, L.D. OSTRANDER, JR., AND F.H. EPSTEIN.
Epidemiological significance of premature systoles in coronary heart disease and sudden death in Tecumseh, Michigan.
Circulation 38(Suppl. 6):54, 1968.

0614

CHIPPERFIELD, B., AND J.R. CHIPPERFIELD.
Heart-muscle magnesium, potassium, and zinc concentrations after sudden death from heart-disease.
Lancet 2:293-295, 1973.

0615

CHOLEWA, L., M. MAGDON, K. MURK, AND J. SZNAJD.
Serum RNAse activity in patients with myocardial infarction. Part 1. Changes in the first 3 days of the disease.
Polskie Archiwum Medycyny Wewnetrznej 11:1398-1406, 1972.

0616
CHOOK, E.K.
   Criteria for return to work. Case study of hypertensives.
   Internationales Archiv für Arbeitsmedizin 26:103-110, 1970.

0617
CHOQUETTE, G.
   Tobacco and coronary disease.
   Canadian Journal Public Health 64:S25-S31, 1973.

0618
CHOQUETTE, G., R.J. FERGUSON, AND L. CHANIOTIS.
   Changes observed in middle-aged men comprising normal subjects and coronary patients, after a
   six month physical reconditioning program.
   Union Médicale du Canada 101:929, 1972.

0619
CHOPRA, M.P., U. THADANI, C.P. ABER, ET AL.
   Plasma cortisol, urinary 17-hydroxycorticoids, and urinary vanilyl mandelic acid after acute
   myocardial infarction.
   British Heart Journal 34(10):992-997, 1972.

0620
CHRISTAKIS, G.
   Diet and coronary heart disease: A public health viewpoint.
   Academy Medicine New Jersey Bulletin 10(4):262-268, 1964.

0621
CHRISTAKIS, G., AND M. WINSTON.
   Nutritional therapy in acute myocardial infarction.
   Journal American Dietetic Association 63:233, 1973.

0622
CHRISTIAN, P.
   Risk factors and risk personality in myocardial infarct.
   Medizinische Klinik 61:881-882, 1966.

0623
CHRISTIAN, P.
   Occupation and disease.
   Medizinische Klinik 62(20):786-787, 1967.

0624
CHRISTIAN, P., AND P. HAHN.
   Myocardial infarction from the psychosomatic and anthropological viewpoint.
   Internist 13:421-24, 1972.

0625
CHRISTIANSEN, I., K. IVERSEN, AND A.P. SKOUBY.
   Benefits obtained by the introduction of a coronary-care unit.
   Acta Medica Scandinavica 189:285-291, 1971.

0626
CHRISTENSEN, M.S., AND N.J. CHRISTENSEN.
   Plasma catecholamines in hypertension.
   Scandinavian Journal Clinical Laboratory Investigation 30:169-73, 1973.

0627
CHRISTENSSON, B., T. KARLEFORS, AND H. Westling.
   Haemodynamic effects of nitroglycerin in patients with coronary heart disease.
   British Heart Journal 27:511, 1965.

0628
CHRISTENSSON, B., I. NORDENFELT, H. WESTLING, AND T. WHITE.
   Haemodynamic effects of nitroglycerin in normal subjects during supine and sitting exercise.
   British Heart Journal 31:80, 1969.

0629
CHROBOK, H.
   Atrial wall infarction recognized intravitally.
   Wiadomosci Lekarskie 25(16):1451-1453, 1972.

0630
CHUNG, D.K., AND E.K. CHUNG.
   Atrial electrical alternans.
   Postgraduate Medicine 52(6):118-119, 1972.

0631
CHUNG, D.K., ET AL.
   Two-step (Master) exercise test.
   West Virginia Medical Journal 67:375-376, 1971.

0632
CHUNG, E.K.
   Guide to the use of artificial pacemakers. I.
   Postgraduate Medicine 52:137-143, 1972.

0633
CHUNG, E.K.
   Guide to the use of artificial pacemakers. II.
   Postgraduate Medicine 52(3):221-224, 1972.

0634
CHUNG, E.K.
   Prophylactic uses of antiarrhythmic drugs in acute myocardial infarction.
   Postgraduate Medicine 54(4):197, 1973.

0635
CHUNG, E.K., AND E.J. MORGAN.
   Unusually marked sinus arrhythmia as a complication of acute diaphragmatic myocardial infarction.
   Japanese Heart Journal 10(4):363-368, 1969.

0636
CIBULSKI, A.A., P.H. LEHAN, AND H.H. TIMMIS.
Retrograde flow technique versus Krypton 85 clearance technique for estimation of myocardial collaterals.
American Journal Physiology 223:1081, 1972.

0637
CIHAK, J., J. SKACHOVA, AND H. KAFKA.
Influence of the long-term administration of anticoagulants on the mortality from myocardial infarction.
Sbornik Lekarsky 68(10):281-288, 1966.

0638
CLANCY, R.L., T.P. GRAHAM, JR., W.J. POWELL, JR., AND J.P. GILMORE.
Inotropic augmentation of myocardial oxygen consumption.
American Journal Physiology 212(5):1055-1061, 1967.

0639
CLARK, R.J.
Experience of the cardiac work classification unit in Boston, Massachusetts.
In: Rosenbaum, F. and E. Belknap, Eds. Transactions of the first Wisconsin Conference on Work and the Heart, pp. 311-321. New York, Hoeber, 1959.

0640
CLARKE, A.M.
Electromyogram and myogram responses under pre-strain conditions in normal humans as an index of fusimotor sensitization of muscle spindles.
Medical Biological Engineering 10:291-296, 1972.

0641
CLAUSEN, J.P.
Effects of physical conditioning: A hypothesis concerning circulatory adjustment to exercise.
Scandinavian Journal Clinical Laboratory Investigation 24(4):305-313, 1969.

0642
CLAUSEN, J.P., O.A. LARSEN, AND J. TRAP-JENSEN.
Physical training in the management of coronary artery disease.
Circulation 40:143-154, 1969.

0643
CLAUSEN, J.P., AND N.A. LASSEN.
Muscle blood flow during exercise in normal man studied by the ^{133}Xenon clearance method.
Cardiovascular Research 5:245-254, 1971.

0644
CLAUSSEN, J.P., AND J. TRAP-JENSEN.
Effects of training on the distribution of cardiac output in patients with coronary artery disease.
Circulation 42(4):611-624, 1970.

0645
CLAUSEN, J.P., AND J. TRAP-JENSEN.
Regulation and distribution of cardiac output during exercise in patients with coronary artery disease and the effects of training.
In: Larsen, O.A. and R.O. Malmborg, Eds. Coronary heart disease and physical fitness, pp. 74-79. Baltimore, University Park Press, 1971.

0646
CLAUSEN, J.P., J. TRAP-JENSEN, AND N.A. LASSEN.
Evidence that the relative exercise-bradycardia induced by training can be caused by extracardiac factors.
In: Larsen, O.A. and R.O. Malmborg, Eds. Coronary heart disease and physical fitness, pp. 27-28. Baltimore, University Park Press, 1971.

0647
CLEVELAND, S.E., AND D.L. JOHNSON.
Personality patterns in young males with coronary disease.
Psychosomatic Medicine 24(6):600-610, 1962.

0648
CLINE, R.E., R.G. ARMSTRONG, AND W. STANFORD.
Successful myocardial revascularization after ventricular fibrillation induced by treadmill exercise.
Journal Thoracic Cardiovascular Surgery 65:802-05, 1973.

0649
COBB, L.A., H.S. RIPLEY, AND J.W. JONES.
Role of the nervous system in free fatty acid mobilization as demonstrated by hypnosis.
In: Karvonen, M.J. and A.J. Barry, Eds. Physical activity and the heart, pp. 192-199. Springfield, Ill., Thomas, 1967.

0650
COBO, L.
Cardioversion. Results and indications.
Revista Española de Cardiologia 25(5):401-406, 1972.

0651
COCHRANE, R.
High blood pressure as psychosomatic disorder: A selective review.
British Journal Social Clinical Psychology 10(1):61-72, 1971.

0652
COHEN, E., AND I.W.P. OBEL.
Some aspects of potassium and the cardiovascular system.
South African Medical Journal 46(30):11-14, 1972.

0653
COHEN, H., AND C. GOLDBERG.
Effect of physical exercise on alimentary lipaemia.
British Medical Journal 2:509, 1960.

0654
COHEN, H.C., E.G. GOZO, JR., R. LANGENDORF, B.M. KAPLAN, A. CHAN, A. PICK, AND G. GLICK.
Response of resistant ventricular tachycardia to Bretylium. Relation to site of ectopic focus and location of myocardial disease.
Circulation 47:331-340, 1973.

0655
COHEN, R.J., S.E. EPSTEIN, L.S. COHEN, AND L.H. DENNIS.
Alterations of fibrinolysis and blood coagulation induced by exercise, and the role of beta-adrenergic-receptor stimulation.
Lancet 2:1264-1270, 1968.

0656
COHN, L.H., W.W. ANGELL, AND N.E. SHUMWAY.
Body fluid shifts after cardiopulmonary bypass. I. Effects of congestive heart failure and hemo-dilution.
Journal Thoracic Cardiovascular Surgery 62(3):423-430, 1971.

0657
COHN, P.F., AND R. GORLIN.
Abnormalities of left ventricular function associated with the anginal state.
Circulation 46(4):1065-1078, 1972.

0658
COHN, P.F., H.R. HORN, L.E. TEICHOLZ, T.H. KREULEN, M.V. HERMAN, AND R. GORLIN.
Effects of angiographic contrast medium on left ventricular function in coronary artery disease. Comparison with static and dynamic exercise.
American Journal Cardiology 32:31, 1973.

0659
COHN, P.F., P.S. VOKONAS, M.V. HERMAN, AND R. GORLIN.
Postexercise electrocardiogram in patients with abnormal resting electrocardiograms.
Circulation 43(5):648-654, 1971.

0660
COHN, P.F., P.S. VOKONAS, A.S. MOST, M.V. HERMAN, AND R. GORLIN.
Diagnostic accuracy of two-step postexercise ECG: Results in 305 subjects studied by coronary arteriography.
Journal American Medical Association 220:501-506, 1972.

0661
COLAO, G.
On the necessity of occupational rehabilitation of the heart disease patient (with special reference to functional tests).
Rassegna Internazionale di Clinica e Terapia 46:912-937, 1966.

0662
COLBERT, J.N., R.A. KALISH, AND P. CHANG.
Two psychological portals of entry for disadvantaged groups.
Rehabilitation Literature 34:194, 1973.

0663
COLEMAN, A.E., C.L. BURFORD, AND P. KREUZER.
  Aerobic capacity of relatively sedentary males.
  Journal Occupational Medicine 15(8):628-632, 1973.

0664
COLEMAN, A.J., J.W. DOWNING, W.P. LEARY, ET AL.
  The immediate cardiovascular effects of Althesin (Glaxo CT 1341), a steroid induction agent, and
  thiopentone in man.
  Anaesthesia 27(4):373-378, 1972.

0665
COLEMAN, A.J., AND W.P. LEARY.
  Cardiovascular effects of salbutamol: a comparison with isoprenaline.
  South African Medical Journal 46(33):1177-1179, 1972.

0666
COLEMAN, A.J., AND W.P. LEARY.
  Cardiovascular effects of acebutotol (M and B 17803A) in exercising man; a comparative study
  with practolol and propranolol.
  Current Therapeutic Research Clinical Experimental 14(10):673-678, 1972.

0667
COLIN, W.
  Physical training of the cardiac patient.
  Revue de Réadaptation 13:67, 1971.

0668
COLLIGNON, P., J. BOOZ, M. DUBART, H. KULBERTUS, AND L. HUMBLET.
  Recording of electrocardiograms during effort.
  Revue Médicale de Liège 25:234-237, 1970.

0669
COLLINS, F.R., AND S.G. KRAMER.
  Hemodynamic assessment of poor risk and critically ill patients.
  American Journal Surgery 122(4):560-564, 1971.

0670
COLTART, D.J.
  Comparison of effects of propranolol and practolol on exercise tolerance in angina pectoris.
  British Heart Journal 33(1):62-64, 1971.

0671
COLTON, C.K., S. FRIEDMAN, D.E. WILSON, AND R.S. LEES.
  Ultrafiltration of lipoproteins through a synthetic membrane. Implications for the filtration theory
  of atherogenesis.
  Journal Clinical Investigation 51(9):2472-2481, 1972.

0672
CONNELL, M.D.
  Serum D-glutamyl transferase following myocardial infarction.
  Journal Clinical Pathology 26:684, 1973.

0673
CONNOLLY, J.E.
  Studies on mechanical assistance to the failing circulation.
  American Journal Surgery 119:565-569, 1970.

0674
CONOLLY, M.E., D.S. DAVIES, C.T. DOLLERY, ET AL.
  Metabolism of isoprenaline in dog and man.
  British Journal Pharmacology 46(3):458-472, 1972.

0675
CONNOR, W.E.
  The use of drugs and diets in the control of coronary heart disease.
  Journal Iowa Medical Society 56(7):657-660, 1966.

0676
CONNOR, W.E.
  Measures to reduce the serum lipid levels in coronary heart disease.
  Medical Clinics North America 52(5):1249-1260, 1968.

0677
CONNOR, W.E., AND S.L. CONNOR.
  The key role of nutritional factors in the prevention of coronary heart disease.
  Preventive Medicine 1:49-83, 1972.

0678
CONRAD, H.
  Work capacity of hypertensive patients before and after antihypertensive therapy.
  Helvetica Medica Acta 32(3):210-226, 1965.

0679
CONRAD, L.L., G.L. HONICK, C.W. WIGGINS, AND J.D. KYRIACOPOULOS.
  Double-blind study of the effectiveness of long-term anticoagulant therapy in myocardial in-
  farction.
  Circulation 24(4 Part 2):908, 1961.

0680
CONRADI, E.
  Problems of therapeutic training in cardiocirculatory affections.
  Zeitschrift für Ärztliche Fortbildung 66(9):462-466, 1972.

0681
CONRADSSON, T., B. LIANDER, L. RYDEN, ET AL.
  Severe acute aortic regurgitation caused by bacterial endocarditis.
  Lakartidningen 69:5487, 1972.

0682
CONSTANTINIDES, E.D.
  Psychiatric problems during rehabilitation after myocardial infarction.
  Hellenic Armed Forces Medical Review 6(1):29-32, 1972.

0683
CONTI, C.R., R.K. BRAWLEY, L.S.C. GRIFFITH, B. PITT, J. O'NEAL HUMPHRIES, V.L. GOTT, AND R.S. ROSS.
Unstable angina pectoris: morbidity and mortality in 57 consecutive patients evaluated angiographically.
American Journal Cardiology 32:745, 1973.

0684
COODLEY, E.L.
Prognostic value of enzymes in myocardial infarction.
Journal American Medical Association 225:597, 1973.

0685
COOK, K.J., AND N.H. HORWITZ.
An instrument for the evaluation of defibrillator performance.
Journal Association Advancement Medical Instrumentation 6(5):325-329, 1972.

0686
COOK, L.P.
Statistics—magnitude of the problem.
Journal Rehabilitation 32:17, 1966.

0687
COOPER, K.H.
Quantifying Physical Activity – How and Why.
Journal South Carolina Medical Association (Suppl.) 65(12):37-40, 1969.

0688
COOPER, K.H., S.M. FOX, III, H.K. HELLERSTEIN, AND I.M. LEVITAS.
The Fitness Kick: Where do you fit in?
Medical Economics 46:102-126, 1969.

0689
COOPER, K.H., AND A. ZECHNER.
Physical fitness in United States and Austrian military personnel: A comparative study.
Journal American Medical Association 215:931-934, 1971.

0690
COOPER, N., J.R. BRAZLER, C. HOTTENROTT, D.G. MULDER, J.V. MALONEY, JR., AND G.D. BUCKBERG.
Myocardial depression following citrated blood transfusion: an avoidable complication.
Archives Surgery 107:756, 1973.

0691
COOPER, R., ET AL.
Ultrasound determination of mean fiber-shortening rate in man.
American Journal Cardiology 29:257, 1972.

0692
COPE, G.D., B.E. HOPKINS, AND R.R. TAYLOR.
Effects of chronic circulatory volume overload on digitalis intoxication.
Cardiovascular Research 7:638-41, 1973.

0693
COPELAND, G.D., A.B. McEACHRAN, H.W. SMITH, AND D.A. BRODY.
  The McFee-Parungao (axial) vectorcardiogram in normal subjects.
  American Heart Journal 86:42, 1973.

0694
CORCORAN, A.C.
  Changing status of sodium restriction in therapy of hypertension.
  American Journal Cardiology 8:887-889, 1961.

0695
CORDAY, E., H. GOLD, L.B. DEVERA, J.H. WILLIAMS, AND J. FIELDS.
  Effect of the cardiac arrhythmias on the coronary circulation.
  Annals Internal Medicine 50(3):535, 1959.

0696
COREA, L., M. TIMIO, U. BUONCRISTIANI, AND M. TOSO.
  Lidocaine in arrhythmias.
  Folia Cardiologica (Milano) 28:149-156, 1969.

0697
CORNFIELD, J., AND S. MITCHELL.
  Possible effects on coronary heart disease of intervention on selected risk factors.
  Archives Environmental Health 19:382, 1969.

0698
COSBY, R.S., J.A. GIDDINGS, J.R. SEE, AND M. MAYO.
  Clinicoarteriographic correlations in angina pectoris with and without myocardial infarction.
  American Journal Cardiology 30(5):472-475, 1972.

0699
COSBY, R.S., J.A. GIDDINGS, J.R. SEE, AND M. MAYO.
  Variant angina: case reports and critique.
  American Journal Medicine 53(6):739-742, 1972.

0700
COSTEAS, F., G. POULIAS, H. MASTROYANNIS, AND L. SOTIRAKIS.
  Unusual mechanical phenomena directly or indirectly related to cardiac pacing.
  Acta Cardiologica 27(6):698-713, 1972.

0701
COSTILL, D.L.
  Effect of water temperature on aerobic working capacity, central core temperature, and heart
  rate.
  In: Balke, B., Ed., Physiological aspects of sports and physical fitness, p. 66. Athletic Institute,
  1968.

0702
COTES, J.E., ET AL.
  Factors relating to the aerobic capacity of 46 healthy British males and females, ages 18 to 28
  years.
  Proceedings Royal Society London, B. 174:91, 1969.

0703

COTES, J.E., AND J.A. REYNOLDS.
Equipment for monitoring the physiological response to submaximal exercise.
Journal Physiology 213:17p, 1971.

0704

COTTIER, P., AND N.F. ROBERT.
The long-term treatment of hypertension.
Internist 9(3):119-127, 1968.

0705

COUTURIER, Y., M. DUCLOUX, M. BARBOTIN, ET AL.
Coronary artery insufficiency in African Negroes. Fifteen cases observed at the Central Hospital of Dakar.
Médecine Tropicale 32(6):743-753, 1972.

0706

COVELL, J.W.
Mechanics of contraction in the intact heart.
In: Kenedi, R.M., Ed., Biomechanics and related bioengineering topics, pp. 289-302. London, Pergamon, 1965.

0707

COVELL, J.W., AND J. ROSS, JR.
Nature and significance of alterations in myocardial compliance.
American Journal Cardiology 32:449, 1973.

0708

COX, J.L., T.M. DANIEL, AND J.P. BOINEAU.
The electrophysiologic time-course of acute myocardial ischemia and the effects of early coronary artery reperfusion.
Circulation 48:971, 1973.

0709

COX, J.R., G.A.B. DAVIES-JONES, AND P.J. LEONARD.
Sodium content and urinary aldosterone excretion in patients with congestive heart failure before and after treatment and comparison with normal subjects undergoing salt restriction.
Clinical Science 26(1):177-184, 1964.

0710

COX, J.R., JR., AND R.D. LOGUE.
Some observations on the economics of computer systems for monitoring electrocardiographic rhythms.
Computers Biomedical Research 4(5):447-459, 1971.

0711

CRAIG, C.P.
Long term suppression of foreign body endocarditis with cephalexin.
American Heart Journal 84(5):714-715, 1972.

0712

CRAMPTON, R.S.
Bed rest after myocardial infarction.
Annals Internal Medicine 79:449, 1973.

0713
CRAMPTON, R.S., R. STILLERMAN, J.A. GASCHO, ET AL.
Prehospital coronary care in Charlottesville and Albermarle County.
Virginia Medical Monthly 99(11):1191-1196, 1972.

0714
CRAWFORD, M.D.
Hardness of drinking water and cardiovascular disease.
Proceedings Nutrition Society 31:347-353, 1972.

0715
CREDITOR, M.C., AND U.K. LOSCHKY.
Incidence of suppressed renin activity and of normokalemic primary aldosteronism in hypertensive
Negro patients.
Circulation 37:1027-1031, 1968.

0716
CRESS, R.H., F. BURRELL, AND W.C. FLEMING.
A review of the dangers of prolonged bed rest.
Alabama Journal Medical Science 5(4):434-440, 1968.

0717
CRETEANU, G., M. BALAN, V. HURJUI, ET AL.
Digitalis treatment in relation to the patient's age.
Revista Medico-Chirurgicală Societaţii de Medici şi Naturalisti din Iaşi 6(4):897-903, 1972.

0718
CREWS, J., AND E.E. ALDINGER.
Effect of chronic exercise on myocardial infarction.
American Heart Journal 74:536, 1967.

0719
CRISTAL, N., D. SOFFER, AND L. FRIEDMAN.
The prehospital phase of acute myocardial infarction in an urban rural community.
Israel Journal Medical Sciences 8(12):1961-1967, 1972.

0720
CRISTODORESCO, R.
Conversion of auricular fibrillation to sinus rhythm by quinidine after failure of electroshock
therapy.
Revue Roumaine de Médecine Interne 9:359, 1972.

0721
CRITZ, J.B., D.A. CUNNINGHAM, P.A. RECHNITZER, AND M.S. YUHASZ.
Plasma enzyme levels in post-coronary patients after exercise.
Archives Physical Medicine Rehabilitation 53(11):499, 1972.

0722
CROCKETT, L.K., M. THOMPSON, AND A. DEKKER.
A review of cardiac amyloidosis. Report of a case presenting as constrictive pericarditis.
American Journal Medical Sciences 264(2):149-156, 1972.

0723
CRONIN, R.F.P., D.J. MACINTOSH, E.A.S. REID, J.C. SINNOTT, AND J.A. SOSA.
Mechanism of hyperventilation during exercise in mitral stenosis.
Canadian Medical Association Journal 94(13):661-662, 1966.

0724 CROOG, S.H., ET AL.
The heart patient and the recovery process. A review of the directions of research on social and psychological factors.
Social Science Medicine 2:111-164, 1968.

0725
CROOG, S.H., AND S. LEVINE.
Social status and subjective perceptions of 250 men after myocardial infarction.
Public Health Reports 84:989-997, 1969.

0726
CROOG, S.H., AND S. LEVINE.
Religious identity and response to serious illness: a report on heart patients.
Sociology Science Medicine 6:17-31, 1972.

0727
CROOG, S.H., D.S. SHAPIRO, AND S. LEVINE.
Denial among male heart patients: An empirical study.
Psychomatic Medicine 33(5):385-397, 1971.

0728
CROSS, D.F.
Use of atrial pacing and exercise in studying ventricular function during angina.
American Journal Cardiology 26:217-218, 1970.

0729
CUCCHINI, F., P. LEVONI, AND C.D. CARLI.
The lactic dehydrogenase isoenzymes in myocardial infarction study of the behavior of the fast fractions.
Giornale Italiano di Cardiologia 2:379-84, 1972.

0730
CUCHE, J.L., O. KUCHEL, A. BARBEAU, ET AL.
Cardiovascular effects of dopamine: physiopathogenic implications in the regulation of the blood pressure.
Union Médicale du Canada 101:2090, 1972.

0731
CUCURACHI, L., AND V. SALVATORE.
Diet in therapy of atherosclerosis. (Critical review).
Ateneo Parmense 34(5):449-465, 1963.

0732
CULL, J.G., AND R.E. HARDY.
Vocational rehabilitation: profession and process.
Springfield, Ill. Thomas, 1972.

0733
CULLHED, I.
  The effect of alprenolol on hemodynamics in angina pectoris.
  Acta Medica Scandinavica 193:411, 1973.

0734
CULLHED, I., E. NOU, AND A.J. UUSITALO.
  Effect of oxygen administration on blood oxygen in myocardial infarction.
  Acta Societatis Medicorum Upsaliensis 75(1/2):44-52, 1970.

0735
CUMMING, G.R.
  Current levels of fitness.
  Canadian Medical Association Journal 96:868-877, 1967.

0736
CUMMING, G.R.
  Effects of propranolol on the resting and exercise hemodynamics of pulmonary stenosis.
  Circulation 37-38 (Suppl. 6):VI-62, 1968.

0737
CUMMING, G.R.
  Stroke volume during recovery from supine bicycle exercise.
  Journal Applied Physiology 32(5):575-578, 1972.

0738
CUMMING, G.R., L. BORYSYK, AND C. DUFRESNE.
  The maximal exercise ECG in asymptomatic men.
  Canadian Medical Association Journal 106(6):649-653, 1972.

0739
CUMMING, G.R., AND G.H. MIR.
  Effects of propranolol on the resting and exercise hemodynamics of pulmonary stenosis.
  Canadian Journal Physiological Pharmacology 47(2):137-142, 1969.

0740
CUNNINGHAM, D.J.C., E.S. PETERSEN, T.G. PICKERING, AND P. SLEIGHT.
  The effects of hypoxia, hypercapnia, and asphyxia on the baroreceptor cardiac reflex at rest and
  during exercise in man.
  Acta Physiologica Scandinavica 86(4):456-465, 1972.

0741
CURRENS, J.H., AND P.D. WHITE.
  Half a century of running. Clinical, physiologic and autopsy findings in the case of Clarence
  De Mar ("Mr. Marathon").
  New England Journal Medicine 265:988, 1961.

0742
CZAPLICKI, S.
  Application of radioelectrocardiography for exercise tolerance test.
  Polski Tygodnik Lekarski 22(29):1097-1100, 1967.

0743
CZAPLICKI, S.
   Application of radioelectrocardiography for exercise test.
   Polish Medical Journal 7:832-838, 1968.

0744
DADD, M.J., AND D.E.L. WILCKEN.
   Echocardiography in left atrial myxoma: relation to the findings in mitral stenosis.
   Australian New Zeland Journal Medicine 2(2):124-127, 1972.

0745
DAGENAIS, G.R., R.E. MASON, G.C. FRIESINGER, C. WENDER, AND R.S. ROSS.
   Exercise tolerance in patients with angina pectoris: Daily variation and effect of pentaerythritol
   tetranitrate.
   Johns Hopkins Medical Journal 125:301, 1969.

0746
DAGENAIS, G.R., B. PITT, AND R.S. ROSS.
   Exercise tolerance in patients with angina pectoris: Daily variation and effects of erythrityl
   tetranitrate, propranolol and alprenolol.
   American Journal Cardiology 28(1):10-16, 1971.

0747
DAHL, L.K., G. LEITL, AND M. HEINE.
   Influence of dietary potassium and sodium/potassium molar ratios on the development of salt
   hypertension.
   Journal Experimental Medicine 136(2):318-330, 1972.

0748
DAHLBACK, O., I. DAHN, AND H. WESTLING.
   Hemodynamic observations in coarctation of the aorta with special reference to the blood
   pressure above and below the stenosis at rest and during exercise.
   Scandinavian Journal Clinical Laboratory Investigation 16:339-346, 1964.

0749
DAILY, B.N.J.
   Stress and myocardial infarction.
   British Medical Journal 2:420, 1973.

0750
DALDERUP, L.M.
   Ischemic heart disease and vitamin D.
   Lancet II:92, 1973.

0751
DALL, J.L.C.
   Digitalis intoxication in elderly patients.
   Lancet 7378:194-195, 1965.

0752
DALTON, B.
   Anaesthesia and coronary heart disease.
   Journal Irish College Physicians Surgeons 2(2):36-40, 1972.

0753
DALY, E.
  Rehabilitation after cardiac surgery.
  Lancet 2:1150, 1967.

0754
DALY, J.W., A.J. BARRY, AND N.C. BIRKHEAD.
  The physical working capacity of older individuals.
  Journal Gerontology 23:134-139, 1968.

0755
DAMATO, A.N., S.H. LAU, R. HELFANT, E. STEIN, R.D. PATTON, B.J. SCHERLAG, AND W.D.
  BERKOWITZ.
  A study of heart block in man using His bundle recordings.
  Circulation 39:297-305, 1969.

0756
DAMIR, A.M., AND S.I. NECHAEV.
  The work capacity of patients with chronic coronary insufficiency.
  Terapevticheskii Arkhiv 38:18-24, 1966.

0757
DAN, A.J., A.G. BURSTEIN, AND J. NAUGHTON.
  Income and outcome.
  Journal Consulting Clinical Psychology 25:153-156, 1970.

0758
DANIELSON, G.K., R. SHABETAI, AND L.R. BRYANT.
  Failure of endocardial pacemaker due to late myocardial perforation. Successful restoration of
  cardiac pacing by conversion to an epicardial system.
  Journal Thoracic Cardiovascular Surgery 54(1): 42-48, 1967.

0759
DANILOV, IU. E.
  The value of sanatorium-health resort therapy in the neuropsychological, physical and vocational-
  economic rehabilitation of patients with cardiovascular diseases.
  Voprosy Kurortologii Fiziotherapii i Lechebnoi Fizicheskoy Kul'tury 33:108-115, 1968.

0760
DANILOW, J.J.
  The development and the current state of thalassotherapy in the Baltic spas of the Soviet Union.
  Zeitschrift Physiotherapie 23(4):241-243, 1971.

0761
DANILOWICZ, D.A., AND H.P. GABRIEL.
  Post cardiotomy psychosis in non-English speaking patients.
  Psychiatry Medicine 2(4):314-320, 1971.

0762
DANNEMANN, H., P. LUBKE, AND K. RAMAN.
  Physical measurements of the circulation during methohexital anesthesia.
  Zeitschrift für Praktische Anaesthesie und Wiederbelebung 7(5):277-282, 1972.

0763
DAOUD, F.S., B. SURAWICZ, AND L.S. GETTES.
  Effect of isoproterenol on the abnormal I wave.
  American Journal Cardiology 30(8):810-819, 1972.

0764
DARBY, S., M.A. BENNETT, J.C. CRUICKSHANK, AND B.L. PENTECOST.
  Trial of combined intramuscular and intravenous lignocaine in prophylaxis of ventricular tachyarrhythmias.
  Lancet 1:817-819, 1972.

0765
D'ARCY, V.
  Three years' experience of myocardial infarction.
  Journal Irish Medical Association 65(21):532-536, 1972.

0766
DARLING, R.C., J.K. RAINES, B.J. BRENER, AND W.G. AUSTEN.
  Quantitative segmental pulse volume recorder: A clinical tool.
  Surgery 72(6):873-887, 1972.

0767
DARMADY, J.M., A.S. FOSBROOKE, AND J.K. LLOYD.
  Prospective study of serum cholesterol levels during first year of life.
  British Medical Journal 2:685-688, 1972.

0768
DAS, P.C., AND J.D. CASH.
  Fibrinolysis at rest and after exercise in hepatic cirrhosis.
  British Journal Haematology 17:431-43, 1969.

0769
DA SILVA, W.N.
  Principles of a questionnaire for epidemiologic study to promote the early detection of coronary disease.
  Arquivos Brasileiros de Cardiologia 24(Suppl. 1):29, 1971.

0770
DA SILVA, W.N., AND S.P. SPINELLI.
  Some aspects about the epidemiology of ischemic heart disease.
  Arquivos Brasileiros de Cardiologia 24(Suppl. 1):25, 1971.

0771
DATEY, K.K., AND N.C. NANDA.
  Hyperglycemia after acute myocardial infarction.
  New England Journal Medicine 276:262-265, 1967.

0772
DATSENKO, I.I.
  Changes of cardiac activity in experimental chronic carbon monoxide intoxication.
  Gigiena i Sanitariya 31(3):102-105, 1966.

0773
DAVIES, C.T.M., A.C. CHUKWEUMEKA, AND J.P.M. VAN HAAREN.
Iron deficiency anemia, its effect on maximum aerobic power and responses to exercise in African males aged 17-40 years.
Clinical Science 44:555-562, 1973.

0774
DAVIES, C.T.M., H.C. DRYSDALE, AND R. PASSMORE.
Does exercise promote health?
Lancet 2:930, 1963.

0775
DAVIES, C.T.M., A. KITCHIN, AND J.M.M. NEILSON.
Continuous analysis of the electrocardiogram wave form during exercise.
Journal Physiology (London) 198(2):61P-62P, 1968.

0776
DAVIES, M.
Blood pressure and personality.
Journal Psychosomatic Research 14(1):89-104, 1970.

0777
DAVIES, M.H.
Is high blood pressure a psychosomatic disorder? A critical review of the evidence.
Journal Chronic Diseases 24(4):239-258, 1971.

0778
DAVYDOVA, A.A.
Myocardial contractility in elderly patients suffering from chronic pneumonia.
Zdravookhranenie Belorussi (USSR) 19:27, 1973.

0779
DAWIDOWICZ, A.
Atherosclerosis, coronary heart disease and physical activity.
Wiadomosci Lekarskie 24(20):1911, 1971.

0780
DAWBER, T.R., AND H.E. THOMAS, JR.
Prevention of myocardial infarction.
Progress Cardiovascular Diseases 13(4):343-360, 1971.

0781
DAWSON, A.A., AND K.N. PALMER.
A long term follow-up of drug treatment in severe hypertension.
Scottish Medical Journal 11(4):113-118, 1966.

0782
DAY, H.W.
Effectiveness of an intensive coronary care area.
American Journal Cardiology 15:51, 1965.

0783

DE ANGELIS, L., M. PISCAGLIA, AND G. DRAGO.
Study on the vocational rehabilitation following myocardial infarct.
Folia Medica (Napoli) 50:1030-1038, 1967.

0784

DEASY, L.C.
Some reflections on coronary heart disease: socio-medical implications for patients and their families.
Social Science Medicine 3:659-667, 1970.

0785

DE BAKEY, M.E.
Prospects for and implications of the artificial heart and assistive devices.
Journal Rehabilitation 32:106, 1966.

0786

DE BUSK, R.F., A.P. SPIVACK, A. VAN KESSEL, C. GRAHAM, AND D.C. HARRISON.
The coronary care unit activities program: Its role in post-infarction rehabilitation.
Journal Chronic Diseases 24:373-381, 1971.

0787

DECKER, D.D., M.J. GERBRANDT, AND M.I. DUNN.
The exercise phonocardiogram in mitral stenosis.
American Heart Journal 71(4):509-514, 1966.

0788

DEGRE, S., A. DE COSTER, R. MESSIN, AND H. DENOLIN.
Normal pulmonary pressure flow relationship during exercise in the sitting position.
Internationale Zeitschrift für Angewandte Physiologie 31(1):53-59, 1972.

0789

DE LA CHAPELLE, C.E., ET AL.
Treatment of patients after recovery from myocardial infarction. (I).
Modern Concepts Cardiovascular Diseases 33:885-888, 1964.

0790

DE LA CHAPELLE, C.E., ET AL.
Treatment of patients after recovery from myocardial infarction. (II).
Modern Concepts Cardiovascular Diseases 33:889-892, 1964.

0791

DELAHAYE, A.
Occupational reclassification of cardiac patients.
Revue Lyonnaise Médicale 17:443-445, 1968.

0792

DE LA IGLESIA, F.A., AND G. LUMB.
Ultrastructural and circulatory alterations of the myocardium in experimental coronary artery narrowing.
Laboratory Investigation 27(1):17-31, 1972.

0793
DELBUE, C.
   Diet and chemical agents in the prevention and treatment.
   Dia Medico 34(77):2041-2042, 1962.

0794
DELEIXHE, A., AND G. REGINSTER-HANEUSE.
   Medico-social effects of myocardial infarct.
   Archives Belges de Médecine Sociale, Hygiene, Médecine du Travail et Médecine Légale
   28:267-280, 1970.

0795
DELGADO, S.
   Pericardial biopsy.
   Academia Peruana de Cirugia 23(3):123-134, 1971.

0796
DELIUS, L.
   Psychosomatic aspects of cardiovascular disorders.
   Zeitschrift für Psychosomatische Medizin und Psychoanalyse 10:242-253, 1964.

0797
DELIUS, L.
   Rehabilitation, evaluation and course of chronic coronary diseases.
   Medizinische Klinik 61(39):1561, 1966.

0798
DELIUS, L.
   Psychological and psychotherapeutic aspects in the rehabilitation of cardiac patients.
   Zeitschrift für Kreislaufforschung 57:84-97, 1968.

0799
DELIUS, W., I. CULLHED, L. NORDGREN, AND G. STRÖM.
   Diagnostic value of ergometer exercise in coronary disease.
   Zeitschrift für Kreislaufforschung 60(7):669, 1971.

0800
DELIUS, W., I. CULLHED, L. NORDGREN, AND G. STRÖM.
   Diagnostic value of ergometer stress in patients with coronary disease.
   Verhandlungen der Deutschen Gesellschaft für Kreislaufforschung 37:210-213, 1971.

0801
DELIUS, L., AND J. TÄGERT.
   Psychological studies on the rehabilitation of patients with circulatory diseases.
   Zeitschrift für Kreislaufforschung 60(4):281-288, 1971.

0802
DELMAN, A.J., G.M. GORDON, E. STEIN, AND D.J.W. ESCHER.
   The second sound-mitral opening snap (A2-Os) interval during exercise in the evaluation of mitral
   stenosis.
   Circulation 33:399-403, 1966.

0803
DEMANEY, M.A., A. TAMBE, AND H.A. ZIMMERMAN.
  Correlation between coronary arteriography and the postexercise electrocardiogram.
  American Journal Cardiology 19(4):526-530, 1967.

0804
DEMBO, A.G.
  Clinical evaluation of some acute changes in the heart from physical overexertion.
  Kardiologiya 10(5):113-116, 1970.

0805
DEMEDTS, M., AND N.R. ANTHONISEN.
  Effects of increased external airway resistance during steady-state exercise.
  Journal Applied Physiology 35:361, 1973.

0806
DE MELLO, W.C. (ED.)
  Electrical phenomena in the heart.
  New York, Academic Press, 1972.

0807
DE MICHELI, A., G.A. MEDRANO, A. VILLAREAL, AND D. SODI PALLARES.
  Experimental study on acute quinidine poisoning.
  Archivos del Instituto de Cardiologia de Mexico 42:580, 1972.

0808
DENBOROUGH, M.A., A.J. GOBLE, R.R.H. LOVELL, AND P.J. NESTEL.
  A trial of long-term treatments after myocardial infarction. Comparison of heparin and phen-
  procoumon given for six months.
  Medical Journal Australia 50:937-941, 1962.

0809
DE NEVE, M., G. MORTIER, AND L. VAN DEN BERGHE.
  Physical training after myocardial infarction.
  Rheumatology and Physical Medicine 27(2):53-89, 1972.

0810
DENGLER, H.J., G. BODEM, AND K. WIRTH.
  Pharmacokinetic studies on H^3 digoxin and H^3 lanatoside in man.
  Arzneimittel-Forschung 23(1):64-74, 1973.

0811
DENISON, D.M., P.D. WAGNER, G.L. KINGABY, AND J.B. WEST.
  Cardiorespiratory responses to exercise in air and underwater.
  Journal Applied Physiology 33(4):426-430, 1972.

0812
DE PALMA, R.G., C.A. HUBAY, R. BOTTI, AND J.L. PETERKA.
  Treatment of surgical patients with atherosclerosis and hyperlipidemia.
  Surgery Gynecology Obstetrics 131(2):313-322, 1970.

0813
DE QUATTRO, V., AND S. CHAN.
   Raised plasma-catecholamines in some patients with primary hypertension.
   Lancet North American Edition 1(7755):806-809, 1972.

0814
DEREVICI, I., T. VLAD, AND P. MOLDOVEANU.
   Point of view on cardiac psychiatric correlations.
   Archives Union Médicale Balkanique 7(1):87-88, 1969.

0815
DERVILLÉE, E., AND P. DUTASTA.
   Considerations on the reclassification of occupational handicaps of cardiovascular origin in industry.
   Archives des Maladies Professionelles de Médecine du Travail et de Sécurité Sociale 28(9):705-714, 1967.

0816
DERYAGINA, G.P.
   Effect of emotional stress on indices of blood coagulation system, lipid metabolism and functional state of the adrenals in healthy persons and in patients with cardiac ischemia.
   Kardiologiya 11(7):42-46, 1971.

0817
DESANCTIS, R.W., P. BLOCK, AND A.M. HUTTER, JR.
   Tachyarrhythmias in myocardial infarction.
   Circulation 45:681-702, 1972.

0818
DESCHRYVER, C., P. DEHERDT, AND J. LAMMERANT.
   Effect of physical training on cardiac catecholamine concentrations.
   Nature 214:907, 1967.

0819
DETRY, J.M.R.
   Exercise testing and training in coronary heart disease.
   Leiden, The Netherlands, Stenfert-Kroese, 1973.

0820
DETRY, J.M.R., AND R.A. BRUCE.
   Effects of nitroglycerin on "maximal" oxygen intake and exercise electrocardiogram in coronary heart disease.
   Circulation 43(1):155-163, 1971.

0821
DETRY, J.M.R., AND R.A. BRUCE.
   Effects of physical training on exertional S-T-segment depression in coronary heart disease.
   Circulation 44(3):390-396, 1971.

0822
DETRY, J.M.R., F. PIETTE, AND L.A. BRASSEUR.
   Hemodynamic determinants of exercise ST-segment depression in coronary patients.
   Circulation 42(4):593-599, 1970.

0823

DETRY, J.M.R., M. ROUSSEAU, G. VAN DENBROUCKE, F. KUSUMI, L.A. BRASSEUR, AND R.A. BRUCE.
Increased arteriovenous oxygen difference after physical training in coronary heart disease.
Circulation 44(1):109-118, 1971.

0824

DEUTSCH, E.
The conservative therapy of artereosclerotic vascular damage.
Wiener Klinische Wochenschrift 23:421-425, 1969.

0825

DEUSCHLE, K.W.
The concept of community medicine and heart disease.
Bulletin New York Academy Medicine 49(6):451-457, 1973.

0826

DEUTSCHER, S.
Some factors influencing the distribution of premature death from coronary heart disease in Nova-Scotia.
American Journal Public Health 63:150, 1973.

0827

DEVINE, C.E., AND F.O. SIMPSON.
The morphological basis for the sympathetic control of blood vessels.
New Zealand Medical Journal 67:326-334, 1968.

0828

DEWAR, H.A.
Long-term therapy of ischaemic heart disease.
Arzneimittel-Forschung 22(10a):1835-1840, 1972.

0829

DE WEESE, J.A., A.J. MOSS, AND P.N. YU.
Infarctectomy and closure of ventricular septal rupture following myocardial infarction.
Circulation 45 (Suppl.):97-101, 1972.

0830

DE WIJN, J.F.
Medical aspects of the changing pattern of the Dutchman's diet and physical activity in the past 30 years.
Nederlands Milk Dairy Journal 24(2):106-119, 1970.

0831

DHURANDHAR, R.W., R.L. MacMILLAN, AND K.W.G. BROWN.
Primary ventricular fibrillation complicating acute myocardial infarction.
American Journal Cardiology 27(4):347-351, 1971.

0832

DHURANDHAR, R.W., S.J. TEASDALE, AND W.A. MAHON.
Bretylium tosylate in the management of refractory ventricular fibrillation.
Canadian Medical Journal 105:161-173, 1971.

0833

DHURANDHAR, R.W., D.L. WATT, M.D. SILVER, ET AL.
  Prinzmetal's varient from angina with arteriographic evidence of coronary arterial spasm.
  American Journal Cardiology 30(8):902-905, 1972.

0834

DIARD, F., C. LARROUDE, AND J. TAVERNIER.
  Radiology of the mesenteric ischaemias.
  Bordeaux Médical 4(9):2211-2248, 1971.

0835

DIAZ, F.V.
  The rehabilitation and the ergonomy in cardiovascular heart disease.
  Revista Española de Cardiologia 26(2):71, 1973.

0836

DICOVSKY, C., J. POSTIGO, M. APTECAR, ET AL.
  Preliminary report on the treatment of two patients with assisted circulation.
  Revista Argentina de Cardiologia 40(6):438-447, 1972.

0837

DIEHL, H.J., F. SORGE, H. HOFFMANN, ET AL.
  The incidence of hyperlipoproteinemia and other risk factors in chronic and acute phases of patients with myocardial infarction.
  Arzneimittel-Forschung 22(10a):1815-1818, 1972.

0838

DIEKMEIER, L.
  The physical and psychological factors of efficiency of the terrain cure. (Oertel's treatment).
  Archiv für Physikalische Therapie Balneologie und Klimatologie (Leipzig) 18:319-324, 1966.

0839

DIENSTL, F., R. MAUSER, H. SCHWINGSHACKL, AND H. AMOR.
  Hybrid computer for the qualitative analysis of cardiac arrhythmias.
  Verhandlungen der Deutschen Gesellschaft für Kreislaufforschung 38:338-342, 1972.

0840

DIETZMAN, R.H., L.H. ROMERO, C.B. BECKMAN, C.H. SHATNEY, AND R.C. LILLEHEI.
  The influence of the sympathetic nervous system during cardiogenic shock.
  Surgery Gynecology Obstetrics 137:773, 1973.

0841

DI GIORGI, S., R.O. WEST, AND J.O. PARKER.
  Coronary heart disease hemodynamic response to exercise before and after nitroglycerin.
  Malattie Cardiovascolari 9(1):29-50, 1968.

0842

DIJKEMA, F.K., AND G. ELZINGA.
  Integrator for aortic and pulmonary artery flow signals, with automatic zero adjustment and beat-to-beat mean flow computation.
  Cardiovascular Research 7:572, 1973.

0843
DILL, D.B.
Individual variability in the responses of man to heat.
In: Balke, B., Physiological aspects of sports and physical fitness, pp. 47-48. The Athletic Institute, 1968.

0844
DIMITRIU, C.G., A. KARASSI, S. LACK, ET AL.
Rupture of the ventricular wall in myocardial infarct.
Medicina Internă 24(9):1103-1116, 1972.

0845
DIMNIK, R.
Analogous metabolic studies on coronary patients and healthy subjects.
In: Plavšić, C. and M.M. Gertler, Eds., The first international biennial conference on cardiac rehabilitation, Dubrovnik, Yugoslavia, 1969.

0846
DIMOND, G.E.
The exercise test and prognosis of coronary heart disease.
Circulation 24:736-738, 1961.

0847
DIMOND, G.E.
The exercise apex cardiogram: a clinical test in angina pectoris.
American Journal Cardiology 27:120-121, 1971.

0848
DIONISIO, S.D.
A geographic study.
In: Proceedings, Third Asian-Pacific Congress of Cardiology, pp. 94-97. Kyoto, Japan, 1964.

0849
DI PAOLO, E., G.A. PERRONE, AND R. MATTAGE.
Effect of beta-blocking aspects on exercise tests with the cycloergometer evaluated by means of a micro-electrocardiographic method.
Bolletino della Società Italiana di Cardiologia 17:27-35, 1972.

0850
DISTELBRINK, C.A., C.A. ASCOOP, P.A. DE LANG, AND M.A. VAN DEN AKER JANSEN.
The exercise VCG in relation to coronary arteriography in patients with ischaemic heart disease.
Progress Report Medicophysical Institute TNO 3:179, 1972.

0851
DJIANA, P.
Problems arising in the anesthetic and resuscitative management of auriculoventricular blocks.
Corse Méditerranée Médicale 18:99, 1972.

0852
DLIN, B.M., H.K. FISCHER, AND B. HUDDELL.
Psychologic adaptation to pacemaker and open heart surgery.
Archives General Psychiatry 19:599, 1968.

0853
DOAN, A.E., D.R. PETERSON, J.R. BLACKMON, AND R.A. BRUCE.
Myocardial ischemia after maximal exercise in healthy men. A method for detecting potential coronary heart disease.
American Heart Journal 69:11-21, 1965.

0854
DOBROW, R.J., P.A. GORMAN, J.B. CALATAYUD, S. ABRAHAM, A.L. WEIHRER, AND C.A. CACERES.
Accuracy of electrocardiographic measurements by computer.
American Journal Medical Electronics 4:121-126, 1965.

0855
DOBROWOLSKI, L.A.
Arteriosclerosis and calcification.
Giornale di Gerontologia 19:552, 1971.

0856
DOBROWOLSKI, L.A.
Study of aortic calcification in vitro.
Europa Medicophysica 8:43-47, 1972.

0857
DOBRZANSKI, T., AND J. BARTOSZEWSKI.
Painless myocardial infarction in psychiatric patients.
Polish Medical Journal 10(3):590-593, 1971.

0858
DOCK, W.
The evil sequelae of complete bed rest.
Journal American Medical Association 125:1083, 1944.

0859
DOCK, W.
The management of patients with angina and infarction of the heart.
Arizona Medicine 21:876-878, 1964.

0860
DODEK, A., D.G. KASSEBAUM, AND J.D. BRISTOW.
Pulmonary edema without cardiomegaly: Ischemic cardiomyopathy and the small stiff heart.
American Heart Journal 85(2):281-284, 1973.

0861
DODINOT, B., J.P. SAULNIER, J.L. NEIMANN, ET AL.
Dangers of demand pacing in the acute stage of myocardial infarction.
Archives des Maladies du Coeur et des Vaisseaux 65(12):1423-1432, 1972.

0862
DOENECKE, P., L. BETTE, G. HARBAUER, ET AL.
Reduction of the frequency of dislocation by use of newly developed transvenous pacemaker electrodes.
Zeitschrift für Kreislaufforschung 61(10):887-891, 1972.

0863

DOHBA, N., I. CHIBA, T. YAGUCHI, M. USAMI, Y. NAKAMURA, S. MYOJYO, K. KONDO, S. ITAKURA, Y. ANDO, AND A. HIRAI.
Vector cardiographic and cardiac dynamic analyses in exercise by a bicycle ergometer.
Japanese Circulation Journal 33(8):865, 1969.

0864

DOHRENWEND, B.P.
Social stress and cardiac disease. Workshop Summary. Toward the development of theoretical models: I.
Milbank Memorial Fund Quarterly (Suppl.) 45:155-162, 1967.

0865

DOLABCHIAN, Z.L., E.M. KRISHCHIAN, E.KH. SIKUNI, AND N.G. TATINIAN.
Automatic identification of cardiac rhythm and conductivity disturbances with the aid of digital computers.
Akademiia Nauk Armianskoi SSR, Doklady 56(2):123-128, 1973.

0866

DOLLERY, C.T., H.M. PERRY, JR., H.P. DUSTAN, AND R.H. LYONS.
Medical management of hypertension.
Circulation 28(4 Part 1):595-602, 1963.

0867

DOMINIAN, J., AND M. DOBSON.
Study of patients' psychological attitudes to a coronary care unit.
British Medical Journal 4:795-798, 1969.

0868

DONAT, K., AND H. KOEFFLER.
Principles and results of early rehabilitation after cardiac infarction in the hospital.
Zeitschrift für Kreislaufforschung 60(7):670, 1971.

0869

DONGIER, M.
Psychosomatic approach in cardiology: Art, science or pseudoscience? Record of the means of study.
Coeur et Médecine Interne 7(2):229-235, 1968.

0870

DONOSO, H., E. APUD, AND N.P.V. LUNDGREN.
Direct estimation of circulatory fatigue using a bicycle ergometer.
Ergonomics 14(1):53-60, 1971.

0871

DOR, V., G. CHAUVIN, B. MERMET, AND P. KREITMANN.
Emergency extracorporeal circulation in patients aged between 70 and 81 years (with reference to four cases).
Archives des Maladies du Coeur et des Vaisseaux 65(11):1343-1347, 1972.

0872

DOROFEEVA, L.A., AND N.L. DONSKOVA.
Long-range follow-up in myocardial infarction.
Sovetskaya Meditsina 34(4):114-115, 1971.

0873
DOROFEEVA, Z.Z., I.F. IGNATIEVA, U.P. KUMEKIN, AND V.M. SHEREMETA.
Possibilities of vectocardiographic differentiation of two forms of combined hypertrophy of both cardiac ventricles.
Kardiologiya 12(9):89-96, 1972.

0874
DOROSSIEV, D.L.
A method of quantitative evaluation of disturbances in heart rhythm during physical activity.
Malattie Cardiovascolari 10:91, 1969.

0875
DOROSSIEV, D., I. PERTCHEV, A. NIKOV, AND A. TZOLOV.
Limiting factors for physical training after myocardial infarction.
Cor et Vasa 13(1):18-24, 1971.

0876
DOSCHITSIN, V.L., AND V.I. SIMONOV.
The treatment of cardiac arrhythmias with beta-adrenergic blocking agents—propranolol, benzodixin, visken, eraldin and trasicor.
Kardiologiya 11:49-54, 1971.

0877
DOUGLAS, A.H.
Ischaemic heart disease in monozygotic twins.
Diseases Chest 49:522-528, 1966.

0878
DOUGLAS, J.E.
Cardiovascular conditioning and rehabilitation. A mandate for action.
Journal Arkansas Medical Society 69(6):173-177, 1972.

0879
DOVENMUEHLE, R.H.
Death and dying: Attitudes of patient and doctor. II. Affective response to life-threatening cardiovascular disease.
Group for the Advancement of Psychiatry, Symposium 5:607-613, 1965.

0880
DOVENMUEHLE, R.H., AND A. VERWOERDT.
Physical illness and depressive symptomatology. I. Incidence of depressive symptoms in hospitalized cardiac patients.
Journal American Geriatrics Society 10(11):932-947, 1962.

0881
DOVGYALLO, G.K., AND I.S. GULKO.
Interrelation between the shifts of some biochemical and electrophysiological indices in patients with myocardial infarction.
Terapevticheskii Arkhiv 43:43, 1971.

0882
DOWER, G.E., H.E. HORN, AND W.G. ZIEGLER.
The polarcardiograph. Terminology and normal findings.
American Heart Journal 69(3):355-368, 1965.

0883
DOWER, G.E., H.E. HORN, AND W.G. ZIEGLER.
The polarcardiograph. Diagnosis of myocardial infarction.
American Heart Journal 69(3):369-381, 1965.

0884
DOWLING, J.T., R.O. RUSSELL, G.K. MASSING, AND C.E. RACKLEY.
Present-day management of acute myocardial infarction-outline of policy and practice in myocardial infarction research unit at University of Alabama in Birmingham.
Southern Medical Journal 66:518, 1973.

0885
DOWNING, J.W., W.P. LEARY, A.J. COLEMAN, AND D.G. MOYES.
The immediate cardiovascular effects of pancuronium.
South African Medical Journal 46(28):962-966, 1972.

0886
DOYLE, J.T., A.S. HESLIN, H.E. HILLEBOE, P.F. FORMEL, AND R.F. KORNS.
A prospective study of degenerative cardiovascular disease in Albany: report of three years' experience. I. Ischemic heart disease.
American Journal Public Health 47(4 Part 2):25-32, 1957.

0887
DOYLE, J.T., AND W.B. KANNEL.
Coronary risk factors: 10 year findings in 7446 Americans. Pooling Project, Council on Epidemiology, American Heart Association.
Presented at VI World Congress of Cardiology, London, England, September 6-12, 1970.

0888
DOYLE, J.T., AND S.H. KINCH.
The prognosis of an abnormal electrocardiographic stress test.
Circulation 41:545-553, 1970.

0889
DOYLE, J.T., S.H. KINCH, AND D.F. BROWN.
Cardiovascular screening to assess risk of coronary heart disease.
Public Health Reports 83(8):659-667, 1968.

0890
DRAPER, H.W., C.J. PEFFER, F.W. STALLMANN, D. LITTMANN, AND H.V. PIPBERGER.
The corrected orthogonal electrocardiogram and vectorcardiogram in 510 normal men.
Circulation 30:853-864, 1964.

0891
DRAPKIN, A., AND C. MERSKEY.
Anticoagulant therapy after acute myocardial infarction. Relation of therapeutic benefit to patient's age, sex, and severity of infarction.
Journal American Medical Association 222(5):541-548, 1972.

0892
DREIFUS, L.S., B. STALLER, AND M. NAJMI.
Disturbances of impulse formation and conduction in response to measured exercise.
Circulation 33 (Suppl. 3):91, 1966.

0893
DRESZLER, L., AND J. BOHM.
Electrode dislocations in intracardiac pacemaking.
Deutsche Gesundheitswesen 27(40):1896-1899, 1972.

0894
DREYFUSS, F., J. SHANAN, AND M. SHARON.
Some personality characteristics of middle-aged men with coronary artery disease.
Psychotherapy Psychosomatics 14(1):1-16, 1966.

0895
DRORY, Y., Y. ESHCHAR, AND J.J. KELLERMANN.
Use of single-stage exercise test with individually adjusted work load in electrocardiographic diagnosis of ischemic heart disease.
Chest 59:138-145, 1971.

0896
DRUNKENMOELLE, C.
Psychological investigations of the neurotic aspects of the effort syndrome.
Psychotherapy Psychosomatics 22:34, 1973.

0897
DRUSS, R.G., AND D.S. KORNFELD.
The survivors of cardiac arrest. A psychiatric study.
Journal American Medical Association 201(5):291-296, 1967.

0898
DRUT, R.
Fibrocartilaginous nodule in relation to the conduction system of the heart.
Archivos de la Fundacion Roux-Ocefa 6(1-2):69-71, 1972.

0899
DUBIEL, J.P., J.S. DUBIEL, J. SZCZEKLIK, AND T. HORZELA.
Determination of myocardial blood flow in man with the use of the isotope xenon 133.
Polskie Archiwum Medycyny Wewnetrznej 49(4):319-328, 1972.

0900
DUBIEL, J.S.
Behaviour of the cardiac output at rest and during exercise in patients with chronic cardiac failure.
Przeglad Lekarski 28(12):770-775, 1971.

0901
DUBOUCHER, G.
Complete arrhythmia and statistical method.
Archives des Maladies du Coeur 53:1122-36, 1960.

0902
DUCHENE, M.P., G. SCHAFF, AND J. LAVARENNE.
Studies of the Institute of Cardiologic Research at Royat.
Royat, France. Institut de Recherches Cardiologiques, 1971.

0903
DUCHOSAL, P.W., AND J. GONCALVES.
ECG and VCG in ischemic heart disease.
Schweizerische Medizinische Wochenschrift 102:1815, 1972.

0904
DUCLOS, F.
Psychological vectors acting on the heart patient destined for surgery.
Revista Española de Cardiologia 19:231-238, 1966.

0905
DUCLOS, F., AND J. ARMENTA.
Permanent Osborn wave without causal hypothermia.
Revista Española de Cardiologia 25(4):379-382, 1972

0906
DUCLOUX, G., M.O. PONTAC, C. STANOWIAK, AND G. SOOTS.
Ventricular wall aneurysms following myocardial infarction. II. Operative modalities and overall results.
Coeur et Médecine Interne 12:397, 1973.

0907
DUDECK, J., H. VON EGIDY, R. LIPPOLD, AND J. MICHAELIS.
A data recording system for the computerized analysis of phonocardiograms and electro-cardiograms.
Medizinische Technik 92(5):209-215, 1972.

0908
DUGHERA, L., AND M. DI LEO.
Notes on phonocardiography in geriatric medicine.
Archivio per le Scienze Mediche 127(10):418-426, 1971.

0909
DUKE, M.
Bed rest in acute myocardial infarction. A study of physician practices.
American Heart Journal 82(4):486-491, 1971.

0910
DUKE, M.
Atrioventricular block due to accidental digoxin ingestion treated with atropine.
American Journal Diseases Children 124(5):754-756, 1972.

0911
DUKHOVNAYA, O.L.
Effect of metered physical exercise on the functional state of the myocardium in patients with rheumatic heart disease (According to data of tele-electrocardiography).
Voprosy Reumatisma 6(3):54-58, 1966.

0912
DUMOIS, A.O.
  Heart disease in the community.
  Bulletin New York Academy Medicine 49(6):485-491, 1973.

0913
DUNCAN, R.J., AND C.B. NASH.
  Dose response effects of quinidine on electrophysiological properties of the heart.
  Archives Internationales de Pharmacodynamie et de Therapie 199(2):358-367, 1972.

0914
DUNKMAN, W.B., R.C. LEINBACH, M.J. BUCKLEY, ET AL.
  Clinical and hemodynamic results of intraaortic balloon pumping and surgery for cardiogenic
  shock.
  Circulation 46(3):465-477, 1972.

0915
DUNNIGAN, M.G., T. FYFE, M.T. MCKIDDIE, AND S.M. CROSBIE.
  The effects of isocaloric exchange of dietary starch and sucrose on glucose tolerance, plasma
  insulin and serum lipids in man.
  Clinical Science 38:1-9, 1970.

0916
DURBECK, D.C., F. HEINZELMANN, J. SCHACTER, W.L. HASKELL, G.H. PAYNE, R.T. MOX-
  LEY, M. NEMIROFF, D.D. LIMONCELLI, L.B. ARNOLDI, AND S.M. FOX, III.
  The NASA-USPHS health evaluation and enhancement program.
  American Journal Cardiology 30:784-790, 1972.

0917
DURNIN, J.V.G.A.
  The influence of nutrition.
  Canadian Medical Association Journal 96:715-718, 1967.

0918
DUSSART, P.
  Vocational guidance of young cardiac patients.
  Archives des Maladies Professionelles, de Médecine du Travail et de Sécurité Sociale 27:147-151,
  1966.

0919
DWYER, E.M., JR., L. WIENER, AND J.W. COX.
  Effects of beta-adrenergic blockage (propranolol) on left ventricular hemodynamics and the
  electrocardiogram during exercise-induced angina pectoris.
  Circulation 38(2):250-260, 1968.

0920
EARLEY, L.E., M.H. HUMPHREYS, AND E. BARTOLI.
  Capillary circulation as a regulator of sodium reabsorption and excretion.
  Circulation Research 31(Supl. II):1-18, 1972.

0921
EBERT, R.V.
  A critical review of studies on long-term anticoagulant therapy after myocardial infarction.
  Annals Internal Medicine 60(4):709, 1964.

0922

EBERT, R.V., C.W. BORDEN, H.R. HIPP, D. HOLZMAN, A.F. LYON, AND H. SCHNAPER.
Long-term anticoagulant therapy after myocardial infarction. Final report of the Veterans Administration cooperative study [bishydroxycoumarin].
Journal American Medical Association 207(2):2263-2267, 1969.

0923

ECKER, R.R., C.B. MULLINS, J.C. GRAMMER, W.J. REA, AND J.M. ATKINS.
Control of intractable ventricular tachycardia by coronary revascularization.
Circulation 44:666-670, 1971.

0924

ECKSTEIN, R.W.
Effect of exercise and coronary artery narrowing on coronary collateral circulation.
Circulation Research 5:230, 1975.

0925

EDDY, J.D., AND S.P. SINGH.
Treatment of cardiac arrhythmias with phenytoin.
British Medical Journal 4:270-273, 1969.

0926

EDERER, F.
Serum cholesterol changes: Effects of diet and regression toward the mean.
Journal Chronic Diseases 25:277-289, 1972.

0927

EDHAG, O., AND S. ZETTERQUIST.
Peripheral circulatory adaptation to exercise in restricted cardiac output. A hemodynamic and metabolic study in patients with complete heart block and artificial pacemaker.
Scandinavian Journal Clinical Laboratory Investigation 21(2):123-135, 1968.

0928

EDWARDS, R.H.T., A. KRISTINSSON, D.A. WARRELL, AND J.F. GOODWIN.
Effects of propranolol on response to exercise in hypertrophic obstructive cardiomyopathy.
British Heart Journal 32(2):219-225, 1970.

0929

EGEBERG, O.
The effect of exercise on the blood clotting system.
Scandinavian Journal Clinical Laboratory Investigation 15:8-13, 1963.

0930

EICHHORN, R.L., AND R.M. ANDERSEN.
Changes in personal adjustment to perceived and medically established heart disease: A panel study.
Journal Health Human Behavior 3(4):242-249, 1962.

0931

EISENBERG, H., J.J. KULA, AND D.F. ODOARDO.
Epidemiology of coronary heart disease in Middlesex County, Conn. Pilot study of dietary assessment of patients with primary myocardial infarction.
Journal American Dietetic Association 47:391-395, 1965.

0932
EISENREICH, R., AND H. WALTHER.
  Myocardial infarction as a consequence of accident. Part 2. Medically connected questions.
  Zeitschrift für Aerztliche Fortbildung 66:518-522, 1972.

0933
EKBLOM, B.
  Effect of physical training on oxygen transport system in man.
  Acta Physiologica Scandinavica (Suppl.) 328:9-45, 1969.

0934
EKBLOM, B., AND L. HERMANSEN.
  Cardiac output in athletes.
  Journal Applied Physiology 25:619-625, 1968.

0935
EKBLOM, B., P. ÅSTRAND, B. SALTIN, J. STENBERG, AND B. WALLSTRÖM.
  Effect of training on circulatory response to exercise.
  Journal Applied Physiology 24:518-528, 1968.

0936
EKELUND, L-G.
  Exercise, including weightlessness.
  Annual Review Physiology 31:85-116, 1969.

0937
ELIAKIM, M.
  Atrial parasystole. Effect of carotid sinus stimulation, valsalva maneuver and exercise.
  American Journal Cardiology 16:457-461, 1965.

0938
ELIAKIM, M., AND H.N. NEUFELD, EDS.
  Cardiology current topics and progress. Sumposia of the fourth Asian Pacific Congress of
  Cardiology, Israel, 1968. New York, Academic Press, 1969.

0939
ELIOT, R.S.
  Mysteries of sudden death and myocardial infarction.
  Chest 62(6):657, 1972.

0940
ELIOT, R.S., J.W. HOLSINGER, H.M. HAWKINS, AND J.M. SALHANY.
  Relief of myocardial ischemia associated with increased blood oxygen release.
  Clinical Research 20(1):67, 1972.

0941
ELISEO, V., ET AL.
  Work activity and survival of patients with myocardial infarct. (Study conducted for a period of
  ten years, 1946-1955, on 279 subjects.)
  Folia Medica 50:810-819, 1967.

0942

ELKELES, R.S., C. LOWY, A.D.H. WYLLIE, J.L. YOUNG, AND T.R. FRASER.
Serum insulin, glucose, and lipid levels among mild diabetics in relation to incidence of vascular complications.
Lancet 1:880-883, 1971.

0943

ELLESTAD, M.H., W. ALLEN, M.C.K. WAN, AND G.L. KEMP.
Maximal treadmill stress testing for cardiovascular evaluation.
Circulation 39(4):517-522, 1969.

0944

ELMFELDT, D., G. TIBBLIN, J.A. VEDIN, ET AL.
Sudden death from heart disease. Identification of high risk subjects.
Lakartidningen 69:5201, 1972.

0945

EL-SHERIF, N.
Tachycardia-dependent versus bradycardia-dependent intermittent bundle-branch block.
British Heart Journal 34:167-176, 1972.

0946

EL-SHERIF, N.
Paroxysmal atrial flutter and fibrillation: induction by carotid sinus compression and prevention by atropine.
British Heart Journal 34(10):1024-1028, 1972.

0947

ENDERLE, J., J. STRUYVEN, G. PRIMO, ET AL.
Personal experience of coronarography and of the revascularization of the myocardium by surgery.
Bruxelles Médical 51:557, 1971.

0948

ENESCO, I., V. TACOU, R. FRIEDMAN, AND E. BABEI.
Efficiency of physical work in cardiac patients and work capacity of cardiac patients, determined by ergospyrometric methods.
Revue Roumaine Médecine Interne 4(2):93-105, 1967.

0949

ENGEL, G.L.
Sudden and rapid death during psychological stress: Folklore or folk wisdom?
Annals Internal Medicine 74(5):771-782, 1971.

0950

ENGELHARDT, K.
Sociopsychological stress factors.
Medizinische Klinik 60:338-340, 1965.

0951

ENGER, S.C., AND S. RITLAND.
Glucose tolerance, insulin release and lipoprotein pattern in patients after myocardial infarction.
Acta Medica Scandinavica 194:97, 1973.

0952
ENGLISH, T.A.H., AND J.K. ROSS.
Surgical aspects of bacterial endocarditis.
British Medical Journal 4:598-602, 1972.

0953
ENGSTEDT, L., G. KALLNER, J. KARNELL, AND G. MATELL.
Treatment of myocardial infarction at Sodersjukhuset, Stockholm. Part II. Analyses of 357 patients with suspected but not verified myocardial infarction.
Opuscula Medica 16(3):92-96, 1971.

0954
EPOIS, A., P. ROCHA, G. ROUDY, ET AL.
Haemodynamic effects of selective beta adrenergic blockade during acute stage of myocardial infarction.
British Heart Journal 34(12):1295-1301, 1972.

0955
EPSTEIN, F. H.
The epidemiology of coronary heart disease: A review.
Journal Chronic Diseases 18:735-774, 1965.

0956
EPSTEIN, F.H.
International trends in coronary heart disease epidemiology.
Annals Clinical Research 3(6):293-299, 1971.

0957
EPSTEIN, F.H.
An epidemiologist's conclusion.
Milbank Memorial Fund Quarterly 59(Suppl. 2):249-255, 1972.

0958
EPSTEIN, F.H.
Introduction to coronary heart disease. Prevention forum.
Preventive Medicine 1:23-26, 1972.

0959
EPSTEIN, F.H.
Epidemiology of cardiovascular disease: Respective role of neural and non-neural factors.
In: Zanchetti, A., Ed. Symposium on neural and psychological mechanisms in cardiovascular disease. Milan, International Soćiety of Cardiology and Il Ponte, 1972.

0960
EPSTEIN, F.H.
Coronary heart disease epidemiology revisited. Clinical and community aspects.
Circulation 48:185, 1973.

0961
EPSTEIN, F.H.
Glucose intolerance and cardiovascular disease.
Triangle 12(1):3-8, 1973.

0962
EPSTEIN, F.H., ET AL.
Epidemiological studies of cardiovascular disease in a total community—Tecumseh, Michigan.
Annals Internal Medicine 62:1170-1187, 1965.

0963
EPSTEIN, F.H., ET AL.
The Tecumseh Study. Design, progress and perspectives.
Archives Environmental Health 21:402-407, 1970.

0964
EPSTEIN, S.E.
Hypotension, nitroglycerin, and acute myocardial infarction.
Circulation 47(2):217-219, 1973.

0965
EPSTEIN, S.E., G.D. BEISER, AND M. STAMPFER.
Exercise in patients with heart disease: Effects of body position and type and intensity of exercise.
American Journal Cardiology 23(4):572-576, 1969.

0966
EPSTEIN, S.E., G.D. BEISER, M. STAMPFER, B.F. ROBINSON, AND E. BRAUNWALD.
Characterization of the circulatory response to maximal upright exercise in normal subjects and patients with heart disease.
Circulation 35(6):1049-1062, 1967.

0967
EPSTEIN, S.E., ET AL.
Effects of a cold environment on the circulatory response to exercise: implications concerning angina pectoris.
Clinical Research 16(2):228, 1968.

0968
EPSTEIN, S.E., D.R. REDWOOD, R.E. GOLDSTEIN, G.D. BEISER, D.R. ROSING, D.L. GLANCY, R.L. REIS, AND E.B. STINSON.
Angina pectoris: pathophysiology, evaluation and treatment.
Annals Internal Medicine 75(2):263-296, 1971.

0969
EPSTEIN, S.E., B.F. ROBINSON, R.L. KAHLER, AND E. BRAUNWALD.
Effects of beta-adrenergic blockade on the cardiac response to maximal and submaximal exercise in man.
Journal Clinical Investigation 44(11):1745-1753, 1965.

0970
EPSTEIN, S.E., D.R. ROSING, P. BRAKMAN, D.R. REDWOOD, AND T. ASTRUP.
Impaired fibrinolytic response to exercise in patients with type-IV hyperlipoproteinaemia.
Lancet 2:631-634, 1970.

0971

EPSTEIN, S.E., M. STAMPFER, G.D. BEISER, R.E. GOLDSTEIN, AND E. BRAUNWALD.
Effects of a reduction in environmental temperature on the circulatory response to exercise in man. Implications concerning angina pectoris.
New England Journal Medicine 280(1):7-11, 1969.

0972

ERBSTOESSER, H.
Determination of heart diseases by the x-ray mass survey evaluation of cardiosurgical material of patients.
Zeitschrift für Erkrankungen der Atmungsorgane 133(1-3):202-205, 1970.

0973

ERICKSON, L., E. SIMONSON, H.L. TAYLOR, H. ALEXANDER, AND A. KEYS.
The energy cost of horizontal and grade walking on the motor driven treadmill.
American Journal Physiology 145:391, 1946.

0974

ERICSSON, M., A. GRANATH, P. OHLSEN, T. SODERMAR, AND U. VOLPE.
Arrhythmias and symptoms during treadmill testing 3 weeks after myocardial infarction in 100 patients.
British Heart Journal 35:787, 1973.

0975

ERICSSON, B., K. HAEGER, AND S.E. LINDELL.
Effect of physical training on intermittent claudication.
Angiology 21(3):188-192, 1970.

0976

ERIKSSEN, J., AND C. MULLER.
Quinidine in acute myocardial infarction.
Geriatrics 26:160, 1971.

0977

ESKWITH, I.S., J.J. LAWRENCE, AND T. MCLOUGHLIN.
The relationship of urinary potassium excretion to dietary sodium content in cardiac patients receiving oral diuretics.
American Journal Cardiology 9(2):194-202, 1962.

0978

ETTINGER, P.O., M.J. FRANK, AND G.E. LEVINSON.
Hemodynamics at rest and during exercise in combined aortic stenosis and insufficiency.
Circulation 45(2):267-276, 1972.

0979

EVANG, K., AND K.L. ANDERSEN.
Physical activity in health and disease.
Baltimore, Williams and Wilkins, 1966.

0980

EVANS, R.B., AND J. MARMORSTON.
Improved mental functioning with premarin therapy in atherosclerosis.
Proceedings Society Experimental Biology Medicine 113(3):698, 1963.

0981
EVANS, W.
  After heart disease.
  Nursing Times 62:180-181, 1966.

0982
EWING, D.J., ET AL.
  Static exercise in untreated systemic hypertension.
  British Heart Journal 35(4):413, 1973.

0983
FABIAN, J., E.J. EPSTEIN, AND N. COULSHED.
  Polygraphic recording of systolic phases of the left ventricle. I. Control group.
  Casopis Lekaru Ceckych 111(46):1079-1086, 1972.

0984
FABIAN, J., E.J. EPSTEIN, AND N. COULSHED
  Duration of phases of left ventricular systole using indirect methods. I. Normal subjects.
  British Heart Journal 34(9):874-881, 1972.

0985
FABIAN, J., E.J. EPSTEIN, N. COULSHED, AND C.S. McKENDRICK.
  Duration of phases of left ventricular systole using indirect methods. II. Acute myocardial infarction.
  British Heart Journal 34(9):882-889, 1972.

0986
FAERCHTEIN, I., A.F. ROQUE, AND I. KASTANSKY.
  The use of the beta-adrenergic blocking agent LB-46 (pindolol) in the treatment of angina pectoris.
  Arquivos Brasileiros de Cardiologia 25(4):299-305, 1972.

0987
FAGRAEUS, L., J. KARLSSON, D. LINNARSSON, AND B. SALTIN.
  Oxygen uptake during maximal work at lowered and raised ambient air pressures.
  Acta Physiologica Scandinavica 87:411, 1973.

0988
FAHRENBERG, J., AND M. MYRTEK.
  A critical contribution to psychophysiological personality research.
  Zeitschrift für Experimentelle und Angewandte Psychologie (Göttingen) 13:222-247, 1966.

0989
FAIDUTTI, B., AND C. HAHN.
  Immediate and medium term results of direct coronary surgery and preoperative evaluation of surgical risk.
  Schweizerische Medizinische Wochenschrift 102(47):1736-1738, 1972.

0990
FALLS, H.B.
  The relative energy requirements of various physical activities in relation to physiological strain.
  Journal South Carolina Medical Association (Suppl.) 65(12):8-11, 1969.

0991
FALZI, G., A. RITUCCI, AND A. LIBERATORE.
Traumatic lesions produced by external cardiac massage (review of the literature and personal patient material).
Anestesia e Rianimazione 13(1):35-65, 1972.

0992
FARBEROW, N.L., J.W. MCKELLIGOTT, S. COHEN, AND A. DARBONNE.
Suicide among patients with cardiorespiratory illnesses.
Journal American Medical Association 195(6):422, 1966.

0993
FAREEDUDDIN, K., AND W.H. ABELMANN.
Impaired orthostatic tolerance after bed rest in patients with myocardial infarction.
New England Journal Medicine 280(7):345, 1969.

0994
FARHAD, D., J. BARDET, G. ROUDY, ET AL.
Comparative study of two methods of simplified calculation of cardiac output by indicator dilution technique.
Archives des Maladies du Coeur et des Vaisseaux 65(7):827-835, 1972.

0995
FARRER BROWN, G., AND M.H. TARBIT.
What is the spectrum of endomyocardial fibrosis?
Tropical Geographical Medicine 24(3):208-218, 1972.

0996
FARRONI, A., AND P. POGGI.
Social aspects of the rehabilitation of heart disease patients. Statistical study of heart diseases detected at the Poliambulatorio-Sezione Cardiologica INAM, Piacenza.
Minerva Cardioangiologica 13:843-847, 1965.

0997
FASOLA, A.F., AND B.L. MARTZ.
Peripheral venous renin activity during $70°$ tilt and lower body negative pressure.
Aerospace Medicine 43(7):713-715, 1972.

0998
FASOLA, A.F., B.L. MARTZ, AND O.M. HELMER.
Renin activity during supine exercise in normotensives and hypertensives.
Journal Applied Physiology 21(6):1709-1712, 1966.

0999
FASSATI, P., M. FASSATI, J. SONKA, AND K. LESENSKY.
New approach to the treatment of angina pectoris by dehydroepiandrosterone sulphate.
Casopis Lekaru Ceskych 110(26):606-609, 1971.

1000
FAVARA, B.E., AND R.A. FRANCIOSI.
Diphtherial myocardiopathy.
American Journal Cardiology 30(4):423-426, 1972.

1001

FAZEKAS, I.G., AND A.M. DEKOVA.
  Corticosteroid fractions of the normal heart muscle and of myocardial infarction.
  Rheumatologia Balneologia Allergologia 13(3):170-179, 1972.

1002

FEARNLEY, G.R., AND R. LACKER.
  The fibrinolytic activity of normal blood.
  British Journal Hematology 1:189-198, 1955.

1003

FEDOROV, G.I.
  Some biochemical and instrumental indices in patients having atherosclerosis, hypertension, and in
  practically healthy people engaged in mental and physical work.
  Kardiologiya 8(8):17-26, 1968.

1004

FEDOSEEV, A.A.
  The ballistocardiogram in patients with coronary failure.
  Abstracts Soviet Medicine 5:1431, 1961.

1005

FEEST, T.G., G.C. SUTTON, R.J. VECHT, AND R.V. GIBSON.
  Signs of pericardial constriction in rupture of ventricular septum complicating myocardial in-
  farction.
  British Heart Journal 34(11):1176-1180, 1972.

1006

FEIFEL, H., J. FREILICH, AND L.J. HERMANN.
  Death fear in dying heart and cancer patients.
  Journal Psychosomatic Research 17:161-166, 1973.

1007

FEINGOLD, R.S.
  Heart rates and predicted maximal oxygen uptake following training at low to moderate duration
  and intensity.
  Ph.D. Dissertation, New Mexico University (Albuquerque), 1972.

1008

FEJFAR, Z.
  Risk Factors in ischemic heart disease.
  Acta Cardiologica (Suppl.) 27(15):7-35, 1972.

1009

FEJFAR, Z., ET AL.
  Ischemic heart disease, Prognosis, therapy, rehabilitation and prevention.
  Casopis Lekaru Ceskych 109:477-482, 1970.

1010

FEJFAR, Z., AND Z. PISA.
  Ischaemic heart disease prognosis, treatment, rehabilitation and prevention.
  Cor et Vasa 13(1):1-17, 1971.

1011
FELDER, O.
The functional test of the cardiorespiratory system as the basis for selected, professional rehabilitation.
Münchener Medizinische Wochenschrift 107:1247-1254, 1965.

1012
FELDMAN, D.J.
Rehabilitation of the cardiac patient.
Modern Treatment 5:931-941, 1968.

1013
FELLIN, R., D. FEDELE, G. BAGNARIOL, ET AL.
Treatment of primary hyperlipidemias with a tetrahydronaphthalene derivative.
Gazzetta Italiana di Cardiologia 2(6A):863-870, 1972.

1014
FELTON, J.S., AND H.R. VOSS.
Cardiopulmonary evaluation studies in an occupational health program.
Journal Occupational Medicine 14(7):552-555, 1972.

1015
FENZ, W.D., AND J.M. PLAPP.
Voluntary control of heart rate in a practitioner of yoga: Negative findings.
Perceptual Motor Skills 30:493-494, 1970.

1016
FERNANDEZ, F., AND J. LENEGRE.
Intracardial conduction disturbances. Tentative classification.
Archives des Maladies du Coeur et des Vaisseaux 65(12):1381-1388, 1972.

1017
FERRER, M.I., AND R.M. HARVEY.
Some hemodynamic aspects of cardiac arrhythmias in man: A clinicophysiologic correlation.
American Heart Journal 68(2):153-165, 1964.

1018
FILER, L.J., JR., L.A. BARNESS, R.B. GOLDBLOOM, ET AL.
Childhood diet and coronary heart disease.
Pediatrics 49(2):305-307, 1972.

1019
FILIPECKI, R.
Effect of propranolol on the ballistocardiographic curve in healthy subjects.
Polski Tygodnik Lekarski 27:1307, 1972.

1020
FINAGIN, L.K., V.F. ZATOKOVENKO, AND R.T. NOVIKOVA.
Influence of electric stimulation of the hypothalamus on catecholamine, phosphorated compound, and cholesterol levels.
In: Role of the hypothalamus and the limbic system of the brain in regulating vegetative functions, pp. 136-142. Kiev, Izdatelśtvo Kievskogo Universiteta, 1973.

1021
FINN, F., N. HICKEY, E.F. O'DOHERTY, AND R. MULCAHY.
   The psychological profiles of male and female patients with coronary heart disease.
   Irish Journal Medical Science, Seventh Series 2:339-341, 1969.

1022
FINN, F., R. MULCAHY, AND E.F. O'DOHERTY.
   The psychological assessment of patients with coronary heart disease.
   Irish Journal Medical Science, Sixth Series (489):399-404, 1966.

1023
FINNERTY, F.A., JR.
   Critical considerations in the treatment of arterial hypertension.
   Modern Concepts Cardiovascular Disease 42:37, 1973.

1024
FINNERTY, F.A., JR., E.C. MATTIE, AND F.A. FINNERTY, III.
   Hypertension in the inner city. I. Analysis of clinic dropouts.
   Circulation 47:73-75, 1973.

1025
FINNERTY, F.A., JR., L.W. SHAW, AND C.K. HIMMELSBACH.
   Hypertension in the inner city. II. Detection and follow-up.
   Circulation 47:76-78, 1973.

1026
FIORE, C.E., C. CATALIOTTI, AND G. TAMBURINO.
   High frequency paroxysmal tachycardia with mechanical hyperhemolysis.
   Haematologica 56(11):471-478, 1971.

1027
FISCH, C.
   Digitalis intoxication.
   Journal American Medical Association 216(11):1770-1773, 1971.

1028
FISCH, C.
   Relations of electrolyte disturbances to cardiac arrhythmias.
   Circulation 47:408-419, 1973.

1029
FISCH, C. AND S.B. KNOEBEL.
   Recognition and therapy of digitalis toxicity.
   Progress Cardiovascular Disease 12:71, 1970.

1030
FISCH, S.
   Status of propranolol.
   Journal American Medical Association 226:1009, 1973.

1031
FISCHER, H., AND R. MULLER.
   Results of qualitative and quantitative measurements of edema.
   Folia Angiologica 20(4-5):180-184, 1972.

1032
FISCHER, H.K., ET AL.
  Emotional factors in coronary occlusion. II. Time patterns and factors related to onset.
  Psychosomatics 5:280-291, 1964.

1033
FISH, P.J., ET AL.
  Arteriography using ultrasound.
  Lancet 1:1269, 1972.

1034
FISHER, M., D. NUTTER, AND R. SCHLANT.
  Hemodynamic evaluation of isometric exercise testing in cardiac patients.
  Circulation 43-44(Suppl. II):50, 1971.

1035
FISHER, M.L., D.O. NUTTER, W. JACOBS, AND R.C. SCHLANT.
  Haemodynamic responses to isometric exercise (handgrip) in patients with heart disease.
  British Heart Journal 35:422-432, 1973.

1036
FISHER, S.
  The cardiac work evaluation unit.
  Malattie Cardiovascolari 10(1-2):465-472, 1969.

1037
FISHER, S.
  Impact of physical disability on vocational activity: Work status following myocardial infarction.
  Scandinavian Journal Rehabilitation Medicine 2(2/3):65-70, 1970.

1038
FISHER, S.
  International survey on the psychological aspects of cardiac rehabilitation.
  Scandinavian Journal Rehabilitation Medicine 2(2/3):71-77, 1970.

1039
FISHER, S.H.
  The cardiac homemaker.
  Journal Rehabilitation 32:74, 1966.

1040
FISHMAN, N.H., L.H. EDMUNDS, J.C. HUTCHINSON, AND B.B. ROE.
  Five year experience with the Smeloff Cutter mitral prosthesis.
  Journal Thoracic Cardiovascular Surgery 62(3):345-356, 1971.

1041
FITZGIBBON, G.M., G.W. BURGGRAF, T.D. GROVES, AND P.O. PARKER.
  A double Master's two-step test: Clinical, angiographic, and hemodynamic correlations.
  Annals Internal Medicine 74:509, 1971.

1042
FITZPATRICK, G.F., L.G. HAMPSON, AND J.H. BURGESS.
  Bedside determination of left atrial pressure.
  Canadian Medical Association Journal 106(12):1293-1298, 1972.

1043
FLAMM, M.D., K.E. COHN, AND E.W. HANCOCK.
   Measurement of systemic cardiac output at rest and exercise in patients with atrial septal defect.
   American Journal Cardiology 23(2):258-265, 1969.

1044
FLANDROIS, R., ET AL.
   Evaluation tests of physical fitness and their use with cardiac patients.
   Malattie Cardiovascolari 9:269-284, 1968.

1045
FLEISCH, A.O.
   Spirometry with different concentrations of oxygen and during work in left heart insufficiency.
   Cardiologia 38(3): 172-182, 1961.

1046
FLEISCH, A.O.
   Clinical significance of bifid T waves in the electrocardiogram taken at rest and during stress.
   Cardiologia 44(3):177-186, 1964.

1047
FLEISCHMAN, A.I., B. GITTLEMAN, AND M.L. BIERENBAUM.
   Effect of a polyunsaturated diet upon adipose tissue fatty acids in young coronary males: A five year cohort study.
   Circulation 33-34(Suppl. III):10, 1966.

1048
FLEISCHMAN, A.I., T. HAYTON, AND M.L. BIERENBAUM.
   Serum lipids and certain dietary factors in young men with coronary heart disease.
   Journal American Dietetic Association 50(2):112-115, 1967.

1049
FLEISCHMANN, D., S. EFFERT, W. BLEIFELD, ET AL.
   Incidence and prognosis of intraventricular conduction disturbances in patients with chronic heart block and Adams Stokes syndrome.
   Klinische Wochenschrift 50(16):768-775, 1972.

1050
FLETCHER, G.F.
   Submaximal treadmill exercise evaluation in patients with symptoms of cardiovascular disease: an aid to rehabilitation and reemployment.
   Chest 63:153, 1973.

1051
FLETCHER, G.F., AND J.D. CANTWELL.
   Exercise in the management of coronary heart disease. A guide for the practicing physician.
   Springfield, Ill. Thomas, 1971.

1052
FLOOK, V., AND G.R. KELMAN.
   Submaximal exercise with increased inspiratory resistance to breathing.
   Journal Applied Physiology 35:379, 1973.

1053
FLOREY, C.D., H. McDONALD, W.E. MIALL, AND R.D.G. MILNER.
Serum lipids and their relation to blood glucose and cardiovascular measurements in a rural population of Jamaican adults.
Journal Chronic Diseases 26:85, 1973.

1054
FLORIN, A.A., J.P. HARKNESS, J.G. COLLINS, AND H. BURTON.
Heart screening in the Newark model cities area: a feasibility study.
American Journal Public Health 61:1130-1139, 1971.

1055
FLOWERS, N.C., AND L.G. HORAN.
Comparative surface potential patterns in obstructive and nonobstructive cardiomyopathy.
American Heart Journal 86:196, 1973.

1056
FLYNN, R.L., AND S.M. FOX, III.
A coronary care concept.
Proceedings New England Cardiovascular Society 24:24-26, 1966.

1057
FLYNN, R.L., AND S.M. FOX, III.
Coronary care units: Coronary care programs in the United States.
Israel Journal Medical Sciences 3:279, 1967.

1058
FOGELMAN, A.M., A.S. ABBASI, M.L. PEARCE, AND A.A. KATTUS.
Echocardiographic study of the abnormal motion of the posterior left ventricular wall during angina pectoris.
Circulation 46(5):905-913, 1972.

1059
FOGELSON, L.I.
Rehabilitation of patients who have suffered myocardial infarction.
Sovetskaya Meditsina 34(4):16-23, 1971.

1060
FOGELSON, L.I., ET AL.
Temporary loss of working capacity in myocardial infarction.
Kardiologiya 7:50-54, 1967.

1061
FOLKINS, C.H., S. LYNCH, AND M.M. GARDNER.
Psychological fitness as a function of physical fitness.
Archives Physical Medicine Rehabilitation 53(11):503, 1972.

1062
FOLLATH, F.
Venous pressure and heart minute volumes during work in coronary heart disease.
Cardiologia 48(4):366-368, 1966.

1063
FOLLE, L.E., J. DIGHIERO, I. SADI, D. POMMERENCK, AND R. ELENA.
Hemodynamic response to exercise after beta-adrenergic blockade in normal and labile hypertensive patients.
Cardiologia 55(2):105-113, 1970.

1064
FOLLI, G., G. BINAGHI, AND P. GIANI.
Aptitude to exercise in patients with previous myocardial infarction.
Acta Cardiologica (Bruxelles) 23:273-287, 1968.

1065
FOLLI, G., G. BINAGHI, P. GIANI, AND L. ONIDA.
The electrocardiogram during effort: technique and first results of a test with the cycloergometer.
Malattie Cardiovascolari 6:211, 1965.

1066
FOLSE, R.
Alterations in femoral blood flow and resistance during rhythmic exercise and sustained muscular contractions in patients with arteriosclerosis.
Surgery Gynecology Obstetrics 121(4):767-776, 1965.

1067
FONTANA, A., AND S. LUSENA.
A clinical study of the effect of creatinolfosfate in heart patients receiving digitalis treatment.
Minerva Medica 63(82):4470-4481, 1972.

1068
FONTENIER, G.
A sensitive, high impedance cardiac rhythm follower.
Medical Biological Engineering 10:175-178, 1972.

1069
FORESTI, A., G. SALA, E.M. BIANCHI, AND D. RIVA.
Evaluation of coronary insufficiency in patients affected by myocardial infarction.
Bollettino della Società Italiana di Cardiologia 14(6):969-975, 1969.

1070
FORMGREN, H.
Practolol in the treatment of tachyarrhythmias in patients with bronchial asthma.
American Heart Journal 84(5):710-712, 1972.

1071
FORNOL, F.G., AND J.A. KOHLER.
Frequency of myocardial infarction in preexisting hepatic diseases.
Münchener Medizinische Wochenschrift 115(3):72-75, 1973.

1072
FORRESTER, J.S., R.H. HELFANT, A. PASTERNAC, E.A. AMSTERDAM, A.S. MOST, H.G. KEMP, AND R. GORLIN.
Atrial pacing in coronary heart disease: Effect on hemodynamics, metabolism and coronary circulation.
American Journal Cardiology 27(3):237-243, 1971.

1073
FORTE, I., J.H. HAFKENSCHIEL, J.E. SCHMITTHENNER, H. NEAL, AND E.A. DAUGHERTY.
The role of exercise tests in the diagnosis of coronary artery insufficiency. Pulmonary and cardiac response to a treadmill work capacity test applicable to patients convalescing from acute myocardial infarction.
American Heart Journal 61(6):756-762, 1961.

1074
FORTUIN, N.J., AND G.C. FRIESINGER.
Exercise-induced S-T segment elevation: Clinical, electrocardiographic and arteriographic studies in twelve patients.
American Journal Medicine 49(4):459-464, 1970.

1075
FORTUIN, N.J., W.P. HOOD, JR., AND E. CRAIGE.
Evaluation of left ventricular function by echocardiography.
Circulation 46(1):26-35, 1972.

1076
FORWARD, E.
Patient evaluation with an audioelectromyogram monitor: the Muscle Whistler.
Physical Therapy 52:402, 1972.

1077
FOSTER, G.L., AND T.I. REEVES.
Cardiovascular response to exercise in patients with angina pectoris.
Circulation 24(4 Part 2):934-935, 1961.

1078
FOSTER, G.L., T.J. REEVES, AND J.H. MEADE, JR.
Hemodynamic responses to exercise in clinically normal middle-aged men and in those with angina pectoris.
Journal Clinical Investigation 43:1758-1768, 1964.

1079
FOSTER, S., AND K.G. ANDREOLI.
The postcoronary patients. Behavior following acute myocardial infarction.
American Journal Nursing 70:2344-2347, 1970.

1080
FOUCHARD, J., C. FOURNIER, J. FORMAN, ET AL.
Rupture of an aneurysm of the ventricle after myocardial infarction with formation of a false aneurysm compressing the right heart chambers.
Archives des Maladies du Coeur et des Vaisseaux 65(10):1251-1260, 1972.

1081
FOUCHÉ, S., AND J. DELAMARE.
Occupational adjustment of cardiac patients. Experience of the Ligue pour l'Adaptation du Diminué Physique au Travail (L.A.D.A.P.T.).
Gazette Médicale de France 72:3005-3023, 1965.

1082
FOX, A.C.
Regulation of myocardial function.
In: Plavšić, C. and M.M. Gertler, Eds. The first international biennial conference on cardiac rehabilitation, Dubrovnik, Yugoslavia, 1969.

1083
FOX, E.L., R.L. BARTELS, C.E. BILLINGS, D.K. MATHEWS, ET AL.
Intensity and distance interval training programs and changes in aerobic power.
Medicine Science Sports 5:18, 1972.

1084
FOX, E.L., D.K. MATHEWS, W.S. KAUFMAN, AND R.W. BOWERS.
The effects of football equipment on thermal balance and energy cost during exercise.
In: Balke, B., (Ed.) Physiological aspects of sports and physical fitness, pp. 41-44. The Athletic Institute, 1968.

1085
FOX, S.M., III.
Questions and Answers: Exercise and heart disease.
Journal American Medical Association 195:1161-1162, 1966.

1086
FOX, S.M., III.
Federal agencies and the clinical investigator. Fourth Bethesda Conference, American College Cardiology.
American Journal Cardiology 19:899-907, 1967.

1087
FOX, S.M., III.
Commentary on physical activity and the coronary circulation.
Canadian Medical Association Journal 96:860, 1967.

1088
FOX, S.M., III.
Policy and future of intensive coronary care.
In: Julian, D.G., and M.F. Oliver, Eds. Acute Myocardial Infarction, pp. 328-339. Baltimore, Williams and Wilkins, 1968.

1089
FOX, S.M., III.
The incidence, prevalence and death rates of cardiovascular disease; Some practical implications.
In: Hurst, J.W., and R.B. Logue, Eds. The Heart, Arteries, and Veins, (2nd ed.), pp. 567-570. New York, McGraw-Hill, 1969.

1090
FOX, S.M., III.
Epidemiological studies on physical activity and coronary heart disease.
Klinische Wochenschrift 49:1038-1039, 1971.

1091
FOX, S.M., III.
  Priorities in funding for heart disease programs.
  American Journal Cardiology 30:110, 1972.

1092
FOX, S.M., III.
  National cardiovascular disease program goals for 1976.
  American Journal Cardiology 30:709-710, 1972.

1093
FOX, S.M., III.
  Remarks on assuming the presidency, American College Cardiology.
  American Journal Cardiology 29:739, 1972.

1094
FOX, S.M., III.
  Relationship of activity habits to coronary heart disease.
  In: Naughton, J., and H.K. Hellerstein, Eds. Exercise testing and exercise training in coronary heart disease, pp. 3-21. New York, Academic Press, 1973.

1095
FOX, S.M.
  Graded exercise testing in the diagnosis of latent heart disease.
  Proceedings of the Midwest Regional Medical Symposium: Exercise and the Heart, pp. 43-49. University of Wisconsin, La Crosse, August 1973.

1096
FOX, S.M.
  Arteriosclerotic heart disease and its relationship to physical exercise.
  Proceedings of the Midwest Regional Medical Symposium: Exercise and the Heart, pp. 8-11. University of Wisconsin, La Crosse, August 1973.

1097
FOX, S.M.
  A national program for cardiovascular health.
  In: Vogel, J.H.K., Ed. Myocardial infarction: A new look at an old subject. Advances Cardiology, Vol. 9, pp. 212-219. Basel, Switzerland. S. Karger, 1973.

1098
FOX, S.M., AND J.K. COOPER.
  Legal aspects of allied health personnel in early coronary care.
  In: Corday, E., and H.J.C. Swan, Eds. Myocardial infarction, pp. 225-228. Baltimore, Williams and Wilkins, 1973.

1099
FOX, S.M., III, AND E. CORDAY.
  Early care for the acute coronary suspect. Sixth Bethesda Conference, American College Cardiology.
  American Journal Cardiology 23:603-618, 1969.

1100
FOX, S.M., III, ET AL.
Exercise and stress testing workshop report.
Journal South Carolina Medical Association 65(Suppl.):76, 1969.

1101
FOX, S.M., III, AND W.L. HASKELL.
Physical activity and health maintenance.
Journal Rehabilitation 32:89, 1966.

1102
FOX, S.M., III, AND W.L. HASKELL.
Population studies.
Canadian Medical Association Journal 96:806-811, 1967.

1103
FOX, S.M., AND W. L. HASKELL.
The excerise stress test: needs for standardization.
Proceedings, Fourth Asian-Pacific Congress of Cardiology, Tel-Aviv, Israel, September 1-7, 1968.

1104
FOX, S.M., III, AND W.L. HASKELL.
The detection of coronary heart disease as a challenge to the work physiologist.
In: Proceedings of the research conference on Applied Work Physiology, New York University, Medical Center, April 10-11, 1968, pp. 283-307.

1105
FOX, S.M., III, AND W.L. HASKELL.
Physical activity and the prevention of coronary heart disease.
Bulletin New York Academy Medicine 44:950, 1968.

1106
FOX, S.M., III, AND W.L. HASKELL.
The exercise stress test: Needs for standardization.
In: Eliakim, M. and H.N. Neufeld, Eds. Cardiology, current topics and progress, pp. 149-154. New York, Academic Press, 1969.

1107
FOX, S.M., III, S.N. JONES, AND R.J. GERSHEN.
Integration of early coronary care into existing rescue systems.
In: Corday, E., and H.J.C. Swan, Eds. Myocardial infarction, pp. 215-224. Baltimore, Md. Williams and Wilkins, 1973.

1108
FOX, S.M., III, AND J.P. NAUGHTON.
Physical activity and the prevention of coronary heart disease.
Preventive Medicine 1:92-120, 1972.

1109
FOX, S.M., III, J.P. NAUGHTON, AND P.A. GORMAN.
Physical activity and cardiovascular health. I. Potential for prevention of coronary heart disease and possible mechanisms. II. The exercise prescription: Intensity and duration. III. The exercise prescription: Frequency and type of activity.
Modern Concepts Cardiovascular Disease 41:17-30, 1972.

1110
FOX, S.M., III, J.P. NAUGHTON, AND W.L. HASKELL.
Physical activity and the prevention of coronary heart disease.
Annals Clinical Research 3(6):404-432, 1971.

1111
FOX, S.M., III, AND O. PAUL.
Physical activity and coronary heart disease. I.
American Journal Cardiology 23:298-303, 1969.

1112
FOX, S.M., III, AND J.S. SKINNER.
Physical activity and cardiovascular health.
American Journal Cardiology 14:731-746, 1964.

1113
FOX, S.M., III, AND J.S. SKINNER.
Some planning in the United States for further studies to define the relationship between physical activity and coronary heart disease.
In: Karvonen, M.J., and A.J. Barry, Eds. Physical activity and the heart. Springfield, Ill., Thomas, 1967.

1114
FOX, S.M., III, AND J.S. SKINNER.
On the relationship between bodily activity and coronary heart disease.
Verhandlungen der Deutschen Gesellschaft für Kreislaufforschung, 38:82-93, 1971.

1115
FOZZARD, H.
Computer handling of coronary care unit data.
Medical Clinics North America 57(1):143-154, 1973.

1116
FRADA, G.
Present orientation on the subject of recovery for work of heart disease patients.
Minerva Medica 56:4385-4391, 1965.

1117
FRANCISCIS, DE P., C. AUFIERO, G. CORSINI, ET AL.
Correlation between spleen and cardiac function.
Rassegna di Medicina Sperimentale 18(5):166-172, 1971.

1118
FRANK, C.W., ET AL.
Myocardial infarction in men: role of physical activity and smoking in incidence and mortality.
Journal American Medical Association 198:1241, 1968.

1119
FRANK, C.W., E. WEINBLATT, AND S. SHAPIRO.
Angina pectoris in men: prognostic significance of selected medical factors.
Circulation 47(3):509-517, 1973.

1120
FRANK. C.W., E. WEINBLATT, S. SHAPIRO, AND R.V. SAGER.
Physical inactivity as a lethal factor in myocardial infarction among men.
Circulation 34:1022-1033, 1966.

1121
FRANK, F.D., AND J. WEINTRAUB.
Job satisfaction and mortality from coronary heart disease: Critique of some of the research.
Journal Chronic Diseases 26:351, 1973.

1122
FRANK, K.A., S.S. HELLER, AND D.S. KORNFELD.
A survey of adjustment to cardiac surgery.
Archives Internal Medicine 130(5):735-738, 1972.

1123
FRANK, M.J., AND G.E. LEVINSON.
Measurement of myocardial contractility in man.
Clinical Research 12:182, 1964.

1124
FRANK, M.J., AND G.E. LEVINSON.
An index of the contractile state of the myocardium in man.
Journal Clinical Investigation 47:1615, 1968.

1125
FRANKEL, E.
Coronary disease and personality.
British Medical Journal 1:382-383, 1969.

1126
FRANKL, W.S., R.D. DEITZ, AND L. SOLOFF.
The Q-T ratio as a guide to the exercise test in the digitalized subject.
Diseases Chest 54(2):119-21, 1968.

1127
FRANKL, W.S., W.L. WINTERS, AND L.A. SOLOFF.
The effects of smoking on the cardiac output at rest and during exercise in patients with healed myocardial infarction.
Circulation 31:42-44, 1965.

1128
FRANKL, W.S., W.L. WINTERS, AND L.A. SOLOFF.
Cardiac output at rest and during exercise in patients with healed myocardial infarction.
American Journal Medical Sciences 249:676-681, 1965.

1129
FRANKLIN, M., M.V. O'REILLY, AND M.J. KRAUTHAMER.
    The bearing of collaterals on prognosis in ischaemic heart disease.
    Journal Irish College Physicians Surgeons 2(1):15-18, 1972.

1130
FRANKLIN, M.A.
    Patient education in diet therapy.
    Academy Medicine New Jersey, Bulletin 10(4):287-294, 1964.

1131
FRANTSEV, V.I., S.M. ARONOV, AND V.T. SELIVANENKO
    Regulation of the renal circulation in patients with congenital diseases of the heart and major
    vessels.
    Kardiologiya 11:69-75, 1971.

1132
FREDELL, C.H.
    Arterial surgery in the small hospital.
    Arizona Medicine 29(9):709-714, 1972.

1133
FREDMAN, J.T.
    Sexual capacities in the aging male.
    Geriatrics 16:37-43, 1961.

1134
FREDRICKSON, D.S.
    Mutants, hyperlipoproteinemia and coronary artery disease.
    British Medical Journal 2:187, 1971.

1135
FREDRICKSON, D.S., R.I. Levy, AND R.S. LEES.
    Fat transport in lipoproteins—an integrated approach to mechanisms and disorders.
    New England Journal Medicine 276:34-44, 94-103, 148-156, 215-225, 273-281, 1967.

1136
FREEMAN, D.J., AND M. MUCKERHEIDE.
    A practical method of recording electrocardiograms during the exercise.
    Vascular Diseases 4(3):150-158, 1967.

1137
FREEMAN, J.A., M. CORBIN, M. DUNN, AND W. GRAY.
    Correlation of single lead telemetric treadmill exercise testing with coronary angiography.
    Journal Electrocardiology (San Diego) 6:231, 1973.

1138
FREEMAN, Z.
    The present status of the exercise electrocardiogram.
    Medical Journal Australia 2:672-676, 1967.

1139
FREENY, P.C., T.T. SCHATTENBERG, G.K. DANIELSON, D.C. McGOON, AND B.H. GREEN-
BERG.
Ventricular septal defect and ventricular aneurysm secondary to acute myocardial infarction.
Report of four cases with successful surgical treatment.
Circulation 43:360-364, 1971.

1140
FREIS, E.D.
The treatment of hypertension. Why, when and how.
American Journal Medicine 52(5):664-671, 1972.

1141
FREIS, E.D.
Hypertension. A challenge in preventive cardiology.
Circulation 47(1):1-2, 1973.

1142
FREIS, E.D., AND M.C. KYLE.
Computer analysis of carotid and brachial pulse waves. Effects of age in normal subjects.
American Journal Cardiology 22:691-695, 1968.

1143
FRENCH, J.R.P., JR., AND R.D. CAPLAN.
Psychosocial factors in coronary heart disease.
Industrial Medicine Surgery 39(9):383-397, 1970.

1144
FRIC, J., L. MIHULOVA, Z. CERNOCHOVA, AND J. VYCICHL.
Physical activity and diet of persons threatened by myocardial infarction.
Rehabilitacia (Bratislava) 5:21, 1972.

1145
FRICK, M.H.
Significance of bradycardia in relation to physical training.
In: Karvonen, M.J., and A.J. Barry, Eds. Physical activity and the heart, pp. 33-41. Springfield,
Ill. Thomas, 1967.

1146
FRICK, M.H.
Coronary implications of hemodynamic changes caused by physical training.
American Journal Cardiology 22:417-425, 1968.

1147
FRICK, M.H.
Some aspects of fitness testing.
In: Eliakim, M., and H.N. Neufeld, Eds. Cardiology, current topics and progress, p. 155. New
York, Academic Press, 1969.

1148
FRICK, M.H.
The effect of physical training in manifest ischemic heart disease.
Circulation 40:433-435, 1969.

1149
FRICK, M.H.
The response of heart volume and ventricular functions to physical training in coronary heart disease.
Malattie Cardiovascolari 10(1-2):331-339, 1969.

1150
FRICK, M.H.
Testing of exercise tolerance in patients with coronary artery disease.
Scandinavian Journal Clinical Laboratory Investigation Suppl. 24(110):109, 1969.

1151
FRICK, M.H.
The effect of physical training in manifest ischemic heart disease.
Circulation 40:433-435, 1969.

1152
FRICK, M.H.
Effects of physical training in coronary heart disease.
Verhandlungen der Deutschen Gesellschaft für Kreislaufforschung 37:94, 1971.

1153
FRICK, M.H.
Management of angina pectoris by drugs.
Duodecim 88:1362, 1972.

1154
FRICK, M.H., AND M. KATILA.
Hemodynamic consequences of physical training after myocardial infarction.
Circulation 37(2):192-202, 1968.

1155
FRICK, M.H., AND M. KATILA.
The effect of physical exercise in patients with coronary diseases.
Zeitschrift für Kreislaufforschung 60(7):666, 1971.

1156
FRICK, M.H., M. KATILA, AND A.-L. SJÖGREN.
Cardiac function and physical training after myocardial infarction.
In: Larsen, O.A. and R.O. Malmborg, Eds. Coronary heart disease and physical fitness, pp. 43-47. Baltimore, University Park Press, 1971.

1157
FRICK, M.H., A. KONTTINEN, AND H.S.S. SARAJAS.
Effects of physical training on circulation at rest and during exercise.
American Journal Cardiology 12:142-147, 1963.

1158
FRICK, M.H., AND S. PUNSAR.
Physical fitness of patients with left to right shunts (anomaly).
In: Karvonen, M.J. and A.J. Barry, Eds. Physical activity and the heart, pp. 42-50. Springfield, Ill. Thomas, 1967.

1159
FRICK, M.H., AND T. SOMER.
Assessment of the effect of long-term dipyridamole in angina pectoris by atrial pacing and physical exercise.
Annals Clinical Research 3(3):143-149, 1971.

1160
FRICK, M.H., K. VIRTANEN, AND J. SAVELA.
Modification of digitalis induced electrocardiographic changes by propranolol and potassium.
Annals Clinical Research 4(4):213-218, 1972.

1161
FRIEDBERG, C.K.
Some comments and reflections on changing interests and new developments in angina pectoris.
Circulation 46(6):1037-1047, 1972.

1162
FRIEDBERG, C.K.
Angina pectoris.
American Heart Association Monograph 37:1035, 1972.

1163
FRIEDBERG, C.K.
Early diagnosis of coronary heart disease. Critical review.
In: Halonen, P. and A. Louhija, Eds. Early diagnosis of coronary heart disease, pp. 1-24. Basel, Switzerland. S. Karger, 1973.

1164
FRIEDBERG, C.K., ET AL.
The two-step exercise electrocardiogram: A double-blind evaluation of its use in the diagnosis of angina pectoris.
Circulation 26:1254, 1962.

1165
FRIEDBERG, H.D.
Atrial fibrillation and digitalis toxicity.
American Heart Journal 77:429, 1969.

1166
FRIEDMAN, E.H.
Personality types and coronary artery disease.
Journal American Medical Association 219:385, 1972.

1167
FRIEDMAN, E.H., AND H.K. HELLERSTEIN.
Occupational stress, law school hierarchy, and coronary artery disease in Cleveland attorneys.
Psychosomatic Medicine 30:72-86, 1968.

1168
FRIEDMAN, E.H., H.K. HELLERSTEIN, G.L. EASTWOOD, AND S.E. JONES.
Behavior patterns and serum cholesterol in two groups of normal males.
American Journal Medical Sciences 255:237-244, 269-271, 1968.

1169
FRIEDMAN, E.H., H.K. HELLERSTEIN, AND B.P. HSI.
Validation of behavior pattern A.
Circulation 43-44(Suppl. II):166, 1971.

1170
FRIEDMAN, E.H., AND H.K. HELLERSTEIN.
Influence of psychosocial factors on coronary risk and adaptation to a physical fitness evaluation program.
In: Naughton, J.P., H.K. Hellerstein, and I.C. Mohler, Eds. Exercise testing and exercise training in coronary heart disease, pp. 225-235. New York, Academic Press, 1973.

1171
FRIEDMAN, G.D., H.K. URY, A.L. KLATSKY, AND A.B. SIEGELAU.
Psychological questionnaire predictive of myocardial infarction.
Circulation 48(4):23, 1973.

1172
FRIEDMAN, L.D., E. GOLDBERGER, AND M.R. SCHOENFELD.
The long-term effect of dipyridamole on anginal pain.
Journal New Drugs 4(3):162-165, 1964.

1173
FRIEDMAN, M., A.E. BROWN, AND R.H. ROSENMAN.
Voice analysis test for detection of behavior pattern: Responses of normal men and coronary patients.
Journal American Medical Association 208(5):828-836, 1969.

1174
FRIEDMAN, M., AND R.H. ROSENMAN.
Association of specific overt behavior pattern with blood and cardiovascular findings.
Journal American Medical Association 169:1286-1296, 1959.

1175
FRIEDMAN, M., AND R.H. ROSENMAN.
Overt behavior patterns in coronary disease. Detection by a new psychophysiological procedure.
Journal American Medical Association 173:1320, 1966.

1176
FRIEDMAN, M., AND R.H. ROSENMAN.
Type A behavior pattern: Its association with coronary heart disease.
Annals Clinical Research 3(6):300-312, 1971.

1177
FRIEDMAN, M., AND R.H. ROSENMAN.
The prudent management of the coronary-prone individual.
Geriatrics 27(5):74-79, 1972.

1178
FRIEDMAN, M., AND H.N. UHLEY.
Management of coronary artery disease.
Postgraduate Medicine 42(3):155-164, 1967.

1179
FRIEDRICH, G., R. JAKOB, AND H.T. KOCH.
Myocardial infarction from the viewpoint of the hospital.
Zeitschrift für die Gesamte Innere Medizin und Ihre Grenzgebiete 26(1):11-18, 1971.

1180
FRIESEN, W.J., ET AL.
Effects of digoxin on the oxygen debt and the exercise electrocardiogram in normal subjects.
Canadian Medical Association Journal 97:960-64, 1967.

1181
FRIESINGER, G.C., R.O. BIERN, I. LIKAR, AND R.E. MASON
Exercise electrocardiography and vasoregulatory abnormalities.
American Journal Cardiology 30(7):733-740, 1972.

1182
FRITZ, P.J., M. FRANK, AND W.S. SIMMONS.
Effects of a cardiac glycoside on plasma phospholipid levels in man.
Research Communications Chemical Pathology Pharmacology 4(2):439-448, 1972.

1183
FROELICHER, V.F., AND A. OBERMAN.
Analysis of epidemiologic studies of physical inactivity as risk factor for coronary artery disease.
Progress Cardiovascular Diseases 15(1):41-65, 1972.

1184
FROELICHER, V.F., F.G. YANOWITZ, A.J. THOMPSON, AND M.C. LANCASTER.
The correlation of coronary angiography and the electrocardiographic response to maximal tread-mill testing in 76 asymptomatic men.
Circulation 48:597-604, 1973.

1185
FROHLICH, E.D., R.C. TARAZI, H.P. DUSTAN, AND I.H. PAGE.
Reduced resting cardiac output in compensated hypertensive heart disease.
Clinical Research 15(3):406, 1967.

1186
FROMENT, A., H. MILON, AND R. FROMENT.
Arterial hypertension in patients over sixty years of age.
Bordeaux Médical 4(6):1885-1893, 1971.

1187
FROMENT, R.
Occupational readjustment of cardiac patients. Introduction.
Gazette Médicale de France 72:2933-2934, 1965.

1188
FROST, H., H. MALINOWSKY, AND J. RUTENFRANZ.
Continuous radiotelemetric recording of precordial leads (after Wilson) in long term electro-cardiograms of radar control operators during working hours.
Internationales Archiv für Arbeitsmedizin 30:49, 1972.

1189
FROUFE, D.J., F. MALPARTIDA, AND A. ESTANDIA.
Indications for temporary pacemaker in acute myocardial infarction. Study of 100 consecutive cases.
Archivos del Instituto de Cardiologia de Mexico 42(5):726, 1972.

1190
FROYSAKER, T., K.V. HALL, E. SKAGSETH, AND L. EFSKIND.
Surgery in myocardial infarction.
Scandinavian Journal Thoracic Cardiovascular Surgery 6:159-163, 1972.

1191
FUCCELLA, L.M., AND P. IMHOF.
Experience with a new beta-receptor blocking agent (Trasicor) in the management of cardiac arrhythmias.
Pharmacologia Clinica 1(3):123-130, 1969.

1192
FUJINAMI, T., K. OKADO, K. SENDA, M. SUGIMURA, AND M. KISHIKAWA.
Experimental atherosclerosis with ascorbic acid deficiency.
Japanese Circulation Journal 35:1559-1565, 1971.

1193
FUJITA, Y.
Studies on the evaluation of cardiac function in patients with cardiovascular diseases. (I). Comparison of 3 and 10 minutes exercise loading with treadmill.
Japanese Circulation Journal 37(7):819-825, 1973.

1194
FUJITA, Y.
Studies on the evaluation of cardiac function in patients with cardiovascular diseases. (II). Multiple load test with treadmill.
Japanese Circulation Journal 37(7):821-838, 1973.

1195
FUNG, Y-C.
Mathematical representation of the mechanical properties of the heart muscle.
Journal Biomechanics 3:381-404, 1970.

1196
FUNKE, H.D.
The threshold regulated pacemaker—novel principle of electrical stimulation of the myocardium.
Zeitschrift für Kreislaufforschung 61:853, 1972.

1197
FURBERG, C.
Adrenergic beta-blockade and physical working capacity.
Acta Medica Scandinavica 182(1):119-127, 1967.

1198
FURBERG, C.
Effects of repeated work tests and adrenergic beta-blockade on electrocardiographic ST and T changes.
Acta Medica Scandinavica 183:153-161, 1968.

1199
FURBETTA, D.
  Reasons why subjects with heart disease quit their work.
  Cardiologia Pratica 21:155-163, 1970.

1200
FURMAN, R.H.
  Diet and coronary artery disease.
  Postgraduate Medicine 42(3):172-182, 1967.

1201
FURUYA, H., Y. KATSUMARO, M. KAZUTOSHI, Y. YOSHITADA, K. KAZUO, AND Y. KUNIO.
  The clinical evaluation of the exercise-test by the use of radioelectrocardiography.
  Japanese Heart Journal 4(1):81-91, 1963.

1202
GABOR, G., I. PORUBSZKY, AND P. KALMAN.
  Determination of systolic time intervals using the apex cardiogram and its first derivative.
  American Journal Cardiology 30(3):217-221, 1972.

1203
GADERMANN, E., H. JUNGMANN, AND G. STEIN.
  Use of cold in the early rehabilitation of infarct patients.
  Zeitschrift für Kreislaufforschung 60:676, 1971.

1204
GADZHIEV, S.A., AND A.Y. RYVKIN.
  The use of functional tests in clinical phonocardiography of cardiac failure.
  Kardiologiya 11(1):23-30, 1971.

1205
GALAZKA, A., Z. CHECINSKA, AND D. SILBER.
  A case of pulseless disease of lupous artiology.
  Polski Tygodnik Lekarski 27(34):1320-1321, 1972.

1206
GALBRAITH, A., AND F.T. HATCH.
  A system of proportioned fat diets for clinical use.
  American Journal Clinical Nutrition 16(6):480-491, 1965.

1207
GALEA, E.G.
  Delayed convalescence after initial cardiac infarction.
  Medical Journal Australia 53:238-239, 1966.

1208
GALLAGHER, J.J., A.N. DAMATO, S.H. LAU, ET AL.
  Antecubital vein approach for recording His bundle activity in man.
  American Heart Journal 85:199, 1973.

1209
GALLAGHER, P.J., AND G.A. GRESHAM.
  Heart block with infected cardiac rheumatoid arthritis.
  British Heart Journal 35(1):110-112, 1973.

1210

GAMBOA, R., J.D. KLINGEMAN, AND H.V. PIPBERGER.
Computer diagnosis of biventricular hypertrophy from the orthogonal electrocardiogram.
Circulation 39:72-82, 1969.

1211

GANASSI, M.
Motor reeducation of the patient with vascular hemiplegia and cardiac insufficiency.
Europa Medicophysica 7(4):195-198, 1971.

1212

GANDJOUR, A., J. STOERMER, AND C. SCHMIDT'
Vectorcardiographic findings in idiopathic hypertrophic subaortic stenosis.
Zeitschrift für Kreislaufforschung 61(10):918-933, 1972.

1213

GANELINA, I.E., R.D. DIBNER, V.F. LUTKOV, L.I. KARPENKO, L.I. ROZENBERG, T.A. STENA-
NOVA, V.V. VEDERNIKOV, AND A.S. PROKOPENKO.
Physical rehabilitation of patients in the acute period of myocardial infarction. Part I. An
experiment using a 3-week program for rehabilitation of patients during the acute period of
myocardial infarction.
Kardiologiya 12:18, 1972.

1214

GANELINA, I.E., S.I. KALYAEVA, B. LUKACHEV, M. SEMENOV, Y.L. SEGAL, AND A.S.
PROKOPENKO.
Physical rehabilitation of patients in acute period of myocardial infarction. Part II.
Kardiologiya 12:20, 1972.

1215

GANELINA, I.E., AND Y.M. KRAEVSKY.
Premorbid personality peculiarities in patients with cardiac ischemia.
Kardiologiya 11(2):40-45, 1971.

1216

GANELINA, I.E., AND K.K. RESSER.
Arrhythmic collapse (shock) in acute myocardial infarction.
Kardiologiya 12:16, 1972.

1217

GANTEN, D., U. GANTEN, P. GRANGER, ET AL.
Renin in heart muscle and arterial tissue.
Verhandlungen der Deutschen Gesellschaft für Kreislaufforschung 38:268-272, 1972.

1218

GANZ, W., AND H.S. MARCUS.
Failure of intracoronary nitroglycerin to alleviate pacing induced angina.
Circulation 46(5):880-889, 1972.

1219

GARCÍA-PALMIERI, M., R. COSTAS, JR., M. CRUZ-VIDAL, M. CORTES-ALICEA, A.A. COLÓN,
M. FELIBERTI, A.M. AYALA, D. PATTERNE, R. SOBRINO, R. TORRES, AND E. NAZARIO.
Risk factors and prevalence of coronary heart disease in Puerto Rico.
Circulation 42(3):541-549, 1970.

1220
GARCÍA-PALMIERI, M.R., R. COSTAS, JR., J. SCHIFFMAN, A.A. COLÓN, R. TORRES, AND E. NAZARIO.
Interrelationship of serum lipids with relative weight, blood glucose, and physical activity.
Circulation 45:829-836, 1972.

1221
GARELLO, L., F.M. CHIOSSI, AND D. RIBALDONE.
A case of chickenpox myocarditis.
Gaslini 3(1):26-30, 1971.

1222
GARFINKEL, H.J., AND R.G. O'DRISCOLL.
Control of paroxysmal ventricular tachycardia with oral contraceptives.
Chest 64:379, 1973.

1223
GARRETT, H.L., R.V. PRANGLE, AND G.V. MANN.
Physical conditioning and coronary risk factors.
Journal Chronic Diseases 19:899, 1966.

1224
GARRISON, G.E., AND W.H. GULLEN.
Postexercise electrocardiograms, coronary heart disease, and airline pilots.
Aerospace Medicine 43(1):86-91, 1972.

1225
GARRITY, T.F.
Social involvement and activeness as predictors of morale six months after first myocardial infarction.
Social Science Medicine 7:199-207, 1973.

1226
GARRITY, T.F.
Vocational adjustment after first myocardial infarction; comparative assessment of several variables suggested in the literature.
Social Science Medicine 7(9):705, 1973.

1227
GARRITY, T.F., AND R.F. KLEIN.
A behavioral predictor of survival among heart attack patients.
In: Palmore, D. and F.C. Jeffers, Eds. Prediction of life span, recent finding, pp. 215-222. Lexington, Mass., Heath, 1971.

1228
GASPARY, F., AND A.J. GUIMPEL.
Severe hypoglycemia associated with an intrauricular rhabdomyosarcoma.
Malattie Cardiovascolari 10(3):605-615, 1969.

1229
GATTHEINER, V.
Long range strenuous sports training for cardiac reconditioning and rehabilitation.
American Journal Cardiology 22:426-435, 1968.

1230
GAU, G.T.
  Coronary artery disease.
  Minnesota Medicine 56:968, 1973.

1231
GAVRILESCU, S., S. COTOI, AND T. POP.
  Hemodynamic monitoring methods for patients with critical states of the cardiovascular system.
  Viața Medicală 19:885, 1972.

1232
GAVRILESCU, S., AND T. POP.
  The utility of beta-adrenergic stimulating medication in the therapy of chronic atrioventricular block.
  Viața Medicală 19(22):1021-1024, 1972.

1233
GAVRILESCU, S., AND C. STREIAN.
  Action of lanatoside C during the acute stage of myocardial infarction. Hemodynamic study of 14 patients with sinus rhythm.
  Revue Roumaine de Médecine Interne 9:271, 1972.

1234
GAZES, P.C.
  Treatment of acute myocardial infarction. 2. Ventricular ectopic arrhythmias.
  Postgraduate Medicine 48(1):168-172, 1970.

1235
GAZES, P.C.
  The diagnosis of angina pectoris.
  Postgraduate Medicine 47(4):176-179, 1970.

1236
GAZETOPOULOS, N., AND H. DAVIES.
  Ventilatory response to exercise in patients with left-to-right shunts.
  British Heart Journal 28(5):590-598, 1966.

1237
GEARY, F.J., M.J. SCHWARTZ, AND A.L.L. BELL.
  Postmyocardial infarction ventricular aneurysm septal tear syndrome.
  Chest 60(6):583-586, 1971.

1238
GEDDES, J.S., A.A.J. ADGEY, AND J.F. PANTRIDGE.
  Prognosis after recovery from ventricular fibrillation complicating ischemic heart-disease.
  Lancet 2:273-275, 1967.

1239
GEDDES, L.A.
  Electrical ventricular defibrillation.
  Cardiovascular Research Center Bulletin 10(1):3-42, 1971.

1240

GEDDES, L.A., AND L.E. BAKER.
Thoracic impedance changes following saline injection into right and left ventricles.
Journal Applied Physiology 33(2):278-281, 1972.

1241

GEISMAR, P., F. IVERSEN, J. MOSBECH, AND K. DEYER.
Long-term survival after myocardial infarction. A national follow-up study on 642 patients in Denmark.
International Journal Epidemiology 2:257, 1973.

1242

GEISSLER, W.
Rehabilitation of patients following heart surgery.
Zeitschrift für Aerztliche Fortbildung 59:833-835, 1965.

1243

GEIVERS, H., J.M. VAN NUETEN, AND W. SCHAPER.
The measurement of the refractory period of heart muscle by programmed and automated paired-pulse stimulation.
Medical Biological Engineering 10:193-199, 1972.

1244

GEIZEROVA, H., D. GRAFNETTER, AND G. TIBBLIN.
Prevalence of ischemic heart disease in men in the sixth decade in Prague and Gothenburg.
Casopis Lekaru Ceckych 111(51):1195-1200, 1972.

1245

GELERNTER, H.L., J.C. SWIHART, AND M.A.K. ANGELL.
The use of a mathematical model in the study of the properties of the full-surface electro-cardiogram. I. Scher generators in a homogeneous torso. II. "Enlarged heart" potentials.
Annals New York Academy Sciences 128:1069-1084, 1966.

1246

GELFAND, D.
The diagnosis of coronary heart disease.
Journal Rehabilitation 32:26, 1966.

1247

GELFAND, D., J.E. ACKER, JR., AND H.K. HELLERSTEIN.
Rehabilitation of patients with cardiovascular disease other than stroke—community service.
In: Andrus, E.C., Ed. The heart and circulation: Second annual conference on cardiovascular disease, pp. 820-826. Washington, D.C. Federation American Societies for Experimental Biology, 1965.

1248

GENDA, A., H.YAMAGUCHI, T. WATANABE, Z. ISHIMI, T. NAKAYAMA, K. HARADA, AND M. YOSHIDA.
Studies on serum enzyme alterations in acute myocardial infarction with special reference to LDH and CPK isoenzyme patterns.
Japanese Circulation Journal 37(8):905-906, 1973.

1249
GENSINI, G.G., AND A.E. KELLY.
Incidence and progression of coronary artery disease. An angiographic correlation in 1,263 patients.
Archives Internal Medicine 129(5):814-827, 1972.

1250
GENTRY, W.D., S. FOSTER, AND T. HANEY.
Denial as a determinant of anxiety and perceived health status in the coronary care unit.
Psychosomatic Medicine 34(1):39-44, 1972.

1251
GEORGE, C.F., M.E. CONOLLY, T. FENYVESI, ET AL.
Intravenously administered isoproterenol sulfate, dose response curves in man.
Archives Internal Medicine 130(3):361-364, 1972.

1252
GERAMI, S., B.J. MESSMER, G.L. HALLMAN, AND D.A. COOLEY.
Open mitral commissurotomy. Results of 100 consecutive cases.
Journal Thoracic Cardiovascular Surgery 62(3):366-370, 1971.

1253
GERASIMENKO, YU. A.
Significance of health resort treatment in rehabilitation of patients with hypertensive disease.
Vrachebnoe Delo 2:22-24, 1971.

1254
GERASIMENKO, IU. A., ET AL.
The role of sanatorium treatment in the rehabilitation of cardiovascular patients.
Voprosy Kurortologii Fizioterapii i Lechebnoi Fizicheskoi Kul'tury 35:7-10, 1970.

1255
GERO, S., L. KELLER, AND D. RETSAGY.
Catamnesis in patients who have sustained myocardial infarction.
Kardiologiya 12(2):20-23, 1972.

1256
GERSH, B.J., C. PRYS ROBERTS, S.R. REUBEN, AND D.L. SCHULTZ.
The effects of halothane on the interactions between myocardial contractility, aortic impedance and left ventricular perfoimance. II. Aortic input impedance, and the distribution of energy during ventricular ejection.
British Journal Anesthesia 44(8):767-775, 1972.

1257
GERSHBERG, A.L.
On the fate and rehabilitation in myocardial infarction.
Terapevticheskii Arkhiv 37:94-96, 1965.

1258
GERSHBERG, A.L.
The prognosis of myocardial infarction in lesions of the interventricular septum of the heart.
Kardiologiya 12(11):61-64, 1972.

1259
GERTLER, M.M.
   Differences in efficiency of energy transfer in mitochondrial systems derived from normal and failing hearts.
   Proceedings Society Experimental Biology Medicine 106:109-112, 1961.

1260
GERTLER, M.M.
   Ischemic heart disease, heredity and body build as affected by exercise.
   Canadian Medical Association Journal 96:728-730, 1967.

1261
GERTLER, M.M.
   Physical activity and aging.
   Medicine Sport 4:89-91, 1970.

1262
GERTLER, M.M., L.D. CADY, H.H. WHITER, AND P.D. WHITE.
   Profile of the coronary prone person.
   Modern Medicine 33(5):95, 1965.

1263
GERTLER, M.M., AND H.E. LEETMA.
   Risk factors of ischemic heart and cerebrovascular disease in the United States.
   In: Plavśić, C. and M.M. Gertler, Eds. The first international biennial conference on cardiac rehabilitation, Dubrovnik, Ygoslavia, 1969.

1264
GERTLER, M.M., AND H.E. LEETMA.
   Biochemical adaptation in the heart, secondary to physical effort.
   In: Naughton, J.P., H.K. Hellerstein, and I.C. Mohler, Eds. Exercise testing and exercise training in coronary heart disease, pp. 199-209. New York, Academic Press, 1973.

1265
GERTLER, M.M., H.E. LEETMA, H.A. RUSK, D.A. COVALT, E. SALUSTE, AND J. ROSEN-BERGER.
   Profile of covert ischemic heart and ischemic thrombotic cerebrovascular diseases.
   New York State Journal Medicine 69:2664-2666, 1969.

1266
GERTLER, M.M., H.E. LEETMA, E. SALUSTE, D.A. COVALT, AND J. ROSENBERGER.
   Specificity of risk factors in ischemic cerebrovascular disease.
   Circulation 40(Suppl. III):87, 1969.

1267
GERTLER, M.M., H.E. LEETMA, E. SALUSTE, AND J. ROSENBERGER.
   Coagulability and lipid correlations in ischemic heart disease (IHD), ischemic thrombotic cerebro-vascular disease (ITCVD), and control subjects.
   Circulation 40(Suppl. III):9, 1969.

1268
GERTLER, M.M., H.E. LEETMA, E. SALUSTE, AND J. ROSENBERGER.
   Free fatty acid (FFA) response in ischemic thrombotic cerebrovascular (ITCVD) and heart diseases (IHD).
   Circulation 41(Suppl. III):119, 1970.

1269
GERTLER, M.M., H.E. LEETMA, E. SALUSTE, J.J. WELSH, H.A. RUSK, D.A. COVALT, AND J. ROSENBERGER.
Carbohydrate, insulin, and lipid interrelationship in ischemic vascular disease.
Geriatrics 25:134-148, 1970.

1270
GERTLER, M.M., M. PLECHATY, AND R.G. GUTHRIE.
Differences in ADP and ATP in mitochondria derived from failing hearts.
Federation Proceedings 24:147, 1965.

1271
GERTLER, M.M., M. PLECHATY, AND R.G. GUTHRIE.
Differences in levels of ATP and ADP in normal and failing guinea pig heart mitochondria.
Physiologist 8:172, 1965.

1272
GERTLER, M.M., M. PLECHATY, AND R.G. GUTHRIE.
The effect of digitalis on the level of ATP in mitochondria derived from failing hearts.
Federation Proceedings 25:2560, 1966.

1273
GERTLER, M.M., AND H.A. RUSK.
Rehabilitation principles in congestive heart failure.
American Heart Association Monograph 1 (Edition 2), pp. 116-120, 1966.

1274
GERTLER, M.M., H.A. RUSK, H.H. WHITER, H.E. LEETMA, AND M. EHRENKRANZ.
Ischemic cerebrovascular disease. The assessment of risk factors.
Geriatrics 23:135-141, 1968.

1275
GERTLER, M.M., AND E. SALUSTE.
The treatment of refractory congestive heart failure with 3′,5′-adenosine monophosphate.
In: Sixth World Congress of Cardiology, London. Abstracts of Papers G-147, September 1970.

1276
GERTLER, M.M., E. SALUSTE, AND F. SPENCER.
Biochemical determinations and inferences of human papillary muscles biopsies.
Federation Proceedings 28:1089, 1969.

1277
GERTLER, M.M., E. SALUSTE, AND F. SPENCER.
Biochemical analyses of human papillary muscles and guinea pig ventricles in failure.
Proceedings Society Experimental Biology Medicine 135:817-824, 1970.

1278
GERTLER, M.M., E. SALUSTE, F. SPENCER, AND R. GUTHRIE.
3′,5′-Cyclic AMP (CAMP) influences in congestive heart failure (CHF).
Circulation 40(Suppl. III):87, 1969.

1279
GERTLER, M.M., J.J. WELSH, AND H.H. WHITER.
Early diagnosis of coronary disease and stroke. Early recognition and prevention.
New York State Journal Medicine 66:2765-2771, 1966.

1280
GERTLER, M.M., P.D. WHITE, L.D. CADY, AND H.H. WHITER.
Coronary heart disease—A prospective study.
American Journal Medical Sciences 248:377-398, 1964.

1281
GERTLER, M.M., P.D. WHITE, R. SIMON, AND L.G. GOTTSCH.
Long-term follow-up study of young coronary patients.
American Journal Medical Sciences 247:145-155, 1964.

1282
GERTLER, M.M., AND H.H. WHITER.
Does hypertension truly increase the risk rate of ischemic heart disease^
Circulation 32(Suppl. II):95-96, 1965.

1283
GERTLER, M.M., AND H.H. WHITER.
Individual differences relating to coronary artery disease.
Annals New York Academy Sciences 134:1041-1045, 1966.

1284
GERTLER, M.M., AND H.H. WHITER.
Development of a profile of the coronary prone individual.
Journal American Statistical Association. First annual proceedings on simulation in business and public health, pp. 211-216, 1966.

1285
GERTLER, M.M., AND H.H. WHITER.
Early recognition of covert ischemic heart disease.
In: Raab, W., Ed. Prevention of ischemic heart disease: Principles and practices, pp. 179-185. Springfield, Ill. Thomas, 1966.

1286
GERTLER, M.M., H.H. WHITER, AND S.P. CHAN.
Enzymatic differences in most prone and least prone coronary candidates.
Circulation 34(Suppl. III):11, 1966.

1287
GERTLER, M.M., H.H. WHITER, AND J.J. WELSH.
Assessing the coronary profile.
Geriatrics 2:121-132, 1967.

1288
GESER, H., AND E. ZBINDEN.
Some socio-psychological correlates of high blood pressure in a factory.
Zeitschrift für Praeventiv Medizin 15(4):303-317, 1970.

1289
GETTES, L.S., AND B. SURAWICZ.
   Propranolol: its use in the long-term management of life-threatening arrhythmias and its effect on
   the electrocardiogram.
   Circulation 33(Suppl. III):109-110, 1966.

1290
GETTES, L.S., AND B. SURAWICZ.
   Analysis of paroxysmal life-threatening arrhythmias controlled by long term beta-adrenergic
   blockade: indications for prolonged oral propranolol therapy.
   American Journal Cardiology 19(1):130, 1967.

1291
GEY, G., G. PETTET, AND R.A. BRUCE.
   Prevalence, repeatability and relationship to future cardiovascular events of exertional arrhythmias
   in middle-aged men.
   Clinical Research 20(2):205, 1972.

1292
GHOSE, J.C., K. SARKER, AND A. BANERJEE.
   Physiologic approach to the management of angina pectoris.
   Indian Medical Forum 23(7):261-265, 1972.

1293
GIALLO, P. DEL, AND M. VALIENSI.
   Controlled clinical study of a coronaroactive drug (etafenone hydrochloride).
   Minerva Cardioangiologica 20:642, 1972.

1294
GIANELLY, R.E., B.L. TREISTER, AND D.C. HARRISON.
   The effect of propranolol on exercise-induced ischemic S-T segment depression.
   American Journal Cardiology 24(2):161-165, 1969.

1295
GIANI, P., G. BINAGHI, G. FOLLI, L. BANDERA, AND G. MORTARINO.
   The study of "coronary reserve" in clinical diagnosis.
   Malattie Cardiovascolari 9(1):51-67, 1968.

1296
GIANI, P., G. MORTARINO, L. BRUNO, L. BANDERA, G. BINAGHI, AND G. FOLLI.
   The effect of beta-blocking on the basic ECG, on the ECG of effort and of hyperventilation.
   Bollettino della Società Italiana di Cardiologia (Roma) 14(3):301-308, 1969.

1297
GIANNINI, S.D.
   Coronary risk factors.
   Arquivos Brasileiros de Cardiologia 23(5):345-352, 1970.

1298
GIARD, P.
   Readjustment of the patient with a myocardial infarct.
   Journal des Sciences Médicales de Lille 83:223-230, 1965.

1299
GIARDINA, E-G.V., AND J.T. BIGGER, JR.
   Procaine amide against re-entrant ventricular arrhythmias: lengthening R-V intervals of coupled ventricular premature depolarizations as an insight into the mechanism of action of procaine amide.
   Circulation 48:959, 1973.

1300
GIBBY, R.G., SR, R.G. GIBBY, JR., AND J.C. TOWNSEND.
   Effect of stress upon rate of change of heart-beat rate.
   Perceptual Motor Skills 29:463-466, 1969.

1301
GIBELLI, A., M. MORPURGO, P. GIAROLA, G. BEULCKE, M. CASACCIA, C. PETRINI, AND C. RAMPULLA.
   Comparative study of coagulation, fibrinolysis and cardiorespiratory function in elderly and young subjects after exercise.
   Journal American Geriatrics Society 20(2):59-62, 1972.

1302
GIBSON, T.C.
   Community health services in the management of congestive heart failure.
   Journal Chronic Diseases 19:133-140, 1966.

1303
GIEGLER, I.
   On the clinical significance of vectorcardiography in congenital heart defects. Studies on loading of the heart.
   Basic Research Cardiology 68:277, 1973.

1304
GIESE, W.K.
   Exercise programs: types, directions, and dangers.
   Journal South Carolina Medical Association (Suppl. 1) 65(12):34-37, 1969.

1305
GIESE, W.K.
   Starter Program (Exercise).
   Journal South Carolina Medical Association (Suppl. 1) 65(12):100-101, 1969.

1306
GIFFORD, R.W., JR., AND D.C. HUMPHREY.
   Drug management of the ambulatory patient with hypertension.
   In: Brest, A.N. and J.H. Moyer, Eds. Cardiovascular drug therapy: The eleventh Hahnemann symposium, pp. 52-65. New York, Grune and Stratton, 1965.

1307
GIKNIS, F.L., D.E. HOLT, H.W. WHITEMAN, M.D. SINGH, A. BENCHIMOL, AND E.G. DIMOND.
   Myocardial infarction in 20-year-old identical twins.
   In: Jokl, E., and J.T. McClellan, Eds., Medicine and Sport 5:159-165. Basel, Karger, 1971.

1308
GILBERT, R., AND J.H. AUCHINCLOSS, JR.
Cardiac function during exercise.
Heart Bulletin 14(1):6-8, 1965.

1309
GILBERT, R., AND J.H. AUCHINCLOSS, JR.
Cardiac and pulmonary function at the exercise breaking point in cardiac patients.
American Journal Medical Sciences 257:370-381, 1969.

1310
GILBERT, R., ET AL.
Exercise performance before and after conversion from atrial fibrillation to sinus rhythm.
Circulation 24(4 Part 2):939, 1961.

1311
GILBERSTADT, H., AND Y. SAKO.
Intellectual and personality changes following open-heart surgery.
Archives General Psychiatry 16(2):210-214, 1967.

1312
GILLIES, D.D., D.L. GRAHAM, R.A.G. HOLMES, F.A. POWELL, AND M. TARLINTO.
Myocardial infarction in Fiji.
Medical Journal Australia 2:1027, 1973.

1313
GILLMANN, H.
After care in heart infarct.
Deutsche Medizinische Wochenschrift 95:1083, 1970.

1314
GILSON, J.S.
Anticoagulants in infarction.
Journal American Medical Association 226:1010, 1973.

1315
GINN, W.M., R.W. SHERWIN, W.K. HARRISON, AND B.M. BAKER.
Apexcardiography: Use in coronary heart disease and reproducibility.
American Heart Journal 73(2):168-180, 1967.

1316
GISOLFI, C.V.
Work-heat tolerance derived from interval training.
Journal Applied Physiology 35:349, 1973.

1317
GJOL, N.
Cardiac rupture and acute myocardial infarction.
Geriatrics 27(11):126-137, 1972.

1318
GLAGOV, S., D.A. ROWLEY, D.B. CRAMER, AND R.G. PAGE.
Heart rates during 24 hours of usual activity for 100 normal men.
Journal Applied Physiology 29(6):799-805, 1970.

1319
GLANCY, D.L., L.M. HIGGS, K.P. O'BRIEN, AND S.E. EPSTEIN.
The effects of digitalis on left ventricular response to exercise in patients with angina.
Circulation 39-40(Suppl. III):89, 1969.

1320
GLANCY, D.L., M. HIGGS, K.P. O'BRIEN, AND S.E. EPSTEIN.
Effects of ouabain on the left ventricular response to exercise in patients with angina pectoris.
Circulation 43(1):45-47, 1971.

1321
GLANCY, D.L., PH. YARNELL, AND W.C. ROBERTS.
Traumatic left ventricular aneurysm.
In: Jokl, E. and J.T. McClellan, Eds. Medicine and Sport, 5:71-81. Basel, Karger, 1971.

1322
GLAZUNOV, I.S., ET AL.
Ischaemic heart disease and occupation.
Cor et Vasa 6:274-280, 1964.

1323
GLUECK, C.J., R. FALLAT, AND R. TSANG
Hyperlipidemia in progeny of parents with myocardial infarction before age 50.
Circulation 48(4):15, 1973.

1324
GLUECK, C.J., R. FALLAT, C.R. BUNCHER, R. TSANG, AND P. STEINER.
Familial combined hyperlipoproteinemia: Studies in 91 adults and 95 children from 33 kindreds.
Metabolism 22:1403, 1973.

1325
GOCH, J.H.
Polycardiographic evaluation of the circulatory system in obesity.
Wiadomosci Lekarskie 26(1):1-4, 1973.

1326
GOCH, J.H., AND H. ADAMSKA DYNIEWSKA.
Assessment of the effect of LB 46 on myocardial contractility by the polycardiographic method.
Polski Tygodnik Lekarski 27(25):946-948, 1972.

1327
GODDARD, R.F. (ED.)
The effects of altitude on physical performance.
The Athletic Institute, 1967.

1328
GOENEN, M., H. FERNANDEZ, AND L. BRASSEUR.
Value of the progressive exercise test in the electrocardiographic diagnosis of angina pectoris.
Acta Cardiologica (Bruxelles) 25:1-28, 1970.

1329
GOLD, H.K., R.C. LEINBACH, AND C.A. SANDERS.
Use of sublingual nitroglycerin in congestive failure following acute myocardial infarction.
Circulation 46(5):839-845, 1972.

1330
GOLD, W.M., L.F. MATTIOLI, AND A.C. PRICE.
  Response to exercise in patients with tetralogy of Fallot with systemic-pulmonary anastomoses.
  Pediatrics 43(5):781-793, 1969.

1331
GOLDBARG, A.N.
  Rehabilitation of the coronary patient.
  Medical Clinics North America 57:231, 1973.

1332
GOLDBARG, A.N.
  The effects of pharmacological agents on human performance.
  In: Naughton, J.P., H.K. Hellerstein, and I.C. Mohler, Eds. Exercise testing and exercise training
  in coronary heart disease, pp. 119-128. New York, Academic Press, 1973.

1333
GOLDBARG, A.N., J.F. MORAN, AND R.R. BLOUGH.
  Therapy of angina pectoris with propranolol and long acting nitrates.
  Circulation 39-40(Suppl. III):91, 1969.

1334
GOLDBARG, A.N., J.F. MORAN, AND L. RESNEKOV.
  Multistage electrocardiographic exercise tests: Principles and clinical applications.
  American Journal Cardiology 26(1):84-92, 1970.

1335
GOLDBERG, L.I., D. HORWITZ, AND A. SJOERDSMA.
  Attenuation of cardiovascular responses to exercise as a possible basis for effectiveness of
  monoamine oxidase inhibitors in angina pectoris.
  Journal Pharmacology Experimental Therapy 137(1):39-46, 1962.

1336
GOLDBERG, R.T., AND H.T. SPECTOR.
  Rehabilitation of patients after cardiac surgery. A follow-up study.
  Archives Physical Medicine Rehabilitation 46(5):374-377, 1965.

1337
GOLDBERG, S.J., F.H. ADAMS, AND R.A. HURWITZ.
  Effect of cardiac surgery on exercise performance.
  Journal Pediatrics 71(2):192-197, 1967.

1338
GOLDMAN, M.J., AND H.V. PIPBERGER.
  Analysis of the orthogonal electrocardiogram and vectorcardiogram in ventricular conduction
  defects with and without myocardial infarction.
  Circulation 39:243-250, 1969.

1339
GOLDREYER, B.N.
  Intracardiac electrocardiography in the analysis and understanding of cardiac arrhythmias.
  Annals Internal Medicine 77(1):117-136, 1972.

1340
GOLDSCHLAGER, N., F.J. SAKAI, K.E. COHN, AND A. SELZER.
Hemodynamic abnormalities in patients with coronary artery disease and their relationship to intermittent ischemic episodes.
American Heart Journal 80(5):610-618, 1970.

1341
GOLDSMITH, R.
Activity patterns and coronary heart disease: A hypothesis.
In: Larsen, O.A. and R.O. Malmborg, Eds. Coronary heart disease and physical fitness, pp. 235-239. Baltimore, University Park Press, 1971.

1342
GOLDSTEIN, J.L., W.R. HAZZARD, H.G. SCHROTT, E.L. BIERMAN, AND A.G. MOTULSKY.
Hyperlipidemia in coronary heart disease. I. Lipid levels in 500 survivors of myocardial infarction.
Journal Clinical Investigation 52:1533-1543, 1973.

1343
GOLDSTEIN, J.L., H.C. SCHROTT, W.R. HAZZARD, E.L. BIERMAN, AND A.G. MOTULSKY.
Hyperlipidemia in coronary heart disease. II. Genetic analysis of lipid levels in 176 families and delineation of a new inherited disorder, combined hyperlipidemia.
Journal Clinical Investigation 52:1544-1568, 1973.

1344
GOLDSTEIN, R.E., AND S.E. EPSTEIN.
Medical management of patients with angina pectoris.
Progress Cardiovascular Diseases 14(4):360-398, 1972.

1345
GOLDSTEIN, R.E., C.A. HALL, AND S.E. EPSTEIN.
Comparison of relative inotropic and chronotropic effects of propranolol, practolol and sotalol.
Chest 64:619, 1973.

1346
GOLDSTEIN, R.E., G.D. BEISER, D.R. REDWOOD, D.R. ROSING, M. STAMPFER, AND S.E. EPSTEIN.
Clinical and circulatory effects of isosorbide dinitrate (Isordil) during exercise in patients with angina pectoris.
Circulation 39-40(Suppl. III):92, 1969.

1347
GOLDSTEIN, R.E., D.R. REDWOOD, D.R. ROSING, G.D. BEISER, AND S.E. EPSTEIN.
Alterations in the circulatory response to exercise following a meal and their relationship to postprandial angina pectoris.
Circulation 44(1):90-100, 1971.

1348
GOLDSTEIN, R.E., D.R. ROSING, D.R. REDWOOD, G.D. BEISER, AND S.E. EPSTEIN.
Clinical and circulatory effects of isosorbide dinitrate: Comparison with nitroglycerin.
Circulation 43(5):629-640, 1971.

1349
GOLDSTEIN, S., A.J. MOSS, AND W. GREENE.
Sudden death in acute myocardial infarction. Relationship to factors affecting delay in hospitalization.
Archives Internal Medicine 129(5):720-724, 1972.

1350
GOLLNICK, P.D.
Energy production and lactic acid formation.
In: Balke, B. (Ed.). Physiological aspects of sports and physical fitness, p. 16. The Athletic Institute, 1968.

1351
GOLUBEV, I.S., E.A. GRIGORYAN, V.I. MAKOLKIN, AND N.N. NOVGORODSKAYA.
Remote results of mitral commissurotomy in patients with calcinosis of the mitral valve.
Sovetskaya Meditsina 35(12):76-80, 1972.

1352
GONIN, A., J.D. BERTHOU, J. DELAYE, ET AL.
Prinzmetal's angina pectoris: experience with fifteen cases. Results of coronary arteriography (12 cases) and surgical revascularization (10 cases).
Lyon Médical 228(17):413-420, 1972.

1353
GONZALEZ-LAVIN, L., AND R. ZAJTCHUCK.
Surgical considerations in the treatment of acute acquired ventricular septal defect.
Thorax 26:610-614, 1971.

1354
GOOCH, A.S.
Exercise testing for detecting changes in cardiac rhythm and conduction.
American Journal Cardiology 30(7):741-746, 1972.

1355
GOOCH, A.S., AND J.M. EVANS.
Extended applications of exercise electrocardiography.
Medical Annals District of Columbia 38(2):80-85, 1969.

1356
GOOCH, A.S., AND D. McCONNELL.
Analysis of transient arrhythmias and conduction disturbances occurring during submaximal treadmill exercise testing.
Progress Cardiovascular Diseases 13(3):293-307, 1970.

1357
GOODE, R.C., J. FIRSTBROOK, AND R.J. SHEPHARD.
Effects of exercise and a cholesterol-free diet on human serum lipids.
Canadian Journal Physiology Pharmacology 44:575, 1966.

1358
GOODMAN, A.H., J.A. ANGUS, R. EINSTEIN, AND L.B. COBBIN.
A device for measuring myocardial contractility.
Medical Biological Engineering 10:483-495, 1972.

1359
GORDON, E.E.
  The role of the physiatrist in the management of the cardiac patient.
  Archives Physical Medicine Rehabilitation 48:133-135, 1967.

1360
GORDON, T., AND W.B. KANNEL.
  Premature mortality from coronary heart disease.
  Journal American Medical Association 215:1617, 1971.

1361
GORDON, T., AND W.B. KANNEL.
  Predisposition to atherosclerosis in the head, heart and legs. The Framingham study.
  Journal American Medical Association 221(7):661-666, 1972.

1362
GORDON, T., AND W.B. KANNEL.
  Multiple contributors to coronary risk implications for screening and prevention.
  Journal Chronic Diseases 25(10):561-565, 1972.

1363
GORLICH, H.D.
  Life after myocardial infarction. 4. Psychological disturbances after myocardial infarction.
  Herz Kreislauf 5(12):532, 1973.

1364
GORLIN, R.
  Drug management of angina pectoris: Clinical approach.
  In: Brest, A.N. and J.H. Moyer, Eds. Cardiovascular drug therapy: The eleventh Hahnemann symposium, pp. 319-321. New York, Grune and Stratton, 1965.

1365
GORLIN, R., N. KRASNOW, H.J. LEVINE, AND J.V. MESSER.
  Effect of exercise on cardiac performance in human subjects with minimal heart disease.
  American Journal Cardiology 13(3):293-300, 1964.

1366
GORMAN, P.A., W.S. BYERS, AND R. HAIDER.
  Exercise electrocardiography.
  In: Naughton, J.P., H.K. Hellerstein, and I.C. Mohler, Eds. Exercise testing and exercise training in coronary heart disease, pp. 93-102, New York, Academic Press, 1973.

1367
GORMAN, P.A., AND J.M. EVANS.
  Computer analysis of the electrocardiogram: Evaluation of experience in a hospital heart station.
  American Heart Journal 80:515-521, 1970.

1368
GORMAN, P.A., AND J.M. EVANS.
  The effects of chewable isosorbide dinitrate in coronary insufficiency. A report on exercise electrocardiograms in 13 pateints.
  Medical Annals District of Columbia 40:235-238, 1971.

1369
GOTO, N.
Clinical pathophysiologic investigation on the effect of various coronary vasodilators on myocardial carbohydrate metabolism. I. Myocardial carbohydrate metabolism in various diseases in a resting state. II. The effect of various coronary vasodilators on myocardial carbohydrate metabolism in various diseases.
Japanese Circulation Journal 36(8):845-861, 1972.

1370
GOULD, L., M.K. GOSWAMI, C.V.R. REDDY, AND R.F. GOMPRECHT.
The cardiac effects of tea.
Journal Clinical Pharmacology 13:469, 1973.

1371
GOULD, L., C.V.R. REDDY, AND R.F. GOMPRECHT.
Evaluation of digitalis toxicity by salivary electrolytes.
New England Journal Medicine 286:47, 1972.

1372
GOULD, L., C.V.R. REDDY, AND R.F. GOMPRECHT.
Cardiac effects of Chamomile Tea.
Journal Clinical Pharmacology 13:475, 1973.

1373
GOULD, L., F. UMALI, AND R.F. GOMPRECHT.
The presystolic gallop in acute myocardial infarction.
Angiology 23(9):549-553, 1972.

1374
GOULD, L., K. VENKATARAMAN, M. GOSWAMI, AND R.F. GOMPRECHT.
Cardiac effects of two cigarettes.
Journal Clinical Pharmacology 13(2-3):76-82, 1973.

1375
GOULD, L., K. VENKATARAMAN, M. GOSWAMI, ET AL.
Right sided heart failure in aortic stenosis.
American Journal Cardiology 31(3):381-383, 1973.

1376
GOULD, L., M. ZAHIR, M. SHARIFF, R. DE GUIA, AND M. DI LIETO.
Alcoholic heart disease: The hemodynamic effects of digitalis on exercise.
Japanese Heart Journal 11(6):521-532, 1970.

1377
GOULD, L., M. ZAHIR, A. DE MARTINO, ET AL.
Hemodynamic effects of ethanol in patients with cardiac disease.
Quarterly Journal Studies on Alcohol 33:714-721, 1972.

1378
GRACE, W.J.
Mortality rate from acute myocardial infarction—what are we talking about?
American Journal Cardiology 20:301-303, 1967.

1379
GRACE, W.J.
   The management of acute myocardial infarction without complications.
   Geriatrics 27(5):114-119, 1972.

1380
GRACE, W.J., F.A. CHADBOURN, AND R.F. KENNEDY.
   The time of the first abnormal electrocardiogram in patients with acute myocardial infarction.
   Diseases Chest 56(3):251, 1969.

1381
GRACE, W.J., F.A. CHADBOURN, A. MANISCALCO, AND G. D'ONOFRIO.
   Mobile coronary care unit.
   Diseases Chest 56(3):250, 1969.

1382
GRACE, W.J., AND P.M. YARVOTE.
   Acute myocardial infarction: The course of the illness following discharge from the coronary care
   unit. A description of the intermediate coronary care unit.
   Chest 59(1):15-17, 1971.

1383
GRAETTINGER, J.S., R.A. CARLETON, AND J.J. MUENSTER.
   Circulatory consequences of changes in cardiac rhythm produced in patients by transthoracic
   direct current shock.
   Journal Clinical Investigation 43:2280-2302, 1964.

1384
GRAFF, H.
   Emotional aspects of weight loss in the cardiac patient.
   Pennsylvania Medicine 70:68, 1967.

1385
GRAMIAK, R., K.J. CHUNG, N. NANDA, AND J. MANNING.
   Echocardiographic diagnosis of transposition of the great vessels.
   Radiology 106(1):187-189, 1973.

1386
GRANATH, A., R. JONASSON, J. LINDAHL, AND G. MASCHER.
   Circulatory arrest in exercise tests.
   Lakartidningen 68(50):5831-5891, 1971.

1387
GRANDJEAN, E.
   Ergonomics.
   Revue Médicale Suisse Romande 92(3):201-210, 1972.

1388
GRANT, A., AND B.S. COHEN.
   Acute myocardial infarction: Effect of a rehabilitation program on length of hospitalization and
   functional status at discharge.
   Archives Physical Medicine Rehabilitation 54(5):201, 1973.

1389
GRANT, A.F., D. JONES, S.N. HUNYOR, AND D.M. COLES.
Implantation of permanent cardiac pacemakers.
Medical Journal Australia 2:257-261, 1973.

1390
GRANT, R.P., AND S.M. FOX, III.
Cardiovascular diseases (medical).
Annual Review Medicine 9:69-84, 1958.

1391
GRAY, R.M., ET AL.
Psychosocial factors involved in the rehabilitation of persons with cardiovascular diseases.
Rehabilitation Literature 30:354-359, 1969.

1392
GRAY, W., M. CORBIN, J. KING, AND M. DUNN.
Diagnostic value of vectorcardiogram in strictly posterior infarction.
British Heart Journal 34(11):1163-1169, 1972.

1393
GRAYBIEL, A.
Auricular fibrillation in an asymptomatic young man. Effects of exercise, digitalization, atropiniza-
tion, and the restoration of normal rhythm.
American Journal Cardiology 14(6):828-836, 1964.

1394
GRAYZEL, J., AND J. ANGELES.
Sino atrial block in man provoked by quinidine.
Journal Electrocardiology 5(3):289-294, 1972.

1395
GRAYZEL, J., J.R.F. PENIDO, S.G. EDELSTEIN, AND A.S. HARTWELL.
Pacemaker in a centenarian.
Journal American Medical Association 218(1):95-96, 1971.

1396
GREEN, G.E.
Intracoronary pressure and flow in impending myocardial infarction.
Journal Thoracic Cardiovascular Surgery 64(4):625-628, 1972.

1397
GREEN, J.R., L.J. KROVETZ, D.R. SHANKLIN, J.J. DE VITO, AND W.J. TAYLOR.
Sudden unexpected death in three generations.
In: Jokl, E. and J.T. McClellan, Eds., Medicine and Sport 5:166-175. Basel, Karger, 1971.

1398
GREEN, K.G.
Five years follow-up of multicentre trial of clofibrate (Atromid S) in patients with coronary heart
disease.
Prevent 1:77, 1973.

1399
GREENE, W.A., AND A.J. MOSS.
   Psychosocial factors in the adjustment of patients with permanently implanted cardiac pacemakers.
   Annals Internal Medicine 70(5):897-902, 1969.

1400
GREENE, W.A., S. GOLDSTEIN, AND A.J. MOSS.
   Psychosocial aspects of sudden death. A preliminary report.
   Archives Internal Medicine 129(5):725-731, 1972.

1401
GREENE, W.A., A.J. MOSS, S. GOLDSTEIN, A. LEVY, D.S. SCHALCH, AND R.F. KLEIN.
   Psychosocial, hormonal, and arrhythmia precursors of the early prehospital phase of myocardial infarction.
   Psychosomatic Medicine 34:474, 1972.

1402
GREENBERG, B.H., AND S.H. ANTIN.
   Conduction in atrial flutter after intravenous injection of aminophylline.
   Journal Electrocardiology 5(4):391-393, 1972.

1403
GREENBERG, B.H., B.D. McCALLISTER, AND R.L. FRYE.
   Hemodynamic effects of glucagon in patients with coronary artery disease at rest and during mild supine exercise.
   Clinical Research 17(2):243, 1969.

1404
GREENBERG, B.H., B.D. McCALLISTER, AND R.L. FRYE.
   Effects of glucagon on resting and exercise haemodynamics in patients with coronary heart disease.
   British Heart Journal 34(9):924-929, 1972.

1405
GREENBLATT, D.J., AND R.I. SHADER
   Psychopharmacologic management of anxiety in the cardiac patient.
   Psychiatry Medicine 2:55-66, 1971.

1406
GREENFIELD, J.C., JR., D.J. PATEL, G.O. BARNETT, AND S.M. FOX, III.
   Evaluation of the pressure time derivative method for estimating peak blood flow.
   American Heart Journal 64:101-105, 1962.

1407
GREENOUGH, K.
   Iatrogenic cardiac invalidism. Can the coronary care unit be responsible^
   Journal Rehabilitation 34:16-17, 1968.

1408
GREER, W.E.R.
   Rehabilitation and employment of industrial workers with cardiovascular disease.
   American Journal Cardiology 7:350-353, 1961.

1409
GRELLET, J.
   Complications of selective coronary angiography survey of 3,066 examinations.
   Journal de Radiologie et d' Electrologie 53(8-9):635-640, 1972.

1410
GRIEP, A.H.
   An approach to long-term therapy of ischemic heart disease.
   Vascular Diseases 1(6):299-302, 1964.

1411
GRIFFITH, G.C.
   Home care for the aged cardiac patient.
   Geriatrics 22:140-143, 1967.

1412
GRIGOROV, S.S., E. YU. ALEKSEEV, AND G.P. VLASOV.
   Puncture endocardial cardioversion in acute disorders of the cardiac rhythm.
   Kardiologiya 11:59-64, 1971.

1413
GRIMBY, G.
   Studies on exercise physiology as part of the human adaptability program.
   Nordisk Medicin 79(13):415-418, 1968.

1414
GRIMBY, G.
   The physiological background to physical training in cardiac patients.
   Progress Cardiology 2:281-290, 1973.

1415
GRIMBY, G., T. BJURÖ, AND E. HELANDER.
   Radio-transmitted ECG and measurements of energy expenditure during exercise therapy in
   patients with myocardial infarction.
   Malattie Cardiovascolari 10:143-151, 1969.

1416
GRIMBY, G., M. KORSGREN, AND N.J. NILSSON.
   Atrial flutter and maximal exercise: A case studied before and after conversion to sinus rhythm.
   Acta Medica Scandinavica 180(1):17-22, 1966.

1417
GRODEN, B.M.
   Return to work after myocardial infarction.
   Scottish Medical Journal 12(9):297-300, 1967.

1418
GRODEN, B.M.
   The management of myocardial infarction. A controlled study of the effects of early mobilization.
   Cardiac Rehabilitation 1:13-16, 1971.

1419
GRODEN, B.M., A. ALLISON, AND G.B. SHAW.
  Management of myocardial infarction. The effect of early mobilization.
  Scottish Medical Journal 12:435, 1967.

1420
GRODEN, B.M., AND R.I.F. BROWN.
  Differential psychological effects of early and late mobilisation after myocardial infarction.
  Scandinavian Journal Rehabilitation Medicine 2:60-64, 1970.

1421
GRODEN, B.M., AND A.I. CHEYNE.
  Rehabilitation after cardiac illness.
  British Medical Journal 2:700-703, 1972.

1422
GRODEN, B.M., T. SEMPLE, AND G.B. SHAW.
  Cardiac rehabilitation.
  British Heart Journal 33(4):425-427, 1971.

1423
GROEN, J.J.
  The influence of ethnic and psychosocial factors in the pathogenesis of atherosclerosis and
  coronary heart disease and their significance for therapy and prevention.
  Nederlands Tijdschrift voor Geneeskunde 111:1807-1820, 1967.

1424
GROEN, J.J., J.M. VAN DER VALK, A. WELNER, AND D. BEN-ISHAY.
  Psychobiological factors in the pathogenesis of essential hypertension.
  Psychotherapy Psychosomatics 19(1/2):1-26, 1971.

1425
GROOM, D.
  Cardiovascular observations on Tarahumara Indian runners—the modern Spartans.
  American Heart Journal 81:304-314, 1971.

1426
GROOVER, M.E., JR., AND C. STOUT.
  Physiochemical properties of blood in postmyocardial infarction patients and controls.
  Angiology 17(2):85-95, 1966.

1427
GROSS, D.
  The diagnostic significance of the length of the Q-T interval in the lead aVR in cases of angina
  pectoris.
  Experimental Medicine Surgery 24:45-54, 1966.

1428
GROSS, H.
  Rest and ambulation in myocardial infarction: evaluation of current therapy.
  New York State Journal Medicine 73:1778, 1973.

1429
GROSSE, H.
   Myocardial infarction after former gastrectomies.
   Zeitschrift für Gesamte Innere Medizin 27(15):666-668, 1972.

1430
GROSSMAN, K., I. GIEGLER, K. LEHMANN, ET AL.
   Myocardial infarction in Frank's corrected orthogonal ECG.
   Zeitschrift für Gesamte Innere Medizin 28(2):43-48, 1973.

1431
GROZA, P., AND V. BUZOIANU.
   Studies of the exercise electrocardiogram in relation to cardiac function.
   Revue Roumaine de Physiologie 7:281-289, 1970.

1432
GROZA, P., V. BUZOIANU, AND S. IONESCU.
   Aspects of the exercise electrocardiogram.
   Studii și Cercetari de Fiziologie 12:437-446, 1967.

1433
GRUNER, R.
   Rules for the assessment of industrial disability.
   Erfahrungsheilkunde 21(1):8-14, 1972.

1434
GRUPP, I.L., C.A. BUNDE, AND G. GRUPP.
   Effects of perhexiline maleate on exercise-induced tachycardia.
   Journal Clinical Pharmacology New Drugs 10(5):312-315, 1970.

1435
GUBERGRITS, A.YA., AND L.A. LESHCHINSKII.
   Combined use of Adonis vernalis L. with cardiac glycosides, strophanthidin derivatives, during the
   treatment of patients suffering from circulation insufficiency.
   Sovetskaya Meditsina 31(1):23-27, 1968.

1436
GUBNER, R.S.
   New developments in exercise electrocardiography and evaluation of chest pain.
   Transactions Association Life Insurance Medical Directors America 52:125-138, 1968.

1437
GUDBJARNASON, S.
   Acute alterations in energetics of ischemic heart muscle.
   Cardiologia 56(1-2):232-244, 1972.

1438
GUEST, M., AND D. CELANDER.
   Fibrinolytic activity in exercise.
   Physiologist 3:69, 1960.

1439
GUINEY, T.E., AND B. LOWN.
Electrical conversion of atrial flutter to atrial fibrillation. Flutter mechanism in man.
British Heart Journal 34(12):1215-1224, 1972.

1440
GUINEY, T.E., J.J. RUBENSTEIN, C.A. SANDERS, AND E.D. MUNDTH.
Functional evaluation of coronary bypass surgery by exercise testing and oxygen consumption.
Circulation 48(Suppl. III):141, 1973.

1441
GUJRAL, J.S., H.N. KHATTRI, P.S. BIDWAI, ET AL.
Closed mitral valvotomy in mitral stenosis with significant pulmonary hypertension.
Indian Heart Journal 24(1):40-42, 1972.

1442
GULOTTA, S.J., R.I. HAMBY, A.L. ARONSON, AND K. EWING.
Coexistent idiopathic hypertrophic subaortic stenosis and coronary arterial disease.
Circulation 46(5):890-896, 1972.

1443
GUNNING, J.F., G. COOPER, C.E. HARRISON, AND H.N. COLEMAN, III.
Myocardial oxygen consumption in experimental hypertrophy and congestive heart failure due to pressure overload.
American Journal Cardiology 32:427, 1973.

1444
GUNTHER, K.H.
The determination of cardiac function. Methods and criteria.
Deutsche Gesundheitwesen 28:97, 1973.

1445
GUPTA, P.P., R.C. SRIMAL, AND B.N. DHAWAN.
Central cardiovascular effects of 6-hydroxydopamine.
European Journal Pharmacology 20(2):215-223, 1972.

1446
GUREVICH, T.Z., N.I. OVODOVA, F.I. ZISMAN, V.E. LESINA, AND L.I. OSPINA.
Occupational prognosis after repeated myocardial infarction.
Klinicheskaya Meditsina 49(6):21-24, 1971.

1447
GURTNER, H.P.
Clinical findings in coronary disease.
Schweizerische Medizinische Wochenschrift 102(50):1824-1829, 1972.

1448
GUSTAFSON, A.
Effect of training on blood lipids.
In: Larsen, O.A. and R.O. Malmborg, Eds. Coronary heart disease and physical fitness, pp. 125-129. Baltimore, University Park Press, 1971.

1449
GUTIN, B.
Effect of increase in physical fitness on mental ability following physical mental stress.
Research Quarterly American Association Health, Physical Education, Recreation 37:211-220, 1966.

1450
GUTIN, B.
Exercise induced activation and human performance.
Research Quarterly 44:256, 1973.

1451
GUTMANN, J., AND J. KROTZ.
The accuracy of the strain gage method in measurement of venous capacity.
Folia Angiologica 20(3):103-107, 1972.

1452
GUZMAN, S.V.
The electrocardiogram during and after maximal exercise.
Acta Medica Philippina 6(Ser. 2, No. 2):63-66, 1969.

1453
GUZMAN, S.V.
Effects of propranolol on the ischemic T wave inversion after exercise in apparently healthy subjects.
Acta Medica Philippina 7(4):133-137, 1971.

1454
GVOZDOVA, L.G., ET AL.
Level of pyridozalic coenzymes in the plasma of patients with coronary atherosclerosis kept on a curative diet and after an additional intake of vitamin B_6.
Voprosy Pitaniya 25:40-44, 1966.

1455
GYNTELBERG, F.
Physical fitness and coronary heart disease in Copenhagen males aged 40-59. II.
Danish Medical Bulletin 20(4):105, 1973.

1456
GYULAI, F., AND Z. WALSH.
The $Q-A_2$ interval during exercise in assessing severity of aortic stenosis.
Acta Paediatrica Scandinavica 177(Suppl.):34-35, 1967.

1457
HAASIS R., VON, AND W. RÖSCH.
Auscultation phenomena in acute heart infarction.
Fortschritte der Medizin 24:897-899, 1971.

1458
HABER, L.D.
Disabling effects of chronic disease and impairment. II. Functional capacity limitations.
Journal Chronic Diseases 26:127-151, 1973.

1459
HACKETT, T., AND N.H. CASSEM.
Psychological effects of acute coronary care.
*In:*Meltzer, L.E. and A.J. Dunning, Ed. Textbook of coronary care, P. 443. Amsterdam, Netherlands. Excerpta Medica, 1972.

1460
HACKETT, T.P., AND N.H. CASSEM.
White vs. blue collar responses to having a heart attack.
Psychosomatic Medicine 34:475, 1972.

1461
HACKETT, T.P., AND N.H. CASSEM.
Psychological adaptation to convalescence in myocardial infarction patients.
In: Naughton, J., H.K. Hellerstein, and I.C. Mohler, Eds. Exercise testing and exercise training in coronary heart disease, pp. 253-262. New York, Academic Press, 1973.

1462
HADDEN, D.R., D. BOYLE, D.A.D. MONTGOMERY, AND J.A. WEAVER.
Risk factors for myocardial infarction in maturity—onset diabetes mellitus.
Practitioner 210(1259):655, 1973.

1463
HAENNI, B., AND J. CHATILLON.
Permanent cardiac pacemakers, a chapter of geriatric therapy.
Revue Médicale de la Suisse Romande 91:637, 1971.

1464
HAFT, J.I., K. GERSHENGORN, P.D. KRANZ, AND R. OESTREICHER.
Protection against epinephrine induced myocardial necrosis by drugs that inhibit platelet aggregation.
American Journal Cardiology 30(8):838-843, 1972.

1465
HAFT, J.L., P.D. KRANZ, F.J. ALBERT, AND K. FANI.
Intravascular platelet aggregation in the heart induced by norepinephrine. Microscopic studies.
Circulation 46(4):698-708, 1972.

1466
HAGAN, J.
Vocational counseling in heart disease.
Journal Rehabilitation 32:62, 1966.

1467
HAGAN, J.
The cardiac is not at the end of the line.
Industrial Medicine Surgery 35:653-657, 1966.

1468
HAGENFELDT, L., J. PAASIKIVI, AND A. SJÖGREN.
Plasma levels of free polyunsaturated fatty acids in patients with ischemic heart disease.
Metabolism 22:1349, 1973.

1469
HAGENFELDT, L., AND P.O. WESTER.
Plasma levels of individual free fatty acids in patients with acute myocardial infarction.
Acta Medica Scandinavica 194:357, 1973.

1470
HAGHFELT, T.
Acute myocardial infarction in the Copenhagen area in November 1968: Incidence and mortality.
Acta Medica Scandinavica 189(4):279-283, 1971.

1471
HAHN, A., ET AL.
The postcoronary patient. After coronary care—then what?
American Journal Nursing 60:2350-2352, 1970.

1472
HAHN, P.
Psychosomatic aspects of the infarct profile.
Psychotherapy Psychosomatics 16:224-232, 1968.

1473
HAHN, P., AND K.D. HULLEMANN.
Rehabilitation of patients with myocardial infarction by ambulatory group therapy. Good starts in psychodynamic treatment and remedial exercises.
Praxis der Psychotherapie 17(3):96-103, 1972.

1474
HAISTY, W.K., JR., C. BATCHLOR, J. CORNFIELD, AND H.V. PIPBERGER.
Discriminant function analysis of RR intervals: an algorithm for on line arrhythmia diagnosis.
Computers Biomedical Research 5(3):247-255, 1972.

1475
HAKKILA, J.
Coronary heart disease and rehabilitation.
Duodecim 86:370-373, 1970.

1476
HAKKILA, J., E.S. KENTALA, E.J. VALTONEN, AND K. PYÖRÄLÄ.
Control study of effects of early activation in acute myocardial infarction.
Circulation 43-44(Suppl. II):120, 1971.

1477
HALBERSTAM, M.J., J.S. HANSON, B. TABAKIN, AND A.B. SOULE.
Exercise chest x-rays in mitral stenosis.
Circulation 24(4 Part 2):949, 1961.

1478
HALBERSTAM, M.J.
The challenge to medicine—the solo physician's response.
Ohio State Medical Journal 65:459, 1969.

1479
HALBERSTAM, M.J.
   B(ureaucratic) block of propranolol.
   New England Journal Medicine 288:325, 1973.

1480
HALHUBER, M.
   Prevention and rehabilitation in hypertension.
   Wiener Klinische Wochenshrift 81(39):693-694, 1969.

1481
HALHUBER, M.J.
   Current problems of rehabilitation following myocardial infarct.
   Internist (Berlin) 12:233-236, 1971.

1482
HALHUBER, M.J.
   Rehabilitation after myocardial infarct.
   Bulletin der Schweizerischen Akademie der Medizinischen Wissenschaften 28:53-60, 1972.

1483
HALHUBER, M.J.
   Rehabilitation after myocardial infaraction.
   Deutsche Medizinische Wochenschrift 98:1570, 1973.

1484
HALHUBER, M.J., H. HOFMANN, H. KRAMM, AND M. SEUBERLING.
   Two years of early rehabilitation after myocardial infarction in the clinic Hoehenried West
   Germany. Part 1. Definitions and problems of follow-up treatment.
   Fortschritte der Medizin 91:108, 1973.

1485
HALHUBER, M.J., AND H. KIRCHMAIR.
   Cardiac emergency treatment in medical practice.
   Internist 11(2):64-69, 1970.

1486
HALKIN, H., AND E. KAPLINSKY.
   Simultaneous tachycardias associated with acute myocardial infarction.
   Chest 60(4):394-396, 1971.

1487
HALL, R.J.
   Heart disease in industry.
   American Academy Occupational Medicine 17:416-424, 1968.

1488
HALONEN, P., AND A. LOUHIJA.
   Early diagnosis of coronary heart disease: Proceedings of the Second Paavo Nurmi Symposium,
   Porvoo, Finland, September 9-11, 1971.
   Basel, Switzerland. S. Karger, 1973.

1489
HALLORAN, K.H.
  The telemetered exercise electrocardiogram in congenital aortic stenosis.
  Pediatrics 47(1 Part 1):31-39, 1971.

1490
HALLORAN, K.H., M.M. ITHURALDE, AND S.E. DOWNING.
  Relation between acute changes in pH and pCO_2 and inotropic responses to acetyl strophanthidin.
  American Journal Cardiology 30(1):61-66, 1972.

1491
HALPERN, J.W.
  Cardiac research at the heart station.
  Research News (University of Michigan, Ann Arbor, Mich.) 22(6): 1971.

1492
HAM, G.C.
  Psychosomatic perspectives. The cardiovascular system.
  Psychosomatic Medicine 24(1):31-35, 1962.

1493
HAMBY, R.I., M.P. GUPTA, AND M.W. YOUNG.
  Clinical and hemodynamic aspects of single vessel coronary artery disease.
  American Heart Journal 85(4):458-466, 1973.

1494
HAMER, J., J. FLEMING, AND E. SHINEBOURNE.
  Effect of walking on blood-pressure in systemic hypertension.
  Lancet 2:114-118, 1967.

1495
HAMER, J., T. GRANDJEAN, L. MELENDEZ, AND G.E. SOWTON.
  Effect of propranolol (Inderal) on exercise tolerance in angina pectoris.
  British Heart Journal 28(3):414-418, 1966.

1496
HAMER, J., AND E. SOWTON.
  Effects of propranolol on exercise tolerance in angina pectoris.
  American Journal Cardiology 18(3):354-358, 1966.

1497
HAMMER, J., J. FABIAN, J. PAVLOVIC, AND J. SMID.
  Myocardial rupture in acute myocardial infarction.
  Cor Vasa 14(3):180-187, 1972.

1498
HAMMERSEN, F.
  Capillary permeability in dextran edema.
  Pfluegers Archiv: European Journal Physiology 336(Suppl.):S90-S95, 1972.

1499
HAMMETT, V.B.O.
    Psychological changes with physical fitness training.
    Canadian Medical Association Journal 96:764-769, 1967.

1500
HAMMOND, E.
    Smoking in relation to mortality and morbidity. Findings in first thirty-four months of follow-up
    in a prospective study started in 1959.
    Journal National Cancer Institute 32:1161, 1964.

1501
HAMMOND, E.C., L. GARFINKEL, AND H. SEIDMAN.
    Longevity of parents and grandparents in relation to coronary heart disease and associated
    variables.
    Circulation 43(1):31-44, 1971.

1502
HAMPTON, J.R., AND R. GORLIN.
    Drugs for the prevention of myocardial infarction.
    American Journal Medical Sciences 258:1-6, 1969.

1503
HAN, J.
    Mechanisms of ventricular arrhythmias associated with myocardial infarction.
    American Journal Cardiology 24:800-813, 1969.

1504
HAN, J.
    Ventricular vulnerability during acute coronary occlusion.
    American Journal Cardiology 24:857-864, 1969.

1505
HAN, J.
    Cardiac arrhythmias. A symposium.
    Springfield, Ill. Thomas, 1972.

1506
HANDLEY, A.J., P.A. EMERSON, AND P.R. FLEMING.
    Heparin in the prevention of deep vein thrombosis after myocardial infarction.
    British Medical Journal 2:436-438, 1972.

1507
HANRATH, P., W. MERX, W. BLEIFELD, AND K.W. HEINRICH.
    Ballooned catheters, a methodological advance in intracardiac pressure measurement.
    Medizinische Welt 23(40):1367-1368, 1972.

1508
HANSEN, H.W.
    Diagnosis of temporary cardiac arrhythmias with the longtime ECG. Its significance for cerebral
    and coronary circulation.
    Münchener Medizinische Wochenschrift 112(7):276-280, 1970.

1509
HANSEN, P., T. GEILL, AND E. LUND.
  Dietary fats and thrombosis.
  Lancet 7267:1193-1194, 1962.

1510
HANSEN, P.F., P.A. RASMUSSEN, AND G. NYBERG.
  Alprenolol alone and in conjunction with pentanitrol in angina pectoris—a double blind study
  with exercise tests.
  Acta Medica Scandinavica 193:419, 1973.

1511
HANSON, J.S., AND W.H. NEDDE.
  Preliminary observations on physical training for hypertensive males.
  Circulation Research 27(Suppl. 1):149-153, 1970.

1512
HANSON, J.S., AND B. TABAKIN.
  Simultaneous and rapidly. repeated cardiac output determinations by dye-dilution method.
  Journal Applied Physiology 19(2):275-278, 1964.

1513
HANSON, J.S., B.S. TABAKIN, AND A.M. LEVY.
  Comparative exercise-cardiorespiratory performance of normal men in the third, fourth, and fifth
  decades of life.
  Circulation 37:345-350, 1968.

1514
HANSON, J.S., B.S. TABAKIN, A.M. LEVY, AND W. NEDDE.
  Long-term physical training and cardiovascular dynamics in middle-aged men.
  Circulation 38:783-799, 1968.

1515
HANZLIK, J., A. MAJCZAK, AND J. LOPATYNSKI.
  Tentative analysis of an opinion probe on the necessity and merits of psychological rehabilitation
  after heart blocking infarcts.
  Balneologia Polska 16(1/2):93-96, 1971.

1516
HARBURG, E., W.J. SCHULL, J.C. ERFURT, AND M.A. SCHORK.
  A family set method for estimating heredity and stress. I. A pilot survey of blood pressure
  among Negroes in high and low stress areas, Detroit, 1966-67.
  Journal Chronic Diseases 23:69-81, 1970.

1517
HARDYCK, D.C., ET AL.
  Personality and marital-adjustment differences in essential hypertension in women.
  Journal Consulting Psychology 30:459, 1966.

1518
HARKEN, D.E.
  Coronary artery disease. What can be done by whom?
  Delaware Medical Journal 45:298, 1973.

1519
HARLAND, W.A., J.S. ORR, M.G. DUNNIGAN, AND R.F.C. SEQUEIRA.
Thyroxine secretion rate after myocardial infarction.
British Heart Journal 34(10):1072-1074, 1972.

1520
HARPUR, J.E.
Shorter hospitalization for myocardial infarcts.
New England Journal Medicine 289:805, 1973.

1521
HARPUR, J.E., R.J. KELLETT, W.T. CONNER, H.J.B. GALBRAITH, M. HAMILTON, J.J. MURRAY, J.H. SWALLOW, AND G.A. ROSE.
Controlled trial of early mobilisation and discharge from hospital in uncomplicated myocardial infarction.
Lancet 2:1331-1334, 1971.

1522
HARRIS, A.
Long term treatment of paroxysmal cardiac arrhythmias with propranolol.
American Journal Cardiology 18(1):431-437, 1966.

1523
HARRIS, A., J. GIALAFOS, AND K. JEFFERSON.
Transvenous pacing in presence of anomalous venous return to heart.
British Heart Journal 34(11):1189-1191, 1972.

1524
HARRIS, A., AND G. SUTTON.
Second heart sound in normal subjects.
British Heart Journal 30:739-742, 1968.

1525
HARRIS, A.W.
Management of patients with chronic congestive heart failure.
Modern Treatment 2(2):247-269, 1965.

1526
HARRIS, C.N., M.A. Kaplan, D.P. PARKER, ET AL.
Anatomic and functional correlates of intercoronary collateral vessels.
American Journal Cardiology 30(6):611-614, 1972.

1527
HARRIS, P.
Regional metabolism during exercise in heart disease.
Bulletin New York Academy Medicine 42(11):966-981, 1966.

1528
HARRIS, P., M. BATEMAN, AND J. GLOSTER.
Relations between the cardio-respiratory effects of exercise and the arterial concentration of lactate and pyruvate in patients with rheumatic heart disease.
Clinical Science 23(3):531-543, 1962.

1529
HARRIS, P., M. BATEMAN, AND J. GLOSTER.
The regional metabolism of lactate and pyruvate during exercise in patients with rheumatic heart disease.
Clinical Science 23(3):545-560, 1962.

1530
HARRIS, P., J.H. JONES, M. BATEMAN, C. CHLOUVERAKIS, AND J. GLOSTER.
Metabolism of the myocardium at rest and during exercise in patients with rheumatic heart disease.
Clinical Science 26(1):145-156, 1964.

1531
HARRIS, R.
A critique of cardiac rehabilitation.
New York State Journal Medicine 65:1737-1744, 1965.

1532
HARRIS, R.
Managing the geriatric coronary patient.
Journal Rehabilitation 32:98, 1966.

1533
HARRIS, R.
Viewpoint: Geriatric cardiac rehabilitation.
Gerontologist 7:82, passim, 1967.

1534
HARRIS, R.
Rehabilitation of the cardiac patient. Assessing the cardiac patient for rehabilitation.
New York State Journal Medicine 70:511-515, 1970.

1535
HARRIS, W.S., N. AYTAN, AND J.M. POUGET.
Effects of nitroglycerin on responses of the systolic time intervals to exercise.
Circulation 47:499-508, 1973.

1536
HARRIS, W.S., C.D. SCHOENFELD, R.H. BROOKS, AND A.M. WEISSLER.
Effect of beta-adrenergic blockade on the hemodynamic responses to epinephrine in man.
American Journal Cardiology 17:484-491, 1966.

1537
HARRISON, D.C., ET AL.
Effects of muscular exercise.
Circulation Research 13:460, 1963.

1538
HARRISON, S.G.C., AND B.A. SELLICK.
Cardiovascular effects of althesin in patients with cardiac pathology. Preliminary communication.
British Journal Anesthesia 44:1205, 1972.

1539
HARRISON, T.R., AND T.J. REEVES.
The psychologic management of patients with cardiac disease.
American Heart Journal 70:136-138, 1965.

1540
HART, J.T.
Semicontinuous screening of a whole community for hypertension.
Lancet 2:223-226, 1970.

1541
HÄRTEL, G., V. MANNINEN, J. MELIN, AND A. APAJALAHTI.
Serum-digoxin concentrations with a new digoxin derivative, β-methyldigoxin.
Annals Clinical Research 5:87-90, 1973.

1542
HARTLEY, L.H.
Alterations in submaximal stroke volume and heart rate by previous heavier work loads.
Malattie Cardiovascolari 10(1-2):401-407, 1969.

1543
HARTLEY, L.H., G. GRIMBY, A. KILBOM, N.J. NILSSON, I. ÅSTRAND, J. BJURE, B. EKBLOM, AND B. SALTIN.
Physical training in sedentary middle-aged and older men. III. Cardiac output and gas exchange at submaximal and maximal exercise.
Scandinavian Journal Clinical Laboratory Investigation 24:335-344, 1969.

1544
HARTLEY, L.H., J.A. VOGEL, AND M. LANDOWNE.
Central, femoral and brachial circulation during exercise in hypoxia.
Journal Applied Physiology 34(1):87-90, 1973.

1545
HARTUNG, G.H.
Exercise electrocardiography in athletes and nontrained subjects.
Journal Sport Medicine 12:186, 1972.

1546
HARUMI, K.
Further consideration on a theoretic model of T-wave.
Japanese Circulation Journal 31:1616-1623, 1967.

1547
HARVALD, B.
Long-term anticoagulant therapy after myocardial infarction.
Lancet 7267:656-630, 1962.

1548
HARVARD, C.W.
Recovery after myocardial infarction. 1.
British Medical Journal 1:1467, 1966.

1549
HARVARD, C.W.H.
   Recovery after myocardial infarction. 2.
   British Medical Journal 1:1525-1527, 1966.

1550
HARVEY, R.M., W.M. SMITH, J.O. PARKER, AND M.I. FERRER.
   The response of the abnormal heart to exercise.
   Circulation 26:341-362, 1962.

1551
HASHIBA, K., T. KATAYAMA, A. TAKAHASHI, A. ONO, S. MATSUO, N. TAJIMA, Y.
YAMAGUCHI, M. YOSHIOKA, Y. MORI, AND S. MOCHINAGA.
   Effect of exercise and acetylcholine on the pulmonary circulation in mitral and congenital heart
   disease.
   Japanese Circulation Journal 31(2):1890, 1967.

1552
HASHIDA, E., K. RIN, AND T. INOUE.
   Exercise, body build and electrocardiogram. The influences of sports and training on the
   electrocardiogram.
   Japanese Circulation Journal 37(3):305, 1973.

1553
HASHIDA, E., K. RIN, T. INOUE, ET AL.
   Interpretation of the normal electrocardiogram by multivariate statistical analysis.
   Japanese Circulation Journal 36(1):27-33, 1972.

1554
HASHIDA, E., K. RIN, T. INOUE, ET AL.
   A trial and formulation of regression equations of RV_5 on several constitutional variables
   including age. Relationship between electrocardiogram and body build.
   Japanese Circulation Journal 36(4):325-334, 1972.

1555
HASIK, J.
   Nitrogen and electrolytes balance studies in chronic heart failure with edema.
   Bratislavske Lekarske Listy 56(5):605-611, 1971.

1556
HASKELL, W.L.
   Preparation of exercise program directors for cardiac rehabilitation programs.
   In: Naughton, J.P., H.K. Hellerstein, and I.C. Mohler, Eds. Exercise testing and exercise training
   coronary heart disease, pp. 402-404. New York. Academic Press, 1973.

1557
HASKELL, W.L.
   Physical activity and the prevention of coronary heart disease: What type exercise might be
   effective.
   Journal South Carolina Medical Association 65(Suppl. 1):41-45, 1969.

1558
HASKELL, W.L., AND S.M. FOX, III.
The possible place of stress testing to discover, and physical activity to prevent, coronary heart disease.
Southern Medical Journal 59:642-647, 1966.

1559
HASKELL, W.L., AND S.M. FOX, III.
Exercise and heart disease.
Postgraduate Medicine 44:177-182, 1968.

1560
HASKELL, W.L., AND S.M. FOX, III.
Some factors to consider when selecting an exercise stress testing procedure for the detection of myocardial ischemia.
Malattie Cardiovascolari 10:189-200, 1969.

1561
HASPEL, L.U.
Abnormal heart sounds (S_3 and S_4) with acute myocardial infarction. Prognostic significance of changes detected by phonocardiography and auscultation.
Journal American Osteopathic Association 71(9):771-775, 1972.

1562
HASSANEIN, M., AND A. EMARA.
Some aspects of employment of cardiacs.
Journal Egyptian Medical Association 51:665-679, 1968.

1563
HATCHER, C.R., JR., K. MANSOUR, W.D. LOGAN, P.N. SYMBAS, AND O.A. ABBOTT.
Surgical complications of myocardial infarction.
American Surgeon 36:163-170, 1970.

1564
HATT, P.Y., AND J. MORAVEC.
Acute hypoxia of the myocardium. Ultrastructural changes.
Cardiology 56(1):73-84, 1972.

1565
HATTINGBERG, I., VON.
Studies on the medical understanding of fear in cardiac infarct. 1. The many forms of fear phenomena.
Medizinische Klinik 60:1113-1117, 1965.

1566
HATTINGBERG, I., VON.
Studies on the physician's understanding of anxiety in myocardial infarction. 2. The significance of fear for the physician's understanding.
Medizinische Klinik 60:1150-1153, 1965.

1567
HATTINGBERG, I., VON.
The tasks of rehabilitation treatment in social medicine.
Münchener Medizinische Wochenschrift 108:426-430, 1966.

1568
HATTINGBERG, I., VON.
Experiences with group treatments and single sessions in the rehabilitation of infarct patients.
Psychotherapy Psychosomatics 15(1):27, 1967.

1569
HATTINGBERG, I., VON.
Psychological problems and experiences in the rehabilitation and treatment of workers with myocardial infarction.
Psychotherapy Psychosomatics 16(4-5):233-248, 1968.

1570
HATTINGBERG, I., VON.
Psychological methods in rehabilitation after myocardial infarct.
Medizinische Klinik 65:1905-1910, 1969.

1571
HAU, T.F., AND A. RÜPPELL.
Psychodynamics in coronary diseases.
Medizinische Klinik 61:369-371, 1966.

1572
HAVIAR, V.
Rehabilitation of patients with heart disease in East European countries.
Bratislavske Lekarske Listy 45:515-517, 1965.

1573
HAVIAR, V.
Is prolonged bed rest necessary in myocardial infarction.
Evolution Médicale 13(3):256, 1069

1574
HAWKINS, H., F. GOBEL, AND Y. WANG.
The response of the systolic ejection period to exercise in aortic and mitral valvular heart disease.
Circulation 37-38(Suppl. 6):97, 1968.

1575
HAY, D.R., AND S. TURBOTT.
Rehabilitation after myocardial infarction and acute coronary insufficiency.
New Zealand Medical Journal 71:267-272, 1970.

1576
HAY, D.R., AND S. TURBOTT.
Changes in smoking habits in men under 65 years after myocardial infarction and coronary insufficiency.
British Heart Journal 32(6):738-740, 1970.

1577
HAYASE, S., H. ITO, Y. KONDO, ET AL.
Inhibitory action of propranolol and its stereoisomers on epinephrine induced changes in electrocardiogram.
Japanese Circulation Journal 36(10):1065-1088, 1972.

1578
HAYWOOD, L.J., S.A. SALTZBERG, V.K. MURTHY, ET AL.
   Clinical use of R-R interval prediction for ECG monitoring: time series analysis by autoregressive models.
   Journal Association Advancement Medical Instrumentation 6(2):111-116, 1972.

1579
HAYWOOD, J., AND M.G. WYMAN.
   Effects of isoproterenol, ephedrine, and potassium on artificial pacemaker failure.
   Circulation 31(Suppl. 2):110, 1965.

1580
HAZAN, S.J.
   Psychiatric complications following cardiac surgery. II. A working hypothesis: The chemical approach.
   Journal Thoracic Cardiovascular Surgery 51(3):320-325, 1966.

1581
HAZEKI, T.
   Hemodynamic and metabolic effects of activities of the beta-adrenergic receptor in physical exercise.
   Japanese Circulation Journal 37:141, 1973.

1582
HAZZARD, W.R., J.L. GOLDSTEIN, H.G. SCHROTT, A.G. MOTULSKY, AND E.L. BIERMAN.
   Hyperlipidemia in coronary heart disease. Part 3. Evaluation of lipoprotein phenotypes of 156 genetically defined survivors of myocardial infarction.
   Journal Clinical Investigation 52:1569-1577, 1973.

1583
HEATH, M.J.
   Myocardial infarction—a personal account.
   Journal Rehabilitation 32:46, 1966.

1584
HEBERER, G., G. SCHRAMM, AND F.W. SCHILDBERG.
   Surgical treatment of aneurysms of the ventricular wall.
   Chirurg 42(4):181-187, 1971.

1585
HEDVALL, G., I. KJELLMER, AND T. OLSSON.
   An experimental evaluation of the thermodilution method for determination of cardiac output and of intracardiac right to left shunts.
   Scandinavian Journal Clinical Laboratory Investigation 31(1):61-68, 1973.

1586
HEGGE, F.N., N. TUNA, AND H.B. BURCHELL.
   Coronary arteriographic findings in patients with axis shifts or S-T segment elevation on exercise-stress testing.
   American Heart Journal 86:603-615, 1973.

1587
HEHRLEIN, F.W., J. MULCH, P. PAHUTAN, AND M. IIDA.
The advantage of programmable cardiac pacemakers.
Thoraxchirurgie Vaskuläre Chirurgie 21:233, 1973.

1588
HEIDRICH, R., AND J. OTT.
Exogenous psychoses in heart diseases.
Psychiatrie, Neurologie und Medizinische Psychologie (Leipzig) 17:401-404, 1965.

1589
HEIN, C.
Analysis of the current state and the problems of vocational candidacy examinations of
physically disabled persons.
Zeitschrift für die Gesamte Hygiene 18(1):46-49, 1972.

1590
HEINE, B.
Psychosomatic aspects of hypertension.
Postgraduate Medical Journal 47(550):541-548, 1971.

1591
HEINE, H., H. SCHMIDT, E. JAHN, AND M. KORNOTZKI.
Results of long term outpatient treatment with anticoagulants for patients with myocardial
infarction and peripheral arteriosclerosis.
Zeitschrift für Gesamte Innere Medizin 28(2):27-30, 1973.

1592
HEINLE, R.A., ET AL.
Lipid and carbohydrate abnormalities in patients with angiographically documented coronary
artery disease.
American Journal Cardiology 24:178, 1969.

1593
HEINONEN, O.P., K. AHO, K. PYÖRÄLÄ, ET AL.
Symptomless autoimmune thyroiditis in coronary heart disease.
Lancet 1:785-786, 1972.

1594
HEINZ, N.
Studies on the refractory, supernormal and vulnerable phase of the heart in patients with
bradycardic rhythm disorders.
Archiv für Kreislaufforschung 67(3):201-222, 1972.

1595
HEINZELMANN, F.
Social and psychological factors that influence the effectiveness of exercise programs.
In: Naughton, J.P., H.K. Hellerstein, and I.C. Mohler, Eds. Exercise testing and exercise training
in coronary heart disease, pp. 275-287. New York, Academic Press, 1973.

1596
HEINZELMANN, F., AND R.W. BAGLEY.
Response to physical activity programs and their effects on health behavior.
Public Health Reports 85:905-911, 1970.

1597
HELLER, E.M.
Rehabilitation after myocardial infarction: Practical experience with a graded exercise program.
Canadian Medical Association Journal 97(1):22-27, 1967.

1598
HELLER, E.M.
Practical graded exercise program after myocardial infarction.
Archives Physical Medicine Rehabilitation 50:655-662, 1969.

1599
HELLER, E.M.
Exercise in the management of the postcoronary patient. I.
Applied Therapeutics 10:315-319, 1969.

1600
HELLER, E.M.
Four-year experience with a graded exercise program for postcoronary patients.
Applied Therapeutics 11:386-388, 1969.

1601
HELLER, L.J., AND W.V. WHITEHORN.
Age associated alterations in myocardial contractile properties.
American Journal Physiology 222(6):1613-1619, 1972.

1602
HELLERSTEIN, H.K.
Exercise therapy in coronary disease.
Bulletin, New York Academy Medicine 44(8):1028-1047, 1968.

1603
HELLERSTEIN, H.K.
Exercise and the treatment of heart disease. Techniques of exercise prescription and evaluation.
Journal South Carolina Medical Association 65(Suppl. 1)1:46-56, 1969.

1604
HELLERSTEIN, H.K.
Active physical conditioning of subjects with coronary heart disease.
In: Eliakim, M. and H.N. Neufeld, Eds. Cardiology, current topics and progress, pp. 162-165.
New York, Academic Press, 1969.

1605
HELLERSTEIN, H.K.
Relation of exercise to acute myocardial infarction: therapeutic, restorative, preventive, and etiological aspects.
Circulation 40(5 Suppl. 4):124-129, 1969.

1606
HELLERSTEIN, H.K.
Effects of an active physical reconditioning intervention program on the clinical course of coronary artery disease.
Malattie Cardiovascolari 10:461-463, 1969.

1607
HELLERSTEIN, H.K.
    Rehabilitation of the postinfarction patient.
    Hospital Practice 7(7):45-53, 1972.

1608
HELLERSTEIN, H.K., A. BURLANDO, E.Z. HIRSCH, F.H. PLOTKIN, G.H. FEIL, O. WINKLER, S.
MARIK, AND N. MARGOLIS.
    Active physical reconditioning of coronary patients.
    Circulation 31(Suppl. 2):110, 1965.

1609
HELLERSTEIN, H.K., AND A.B. FORD.
    Comprehensive care of the coronary patient. Optimal (intensive) care, recovery, and
    reconditioning. An opportunity for the physician.
    In: Symposium on coronary heart disease , (2nd ed.). New York, American Heart Association,
    1969.

1610
HELLERSTEIN, H.K., AND E.H. FRIEDMAN.
    Sexual activity and the postcoronary patient.
    Medical Aspects Human Sexuality 3(3):70, 1969.

1611
HELLERSTEIN, H.K., AND E.H. FRIEDMAN.
    Sexual activity and the postcoronary patient.
    Scandinavian Journal Rehabilitation Medicine 2-3:109, 1970.

1612
HELLERSTEIN, H.K., AND E.H. FRIEDMAN.
    Sexual activity and the postcoronary patient.
    Archives Internal Medicine 125(6):987-999, 1970.

1613
HELLERSTEIN, H.K., E.H. FRIEDMAN, P.J. BRDAR, M. WEISS, C.W. DUPERTUIS, D.J. TURELL,
AND D. RUMBAUGH.
    Comparison of personality of males with rheumatic heart disease and with arteriosclerotic heart
    disease.
    Circulation 39-40(Suppl. III):11, 1969.

1614
HELLERSTEIN, H.K., E.H. FRIEDMAN, E.H. BRDAR, P.J. WEISS, ET AL.
    A comparison of the personality of adult subjects with rheumatic heart disease and with
    arteriosclerotic heart disease.
    In: Rehabilitation of non-coronary heart disease, pp. 220-282. International Society of
    Cardiology, 1969.

1615
HELLERSTEIN, H.K., ET AL.
    A community program and study among patients and normal coronary prone subjects. The
    effects of physical activity.
    Minnesota Medicine 52:1335, 1969.

1616
HELLERSTEIN, H.K., E.L. HIRSCH, R. ADER, N. GREENBLOT, AND M. SIEGEL.
Principles of exercise prescription for normals and cardiac subjects.
In: Naughton, J.P., H.K. Hellerstein, and I.C. Mohler, Eds. Exercise testing and exercise training in coronary heart disease, pp. 129-167. New York, Academic Press, 1973.

1617
HELLERSTEIN, H.K., AND T.R. HORNSTEN.
Assessing and preparing the patient for return to a meaningful, productive life.
Journal Rehabilitation 32:48, 1966.

1618
HELLERSTEIN, H.K., T.R. HORNSTEN, R.A. BAKER, AND W.L. HOPPES.
Cardiac performance during postprandial lipemia and heparin-induced lipolysis.
American Journal Cardiology 20:525, 1967.

1619
HELLERSTEIN, H.K., T.R. HORNSTEN, A. GOLDBARG, A.G. BURLANDO, E.H. FRIEDMAN, E.Z. HIRSCH, AND S. MARIK.
The influence of active conditioning upon subjects with coronary artery disease: Cardiorespiratory changes during training in 67 patients.
Canadian Medical Association Journal 96:758-763, 1967.

1620
HELLERSTEIN, H.K., T.R. HORNSTEN, A.N. GOLDBARG, A.G. BURLANDO, E.H. FRIEDMAN, E.Z. HIRSCH, AND S. MARIK.
The influence of active conditioning upon subjects with coronary artery disease: A progress report.
Canadian Medical Association Journal 96:901-903, 1967.

1621
HELLERSTEIN, H.K., T.R. HORNSTEN, C. GODFREY, III, AND J. FAIRBANKS.
Work and heart disease. III. An ecological study of anesthesiologists.
Circulation 33-34(Suppl. III):126, 1966.

1622
HELLERSTEIN, H.K., G.B. PROZAN, I.M. LIEBOW, A.E. DOAN, AND J.A. HENDERSON.
Two step exercise test as a test of cardiac function in chronic rheumatic heart disease and in arteriosclerotic heart disease with old myocardial infarction.
American Journal Cardiology 7:234-252, 1961.

1623
HELMUTH, G.A.
Work and heart disease in Wisconsin. II. Workman's compensation rules of practice.
Journal American Medical Association 198(13):1335-1340, 1966.

1624
HELMUTH, G.A.
Medical studies on Workmen's Compensation and the cardiac.
Industrial Medicine Surgery 36:603-606, 1967.

1625
HELLMUTH, G.A.
     Cardiac criteria for Workmen's Compensation Act of Wisconsin.
     Wisconsin Medical Journal 66:263-271, 1967.

1626
HELLMUTH, G.A.
     Whither cardiac work evaluation units?
     Circulation 39:283-285, 1969.

1627
HELLMUTH, G.A.
     Is workmen's compensation a barrier to cardiac employment?
     Archives Environmental Health 20:404-409, 1970.

1628
HELLMUTH, G.A.
     Cardiac employees and their immediate supervisors. Effects on industrial medical programs.
     Journal Occupational Medicine 13:166-174, 1971.

1629
HELLMUTH, G.A.
     A survey of students in a medical school cardiac work classification unit. Implications for
     vocational health in comprehensive medicine.
     Archives Environmental Health 22:505-511, 1971.

1630
HELLMUTH, G.A.
     Teaching behavior and vocational medicine in a cardiac work classification unit.
     Rehabilitation Literature 33:162-165, 1972.

1631
HELLMUTH, G.A.
     Exercise after myocardial infarction.
     American Family Physician 8(4):94, 1973.

1632
HELLMUTH, G.A., ET AL.
     Psychological factors in cardiac patients. Distortion of clinical recommendations.
     Archives Environmental Health 12:771-775, 1966.

1633
HELLMUTH, G.A., AND P.J. HELLMUTH.
     Attorney attitudes on medicolegal criteria proposed for workmen's compensation cardiac claim
     cases.
     Journal Occupational Medicine 11:466-474, 1969.

1634
HELLMUTH, G.A., AND G.E. RODEY.
     Comprehensive evaluation of heart cases under Workmen's Compensation.
     Journal Rehabilitation 34:18-23, 1968.

1635
HELLMUTH, G.A., G. RODEY, W.J. JOHANNSEN, AND E.L. BELKNAP.
Work and heart disease in Wisconsin, I. Medical basis for workmen's compensation awards over ten years.
Journal American Medical Association 198(1):9-15, 1966.

1636
HELLSTROM, R.
Serum lipids in male patients hospitalized for myocardial infarction.
Acta Medica Scandinavica 182(6):727-736, 1967.

1637
HELTMAN, J., AND S. MARKOWSKI.
The postinfarction syndrome of Dressler.
Wiadomosci Lekarskie 25:1325, 1972.

1638
HELTMAN, J., AND S. MARKOWSKI.
Symptomatology of postinfarction syndrome.
Wiadomosci Lekarskie 25(21):1941-1945, 1972.

1639
HENDRICH, F., M. STEJFA, AND V. HULE.
Diagnostic value of serum lactate dehydrogenase isoenzymes in anginal attacks.
Cor Vasa 12(1):8-11, 1970.

1640
HENDRIX, G.H., AND M.E. CLINE.
Effects of an unusually large amount of intravenous lidocaine.
Journal South Carolina Medical Association 68(9):347-349, 1972.

1641
HENNES, A.R., K. AWAI, J.C. JACKSON, AND M.L. ADAMS.
Abnormalities in lipid formation by platelets from young patients with myocardial infarction.
Circulation 31(Suppl. 2):111, 1965.

1642
HENRICHS, T.F., J.W. MacKENZIE, AND C.H. ALMOND.
Psychological adjustment and psychiatric complications following open heart surgery.
Journal Nervous Mental Disease 152(5):332-345, 1971.

1643
HEPBURN, F.
An effective manual unit for external cardiac massage.
Medical Biological Engineering 10:123-124, 1972.

1644
HERD, J.A.
Behavior and cardiovascular function.
Physiologist 14:83-89, 1971.

1645
HERMAN, M.V., M.D. KLEIN, W.C. ELLIOTT, AND R. GORLIN.
Electrocardiographic, metabolic, and anatomic predictions of zonal myocardial ischemia in coronary artery disease.
Circulation 31(Suppl. 2):111, 1965.

1646
HERNBERG, S.
Correlation between physical working capacity and serum cholesterol in leading businessmen.
In: Karvonen, M.J. and A.J. Barry, Eds. Physical activity and the heart, pp. 249-256. Springfield, Ill. Thomas, 1967.

1647
HERNBERG, S., T. PARTANEN, C.H. NORDMAN, AND P. SUMARI.
Coronary heart disease among workers exposed to carbon disulphide.
British Journal Industrial Medicine 27(4):313-325, 1970.

1648
HERTLE, F.H., G. HOFMEIER, AND J. KEUL.
Coronary heart disease. Advanced training course at the German clinic of diagnostics 26-27 February, 1971.
Stuttgart, Schattauer Verlag, 1972.

1649
HEYDEN-STUCKEY, S.
Myocardial infarct and psychic stress.
Schweizerische Medizinische Wochenschrift 95:1045-1050, 1965.

1650
HEYMANS, C., AND E. NEIL.
Reflexogenic areas of the cardiovascular system.
Boston, Mass. Little, Brown, 1958.

1651
HIEBERT, J.B., AND B.D. McCALLISTER.
Left ventricular function during isometric handgrip exercise in patients with angina pectoris.
Clinical Research 19(3):643, 1971.

1652
HIEJIMA, K., F. SUZUKI, H. KUDO, ET AL.
Atrial reciprocal rhythm following DC conversion of atrial flutter.
Japanese Heart Journal 13(4):362-368, 1972.

1653
HIGASHIHARA, Y.
Myocardial lipid metabolism during exercise in clinical cases.
Japanese Circulation Journal 37(6):657, 1973.

1654
HIGGINS, A.C., AND W.S. POOLER.
Myocardial infarction and subsequent reemployment in Syracuse, New York.
American Journal Public Health 58(2):312-323, 1968.

1655

HIGGINS, I.T.T., ET AL.
   Coronary disease in Staveley, Derbyshire, with an international comparison with three towns in Marion County, West Virginia.
   Journal Chronic Diseases 25(10-11):567, 1972.

1656

HIGGS, B.E., M. CLODE, AND E.J.M. CAMPBELL.
   Changes in ventilation, gas exchange, and circulation during exercise after recovery from myocardial infarction.
   Lancet 2:793-795, 1968.

1657

HILGENBERG, F.
   Roentgenologic aspects of cardiac insufficiency.
   Monatsschrift für Kinderheilkunde 120(11):453-454, 1972.

1658

HILL, D.E., ET AL.
   Specialized care for acute myocardial infarction. Four year experience in a community hospital.
   Minnesota Medicine 56:983, 1973.

1659

HILLEBRECHT, J., AND A.H. LEMMERZ.
   Fundamentals and methods of medical rehabilitation of cardiac infarction patients by the practical physician.
   Medizinische Welt 36:2063-2075, 1967.

1660

HILLESTAD, L.F.
   The peripheral blood flow in intermittent claudication. VII. The difference between the hyperemias following free and ischemic exercise and the effect of the included period of ischemia upon the latter. A comparison of the tests for evaluation of the blood flow and of various methods for gauging the hyperemia. A note on the use of plethysmography in clinical studies.
   Acta Medica Scandinavica 174(6):687-700, 1963.

1661

HILLMAN, L.C., W.M. CARROLL, AND M.S.T. HOBBS.
   Mobile coronary care: A survey amongst general practitioners.
   Medical Journal Australia 2:264, 1973.

1662

HILMER, W.
   Myocardial infarction and sport awards.
   Zeitschrift für Kreislaufforschung 61:303-309, 1972.

1663

HILMER, W., AND W. WEISS.
   Evaluation of ventricular extrasystole on the basis of electrocardiographic images.
   Zeitschrift für Kreislaufforschung 59(12):1097, 1970.

1664
HILTY-TAMMIVAARA, R., AND I. CULLHED.
Exercise-released ventricular fibrillation in hypertrophic subaortic stenosis treated with propranolol: A case report.
Acta Medica Scandinavica 187(4):317-322, 1970.

1665
HINKLE, L.E., JR.
Coronary heart disease and sudden death in actively employed American men.
Bulletin New York Academy Medicine 49(6):467-474, 1973.

1666
HINKLE, L.E., L.H. WHITNEY, E.W. LEHMAN, J. DUNN, B. BENJAMIN, R. KING, A. PLAKUN, AND B. FLEHINGER.
Occupation, education, and coronary heart disease.
Science 161:238-246, 1968.

1667
HINOHARA, S.
Psychological aspects in rehabilitation of coronary heart disease.
Scandinavian Journal Rehabilitation Medicine 2-3:53-59, 1970.

1668
HINOHARA, S., T. SHINODA, M. IGARASHI, G. KOJIMA, T. HORIBE, AND M. NOMURA.
Psychosomatic study on the development of myocardial infarction and its rehabilitation.
Japanese Journal Medicine 11:197, 1972.

1669
HIPP, H.R.
Long-term anticoagulant therapy after myocardial infarction. A study of 747 patients in 15 hospitals.
Journal American Medical Association 193(11):929-934, 1965.

1670
HIRAKAWA, S., M. KINOSHITA, K. NAKAO, H. YAGINUMA, K. MURAI, A. SAKAI, A. WAKABYASHI, AND T. OOTA.
Simultaneous measurements of the cardiac output and peripheral venous pressure at rest and during mild supine leg exercise in normal and abnormal heart.
Japanese Circulation Journal 31:1953-1954, 1967.

1671
HIRSCH, E.Z., H.K. HELLERSTEIN, AND C.A. MACLEOD.
Physical straining and coronary heart disease.
In: Morse, R.L., Ed. Exercise and the heart. Guidelines for exercise programs, p. 106. Springfield, Ill. Thomas, 1972.

1672
HISS, R.G., AND L.E. LAMB.
Electrocardiographic findings in 122,043 individuals.
Circulation 25:947, 1962.

1673
HJORT, P.F., AND K. MOLNE.
  Myocardial infarction during long-term anticoagulant therapy.
  Acta Medica Scandinavica 176(6):693-700, 1964.

1674
HLADOVEC, J., I. PŘEROVSKÝ, AND K. ROZTOČIL.
  The influence of inflammation on the ^{125}I-fibrinogen uptake test in experimental thrombosis.
  Angiologica 10:93, 1973.

1675
HLASTALA, M.P., B. WRANNE, AND C.J. LENFANT.
  Single breath method of measuring cardiac output: A reevaluation.
  Journal Applied Physiology 33(6):846-848, 1972.

1676
HOCHBERG, H.M., A.L. WEIHRER, J.W. MCCALLISTER, J.B. CALATAYUD, A.K. ZIMMERMAN,
AND C.A. CACERES.
  Monitoring of electrocardiograms in a coronary care unit by digital computer.
  Journal American Medical Association 207(13):2421-2424, 1969.

1677
HOCHMAN, L.
  Psychology level of aspiration and need achievement in employed and unemployed coronary
  patients.
  Dissertation Abstracts 28(11):4757-B, 1968.

1678
HOCHREIN, M., AND I. SCHLEICHER.
  Myocardial infarction in cases of diabetes mellitus.
  Medizinische Monatsschrift 24(10):444-448, 1970.

1679
HODGKIN, G.K.H.
  Acute chest pain in the community.
  In: Preventive Techniques for the Modern Community. The Chest and Heart Association, pp.
  6-11. London, England, 1971.

1680
HOEL, B.L., E. LORENTSEN, AND P.G. LUND-LARSEN.
  Haemodynamic responses to sustained hand-grip in patients with hypertension.
  Acta Medica Scandinavica 188(6):491-495, 1970.

1681
HOFMANN, H., AND M. SEUBERLING.
  2 Years of early rehabilitation after myocardial infarction in the clinic Hoehenried West
  Germany. Part 3. Medical aspects of follow-up measures of treatment after myocardial infarction.
  Fortschritte der Medizin 91:114, 1973.

1682
HOFFMAN, B.F., AND P.F. CRANEFIELD.
  Electrophysiology of the heart.
  New York, McGraw-Hill, 1960.

1683
HOFFMAN, B.F., AND P.F. CRANEFIELD.
The physiological basis of cardiac arrhythmias.
American Journal Medicine 37:670, 1964.

1684
HOFFMAN, H.H., W.R. NELSON, AND F.A. GROSS.
Effects of an exercise program on plasma lipids of senior air force officers.
American Journal Cardiology 20:516-24, 1967.

1685
HOLLMAN, W., AND B. GRÜNEWALD.
The elderly man and sport.
Zeitschrift für Allgemeine Medizin der Landarzt 43:649-654, 1967.

1686
HOLLOSZY, J.O.
The epidemiology of coronary heart disease: National differences and the role of physical activity.
Journal American Geriatrics Society 11:718, 1963.

1687
HOLLOSZY, J.O.
Biochemical adaptations in muscle: effects of exercise on mitochondrial oxygen uptake and respiratory enzyme activity in skeletal muscle.
Journal Biological Chemistry 242(9):2278, 1967.

1688
HOLLOSZY, J.O.
Morpholological and enzymatic adaptations to training. A review.
In: Larson, O.A. and R.O. Malmborg, Eds. Coronary heart disease and physical fitness, pp. 147-151. Copenhagen, Munksgaard, 1971.

1689
HOLLOSZY, J.O.
Long-term metabolic adaptation in muscle to endurance exercise.
In: Naughton, J.P., H.K. Hellerstein, and I.C. Mohler, Eds. Exercise testing and exercise training in coronary heart disease, pp. 211-222. New York, Academic Press, 1973.

1690
HOLLOSZY, J.O., J. SKINNER, G. TORO, AND T. CURETON.
Effects of a six-month program of endurance exercise on the serum lipids of middle-aged men.
American Journal Cardiology 14:753, 1964.

1691
HOLM J., A-G DAHLLÖF, P. BJÖRNTORP, AND T. SCHERSTÉN.
Glucose tolerance, plasma insulin, and lipids in intermittent claudication with reference to muscle metabolism.
Metabolism 22:1395, 1973.

1692
HOLMBERG, S.
Effect of severe muscular work on total and coronary circulation in man in relation to findings in the coronary arteriogram.
In: Marchetti, G. and B. Taccardi, Eds. Coronary circulation and energetics of the myocardium, pp. 268-279. New York, S. Karger, 1967.

1693
HOLMBERG, S., R. LUEPKER, AND E. VARNAUSKAS.
Influence of recirculation on myocardial clearance curves with xenon-133.
Acta Medica Scandinavica 189:241-250, 1971.

1694
HOLMBERG, S., W. SERZYSKO, AND E. VARNAUSKAS.
Coronary circulation during heavy exercise in control subjects and patients with coronary heart disease.
Acta Medica Scandinavica 190(6):465-480, 1971.

1695
HOLMGREN, A.
Cardiorespiratory determinants of cardiovascular fitness.
Canadian Medical Association Journal 96:697-705, 1967.

1696
HOLMGREN, A., ET AL.
ECG changes in vasoregulatory asthenia and the effect of physical training.
Acta Medica Scandinavica 165:259-271, 1959.

1697
HOLTZ, H., W. KEYLING, H. TAUSCH, G. STRECKARDT, R. SCHMIDT, AND I. EXNER.
Initial results of an outpatient training treatment after myocardial infarction.
Deutsche Gesundheitswesen 28:2023, 1973.

1698
HOLZER, J., ET AL.
Effectiveness of dopamine in patients with cardiogenic shock.
American Journal Cardiology 32:79, 1973.

1699
HOLZER, J., J.S. KARLINER, A. O'ROURKE, W. PITT, AND J. ROSS, JR.
Effectiveness of dopamine in patients with cardiogenic shock.
American Journal Cardiology 32:79, 1973.

1700
HOLZMANN, M.
New paths in electrocardiographic diagnosis by means of potential recordings from the bundle of His and by pacing.
Schweizerische Medizinische Wochenschrift 102(43):1529-1534, 1972.

1701
HONEYMAN, M.S., ET AL.
Psychological impact of heart disease in the family of the patient.
Psychosomatics 9:34-37, 1968.

1702
HOOD, W.P., JR.
  And the rhythms and combinations are somewhat different when there's no infarction in the background.
  Emergency Medicine 5:32, 1973.

1703
HOPEWELL, W.S.
  Postprandial T-wave changes. Relationship to serum potassium, age, and exercise electrocardiograms.
  Journal Medical Society New Jersey 70(1):39-42, 1973.

1704
HORAN, L.G., N.C. FLOWERS, AND C.B. MILLER.
  A rapid assay of dipolar and extradipolar content in the human electrocardiogram.
  Journal Electrocardiology 5(3):211-223, 1972.

1705
HORGAN, J.H.
  Rehabilitation after myocardial infarction.
  Journal Irish Medical Association 66(23):661-64, 1973.

1706
HORNBAKER, J.H., JR., J.O. HUMPHRIES, AND R.S. ROSS.
  Permanent pacing in the absence of heart block. An approach to the management of intractable arrhythmias.
  Circulation 39(2):189-196, 1969.

1707
HORNSTEN, T.R., AND R.A. BRUCE.
  Stress testing, safety precautions, and cardiovascular health.
  Journal Occupational Medicine 10(11):640-648, 1968.

1708
HORNSTEN, T.R., AND R.A. BRUCE.
  Effects of atrial fibrillation on exercise performance in patients with cardiac disease.
  Circulation 37(4):543-548, 1968.

1709
HORNSTEN, T.R., AND R.A. BRUCE.
  Sustained altered intraventricular conduction during exercise.
  Circulation 37-38(Suppl. 6):102, 1968.

1710
HORNSTEN, T.R., AND R.A. BRUCE.
  Computer analysis of ST responses to submaximal exercise.
  Circulation 37-38(Suppl. 6):102, 1968.

1711
HORNSTEN, T.R., AND R.A. BRUCE.
  Computed ST forces of Frank and bipolar exercise electrocardiograms.
  American Heart Journal 78(3):346-357, 1969.

1712
HORVATH, M., T. DEBROCZI, AND K. LUDVIGH.
Complex cardiorespiratory investigations with minimal ergometric load for screening of patients in cardiac rehabilitation.
Acta Medica Academiae Scientiarum Hungaricae 28(1):37-46, 1971.

1713
HORVATH, S.M.
The physiological stimuli to training in a normal climate.
Canadian Medical Association Journal 96:791-793, 1967.

1714
HORWITZ, D., S.M. FOX, III, AND L.I. GOLDBERG.
Cardiovascular effects of a naturally occurring catecholamine, dopamine, in man.
Clinical Research 8(2):184, 1960.

1715
HOSONO, K.
Prognosis and rehabilitation of myocardial infarction.
Naika, 21:463-471, 1968.

1716
HOWARD, D., C.I. SMITH, G. STEWART, M. VADAS, ET AL.
A prospective survey of the incidence of cardiac intoxication with digitalis in patients being admitted to hospital and correlation with serum digoxin levels.
Australian New Zealand Journal Medicine 3:279, 1973.

1717
HOWARD, E.J.
Chronic atrial fibrillation unrelated to organic heart disease. Follow-up study of five cases.
American Heart Journal 59(3):343-346, 1960.

1718
HOWARD, J., AND B.L. HOLMAN
The effects of race and occupation on hypertension mortality.
Milbank Memorial Fund Quarterly 48(3):263-296, 1970.

1719
HOWARD, J.C., JR.
Psychotropic agents in the coronary patient: What and when.
Psychosomatics 11:335-338, 1970.

1720
HOWELL, M.L., AND R.B. ALDERMAN.
Psychological determinants of fitness.
Canadian Medical Association Journal 96:721-726, 1967.

1721
HOWELL, R.W., AND S. CROWN.
Sickness absence levels and personality inventory scores.
British Journal Industrial Medicine 28(2):126-130, 1971.

1722
HOYT, W.F.
Retinal ischemic symptoms in cardiovascular diagnosis.
Postgraduate Medicine 52(4):85-90, 1972.

1723
HRUBEC, Z., AND W.J. ZUKEL.
Socioeconomic differentials in prognosis following episodes of coronary heart disease.
Journal Chronic Diseases 23:881-889, 1971.

1724
HUBNER, P.J.B., G.M. ZLADY, G.K. LANE, T. HARDARSON, ET AL.
Double-blind trial of propranolol and practolol in hypertrophic cardiomyopathy.
British Heart Journal 35:1116, 1973.

1725
HUEBSCHMANN, H.
On anxiety and compulsive symptoms in patients with heart infarct.
Medizinische Klinik 59:893-894, 1964.

1726
HUEBSCHMANN, H.
Risk situations for cardiac infarction.
Verhandlungen der Deutschen Gessellshaft für innere Medizin 77:867-869, 1971.

1727
HUEP, W.W.
The reaction of Bendigon as dependent on hemodynamics.
Herz/Kreislauf 5:296, 1973.

1728
HUGUES, F.C., D. JULIEN, B. AUFAUVRE, AND J. MARCHE.
Clinical pharmacology of β-adrenergic agonists and antagonists. 2. Adrenergic drugs: the tests with propranolol and terbutaline.
Coeur et Médecine Interne 12:417-423, 1973.

1729
HULL, R., L. BJORK, I. CULLHED, AND T. LONNERHOLM.
Clinical and radiological signs of left ventricular failure in acute myocardial infarction.
Acta Medica Scandinavica 192(3):189-196, 1972.

1730
HULTMAN, E.
Physiological role of muscle glycogen in man with special reference to exercise.
Circulation Research 20(Suppl. 1):99-114, 1967.

1731
HULTMAN, E., J. BERGSTROM, AND A.E. ROCH-NORLUND.
Glycogen storage in human skeletal muscle.
In: Pernow, B. and B. Saltin, Eds. Muscle metabolism during exercise, pp. 273-288. New York, Plenum Press, 1971.

1732
HULTMAN, E., AND N.H. NILSSON.
Liver glycogen in man. Effect of different diets and muscular exercise.
In: Pernow, B. and B. Saltin, Eds. Muscle metabolism during exercise, pp. 143-151. New York, Plenum Press, 1971.

1733
HUME, R., AND M. GEOGHEGAN.
Fibrinolytic activity in patients receiving long-term anticoagulants for myocardial infarction.
Scottish Medical Journal 11(4):128-131, 1966.

1734
HUNTINGTON, C.S., AND W.B. THOMPSON.
Effect of employment on heart disease.
Circulation 24(4 Part 2):962, 1961.

1735
HUPKA, K.
Rehabilitation of patients following myocardial infarction.
Medizinische Welt 21:1181-1182, 1966.

1736
HURZELER, P.A., AND L.R. ZOHMAN.
Practical considerations concerning exercise ECG telemetry equipment.
Medical Research Engineering 10(5):14-18, 1971.

1737
HUTTER, A.M.
Shorter hospitalization for myocardial infarcts.
New England Journal Medicine 289:805, 1973.

1738
HUTTER, A.M., JR., V.W. SIDEL, K.I. SHINE, AND R.W. DE SANCTIS.
Early hospital discharge after myocardial infarction.
New England Journal Medicine 288(22):1141, 1973.

1739
HUTTON, I., A.R. LORIMER, W.S. HILLIS, ET AL.
Haemodynamics and myocardial function after sotalol.
British Heart Journal 34(8):787-790, 1972.

1740
HYATT, K.H., R.W. SULLIVAN, W.R., SPEARS, AND W.R. VETTER.
A study of ventricular contractility and other parameters possibly related to vasodepressor syncope.
NASA CR-128968. Springfield, Va. National Technical Service, 1973.

1741
IATRIDIS, S.G., AND J.H. FERGUSON.
Effect of physical exercise on blood clotting and fibrinolysis.
Journal Applied Physiology 18(2):337-344, 1963.

1742
IBRAHIM, M.A., ET AL.
Personality traits and coronary heart disease. Utilization of a cross-sectional study design to test whether a selected psychological profile precedes or follows manifest coronary heart disease.
Journal Chronic Diseases 19:255-271, 1966.

1743
IBRAHIM, M.A., ET AL.
Psychological patterns and coronary heart disease: An appraisal of the determination of etiology by means of a stochastic process.
Journal Chronic Diseases 20:931-940, 1968.

1744
IBRAHIM, M., M. SILIE, J.P. DELAHAYE, AND R. FROMENT.
Systolic time intervals in valvular aortic stenosis and idiopathic hypertrophic subaortic stenosis.
British Heart Journal 35(3):276-283, 1973.

1745
IDA, M., Y. TAKAHASHI, AND C. KEIHARA.
Psychosomatic correlations in hypotension.
Journal Japanese Psychosomatic Society 12:314-315, 1972.

1746
IIMURA, O., AND M. MIYAHARA.
Ischemic heart disease and catecholamines.
Japanese Circulation Journal 35:973-978, 1971.

1747
IKKALA, E., G. MYLLYLÄ, AND H.S. SARAJAS.
Platelet adhesiveness and ADP induced platelet aggregation in exercise.
Annales Medicinae Experimentalis et Biologiae Fenniae 44:88-92, 1966.

1748
IKKALA, E., G. MYLLYLÄ, AND H.S.S. SARAJAS.
Hemostatic effect of short term muscular exercise in man.
In: Karvonen, M.J. and A.J. Barry, Eds. Physical activity and the heart, pp. 200-207. Springfield, Ill. Thomas, 1967.

1749
IKKOS, D., AND J.S. HANSON.
Response to exercise in congenital, complete atrioventricular block.
Circulation 22:583, 1960.

1750
ILMURZYNSKA, K., AND J. KOMPIEL.
Diagnostic significance of mitral ultrasonography in hypertrophic stenosing cardiomyopathy.
Polski Tygodnik Lekarski 27(30):1156-1158, 1972.

1751
IMPARATO, A.M., AND G.E. KIM.
Electrode complications in patients with permanent cardiac pacemakers.
Archives Surgery 105:705, 1972.

1752
IMURA, N., ET AL.
Population survey on cerebrovascular and cardiovascular diseases: The ten years experience in the farming village of Tanushimaru and the fishing village of Ushibuka.
Japanese Heart Journal 13(2):118-127, 1972.

1753
INAMA, K.
Therapy in the high mountains for diseases of heart and circulation especially in hypertonia and myocardial infarction.
Zeitschrift für Physiotherapie 23(3):220, 1971.

1754
INGRAM, G.I.C., AND J. RICHARDSON.
Anticoagulant prophylaxis and treatment: The new emphasis in management.
Springfield, Ill. Thomas, 1965.

1755
IONESCU, V.
Cardiovascular disorders and the borderland between the pathologic and the normal.
Bucuresti, Romania. Editura Academia RSR, 1972.

1756
IRISAWA, H., AND I. SEYAMA.
The configuration of the P wave during mild exercise.
American Heart Journal 71:467, 1966.

1757
IRISAWA, H., A. IRISAWA, AND N. SHIGETO.
Physiological and morphological correlation of the functional syncytium in the bivalve myocardium.
Comparative Biochemistry and Physiology A: Comparative Physiology 44:207, 1972.

1758
IRVINE, R.O.H., AND J.W. DOW.
Potassium depletion: effects on intracellular pH and electrolyte distribution in skeletal and cardiac muscle.
Australasian Annals Medicine 17:206-213, 1968.

1759
ISAACS, J.H., M. WILBURNE, H. MILLS, AND R. KUHN.
Vector-electrocardiographic exercise test in ischemic heart disease. A more objective measure of exercise tolerance.
Journal American Medical Association 198(10):1065-1070, 1966.

1760
ISERI, L.T., E.L. BALATONY, J.R. EVANS, AND M.G. CRANE.
Pathogenesis of congestive heart failure. Effect of posture and exercise on plasma volume and plasma constituents.
Annals Internal Medicine 55(3):384-394, 1961.

1761
ISHII, Y.
  Measurement of myocardial blood flow by means of external counting method using 86-Rubidium.
  Japanese Circulation Journal 37:163, 1973.

1762
ISHIKAWA, H., I. TAWARA, H. OHTSUKA, M. TAKEYAMA, AND T. KOBAYASHI.
  Psychosomatic study of angina pectoris.
  Psychosomatics 12(6):390-397, 1971.

1763
ISHIKAWA, K., P.M. KINI, AND H.V. PIPBERGER.
  P wave analysis in 2464 orthogonal electrocardiograms from normal subjects and patients with atrial overload.
  Circulation 48:565-574, 1973.

1764
ISHIKO, T.
  Aerobic capacity and external criteria of performance.
  Canadian Medical Association Journal 96:746-750, 1967.

1765
ISHISE, S., K. MORI, S. KAWASAKI, T. FUNATSU, ET AL.
  Influence of exercise on hemodynamics in patients with ischemic heart disease. 2.
  Japanese Circulation Journal 37(8):902-903, 1973.

1766
ISOM, O.W., N.D. KUTIN, E.A. FALK, AND F.C. SPENCER.
  Patterns of myocardial metabolism during cardiopulmonary bypass and coronary perfusion.
  Journal Thoracic Cardiovascular Surgery 66:705, 1973.

1767
ISRAEL, S.
  Traditional standards in present day medicine.
  Medizin und Sport 12(4):114-119, 1972.

1768
ISRAEL, S., AND E. KOHLER.
  The diagnostic value of the quotients of heart rate/systolic blood pressure ratio in graduated exercises.
  Medizin und Sport 12(10):301-304, 1972.

1769
ITASAKA, Y.
  Plasma renin activity in hypertensive diseases.
  Nagoya Journal Medical Science 33(1):31-45, 1970.

1770
IYENGAR, S.R.K., S. RAMCHAND, E.J.P. CHARRETTE, C.K.S. IYENGAR, AND R.B. LYNN.
  Anoxic cardiac arrest: an experimental and clinical study of its effects. Part 1.
  Journal Thoracic Cardiovascular Surgery 66:722, 1973.

1771
JACHUCK, S.J.
    Implanted pacemaker induced dysrhythmia and its management.
    Postgraduate Medical Journal 49:14-17, 1973.

1772
JACKSON, D.H.
    Isometric (Dynamometer) stress testing in coronary heart disease.
    Alabama Journal Medical Sciences 7(3):310-312, 1970.

1773
JACKSON, F.W.
    Cardiac rehabilitation—an alternative approach.
    Pennsylvania Medicine 76:41, 1973.

1774
JACOBS, C.F., AND B.A. LANGDOC.
    Cardiovascular deaths and air pollution in Charleston, S.C.
    Health Service Reports 87(7):623-632, 1972.

1775
JACOBS, D.
    The aetiology and possible prevention of myocardial infarction.
    South African Medical Journal 45(11):275-279, 1971.

1776
JACOBSON, L.B.
    Sinoventricular conduction during atrial arrest.
    Journal Electrocardiology 5(4):385-389, 1972.

1777
JAEGER, M.
    The place of effort tests in cardiovascular diagnosis.
    Schweizerische Zeitschrift für Sportmedizin 20:51, 1972.

1778
JAKUBIK, A.
    Personality of patients with congenital and acquired heart disease.
    Polski Tygodnik Lekarski 26:1039-1041, 1971.

1779
JAKUBIK, A.
    Psychiatric symptoms related to cardiac surgery.
    Kardiologia Polska 16:29-33, 1973.

1780
JAMES, T.N.
    Observations on the cardiovascular involvement, including the cardiac conduction system, in
    progressive muscular dystrophy.
    American Heart Journal 63:48, 1962.

1781
JAMES, T.N.
Arrhythmias and conduction disturbances in acute myocardial infarction.
American Heart Journal 64:416, 1969.

1782
JAMES, T.N.
Order and disorder in the rhythm of the heart. The fifth annual George C. Griffith lecture.
Circulation 47:362-386, 1973.

1783
JAMES, T.N., AND R.E. BIRK.
Pathology of the cardiac conduction system in polyarteritis nodosa.
Archives Internal Medicine 117:561, 1966.

1784
JAMES, T.N., P. FROGGATT, AND T.K. MARSHALL.
Sudden death in young athletes.
Annals Internal Medicine 67:1013, 1967.

1785
JAMES, T.N., AND E.W. REYNOLDS, JR.
Pathology of the cardiac conduction system in a case of diphtheria associated with atrial arrhythmias and heart block.
Circulation 28:263, 1963.

1786
JANKOWSKI, L.W., R.J. FERGUSON, M. LANGELIER, ET AL.
Accuracy of methods for estimating O_2 cost of walking in coronary patients.
Journal Applied Physiology 33(5):672-673, 1972.

1787
JANTSCH, H., J. KRENN, AND M. RADI.
Severe burns at the sites of ECG monitoring electrodes after the use of surgical high frequency apparatus.
Anaesthesist 21(11):482-484, 1972.

1788
JANUSHKEVICHIUS, Z.I., YU. I. BREDEKIS, E.D. RIMSHA, A.S. DUMCHIUS, AND A.V. NORKUS.
Changes in haemodynamics and in myocardial contractile function in patients under paired electric stimulation of heart.
Cor Vasa 13(3):186-193, 1971.

1789
JARLOV, A.L., AND P.M. HOLMKJAER.
A dye densitometer for measuring cardiac output.
Medical Biological Engineering 10:97-100, 1972.

1790
JEFFERSON, G.E.
The social complex.
Journal Rehabilitation 32:59-60, 1966.

1791
JEFFREY, F.E., K. FAREEDUDDIN, AND W.H. ABELMANN.
Increased tolerance of orthostatic stress and resistance to bed rest deconditioning in heart failure.
Clinical Research 17(2):218, 1969.

1792
JELLIFFE, R.W.
Computer-assisted digitalis dosage programs.
Clinical Research 17(2):248, 1969.

1793
JENKINS, C.D.
Psychologic and social precursors of coronary disease. I.
New England Journal Medicine 284(5):244-255, 1971.

1794
JENKINS, C.D.
Psychologic and social precursors of coronary disease. II.
New England Journal Medicine 284(6):307-317, 1971.

1795
JENKINS, C.D., R. H. ROSEMAN, AND S.J. ZYZANSKI.
Cigarette smoking. Its relationship to coronary heart disease and related risk factors in the Western Collaborative Group Study.
Circulation 38:1140, 1968.

1796
JENKINS, C.D., S.J. ZYZANSKI, AND R.H. ROSENMAN.
Progress toward validation of a computer-scored test for the Type A coronary-prone behavior pattern.
Psychosomatic Medicine 33(3):193-202, 1971.

1797
JENKINS, C.D., S.J. ZYZANSKI, R.H. ROSENMAN, AND G.L. CLEVELAND.
Association of coronary-prone behavior scores with recurrence of coronary heart disease.
Journal Chronic Diseases 24:601-611, 1971.

1798
JENKINS, D.H.R., A. MacLEOD, AND S. MacKAY.
The electrocardiogram in swimmers.
Journal Sport Medicine 12:246, 1972.

1799
JENKINS, R.B., S.H. MENDELSON, S. LAMID, AND H.L. KLAWANS.
Levodopa therapy of patients with Parkinsonism and heart disease.
British Medical Journal 3:512-514, 1972.

1800
JENSEN, G., AND B. SIGURD.
Systemic Lupus Erythematosus and acute myocardial infarction.
Chest 64:653, 1973.

1801
JESCHKE, D.
  Rehabilitation of patients with internal diseases by means of physical training with special reference to heart and circulatory diseases.
  Medizinische Welt 35:1822-1829, 1968.

1802
JESCHKE, D., K. CAESAR, AND R. HAASIS.
  Behavior of the maximal pulse frequency in cardiac infarct patients under early regulated physical load: early mobilization.
  Medizinische Welt 23:1135, 1972.

1803
JESSE, M.J., C. HENNEKEN, AND C. FERRER.
  Risk factors in progeny of parents with premature myocardial infarction.
  Circulation 48(4):24, 1973.

1804
JEWITT, D.E., R. BALCON, E.B. RAFTERY, AND S. ORAM.
  Incidence and management of supraventricular arrhythmias after acute myocardial infarction.
  Lancet 7519:734-739, 1967.

1805
JEWITT, D.E., Y. KISHON, M. THOMAS, AND J.P. SHILLINGFORD.
  Lignocaine in management of arrhythmias following acute myocardial infarction.
  British Heart Journal 30(3):427, 1968.

1806
JEWITT, D.E., AND E.B. RAFTERY.
  Incidence and management of supraventricular arrhythmias after acute myocardial infarction.
  American Heart Journal 77(2):290-293, 1969.

1807
JEZEK, V., AND F. SCHRIJEN.
  Effect of exercise on the pulmonary vascular bed.
  Scandinavian Journal Respiratory Disease 52(Suppl. 77):89, 1971.

1808
JEZER, A.
  The workshop in the coronary spectrum.
  Journal Rehabilitation 32:68, 1966.

1809
JICK, H., O.S. MIETTINEN, R.K. NEFF, S. SHAPIRO, O.P. HEINONEN, AND D. SLONE.
  Coffee and myocardial infarction.
  New England Journal Medicine 289:63, 1973.

1810
JIPP, P., M. SCHLAAK, H. GRUNWALD, AND F. SCHAEFER.
  Glucose tolerance and arteriosclerosis.
  Medizinische Klinik 66:1738-1743, 1971.

1811
JOHANNSEN, W.J., G.A. HELLMUTH, AND T. SORAUF.
On accepting medical recommendations. Experiences with patients in a cardiac work classification unit.
Archives Environmental Health 12:63-69, 1966.

1812
JOHNSON, B.C., F.H. EPSTEIN, AND M.O. KJELSBERG.
Distributions and familial studies of blood pressure and serum cholesterol levels in a total community—Tecumseh, Michigan.
Journal Chronic Diseases 18:147, 1965.

1813
JOHNSON, L.C., G. FISHER, L.J. SILVESTER, AND C.C. HOFHEINS.
Anabolic steroid: effects on strength, body weight, oxygen uptake and spermatogenesis upon mature males.
Medicine Science Sports 4:43-45, 1972.

1814
JOHNSON, M.L., J.H. HOLMES, R.D. SPRANGLER, AND B.C. PATON.
Usefulness of echocardiography in patients undergoing mitral valve surgery.
Journal Thoracic Cardiovascular Surgery 64(6):922-934, 1972.

1815
JOHNSON, P.C., R.J. KELLY, W.L. SMITH, A.D. LeBLANC, AND L.E. LAMB.
Cardiac output and coronary blood flow in steady state exercise during steady state hypoxia.
Aerospace Medicine 41(1):12-15, 1970.

1816
JOHNSON, R., J.C. VERGRIETE, AND J. TREMBLAY.
Automatic analysis of electrocardiograms and vectorcardiograms.
L'Union Médicale du Canada 100:1935-1942, 1971.

1817
JOHNSON, R.H., J.L. WALTON, H. KREBS, AND D.H. WILLIAMSON.
Metabolic fuels during and after severe exercise in athletes and nonathletes.
Lancet 2:452, 1969.

1818
JOHNSON, W.P., AND J.A. GROVER.
Hemodynamic and metabolic effects of physical training in four patients with essential hypertension.
Canadian Medical Association Journal 96:842-847, 1967.

1819
JOHNSON, W.P., AND J.W. JONES.
Hemodynamic and oxygen transport responses to exercise in hypertensive and normotensive age peers: Effects on hypotensive drug treatments.
American Journal Medical Sciences 253(2):180-193, 1967.

1820
JOHNSTON, C.I., N.B. PINKUS, AND M. DOWN.
Plasma digoxin levels in digitalized and toxic patients.
Medical Journal Australia 1(17):863-866, 1972.

1821
JOKL, E.
Sudden death after exercise due to myocarditis.
In: Jokl, E. and J.T. McClellan, Eds. Medicine and Sport 5:99-110. Basel, Karger, 1971.

1822
JOKL, E.
Sudden death during exercise due to congenital anomaly of aortic valve.
In: Jokl E. and J.T. McClellan, Eds. Medicine and Sport 5:148-149. Basel, Karger, 1971.

1823
JOKL, E., AND E.H. CLUVER.
Sudden death of a rugby international after a test game.
In: Jokl E. and J.T. McClellan, Eds. Medicine and Sport 5:153-158. Basel, Karger, 1971.

1824
JOKL, E., AND J. GREENSTEIN.
Fatal coronary sclerosis in a boy of ten years.
In: Jokl, E. and J.T. McClellan, Eds. Medicine and Sport 5:64-66. Basel, Karger, 1971.

1825
JOKL, E., AND P. JOKL.
Exercise and altitude.
Medicine and Sport, vol. 1. Basel, Switzerland. S. Karger, 1968.

1826
JOKL, E., AND R.H. MACKINTOSH.
Sudden death of young athlete from rupture of ascending aorta.
In: Jokl, E. and J.T. McClellan, Eds. Medicine and Sport 5:150-152. Basel, Karger, 1971.

1827
JOKL, E., AND J.T. McCLELLAN.
Exercise and cardiac death.
Journal American Medical Association 213(9):1489-1491, 1970.

1828
JOKL, E., AND J.T. McCLELLAN, EDS.
Exercise and cardiac death.
Medicine and Sport, vol. 5. Baltimore, University Park Press, 1971.

1829
JOKL, E., AND T.J. McCLELLAN.
Asymptomatic cardiac disease causing sudden death in association with physical activity.
In: Jokl, E. and J.T. McClellan, Eds. Medicine and Sport 5:1-4. Basel, Karger, 1971.

1830
JOKL, E., AND J.T. McCLELLAN.
Sudden cardiac death of pilots in flight.
In: Jokl, E. AND J.T. McClellan, Eds. Medicine and Sport 5:25-63. Basel, Karger, 1971.

1831
JOKL, E., AND J.T. McCLELLAN.
Sudden cardiac arrest during sports.
Medizinische Welt 22(8):296-298, 1971.

1832
JOKL, E., AND L. MELZER.
   Acute fatal nontraumatic collapse during work and sport.
   In: Jokl, E. and J.T. McClellan, Eds. Medicine and Sport 5:5-18. Basel, Karger, 1971.

1833
JOKL, E., AND B. NEWMAN.
   Death of a wrestler.
   In: Jokl, E. and J.T. McClellan, Eds. Medicine and Sport 5:81-90. Basel, Karger, 1971.

1834
JOKL, E., AND M.M. SUZMAN.
   Mechanisms involved in acute fatal nontraumatic collapse associated with physical exertion.
   In: Jokl, E. and J.T. McClellan, Eds. Medicine and Sport 5:19-24. Basel, Karger, 1971.

1835
JONCKHEERE, P.
   The chronic headache patient: A psychodynamic study of 30 cases, compared with cardiovascular patients.
   Psychotherapy Psychosomatics 19(1/2):53-61, 1971.

1836
JONES, J.H., M. BATEMAN, C. CHLOUVERAKIS, J. GLOSTER, AND P. HARRIS.
   Myocardial metabolism at rest and during exercise in patients with rheumatic heart disease.
   British Heart Journal 24(6):792, 1962.

1837
JONES, R.H., D.C. SABISTON, JR., B.B. BATES, ET AL.
   Quantitative radionuclide angiocardiography for determination of chamber to chamber cardiac transit times.
   American Journal Cardiology 30(8):855-864, 1972.

1838
JONES, R.S.
   Significance of effect of beta blockade on ventilatory function in normal and asthmatic subjects.
   Thorax 27(5):572-576, 1972.

1839
JONES, W.B., AND T.J. REEVES.
   Total cardiac output response during four minutes of exercise.
   American Heart Journal 76(2):209-216, 1968.

1840
JONSSON, B., AND M. LUKIANSKI.
   Systemic arterial pressure during exercise in patients with pulmonary hypertension.
   Acta Medica Scandinavica 173(1):73-81, 1963.

1841
JOOSSENS, J.V.
   Salt and hypertension, water hardness and cardiovascular death rate.
   Triangle 12(1):9-16, 1973.

1842
JOSEPHSON, M.E., A.R. CARACTA, S.H. LAU, ET AL.
Effects of lidocaine on refractory periods in man.
American Heart Journal 84(6):778-786, 1972.

1843
JOSEPHSON, M.E., A.R. CARACTA, J.J. GALLAGHER, AND A.N. DAMATO.
Site of conduction disturbances in a family with myotonic dystrophy.
American Journal Cardiology 32:114, 1973.

1844
JOSHPE, G., A. TOPILOW, B. LEVITT, ET AL.
Recurrent ventricular fibrillation. Treated with countershocks, bretylium tosylate, and rapid cardiac pacing.
New York State Journal Medicine 72(21):2659-2663, 1972.

1845
JOSTEN, J.
Emotional adaptation of cardiac patients.
Scandinavian Journal Rehabilitation Medicine 2-3:49-52, 1970.

1846
JOUANNOT, P., AND P.Y. HATT.
Rehabilitation of cardiac patients principles and practical applications.
Nouvelle Presse Médicale 1:2667-2669, 1972.

1847
JOUVE, A.
The place of psychosomatic medicine in cardiology.
Coeur et Médecine Interne 7(2):327-331, 1968.

1848
JOUVE, A.
The place of psychic factors in the arrhythmias.
Gazzetta Italiana di Cardiologia 2:155-156, 1972.

1849
JOUVE, A., F. PRUDHOMME, J.A. TRIGANO, AND J. TORRESAN.
Is anticoagulant treatment justified on myocardial infarction.
Revue du Praticien 23:5433, 1973.

1850
JUDD, W.T., AND J.L. POLAND.
Myocardial glycogen changes with exercise.
Proceedings Society Experimental Biology Medicine 140(3):955-957, 1972.

1851
JULIUS, S., A. AMERY, AND J. CONWAY.
Blood pressure response to exercise.
Federation Proceedings 25(No. 2 Part 1):393, 1966.

1852
JULIUS, S., A. AMERY, AND J. CONWAY.
Hemodynamic response to exercise in hypertension.
Clinical Research 14(2):251, 1966.

1853
JULIUS, S., A. AMERY, L.S. WHITLOCK, ET AL.
Influence of age on the hemodynamic response to exercise.
Circulation 36:222-230, 1967.

1854
JUNGE-HUELSING, G.
Stress, especially social stress as cause of myocardial infarction.
Therapiewoche 22:3702-3713, 1972.

1855
JUNGMANN, H., AND G. STEIN.
Telemetric ECG studies on infarction patients during cold exposure.
International Journal Biometeorology 16(4):403-408, 1972.

1856
JUNGMANN, H., AND G. STEIN.
Rehabilitation following myocardial infarction.
Arbeitsmedizin Sozialmedizin Arbeitshygiene 7(3):63-67, 1972.

1857
JURCISIN, G.
Physical reconditioning for a Spanish-American war veteran with cardiovascular disease.
Journal American Geriatric Society 14(7):762-767, 1966.

1858
KAHLER, R.L., T.E. GAFFNEY, AND E. BRAUNWALD.
The effects of autonomic nervous system inhibition on the circulatory response to muscular exercise.
Journal Clinical Investigation 41:1981, 1962.

1859
KAHLER, R.L., R.H. THOMPSON, R.E. BUSKIRK, R.L. FRYE AND E. BRAUNWALD.
Reduction of the postexercise oxygen debt by digitalis administration in patients with cardiac disease without heart failure.
Circulation 26(4 Part 2):739, 1962.

1860
KAHLER, R.L., R.H. THOMPSON, R.E. BUSKIRK, R.L. FRYE, AND E. BRAUNWALD.
Studies on digitalis. VI. Reduction of the oxygen debt after exercise digoxin in cardiac patients without heart failure.
Circulation 27:397, 1963.

1861
KAHN, A., Jr.
Hyperlidemia. The coronary problem.
Journal Arkansas Medical Society 70(4):143, 1973.

1862
KAHN, H.A.
The relationship of reported coronary heart disease mortality to physical activity of work.
American Journal Public Health 53:1058, 1963.

1863
KAHN, H.A., J.H. MEDALIE, H.N. NEUFELD, ET AL.
The incidence of hypertension and associated factors: The Israel ischemic heart disease study.
American Heart Journal 84(2):181-182, 1972.

1864
KAJIHARA, T.
A psychosomatic study on acute cardiac deaths.
Journal Japanese Psychosomatic Society 12:310, 1972.

1865
KALMANSON, D.
Venous return, and right heart haemodynamics. II. Bloodflow across the right atrium and the tricuspid valve. Recent data and new concepts.
Nouvelle Presse Médicale 1(23):1569-1572, 1972.

1866
KALTENBACH, M., P. LICHTLEN, AND G.C. FRIESINGER.
Coronary heart disease. Proceedings of the second international symposium. Frankfurt am Main, West Germany, June 1972.
Stuttgart, Georg Thieme Verlag, 1973.

1867
KALTENBACH, M., H. MUELLER, W. ORTMANNS, AND J. VON SCHMIDT.
Have psychotropic drugs a cardiotoxic effect? Investigations on the question of medically caused exercise cardiac insufficiency.
Deutsche Medizinische Wochenschrift 95(44):2214-2217, 1970.

1868
KALTENBACH, M., T. TIEDEMANN, AND W. SCHELLBORN.
The effect of five different long acting nitroglycerin derivatives on angina pectoris.
Deutsche Medizinische Wochenschrift 97:1479, 1972.

1869
KAMENKER, S.M., AND A.S. MELIK-AKHNAZOROV.
Changes of cardiac output after physical exercise in patients with cardiac insufficiency.
Terapevticheskii Arkhiv 39:87-90, 1967.

1870
KAMON, E., K.F. METZ, AND K.B. PANDOLF.
Climbing and cycling with additional weights on the extremities.
Journal Applied Physiology 35:367-370, 1973.

1871
KAMPMEIER, R.H.
Coronary disease—Its emotional impact.
Southern Medical Journal 60:75-76, 1967.

1872
KANNEL, W.B.
   Habitual level of physical activity and risk of coronary heart disease: The Framingham study.
   Canadian Medical Association Journal 96:811-812, 1967.

1873
KANNEL, W.B.
   Habits and heart disease.
   In: Palmore, E. and F.C. Jeffers, Eds. Prediction of life span, recent finding. Lexington, Mass.
   D.C. Heath, 1971.

1874
KANNEL, W.B., W.P. CASTELLI, T. GORDON, AND P.M. MCNAMARA.
   Serum cholesterol, lipoproteins, and the risk of coronary heart disease: The Framingham study.
   Annals Internal Medicine 74:1, 1971.

1875
KANNEL, W.B., W.P. CASTELLI, P.M. MCNAMARA, ET AL.
   Role of blood pressure in the development of congestive heart failure. The Framingham study.
   New England Journal Medicine 287(16):781-787, 1972.

1876
KANNEL, W.B., T.R. DAWBER, G.D. FRIEDMAN, W.E. GLENNON, AND P.M. MCNAMARA.
   Risk factors in coronary heart disease. An evaluation of several serum lipids as predictors of
   coronary heart disease.
   Annals Internal Medicine 61:888, 1964.

1877
KANNEL, W.B., AND M. FEINLEIB.
   Natural history of angina pectoris in the Framingham study.
   American Journal Cardiology 29:154, 1972.

1878
KANNEL, W.B., AND T. GORDON, EDS.
   The Framingham Study: An epidemiological investigation of cardiovascular disease.
   Washington, D.C. U.S. Government Printing Office, 1968.
   Section 24: Diet and the regulation of serum cholesterol. April 1970.
   Section 26: Some characteristics related to the incidence of cardiovascular disease and death.
   December 1970.
   Section 27: Coronary heart disease, atherothrombotic brain infarction, intermittent claudication—a
   multivariate analysis of some factors related to their incidence. May 1971.

1879
KANNEL, W.B., T. GORDON, W.P. CASTELLI, AND J.R. MARGOLIS.
   Electrocardiographic left ventricular hypertrophy and risk of coronary heart disease: The
   Framingham study.
   Annals Internal Medicine 72:813, 1970.

1880
KANNEL, W., A. KAGAN, T.R. DAWBER, AND N. REVOTSKIE.
   Epidemiology of coronary heart disease.
   Geriatrics 17:675, 1962.

1881
KANNEL, W.B., AND P.M. McNAMARA.
   Serum lipid fractions and risk of coronary heart disease: The Framingham study.
   Minnesota Medicine 52:1225, 1969.

1882
KANNEL, W.B., P. SORLIE, AND P. McNAMARA.
   The relation of physical activity to risk of coronary heart disease: The Framingham study.
   In: Larsen, O.A. and R.O. Malmborg, Eds. Coronary heart disease and physical fitness, pp.
   256-260. Baltimore, University Park Press, 1971.

1883
KANTROWITZ, A., AND A.R. KANTROWITZ.
   Design criteria for heart assistance devices.
   In: Segal, B.L. and D.G. Kilpatrick, Eds. Engineering in the Practice of Medicine. Baltimore,
   Williams and Wilkins, 1967.

1884
KAPLAN, B.H., J.C. CASSEL, H.A. TYROLER, J.C. CORNONI, D.G. KLEINBAUM, AND C.C.
   HAMES.
   Occupational mobility and coronary heart disease.
   Archives Internal Medicine 128(6):938-942, 1971.

1885
KAPLAN, M.A., R.E. GRAY, AND L.T. ISERI.
   Hemodynamic and metabolic responses to exercise in atrial fibrillation and sinus rhythm.
   Clinical Research 14(1):125, 1966.

1886
KAPLAN, M.A., C.N. HARRIS, W.S. ARONOW, D.P. PARKER, AND M.H. ELLESTAD.
   Inability of the submaximal treadmill stress test to predict the location of coronary disease.
   Circulation 47:250, 1973.

1887
KAPLAN, S.M.
   Psychosomatic aspects of cardiovascular disease.
   Postgraduate Medicine 47(5):128-132, 1970.

1888
KARAMYCSHEVS, F.I.
   Occupational activity in patients who have had myocardial infarction.
   Klinische Medizin 50:32-36, 1972.

1889
KARDASH, V.A.
   Cardiovascular pathology of Byelorussian railroad workers.
   Zdravookhranenie Belorusskii 18:33-34, 1972.

1890
KARIV, I., AND J.J. KELLERMANN.
   Rehabilitation of cardiac patients under medical supervision. Proceedings of the 9th international
   congress Life Assurance Medicine.
   Tel-Aviv, Israel. March 27-30, 1967.

1891
KARIV, I., AND J.J. KELLERMANN.
Effects of exercise on blood pressure.
Malattie Cardiovascolari 10(1-2):247-252, 1969.

1892
KARIV, I., B. KREISLER, AND S. BEHAR.
Repetitive tachycardia: Effects of exercise tests and amyl nitrite.
British Heart Journal 33(1):115-119, 1971.

1893
KARLINER, J.S., AND J. ROSS, JR.
Evaluation of myocardial contractility in man.
Gazzetta Italiana di Cardiologia 2(5):595-603, 1972.

1894
KARNAFEL, W.
Transient rheoangiographic changes in the forearms in attacks of anginal pain.
Angiologica 9(2):89-91, 1972.

1895
KARNEGIS, J.N.
Experience with the coronary artery bypass graft in a community hospital.
American Heart Journal 86:51, 1973.

1896
KARPATI, P., AND A. ARSANYI.
Normalization of the metabolic acidosis: one of the conditions of successful defibrillation.
Magyar Belorvosi Archiwum 25(5):254-257, 1972.

1897
KARPMAN, V.L., AND G.M. KUKOLEVSKY.
The heart and sports. Essays on Cardiology and Sports. Translation from "Serdtse i Sport; Ocherki Sportivnoy Kardiologii"
Moscow, U.S.S.R. Meditsina Press, 1968. (National Technical Information Service. Springfield, Va.)

1898
KARPOVICH, P.V.
Water resistance and energy expenditure in swimming.
In: Balke, B., Ed. Physiological aspects of sports and physical fitness P. 64. The Athletic Institute, 1968.

1899
KARPPANEN, H., AND P.J. NEUVONEN.
Ischaemic heart-disease and soil magnesium in Finland.
Lancet II: 1390, 1973.

1900
KARSTENS, R., ET AL.
A multidisciplinary approach for the assessment of psychodynamic factors in young adults with acute myocardial infarction.
Psychotherapy Psychosomatics 18:281-285, 1970.

1901
KARVONEN, M.J.
 Modification of the diet in primary prevention trials.
 Proceedings Nutrition Society 31(3):355-362, 1972.

1902
KARVONEN, M.J., AND A.J. BARRY.
 Physical activity and the heart: Proceedings of a Symposium, Helsinki, Finland.
 Springfield, Ill. Thomas, 1967.

1903
KASAHARA, Y.
 Clinical study on ischemic heart disease—study into the long-term prognosis of ischemic heart
 disease in special clinic of circulatory diseases.
 Journal Tokyo Medical College 28:327-341, 1970.

1904
KASALICKY, J., J. HURYCH, J. WIDIMSKY, V. STANEK, ET AL.
 The effect of exercise on left heart hemodynamics in patients with valvular aortic stenosis.
 Cor Vasa 15:81-91, 1973.

1905
KASL, S.V., AND S. COBB.
 Health behavior, illness behavior, and sick-role behavior.
 Archives Environmental Health 12:531-541, 1966.

1906
KASSEBAUM, D.G., AND H.E. GRISWOLD.
 Digitalis in non-failing cardiac diseases.
 Progress Cardiovascular Diseases 12(5):484-492, 1970.

1907
KASSEBAUM, D.G., K.I. SUTHERLAND, AND M.P. JUDKINS.
 A comparison of hypoxemia and exercise electrocardiography in coronary artery disease: diag-
 nostic prevision of the methods correlated with coronary arteriography.
 American Heart Journal 75:759-776, 1968.

1908
KASSER, I.S., AND R.A.BRUCE.
 Maximal exercise responses in coronary heart disease.
 Circulation 37-38(Suppl. 6):111, 1968.

1909
KASSER, I.S., AND R.A. BRUCE.
 Comparative effects of aging and coronary heart disease on submaximal and maximal exercise.
 Circulation 39(6):759-774, 1969.

1910
KASTOR, J.A.
 Digitalis intoxication in patients with atrial fibrillation.
 Circulation 47:888-894, 1973.

1911
KASTOR, J.A., AND P.M. YURCHAK.
   Recognition of digitalis intoxication in the presence of atrial fibrillation.
   Annals Internal Medicine 67:1045, 1967.

1912
KATCH, F.I., W.D. McARDLE, R. CZULA, AND G. PECHAR.
   Maximal oxygen intake, endurance running performance, and body composition of college women.
   Research Quarterly 44:301, 1973.

1913
KATILA, M., AND M.H. FRICK.
   A two-year circulatory follow-up of physical training after myocardial infarction.
   Acta Medica Scandinavica 187:95-100, 1970.

1914
KATO, H., J. TILLOTSON, M.Z. NICHAMAN, G.G. RHOADS, AND H.B. HAMILTON.
   Epidemiologic studies of coronary heart disease and stroke in Japanese men living in Japan,
   Hawaii and California. Serum lipids and diet.
   American Journal Epidemiology 97(6):372-385, 1973.

1915
KATO, K., AND H. WATANABE.
   Hemodynamic responses to exercise in patients with coronary heart disease.
   Japanese Circulation Journal 35(1):29-33, 1971.

1916
KATSILABROS, L., AND N.L. KATSILABROS.
   The arterial steal phenomenon as an explanation of the angina pectoris and the pain of the
   intermittent claudication.
   Angiology 22(10):575-579, 1971.

1917
KATTUS, A.A.
   Exercise testing and therapy in ischemic heart disease.
   Journal South Carolina Medical Association 65(Suppl. 1):57-60, 1969.

1918
KATTUS, A.A., A. ALVARO, AND R.N. MACALPIN.
   Treadmill exercise tests for capacity and adaptation in angina pectoris.
   Journal Occupational Medicine 10:627-635, 1968.

1919
KATTUS, A.A., L.L. BROCK, R.A. BRUCE, S.M. FOX, III, W.L. HASKELL, H.K. HELLERSTEIN,
   J. NAUGHTON, L.F. PARMLEY, JR., H.S. TAYLOR, AND L.R. ZOHMAN.
   Exercise testing and training of apparently healthy individuals: a handbook for physicians.
   New York, American Heart Association, 1972.

1920
KATTUS, A.A., C.R. JORGENSEN, R.E. WORDEN, AND A.B. ALVARO.
   S-T segment depression with near-maximal exercise in detection of preclinical coronary heart
   disease.
   Circulation 44(4):585-595, 1971.

1921
KATTUS, A.A., AND R.N. MACALPIN
Role of exercise in discovery, evaluation and management of ischemic heart disease.
Cardiovascular Clinics 1:255-279, 1969.

1922
KATTUS, A.A., R. MACALPIN, W.P. LONGMIRE, B.J. O'LOUGHLIN, AND H. BISHOP.
Coronary angiograms and the exercise electrocardiogram in the study of angina pectoris.
American Journal Medicine 34:19, 1963.

1923
KATZ, A.M.
Contractile proteins in normal and failing myocardium.
Hospital Practice 7(10):57-69, 1972.

1924
KATZ, L.N.
Psychological aspects of heart disease.
Psychosomatic Medicine 26:413-431, 1964.

1925
KATZ, L.N.
Physical fitness and coronary heart disease: Some basic views.
Circulation 35:405, 1967.

1926
KATZ, L.N., AND A. PICK.
Clinical electrocardiography: I. The arrhythmias.
Philadelphia, Lea and Febiger, 1956.

1927
KATZSCHMANN, R.
Coronary circulatory system during heavy work (Physiology-Pathology-Prophylaxis).
Zeitschrift für die Gesamte Innere Medizin and Ihre Grenzgebiete 25(16):738-746, 1970.

1928
KAUFMAN, J.M., AND R.D. ANSLOW.
Treatment of refractory angina pectoris with nitroglycerin and graded exercise.
Journal American Medical Association 196(2):151-155, 1966.

1929
KAVANAGH, T.
A cold-weather "jogging mask" for angina patients.
Canadian Medical Association Journal 103(12):1290-1291, 1970.

1930
KAVANAGH, T., AND R.J. SHEPHARD.
Immediate antecedents of myocardial infarction in active men.
Canadian Medical Association Journal 109(1):19-22, 1973.

1931
KAVANAGH, T., AND R.J. SHEPHARD.
Antecedents of myocardial infarction.
Canadian Medical Association Journal 109(7):571, 1973.

1932
KAVANAGH, T., R.J. SHEPHARD, H. DONEY, AND V. PANDIT.
  Intensive exercise in coronary rehabilitation.
  Medicine Science Sports 4(1):34-39, 1973.

1933
KAVANAGH, T., R.J. SHEPHARD, V. PANDIT, AND H. DONEY.
  Exercise and hypnotherapy in the rehabilitation of the coronary patient.
  Archives Physical Medicine Rehabilitation 51:578-587, 1970.

1934
KAWAI, C., ET AL.
  The effect of digitalis upon the exercise electrocardiogram.
  American Heart Journal 68:409-420, 1964.

1935
KAWANO, T., AND S. FUKUDA.
  A psychosomatic approach to regional health administration.
  Journal Japanese Psychosomatic Society 12:316, 1972.

1936
KAWANO, T., I. TAKAYAMA, AND T. KANEHISA.
  A study on behavior therapy in internal medicine: 10th report on desensitization of neural
  cardiac diseases.
  Journal Japanese Psychosomatic Society 12:327-328, 1972.

1937
KAZIK, M.
  A case of so-called "exhaustion psychosis."
  Polski Tygodnik Lekarski 22:355-356, 1967.

1938
KEDRA, M.
  Rehabilitation of patients with myocardial infarction.
  Przyglad Lekarski 29(2):269-273, 1972.

1939
KEDRA, M., J. BIELAK, Z. KOZIARA, AND M. TOMASZEK.
  Intravenous propranolol administration in treatment of paroxysmal tachycardia.
  Polski Tygodnik Lekarski 27(18):665-668, 1972.

1940
KEDRA, M., Z. KLEINROCK, B. KOLBER-POSTEPSKA, AND G. SZURSKA.
  Kininogen in plasma of patients with myocardial infarction.
  Polski Tygodnik Lekarski 27:1109-1112, 1972.

1941
KEELAN, P.
  Double-blind trial of propranolol (Inderal) in angina pectoris.
  British Medical Journal 1:897, 1965.

1942
KEENEY, C.E., AND D.W. LARAMIE.
  Effect of exercise on blood coagulation.
  Circulation Research 10:691, 1962.

1943
KEITH, R.A.
  Personality and coronary heart disease: A review.
  Journal Chronic Diseases 19:1231-1243, 1966.

1944
KEITH, R.A., B. LOWN, AND F.J. STARE.
  Coronary heart disease and behavior patterns. An examination of method.
  Psychosomatic Medicine 27:424-434, 1965.

1945
KELLERMANN, J.J.
  Problems of exercise testing.
  Chest 59:124-125, 1971.

1946
KELLERMANN, J.J.
  Rehabilitation following myocardial infarction.
  Journal Indian Medical Association 58:257, 1972.

1947
KELLERMANN, J.J.
  Physical conditioning in patients after myocardial infarction.
  Schweizerische Medizinische Wochenschrift 103(2):79-85, 1973.

1948
KELLERMANN, J.J., ET AL.
  Return to work after myocardial infarction. Comparative study of rehabilitated and nonrehabilitated patients.
  Geriatrics 23:151-156, 1968.

1949
KELLERMANN, J., S. FELDMAN, AND I. KARIV.
  Rehabilitation of the cardiac patient.
  El Torax 14(1):67-73, 1965.

1950
KELLERMANN, J.J., AND I. KARIV.
  Rehabilitation of cardiac patients.
  Israel Journal Medical Sciences 3(2):336-337, 1967.

1951
KELLERMANN, J.J., AND I. KARIV.
  Evaluation of work capacity and physical conditioning of patients with coronary heart disease.
  In: Plavšić, C. and M.M. Gertler, Eds. The first international biennial conference on cardiac rehabilitation. Dubrovnik, Yugoslavia, 1969.

1952
KELLERMANN, J.J., D. LEDERMAN, A. MANN, AND I. KARIV.
Evaluation of physical working capacity and rehabilitation of coronary patients.
In: Eliakim, M. and H.N. Neufeld, Eds. Cardiology, current topics and progress, p. 169. New York, N.Y. Academic Press, 1969.

1953
KELLERMANN, J.J., M. LEVY, S. FELDMAN, AND I. KARIV.
Rehabilitation of coronary patients.
Journal Chronic Diseases 29:815-821, 1967.

1954
KELLERMANN, J.J., A. MANN, D. LEDERMAN, AND I. KARIV.
Functional evaluation of cardiac work capacity by spiro-ergometry in patients with rheumatic heart disease.
Archives Physical Medicine Rehabilitation 50(4):189-193, 1969.

1955
KELLERMANN, J.J., B. MODAN, S. FELDMAN, AND I. KARIV.
Evaluation of physical work capacity in coronary patients after myocardial infarction who returned to work with and without a medically directed RF conditioning program.
In: Brunner, D. and E. Jokl, Eds. Physical activity and aging, pp. 148-155. Baltimore, Md. University Park Press, 1970.

1956
KELLERMANN, J.J., I. WINTNER, AND I. KARIV.
Effect of physical training on neurocirculatory asthenia.
Israel Journal Medical Sciences 5:947-949, 1969.

1957
KELLIHER, G.J., AND J. ROBERTS.
Effect of d(+) and l(-) practolol on ouabain induced arrhythmia.
European Journal Pharmacology 20(2):243-247, 1972.

1958
KELMAN, H.R., M. LOWENTHAL, AND J.N. MULLER.
Community status of discharged patients: results of a longitudinal study.
Archives Physical Medicine Rehabilitation 47:670-675, 1966.

1959
KELSO, G.F., W.J. GALLEN, AND D.Z. FRIEDBERG.
Demography of critical congenital heart disease.
American Heart Journal 86:6, 1973.

1960
KEMP, G.L.
The Q-T ratio in treadmill stress testing.
Angiology 22:523-528, 1971.

1961
KEMP, G.L.
Value of treadmill stress testing in variant angina pectoris.
American Journal Cardiology 30(7):781-783, 1972.

1962

KEMP, G.L., AND M.H. ELLESTAD.
The significance of hyperventilative and orthostatic T-wave changes on the electrocardiogram.
Archives Internal Medicine 121:518, 1968.

1963

KENEDI, P., K. TOTH, AND K. MAJOR.
Electro- and vectorcardiographic examinations of partial intraventricular conduction disturbances (hemiblocks).
Magyar Belorvosi Archiwum 25(5):272-280, 1972.

1964

KENNEDY, O.G., A.R. McKILLOP, AND G.J. RATH.
A systems approach and analysis of physical therapy.
Physical Therapy 52:743, 1972.

1965

KENT, K.M., E.R. SMITH, D.R. REDWOOD, AND S.E. EPSTEIN.
Electrical stability of acutely ischemic myocardium. Influences of heart rate and vagal stimulation.
Circulation 47:291-298, 1973.

1966

KENTALA, E.
Physical fitness and feasibility of physical rehabilitation after myocardial infarction in men of working age.
Annals Clinical Research 4(Suppl. 9):1-84, 1972.

1967

KENTALA, E., J. HEIKKILÄ, AND K. PYÖRÄLÄ.
Variation of QRS amplitude in exercise ECG as an index predicting result of physical training in patients with coronary heart disease.
Acta Medica Scandinavica 194:81, 1973.

1968

KENZLER, W.
Polemic contribution to the psychotherapy of paroxysmal tachycardia.
Acta Psychotherapeutica et Psychosomatica (Basel) 11:333-342, 1963.

1969

KEON, W.J., P. BÉDARD, K.R. SHANKAR, S.Z. ABBAS, ET AL.
Experience with emergency aortocoronary bypass grafts.
Canadian Journal Surgery 16:268, 1973.

1970

KERBER, R.E., AND D.C. HARRISON.
Paradoxical electrocardiographic effects of amyl nitrite in coronary artery disease.
British Heart Journal 34(8):851-857, 1972.

1971

KESHISHIAN, J.M., N.P.D. SMYTH, O.C. HOOD, ET AL.
The behavior of triggered unipolar pacemakers in active magnetic fields.
Journal Thoracic Cardiovascular Surgery 64:772, 1972.

1972
KEYES, J.W.
   Problems in drug management of cardiovascular disorders in geriatric patients.
   Journal American Geriatric Society 13(2):118-124, 1965.

1973
KEYS, A.
   Epidemiological studies related to coronary heart disease. Characteristics of men aged 40-59 in seven countries.
   Acta Medica Scandinavica 180(Suppl. 460), 1967.

1974
KEYS, A.
   Epidemiologic aspects of coronary artery disease.
   Journal Chronic Diseases 6:552, 1967.

1975
KEYS, A.
   A practical, palatable way of eating.
   Minnesota Medicine 52(8):1259-1263, 1969.

1976
KEYS, A.
   Physical activity and the epidemiology of coronary heart disease.
   In: Brunner, D. and E. Jokl, Eds. Physical activity and aging, pp. 250-266. Basel, Switzerland. S. Karger, 1970.

1977
KEYS, A.
   Coronary heart disease in seven countries.
   Circulation 41(Suppl. 1):1, 1970.

1978
KEYS, A., C. ARAVANIS, H. BLACKBURN, F.S.P. VAN BUCHEM, ET AL.
   Probability of middle-aged men developing coronary heart disease in 5 years.
   Circulation 45:815-828, 1972.

1979
KEYS, A., H.L. TAYLOR, H. BLACKBURN, J. BROŽEK, J.T. ANDERSON, AND E. SIMONSON.
   Coronary heart disease among Minnesota business and professional men followed fifteen years.
   Circulation 28:381-395, 1963.

1980
KEZDI, P., W.S. NAYLOR, R. RAMBOUSEK, AND E. STANLEY.
   A practical heart rate and ectopic beat detector.
   Journal Electrocardiology 1(2):213-220, 1968.

1981
KHAJA, F., J.O. PARKER, R.J. LEDWICH, R.O. WEST, AND P.W. ARMSTRONG.
   Assessment of ventricular function in coronary artery disease by means of atrial pacing and exercise.
   American Journal Cardiology 26(2):107-116, 1970.

1982
KHALFEN, E. SH., K.S. IATSENKO, AND D.M. ZAFERMAN.
Prediction of the outcomes of myocardial infarction from formulas derived by the dynamic programming method.
In: Applied mathematics and cybernetics, pp. 279-282. Moscow, USSR. Izdatel'stvo Nauka, 1973.

1983
KHAN, A.H., D.R. BOUGHNER, AND R. HAIDER.
Effect of phentolamine on atrioventricular conduction in man assessed by recording His bundle potential.
British Heart Journal 34(11):1102-1106, 1972.

1984
KHAN, A.H., R. HAIDER, D.R. BOUGHNER, C.M. OAKLEY, AND J.F. GOODWIN.
Sinus rhythm with absent P waves in advanced rheumatic heart disease.
American Journal Cardiology 32:93, 1973.

1985
KHANNA, P.K., P.M. SHAH, D.H. KRAMER, R.A. SCHAEFER, AND I. TAGER.
Effects of altered preload on left ventricular systolic time intervals in acute myocardial infarction.
British Heart Journal 35:1102, 1973.

1986
KHATRI, I.M., AND J.N. COHN.
Effect of post-ganglioni sympathetic blockade on hemodynamic response to exercise.
Federation Proceedings 26(2):287, 1967.

1987
KHOMENOK, V.P.
Sudden death of sportsmen from latent atherosclerosis and hypertensive disease.
Vrachebnoe Delo 12:61-65, 1971.

1988
KHOO, K.L., Y.H. CHONG, AND R.P. PILLAY.
Familial type II hyperlipoproteinaemia in a Chinese family.
Medical Journal Australia 1(21):1048, 1973.

1989
KIDA, H., S. MATSUMOTO, A. NAGATOMO, AND A. TAKEYA.
Glucose tolerance and response to insulin. Free fatty acid and growth hormone in ischemic heart disease.
Japanese Circulation Journal 37(8):887-888, 1973.

1990
KIDSON, M.A.
Personality factors in hypertension.
Australian New Zealand Journal Psychiatry 5(3):139-145, 1971.

1991
KIDSON, M.A.
Personality and hypertension.
Journal Psychosomatic Research 17:35-41, 1973.

1992
KIEF, H.
  Lipid metabolism and arteriosclerosis.
  Naturwissenschaften 57(8):384-387, 1970.

1993
KIENY, R., C. ROOS, R. PETER, AND J.G. LEVY.
  How to supervise a patient with a cardiac pacemaker.
  Journal Médical de Strasbourg 2(10):781-789, 1971.

1994
KILBOM, A.
  Physical training in women.
  Scandinavian Journal Clinical Laboratory Investigation 28(Suppl. 119):1-34, 1971.

1995
KILBOM, A., L.H. HARTLEY, B. SALTIN, J. BJURE, G. GRIMBY, AND I. ÅSTRAND.
  Physical training in sedentary middle-aged and older men. I.
  Scandinavian Journal Clinical Laboratory Investigation 24:315-322, 1969.

1996
KILCOYNE, M.M.
  Hypertension and heart disease in the urban community.
  Bulletin New York Academy Medicine 49(6):501-509, 1973.

1997
KILCOYNE, M.M., P.A. ALSUP, AND R.W. RICHTER.
  Hypertension screening in the central Harlem community.
  Clinical Research 20(3):475, 1972.

1998
KILLIP, T.
  Arrhythmia, sudden death and coronary artery disease.
  American Journal Cardiology 28(5):614-616, 1971.

1999
KILLIP, T.
  Management of arrhythmias in acute myocardial infarction.
  Hospital Practice 7(4):131-140, 1972.

2000
KILPATRICK, D.G.
  Cardiac pacemakers.
  In: Segal, B.L. and D.C. Kilpatrick, Eds. Engineering in the Practice of Medicine, pp. 309-323.
  Baltimore, Md. Williams and Wilkins, 1967.

2001
KIMBALL, R., AND E.W. HANCOCK.
  Left ventricular function in exercise in aortic stenosis.
  Clinical Research 15(1):119, 1967.

2002
KIMERA, Z.
   Recording of the vectorcardiogram during exercise using the telemeter: its methods and clinical results.
   Japanese Circulation Journal 34:359-366, 1970.

2003
KIMURA, E., AND T. KANIE.
   Electrocardiographic diagnosis of left ventricular hypertrophy with the aid of an electronic computer.
   Israel Journal Medical Sciences 5(4):917-919, 1969.

2004
KIMURA, E., Y. MIBUKURA, AND S. MIURA.
   Statistical diagnosis of electrocardiogram by the theorem of Bayes.
   Japanese Heart Journal 4(5):469-488, 1963.

2005
KIMURA, E., K. USHIYAMA, T. YAMAZAKI, K. YOSHIDA, ET AL.
   Effects of some coronary vasodilators on the exercise and anoxia tests, with special reference to the genesis of anginal attack.
   In: Proceedings third Asian Pacific Congress of Cardiology, Kyoto, 10-14 May 1964, pp. 745-747. Kyoto, Japan. Kawakita Printing Co., 1964.

2006
KIMURA, N., K. ABE, H. TOSHIMA, R. TANAKA, ET AL.
   Application of dye dilution method for cardiology. Report III. Electrocardiography and cardiac output after exercise in patients with ischemic heart disease.
   Japanese Circulation Journal 33(8):866, 1969.

2007
KIMURA, N., F. MORI, AND M. YAMADA.
   Problem of dietary treatment for cardiovascular diseases. Dietary treatment for heart disease.
   Japanese Journal Medicine 7(2):108-111, 1968.

2008
KIMURA, N., A. SEKI, S. NAKAKURA, H. TOSHIMA, AND I. FURUKAWA.
   Rehabilitation of acute stage of myocardial infarction by the active exercise treatment. A modified Master's.
   In: Proceedings third Asian Pacific Congress of Cardiology Kyoto, 10-14 May 1964, pp. 1600-1602. Kyoto, Japan, Kawakita Printing Company, 1964.

2009
KIMURA, N., H. TOSHIMA, Y. NAKAYAMA, ET AL.
   Population survey on cerebrovascular and cardiovascular diseases. Ten years experience in the farming village of Tanushimaru and the fishing village of Ushibuka.
   Japanese Heart Journal 13(2):118-127, 1972.

2010
KIMURA, N., N. UTSU, Y. NAKAYAMA, H. TASHIRO, ET AL.
   Correlation between cardiac output and electrocardiogram at rest and after exercise in ischemic heart.
   Japanese Heart Journal 11(4):325-333, 1970.

2011
KINCAID, D.T., AND R.E. BOTTI.
  Significance of isolated left anterior hemiblock and left axis deviation during acute myocardial infarction.
  American Journal Cardiology 30(8):797-800, 1972.

2012
KINCAID, D.T., AND R.E. BOTTI.
  Acute myocardial infarction in the elderly.
  Chest 64(2):170, 1973.

2013
KING, D.J., AND R.F. MANEGOLD.
  Consistency of cardiologists' prognostic judgments in cases of myocardial infarction.
  American Journal Cardiology 15:27-32, 1965.

2014
KING, L.T., D.E. STRANDNESS, JR., AND J.W. BELL.
  The hemodynamic response of the lower extremities to exercise.
  Journal Surgical Research 5(4):167-171, 1965.

2015
KINI, P.M., J.L. WILLEMS, C. BATCHLOR, AND H.V. PIPBERGER.
  St-T changes induced by digitalis and ventricular hypertrophy. Differentiation by quantitative analysis.
  Journal Electrocardiology 5:101, 1972.

2016
KINLEIN, M.L.
  Nursing the coronary patient.
  Journal Rehabilitation 32:39, 1966.

2017
KINLEN, L.J.
  Incidence and presentation of myocardial infarction in an English community.
  British Heart Journal 35:616-622, 1973.

2018
KIRCHEINER, B., AND O. PEDERSEN-BJERGAARD.
  The effect of physical training after myocardial infarction.
  Scandinavian Journal Rehabilitation Medicine 5:105, 1973.

2019
KIRCHOFF, H.W. (ED.)
  Methods of measuring physical fitness.
  In: Physical fitness in flying including the ageing and aged aircrew. Advisory group for aerospace research and development (AGARD), NATO Conference Proceedings No. 81, pp. 1-3. London, 1971.

2020
KIREEV, P.M., Y.G. ALEKSEEVSKIKH, AND E.G. NAVASHINA.
  Changes in the content and distribution of nucleic acids in myocardial infarction.
  Terapevticheskii Arkhiv 44:27, 1972.

2021
KIRKEBY, K.
Disturbances in serum lipids and in their fatty acid composition following acute myocardial infarction.
Acta Medica Scandinavica 192(6):523-528, 1972.

2022
KIRKEBY, K., P. INGVALDSEN, AND I. BJERKEDAL.
Fatty acid composition of serum lipids in men with myocardial infarction.
Acta Medica Scandinavica 192(6):513-519, 1972.

2023
KIRKEBY, K., P. INGVALDSEN, AND I. BJERKEDAL.
Fatty acid composition of serum lipids in wives of men with myocardial infarction.
Acta Medica Scandinavica 192:521-522, 1972.

2024
KIRSTEN, E., M. RODSTEIN, AND Z. IUSTER.
Digoxin in the aged.
Geriatrics 28(1):95-101, 1973.

2025
KISHIMOTO, M.
Prognosis and rehabilitation in bundle block and atrioventricul block in the hospital study.
Japanese Circulation Journal 31(11):1655-1660, 1967.

2026
KISS, E., F. KUBICEK, AND K. POLZER.
Further evaluations with the comprehensive care of patients after myocardial infarction.
Wiener Medizinische Wochenschrift 123:622, 1973.

2027
KITAMURA, K., C.R. JORGENSEN, F.L. GOBEL, ET AL.
Hemodynamic correlates of coronary blood flow and myocardial oxygen consumption during upright exercise.
American Journal Cardiology 26:643, 1970.

2028
KITCHIN, A.H., AND J.M. NEILSON.
The T wave of the electrocardiogram during and after exercise in normal subjects.
Cardiovascular Research 6:143-149, 1972.

2029
KITS VAN HEIJININGEN, H.
Psychodynamic factors in acute myocardial infarction.
International Journal Psycho-Analysis 47:370-374, 1966.

2030
KIVELOFF, B., AND O. HUBER.
Brief maximal isometric exercise in hypertension.
Journal American Geriatric Society 19:1006-1012, 1971.

2031
KIVELOFF, B., AND O. HUBER.
Exercise versus drugs for treatment of hypertension.
Journal American Medical Association 225:314, 1973.

2032
KIVOWITZ, C., W.W. PARMLEY, R. DONOSO, H. MARCUS, ET AL.
Effects of isometric exercise on cardiac performance: The grip test.
Circulation 44(6):994-1002, 1971.

2033
KJELLBERG, S.R., U. RUDHE, AND T. SJOSTRAND.
The amount of hemoglobin (blood volume) in the relation to pulse rate and heart volume during work.
Acta Physiologica Scandinavica 19:152-169, 1949.

2034
KLARMAN, H.E.
Socioeconomic impact of heart disease.
In: Andrus, E.C., Ed. The heart and circulation, pp. 693-707. Washington, D.C. Federation American Societies Experimental Biology, 1965.

2035
KLASSEN, G.A.
Coronary artery disease. A cause of heterogeneous myocardial perfusion.
Cardiologia 56(1-2):343-347, 1972.

2036
KLASSEN, G.A.
Exercise in ischemic heart disease.
Canadian Medical Association Journal 109:9, 1973.

2037
KLASSEN, G.A., G. ANDREW, D.T. ZBOROWSKA-SLUIS, AND M.R. BECKLAKE.
Total and regional blood flow adaptation to training in paddlers.
Federation Proceedings 27(2):231, 1968.

2038
KLATSKY, A.L., G.D. FRIEDMAN, AND A.B. SIEGELAU.
Usage of tobacco, coffee, aspirin, and alcohol as predictors of myocardial infarction.
Circulation 48(4):94, 1973.

2039
KLATSKY, A.L., G.D. FRIEDMAN, AND A.B. SIEGELAU.
Coffee drinking prior to acute myocardial infarction. Results from Kaiser-Permanente Epidemiologic study of myocardial infarction.
Journal American Medical Association 226:540-543, 1973.

2040
KLAUS, A.P., B.L. ZARET, B.L. PITT, AND R.S. ROSS.
Comparative evaluation of sublingual long-acting nitrates.
Circulation 48:519-525, 1973.

2041
KLECZKOWSKI, B.M.
  Epidemiology of cardiovascular diseases: Aims and modern problems.
  Polski Tygodnik Lekarski 24(39):1505-1508, 1969.

2042
KLEIN, H.
  Nonparoxysmal junctional tachycardia complicating acute myocardial infarction.
  Circulation 46:831, 1972.

2043
KLEIN, M.S., W.E. SHELL, AND B.E. SOBEL.
  Serum creatine phosphokinase (CPK) isoenzymes after intramuscular injections, surgery, and
  myocardial infarction—experimental and clinical studies.
  Cardiovascular Research 7(3):412-418, 1973.

2044
KLEIN, R.R., V.A. KLINER, D.P. ZIPES, W.G. TROYER, JR., AND H.G. WALLACE.
  Transfer from a coronary care unit.
  Archives Internal Medicine 122:104, 1968.

2045
KLEIN, W.
  On the quantative diagnosis of mitral stenosis from the ultrasonic echocardiogram.
  Zeitschrift für Kreislaufforschung 58:972-978, 1969.

2046
KLEIN, W.J., JR.
  Whether there's too much or too little, departures from the norm can cause—as well as
  indicate—trouble.
  Emergency Medicine 5:79, 1973.

2047
KLEINBAUM, D.G., L.L. KUPPER, J.C. CASSEL, AND H.A. TYROLER.
  Multivariate analysis of risk of coronary heart disease in Evans County, Georgia.
  Archives Internal Medicine 128(6):943-948, 1971.

2048
KLEINSCHMIDT, T.
  Effects on hypertension by means of socio-psychosomatic relief at "Kuren."
  Psychotherapy Psychosomatics 19(1/2):27-36, 1971.

2049
KLEMM, G.
  Stress ulcer after myocardial infarction.
  Zeitschrift Gesamte Innere Medizin 26:210-213, 1971.

2050
KLINE, E.M.
  Heart disease and employment. The perspective of the occupational physician.
  Journal Occupational Medicine 8:511-513, 1966.

2051
KLISSOURAS, V., F. PIRNAY, AND J.-M. PETIT.
  Adaptation to maximal effort—Genetics and age.
  Journal Applied Physiology 35:288-293, 1973.

2052
KLOSTER, F.E., J.D. BRISTOW, AND H.E. GRISWOLD.
  Cardiac output determination from precordial isotope dilution curves during exercise.
  Journal Applied Physiology 26(4):465-468, 1969.

2053
KLOTZBÜCHER, E., ET AL.
  Controlled training of myocardial infarct patients involving work physiology.
  Zeitschrift für die Gesamte Hygiene und Ihre Grenzbiete 15:654-656, 1969.

2054
KLOTZBÜCHER, E., AND E. GOLETZ.
  The physiologically controlled training of patients after cardiac infarct.
  Zeitschrift für die Gesamte Hygiene and Ihre Grenzgebiete 15(9):654-656, 1969.

2055
KNAPP, E., A. AIGNER, P. BAUMGARTL, AND E. RAAS.
  The correlation of heart rate and systolic circulation times and the indices calculated therefrom.
  Zeitschrift für Kreislaufforschung 61(6):492-497, 1972.

2056
KNAPPE, J., G. KNAPPE, G. STRUBE, K.D. DÜCK, AND W. RELKE.
  Ischemic heart diseases and so-called risk factors. Results of an epidemiological study in Erfurt (Germany).
  Zeitschrift für die Gesamte Innere Medizin und Ihre Grenzgebiete 26(1):18-21, 1971.

2057
KNICK, B., H.-J. LANGE, F. KÖSSLING, D. SKOLUDA, AND G. KREMER.
  Early diabetic and lipid metabolic anomalies in myocardial infarction and in terminal artery disease.
  Deutsche Medizinische Wochenschrift 93:1954-1959, 1968.

2058
KNIPPING, H.W., AND L.H. WORTH.
  Heart infarction. Stuttgart, German Federal Republic. Ferdinand Enke, 1971.

2059
KNOEBEL, S.B., W.C. ELLIOTT, P.L. McHENRY, AND E. ROSS.
  Myocardial blood flow and exercise ECG in cinearteriographically demonstrated coronary artery disease.
  Journal Laboratory Clinical Medicine 74(5):893, 1969.

2060
KNOEBEL, S.B., W.C. ELLIOTT, P.L. McHENRY, AND E. ROSS.
  Myocardial blood flow in coronary artery disease. Correlation with severity of disease and treadmill exercise response.
  American Journal Cardiology 27(1):51-58, 1971.

2061
KNUTTGEN, H.G., AND B. SALTIN.
Oxygen uptake, muscle high-energy phosphates, and lactate in exercise under acute hypoxic conditions in man.
Acta Physiologica Scandinavica 87:368, 1973.

2062
KOATE, P., N. PADONOU, AND M. SANKALE.
Congenital heart diseases in the Senegalese population (in relation with 151 hospital cases in Dakar).
Archives des Maladies du Coeur et des Vaisseaux 66:1345, 1973.

2063
KOATE, P., Y. COUTURIER, AND C. QUENUM.
Ischemic heart disease among Black Africans: About 16 cases of myocardial infarction and 5 cases of coronary angina in Senegalians at Dakar.
Bulletin de la Société Médicale d'Afrique Noire de Langue Française 18(Suppl.):115-121, 1971.

2064
KOBAYASHI, T., ET AL.
Rehabilitation in myocardial infarction.
Japanese Journal Clinical Medicine 23:1782-1790, 1965.

2065
KOBAYASHI, T., ET AL.
Rehabilitation of essential hypertension.
Japanese Journal Clinical Medicine 25:691-696, 1967.

2066
KOBAYASHI, T., ET AL.
Measurement of physical work capacity and its clinical application in cardiac patients.
Japanese Circulation Journal 31(2):231, 1967.

2067
KOBAYASHI, T., ET AL.
Radio-telemetering of electrocardiogram and blood pressure.
Malattie Cardiovascolari 10:129-141, 1969.

2068
KOBAYASHI, T., Y. ITO, T. KISHII, Y. IKEDA, ET AL.
Studies on the rehabilitation of cardiac patients.
Japanese Circulation Journal 29(11):1082, 1965.

2069
KOBAYASHI, T., Y. ITO, K. OTSUKI, ET AL.
Study of actual daily activities and rehabilitation of cardiac outpatients.
Japanese Journal Clinical Medicine 24:2121, 1966.

2070
KOBAYASHI, T., M. TAKEUCHI, Y. IKEDA, A. MORISHIMA, ET AL.
Study on the rehabilitation of cardiac patients.
Japanese Journal Medicine 6(1):28-29, 1967.

2071

KOBAYASHI, T., M. TAKEUCHI, T. KORO, AND Y. IKEDA.
  Rehabilitation and evaluation of patients with ischemic heart disease in Japan.
  In: Eliakim, M. and H.N. Neufeld, Eds. Cardiology, current topics and progress, pp. 166-168. New York, N.Y., Academic Press, 1969.

2072

KOBAYASHI, T., H. ISHIKAWA, AND I. TAWARA.
  Psychosomatic aspects of angina pectoris.
  Scandinavian Journal Rehabilitation Medicine 2-3:87-91, 1970.

2073

KOCH, R.
  Clinical and experimental studies on efficacy and duration of action of N-n-propyl ajmaline hydrogen tartrate in cardiac arrhythmias.
  Arzneimittel-Forschung 22(12):2079-2084, 1972.

2074

KOCH, R., P. TILLMANN, B. WIESZMANN, AND R. WINTER.
  The rontgenographic estimation of the capacity of heart pacemaker.
  Zeitschrift für Kreislaufforschung 61(6):523-528, 1972.

2075

KOCNAR, K., AND J. ROUS.
  Comparison of ECG findings at load in the laboratory and in the field.
  Pracovni Lekarstvi 23(5):165-168, 1971.

2076

KOEHLE, K., E. GAUS, R. KARSTENS, AND D. OHLMEIER.
  Psychotherapy in patients with myocardial infarction during the phase of intensive treatment.
  Therapiewoche 22:4379, 1972.

2077

KOERNER, D.R.
  Cardiovascular benefits from an industrial physical fitness program.
  Journal Occupational Medicine 15:700-707, 1973.

2078

KOFF, A.M., M.E. LYNCH, AND C.E. MCLEAN.
  Classification of cardiac patients and normal subjects by means of maximal exercise treadmill test.
  Angiology 21(1):24-33, 1970.

2079

KOHLHARDT, M., B. BAUER, H. KRAUSE, AND A. FLECKENSTEIN.
  Selective inhibition of the transmembrane Ca conductivity of mammalian myocardial fibres by Ni, Co, and Mn ions.
  Pfluegers Archiv: European Journal Physiology 338(2):115-123, 1973.

2080

KÖHLE, E., AND C. SIMONS.
  Psychodynamic aspects in young patients suffering from peripheral vascular occlusions.
  Psychotherapy Psychosomatics 18:313-320, 1970.

2081
KÖHLER, J.A., ET AL.
  Significance of telemetric transformation of corrected orthogonal leads. XYZ and corrected chest
  wall leads during rest and exertion.
  Verhandlungen der Deutschen Gesellschaft für Kreislaufforschung 37:223-236, 1971.

2082
KOHN, R.M., AND B. CUTCHER.
  Breath-holding time in the screening for rehabilitation potential of cardiac patients.
  Scandinavian Journal Rehabilitative Medicine 2-3:105-107, 1970.

2083
KOHN, R.M.
  Physical reconditioning after myocardial infarction.
  New York State Journal Medicine 70:516-517, 1970.

2084
KOHN, R.M., AND B. CUTCHER.
  The community impact of a work evaluation unit: A controlled study.
  Journal Chronic Diseases 17:659-666, 1964.

2085
KOHNER, E.M., C.T. DOLLERY, C. LOWY, AND B. SCHUMER.
  Effect of diuretic therapy on glucose tolerance in hypertensive patients.
  Lancet 1:986-990, 1971.

2086
KOJI, T.
  Studies on the third heart sound.
  Japanese Circulation Journal 35(10):1253, 1971.

2087
KOLBER-POSTEPSKA, B.
  The influence of exercise and massage on pulse rate, arterial pressure and electrocardiogram in
  patients during cardiological rehabilitation after myocardial infarction.
  Polski Tygodnik Lekarski 24(11):401-403, 1969.

2088
KOLESÁR, J., Z. MIKEŠ, AND E. PARTLOVÁ.
  Studies on the results of rehabilitation of postinfarction conditions by means of spiroergometry.
  Pracovni Lékarstvi 23(5):148-150, 1971.

2089
KOLLAR, E.J.
  Psychological stress: A re-evaluation.
  Journal Nervous Mental Disease 132(5):382-395, 1961.

2090
KOLLAR, J.
  Ultrastructure of the myocardium in alcoholic heart.
  Vnitrni Lekarstvi 18(9):855-862, 1972.

2091
KOLLER, R., J.W. KENNEDY, J.C. BUTLER, AND N.N. WAGNER.
Counseling the coronary patient on sexual activity.
Postgraduate Medicine 51(4):133-136, 1972.

2092
KOMATSU, Y.
Experimental study on the collateral source in coronary occlusion.
Tohoku 84(4):158-196, 1971.

2093
KONECKE, L.L., AND S.B. KNOEBEL.
Nonparoxysmal junctional tachycardia complicating acute myocardial infarction.
Circulation 45:367-374, 1972.

2094
KONES, R.J.
Digitalis and glucagon for acute myocardial infarction—Comparison of an old and a new agent.
Clinical Medicine 80:19-25, 1973.

2095
KONES, R.J., D.H. DOMBECK, AND J.H. PHILLIPS.
Glucagon in cardiogenic shock.
Angiology 23(9):525-535, 1972.

2096
KÖNIG, E. AND N. ZÖLLNER.
Alterations of the plasma volume during leg exercise, idle resting, in people without cardiac failure and people with right heart failure.
Zeitschrift für Gesamte Experimentelle Medizin 140(3):268-286, 1966.

2097
KÖNIG, K.
Physical exercises for diagnostic separation of functional and organic cardiac insufficiency.
Arztliche Forschung 21(7):255-260, 1967.

2098
KÖNIG, K., H. REINDELL, AND O.F. GOLDSCHMIDT.
Comparative long range studies on the effect of exercise and digoxin therapy on patients with healed myocardial infarction.
Medizinische Welt 44:2469-2477, 1965.

2099
KÖNIG, W.
The distortion of electrocardiogram by periodic spontaneous muscular activity.
Zeitschrift für Kreislaufforschung 57:1140-1143, 1968.

2100
KONTOWT, A., AND S. KOZLOWSKI.
Physiological evaluation of the physical capacity of patients with mitral stenosis after commis-surotomy, using the spiroergometric method.
Cor et Vasa 13(1):25-31, 1971.

2101
KONTOWT, A., AND S. KOZLOWSKI.
Tolerance of prolonged physical exercise in acquired valvular heart disease.
Kardiologia Polska 15:47, 1972.

2102
KONTOWT, A., L. ZIOLKOWSKI, AND S. KOZLOWSKI.
Rehabilitation of patients after recent myocardial infarction in recreation training camps.
Polski Tygodnik Lekarski 27(44):1724-1727, 1972.

2103
KONTTINEN, A., AND E.A. NIKKILÄ.
Effect of acute exercise on serum triglycerides and free fatty acids.
In: Karvonen, M.J. and A.J. Barry, Eds. Physical activity and the heart, pp. 208-215. Springfield, Ill. Thomas, 1967.

2104
KONTTINEN, A., AND H. SOMER.
Determination of serum creatine kinase isoenzymes in myocardial infarction.
American Journal Cardiology 29(6):817-820, 1972.

2105
KOPACZYNSKA, K.
Tuberculous myocarditis.
Gruzlica i Choroby Pluc 40(7):607-613, 1972.

2106
KOPPICZ, M., S. LASKOWSKI, AND W. BARCZEWSKI.
Myocardial infarction in a man aged 21 years.
Wiadomosci Lekarskie 25(22):2025-2026, 1972.

2107
KORDENAT, R.K., P. KEZDI, AND D. POWLEY.
Experimental intracoronary thrombosis and selective in situ lysis by catheter technique.
American Journal Cardiology 30(6):640-645, 1972.

2108
KORNEV, M.P., A.P. FILONENKO, B.P. MUKHORIN, AND S.D. FEDOROV.
Wounds of the heart.
Grudnaia Khirurgia 14:28, 1972.

2109
KORNITZER, M., M. DEMEESTER, R. DELCOURT, AND R. BERNARD.
Ischemic cardiopathy in a population of employees in Brussels: Study of the prevalence of ischemic cardiopathies as a function of socioeconomic class.
Revue d'Epidémiologie Médecine Sociale Santé Publique 19(7):599-612, 1971.

2110
KORNITZER, M., M. DEMEESTER, AND A. GOOSSENS.
Comparative study between various cardiovascular studies.
Acta Cardiologica 26(1):11-27, 1971.

2111
KORNREICH, F.
The missing waveform information in the orthogonal electrocardiogram (Frank Leads). I. Where and how can this missing waveform information be retrieved?
Circulation 48:984, 1973.

2112

KORNREICH, F., AND D. BRISMEE.
The missing waveform information in the orthogonal electrocardiogram (Frank Lead). II. Diagnosis of left ventricular hypertrophy and myocardial infarction from "total" surface waveform information.
Circulation 48:996, 1973.

2113
KORO, T.
Study on the voluntary exercise test using radioelectrocardiography and its clinical application. Evaluation of working capacity and the effects of physical training in the rehabilitation of patients with myocardial infarction.
Journal Japanese Society Internal Medicine 59:240-254, 1970.

2114
KORO, T., R. KAMYAR, T. ITO, T. SADA, ET AL.
Ischemic heart disease and exercise test—Application of medical electronics to check-alarm training system.
Japanese Circulation Journal 37(8):903, 1973.

2115
KOROBKINA, G.S., YU. M. NEMENOVA, E.G. PARAMONOVA, L.G. GVOZDOVA, AND Z. YA. GLUSHNEVA.
The effect produced by diets of differing qualitative composition upon the clinical course and lipoid metabolism in patients with coronary atherosclerosis.
Voprosy Pitaniya 22(1):17-22, 1963.

2116
KOROLEV, B.A.
Changes in cardiac activity in prolonged hypokinesia (according to data from vector analysis).
Kosmicheskaya Biologiya i Meditisina 2(5):52-55, 1968.

2117
KOROLKO, A.
Results of long-term administration of anticoagulants in patients with myocardial infarction and coronary arterial disease without infarction.
Polski Tygodnik Lekarski 27(48):1897-1900, 1972.

2118
KORSAN BENGTSEN, K., L. WILHELMSEN, D. ELMFELDT, AND G. TIBBLIN.
Blood coagulation and fibrinolysis in man after myocardial infarction compared with a representative population sample.
Atherosclerosis 16(1):83-88, 1972.

2119
KOSINSKA, D.I.
Legal problems raised by myocardial infarct.
Polski Tydognik Lekarski 26:729-730, 1971.

2120
KOSINSKA, D.I., S. RUDNICKI, AND J. BARYLAK.
Social problems affecting victims of myocardial infarct during hospital rehabilitation.
Polski Tygodnik Lekarski 26:770-772, 1971.

2121
KOSMINSKI, S., AND W. KNAST.
The theoretical bases of arterioplasty and advances in surgical techniques.
Polski Przeglad Chirurgiczny 44:1337, 1972.

2122
KOSOWSKY, B.D., B. LOWN, R. WHITING, AND T. GUINEY.
Occurrence of ventricular arrhythmias with exercise as compared to monitoring.
Circulation 44(5):826-832, 1971.

2123
KOSSLING, F.K., H.H. STELZIG, AND G. WALTHER.
Early diagnosis of myocardial infarction: study on resistance to autolysis of histochemical methods of identification.
Zentralblatt für Allgemeine Pathologie und Pathologische Anatomie 116(1):155-162, 1972.

2124
KOSTIS, J.B., S. GOTZOYANNIS, E. MAVROGEORGIS, ET AL.
The value of the ultrasonic Doppler method and apexcardiography as reference tracings in phonocardiography.
American Heart Journal 84(5):634-642, 1972.

2125
KOTHARI, L.K., A. BORDIA, AND O.P. GUPTA.
The Yogic claim of voluntary control over the heart beat: an unusual demonstration.
American Heart Journal 86:282, 1973.

2126
KOTOV, A.P., ET AL.
Occupational rehabilitation of disabled persons with diseases of circulatory organs.
Vrachebnoe Delo 10:107-111, 1969.

2127
KOTTKE, F.J.
Deterioration of the bedfast patient.
Public Health Reports 80:437, 1965.

2128
KOTTKE, F.J., W.G. KUBICEK, AND M.E. OLSON.
Evaluation of cardiac competence during rehabilitation following myocardial infarction.
Israel Journal Medical Sciences 9(5):568-577, 1973.

2129
KOWAL, S.J.
Anger and angina pectoris.
American Practitioner Digest Treatment 12(8):595-599, 1961.

2130
KOYAMA, S., K. KATO, K. SUZUKI, A. OHTA, ET AL.
Hemodynamics in coronary sclerosis. (I). Effect of exercise on cardiac performance in subjects with angina pectoris.
Japanese Circulation Journal 29(11):82, 1965.

2131
KOYAMA, S., K. KATO, A. OHTA, K. SUZUKI, ET AL.
Studies on hemodynamic consequences in patients with coronary heart disease.
Japanese Journal Medicine 6(1):21-22, 1967.

2132
KOYANAGI, T.
Studies on the anginal attack and catecholamines.
Sapporo Medical Journal 38(3/4):122-136, 1970.

2133
KOZLOVA, Z.P.
Long-term follow-up observations on patients with angina pectoris treated with procaine blockade.
Trudy Khabarovskogo Meditsinskogo Instituta 24:49, 1964.

2134
KOZUKA, T., K. SATO, M. FUJINO, ET AL.
Angiographic studies on a single ventricle.
Nippon Acta Radiologica 32(3):185-195, 1972.

2135
KOZUL, V.
Some aspects of myocardial infarction.
Lijecnicki Vjesnik 87(1):17-23, 1965.

2136
KRACHENBUHL, J.R., D. AUCANT, AND J.P. MAURAT.
Morphological study of the great venous trunks by tomo-echography.
Coeur et Médecine Interne 12:431, 1973.

2137
KRAMER, J.C.
Normal serum cholesterol values.
Journal American Medical Association 226:1011, 1973.

2138
KRAMER, K.D., AND H. HOCHREIN.
The determination of the absorption and disappearance rate of the dose of subtoxicity and maintenance of beta-methyldigoxin in patients with heart failure.
Klinische Wochenschrift 50(21):1009-1014, 1972.

2139
KRAMER, P., AND F. SCHELER.
Kinetics of renal elimination of several cardiac glycosides.
Deutsche Medizinische Wochenschrift 97(40):1485-1490, 1972.

2140
KRAMM, H.
Two years of early rehabilitation after myocardial infarction in the clinic Hoehenried, West Germany. Part 2. Organizational aspects, medical and social cooperation as requirement for follow-up measures of treatment presented on the model Hoehenried.
Fortschritte der Medizin 91:109-113, 1973.

2141
KRASEMANN, E.O.
Coordination of therapeutic measures following myocardial infarct, necessity and possibilities of relief.
Öffentliche Gesundheitswesen 33:737-747, 1971.

2142
KRASNO, L.R., AND G.J. KIDERA.
Continuous electrocardiographic recording during exercise. Its use in evaluating the effect of pentaerythritol tetranitrate.
Angiology 14(8):417-425, 1963.

2143
KRASNOW, N., E.L. ROLETT, P.M. YURCHAK, W.B. HOOD, JR., AND R. GORLIN.
Isoproterenol and cardiovascular performance.
American Journal Medicine 37:514, 1964.

2144
KRAUS, H.
Effects of training on skeletal muscle.
In: Larsen, O.A. and R.O. Malmborg, Eds. Coronary heart disease and physical fitness, pp. 134-137. Baltimore, University Park Press, 1971.

2145
KRAUS, H.
Evaluation of muscular and cardiovascular fitness.
Preventive Medicine 1:178-184, 1972.

2146
KRAUSE, E.G., M. BOHM, H. WILL, AND A. WOLLENBERGER.
Glycogenphosphorylase b: A new serum enzyme test for myocardial infarction.
Deutsche Gesundheitswesen 27(19):903-904, 1972.

2147
KRAUSMAN, D.T.
A system for providing an on-line analogue display of beat-by-beat cardiac output.
Medical Biological Engineering 10:81-88, 1972.

2148
KRAUSS, K.R., A.M. HUTTER, JR., AND R.W. DESANCTIS.
Acute coronary insufficiency. Course and follow-up.
Archives Internal Medicine 129(5):808-813, 1972.

2149
KRAVITZ, A.R., AND D.P. THOMAS.
Emotional reactions to long-term anticoagulant therapy.
Archives Internal Medicine 114(5):663-668, 1964.

2150
KRAYENBUHL, H.P., W. MEIER, AND W. BURIAN.
  Treatment of angina pectoris by electrical stimulation of carotid sinus nerves.
  Schweizerische Medizinische Wochenschrift 102:1739-1740, 1972.

2151
KREBS, H.
  The Croonian Lecture, 1963. Gluconeogenesis.
  Proceedings Royal Society (Biology) 159:545, 1964.

2152
KRETSCHMER, W.
  Problems of the personality in pharmaco-physical treatment.
  Medicinski Arhiv 19:5-11, 1965.

2153
KREUZER, H., A. BOTH, AND L. SEIPEL.
  Stress tests in patients with congenital and acquired cardiac valvular disease after surgery.
  Verhandlungen der Deutschen Gesellschaft für Kreislaufforschung 37:122-132, 1971.

2154
KRIKLER, D.M., AND B. LEWIS.
  Coronary artery disease in a young man with normal serum lipids.
  British Heart Journal 34(11):1186-1188, 1972.

2155
KROTKIEWSKI, M., ET AL.
  Obesity and arterial hypertension. II. Effect of a reducing diet and fasting.
  Bulletin Polish Medical Science History 10:58-62, 1967.

2156
KRUCHININA, N.A., AND S.V. CHERNIGOVSKAYA.
  Role of manic depressive states in the development of ischemic heart disease.
  Kardiologiya 13:56, 1973.

2157
KRUG, A., G. DRUSCHEL, H. BUCHHEIT, AND A. BERNHARD.
  The influence of total heart lung bypass on infarct size following permanent and temporary
  coronary occlusion.
  European Surgical Research 4(6):384-392, 1972.

2158
KRÜGER, K.
  Myocardial infarction a modern disease? Contemplations and facts on prophylaxis.
  Fortschritte der Medizin 90(3):85-87, 1972.

2159
KRUGER, R.P., ET AL.
  Automated radiographic diagnosis via feature extraction and classification of cardiac size and
  shape descriptors. Institute Electrical Electronics Engineers Transactions Biomedical Engineering
  BME-19:174, 1972.

2160
KRUTOVSKAYA, O.V., N.B. ZALADINOVA, V.I. AFAUNOVA, ET AL.
Shifts in coagulating and fibrinolytic activity of the blood after administration of metandienone in patients with coronary atherosclerosis.
Terapevticheskii Arkhiv 44:29, 1972.

2161
KRYLOV, A.A., AND A.N. TARASOV.
Changes in properties of erythrocytes following myocardial infarction as evidenced by the saponine test and investigations with radioactive chromium.
Terapevticheskii Arkhiv 43(7):37-39, 1971.

2162
KUBICEK, F.
Methodical procedures involved in the ergometric exercise test.
Wiener Klinische Wochenschrift 84(33):522-526, 1972.

2163
KUBICEK, F.
Exercise testing of patients with coronary heart disease.
Correlation to coronary angiography.
Herz/Kreislauf 5(9):363, 1973.

2164
KUBLER, W.
Hemodynamic and metabolic alterations in the angina pectoris attack.
Zeitschrift für Kreislaufforschung 61(9):769-780, 1972.

2165
KUCHIN, N.N., AND YE. V. KOLOMEYETS.
Ischemic heart disease and cosmic radiation.
Zdravookhranenie Kazakhstana 3:19-22, 1973.

2166
KUHN, E., AND V. BRODAN.
Experimental procedures used in studies on psychotropic drug-induced changes in physical fitness.
Activitas Nervosa Superior (Praha) 7:268, 1965.

2167
KUHN, F.M.
Psychopharmaca in heart treatment.
Medizinische Welt 28:1551-1559, 1965.

2168
KUHN, P.
Rehabilitation following acute myocardial infarction.
Wiener Klinische Wochenschrift 84(29):471-474, 1972.

2169
KUHN, P.
Prognosis after acute myocardial infarction.
Wiener Klinische Wochenschrift 85:505, 1973.

2170
KUKUSHKIN, N.I., AND M.YE. SAKSON.
Prediction of the vulnerability of the ventricle to arrhythmia with latency and the duration of the extrasystolic response.
Biophysics 16:941-947, 1971.

2171
KULAK, L.L., R.L. WICK, AND C.E. BILLINGS.
Epidemiological study of in-flight airline pilot incapacitation.
Aerospace Medicine 42(6):670-672, 1971.

2172
KULBERTUS, H.E.
The magnitude of risk of developing complete heart block in patients with LAD-RBBB.
American Heart Journal 86:278, 1973.

2173
KULLER, L., M. COOPER, AND J. PERPER.
Epidemiology of sudden death.
Archives Internal Medicine 129:714, 1972.

2174
KULLER, L.H., M. COOPER, J. PERPER, AND R. FISHER.
Myocardial infarction and sudden death in an urban community.
Bulletin New York Academy Medicine 49:532-543, 1973.

2175
KULLER, L., A. LILIENFELD, AND R. FISHER.
Epidemiological study of sudden and unexpected deaths due to arteriosclerotic heart disease.
Circulation 34:1056-1068, 1966.

2176
KUNZE, D., AND G. LEUSCHNER.
The fatty acid pattern of the phosphatides of serum and erythrocytes in patients with angina pectoris with and without coronary arteriosclerosis demonstrable by coronary angiography.
Cor et Vasa 14(3):169-170, 1972.

2177
KUO, P.T.
Hyperglyceridemia in coronary artery disease and its management.
Journal American Medical Association 201(2):87-94, 1967.

2178
KUPLIC, J.B., AND M.H. LURIA.
Dynamic electrocardiography. A study of patients recovering from acute myocardial infarction.
Ohio State Medical Journal 68(10):950-953, 1972.

2179
KURAMOTO, K., M. IKAI, K. ASAHINA, Y. KURODA, ET AL.
Strenuous exercise electrocardiogram of top class swimmers in Mexico City.
Japanese Heart Journal 8(3):291-299, 1967.

2180
KURUCZ, R.L., E.L. FOX, AND D.K. MATHEWS.
Construction of a submaximal cardiovascular step test.
Research Quarterly American Association Health, Physical Education Recreation 40(1):115-122, 1968.

2181
KUSA, O.
Adhesiveness of platelets in acute myocardial infarction.
Bratislavske Lekarske Listy 58(5):590-593, 1972.

2182
KUSTER, J.
Creatine kinase and myocardial infarction. Complication of differential diagnosis after intramuscular injection of diazepam solution.
Münchener Medizinische Wochenschrift 114(45):1972-1976, 1972.

2183
KUTNER, B.
Social barriers to cardiac rehabilitation.
New York State Journal Medicine 70:517-521, 1970.

2184
KUZKO, N.V.
Efficacy of the use of verapamil in patients with angina pectoris.
Vrachebnoe Delo 10:48-50, 1972.

2185
KUZNETSOV, J.I., AND K.M. KOCHIEV.
The response of patients with mitral stenosis to medical physical exercises according to mechanocardiography data.
Vestnik Khirurgii Imenii I.I. Grekova 110(2):67-70, 1973.

2186
KYPKE, W., AND W. EHRENSTEIN.
Training on the bicycle ergometer in middle age: A ten week longitudinal study.
Zeitschrift für Kreislaufforschung 59(6):534-559, 1970.

2187
LABHARDT, F.
Psychic factors in coronary heart disease.
Münchener Medizinische Wochenschrift 108:1223, 1966.

2188
LACHMANN, W., ET AL.
Experience in the rehabilitation of myocardial infarct.
Journal Bone Joint Surgery 50:113-115, 1968.

2189
LADDU, A.R., S. KUMAKURA, AND P. SOMANI.
Antagonism of cardiac arrhythmias by beta-adrenoreceptor blocking agents.
Archives Internationales de Pharmacodynamie et de Therapie 200:168-181, 1972.

2190
LADIMER, I.
   Professional liability in exercise testing for cardiac performance.
   American Journal Cardiology 30(7):753-756, 1972.

2191
LAHAM, J.
   Peri-infarction blocks and segmentary blocks.
   Archives des Maladies du Coeur et des Vaisseaux 66:1267, 1973.

2192
LAJOS, T.Z., D.G. GREENE, I.L. BUNNELL, H.L. FALSETTI, ET AL.
   Surgery for acute myocardial infarction.
   Annals Thoracic Surgery 8(5):452-457, 1969.

2193
   LAKIER, J.B., W.A. POCOCK, G.E. GALE, AND J.B. BARLOW.
   Haemodynamic and sound events preceding first heart sound in mitral stenosis.
   British Heart Journal 34(11):1152-1155, 1972.

2194
LAMB, L.E.
   Pathogenesis of coronary atherosclerosis.
   Presented at American College of Cardiology Symposium, Nashville, Tenn. Jan. 20, 1969.

2195
LAMB, L.E., AND R.G. HISS.
   Influence of exercise on premature contractions.
   American Journal Cardiology 10:209-216, 1962.

2196
LAMB, L.E., A.D. LeBLANC, W.L. SMITH, R.J. KELLY, AND P.C. JOHNSON.
   Cardiac output and coronary blood flow during steady state recumbent exercise.
   Aerospace Medicine 41:132-134, 1970.

2197
LAMB, L.E., W.L. SMITH, R.J. KELLY, A.D. LeBLANC, AND P.C. JOHNSON.
   Cardiac output and coronary blood flow during progressive recumbent exercise.
   Aerospace Medicine 40:1238-1243, 1969.

2198
LAMBERT, C.J., B.F. MITCHEL, JR., G.F. GEISLER, AND M. ADAM.
   A simple method for aortic cannulation.
   Chest 64:274, 1973.

2199
LAMBERT, E.C., AND A.R. HOHN.
   The pediatrician and congenital heart disease.
   Journal Pediatrics 70(5):833-847, 1967.

2200
LAMBIC, I., ET AL.
   An assessment of the success in the rehabilitation of patients who had suffered myocardial
   infarct.
   Medicinski Glasnik 24:309-315, 1970.

2201
LAMBOURN, R.A.
    Religious identity and response to serious illness: A report on heart patients.
    Social Science Medicine 6:33-34, 1972.

2202
LAMID, S., AND F.W. WOLFF.
    Drug failure in reducing pressor effect of isometric handgrip stress test in hypertension.
    American Heart Journal 86:211, 1973.

2203
LAMONT, N. MCE., AND K. POSEL.
    Myocardial infarction: A hypothesis.
    South African Medical Journal 44(5):123-125, 1970.

2204
LANE, F.M.
    Mental mechanisms and the pain of angina pectoris.
    American Heart Journal 85:563-568, 1973.

2205
LANG, E.
    The heart of aging man. Peculiarities of prophylaxis and therapy.
    Zeitschrift für Allgemeine Medizin, der Landarzt 47(24):1233-1237, 1971.

2206
LANG, E.
    Small ECG seminary. Introductory course in practical electrocardiography.
    Basel, Switzerland. S. Karger, 1972.

2207
LANG, E., K. HECK, J.A. KÖHLER, M. MEYTHALER, AND W. HAAS.
    The behavior of contraction times of the heart during physical stress in healthy people and heart
    patients.
    Zeitschrift für Kreislaufforschung 60(7):669, 1971.

2208
LANG, E., AND B. KRAUSS.
    Time intervals of cardiac dynamics during physical working in patients with acquired or congenital
    cardiac defects.
    Zeitschrift für Kreislaufforschung 59(2):145-152, 1970.

2209
LANG, E., R. WEINZIERL, D. SCHILLING, ET AL.
    Study of a new method of rating arterial walls.
    Actuelle Gerontologie 2:17, 1972.

2210
LANG, S.
    Appraisal of 90 cases of myocardial infarction treated in the years 1958-1969 in the District
    Hospital at Brzozow.
    Wiadomosci Lekarskie 24(6):595-596, 1971.

2211
LANGE, R.L., M.S. REID, D.D. TRESCH, ET AL.
Nonatheromatous ischemic heart disease following withdrawal from chronic industrial nitroglycerin exposure.
Circulation 46(4):666-678, 1972.

2212
LANGE-ANDERSEN, K.
The effect of physical training with and without cold exposure upon physiological indices of fitness for work.
Canadian Medical Association Journal 96:801-804, 1967.

2213
LANGE-ANDERSEN, K.
The determinants of physical performance capacity in health and disease.
In: Naughton, J., H.K. Hellerstein, and I.C. Mohler, Eds. Exercise testing and exercise training in coronary heart disease, pp. 33-44. New York, Academic Press, 1973.

2214
LANGE-ANDERSEN, K., R.J. SHEPHARD, H. DENOLIN, E. VARNAUSKAS, AND R. MASIRONI.
Fundamentals of exercise testing.
World Health Organization. Geneva, Switzerland, 1971.

2215
LANGER, G.A.
Effects of digitalis on myocardial ionic exchange.
Circulation 46(1):180-187, 1972.

2216
LANIADO, S., P. SEGAL, AND B. ESRIG.
Role of glucagon hypersecretion in pathogenesis of hyperglycemia following acute myocardial infarction.
Circulation 48(4):797-800, 1973.

2217
LAPICCIRELLA, V.
Anxiety states, altered diaphragmatic breathing, coronary disease.
Japanese Heart Journal 9(4):321-331, 1968.

2218
LAPITZKY, F.G., AND N.V. SHTEIN.
Sudden death in apparently healthy sporting teenagers in the course of usual physical stress.
Sudebno-Meditsinskaia Ekspertiza 13(2):16-18, 1970.

2219
LARINA, T.F.
Dynamics of contractile capacity of the heart in patients with postinfarction myocardiosclerosis.
Terpevticheskii Arkhiv 44(8):58-61, 1972.

2220
LaROSA, J.C.
Hyperlipoproteinemia. I. Diagnosis and clinical significance.
Postgraduate Medicine 51:62, 1972.

2221
LA ROSA, J.C.
  Hyperlipoproteinemia. II. Dietary management. III. Drug therapy.
  Postgraduate Medicine 52(1):75, 128, 1972.

2222
LARSEN, O.A., AND N.A. LASSEN.
  Medical treatment of occlusive arterial disease of the legs. Walking exercise and medically induced hypertension.
  Angiologica 6(5):288-301, 1969.

2223
LARSEN, O.A., AND R.O. MALMBORG, EDS.
  Coronary heart disease and physical fitness.
  Copenhagen, Denmark, Munksgaard and Baltimore, University Park Press, 1971.

2224
LASKOWSKI, S., J. STASZEWSKI, AND T. KARCZEWSKI.
  Acute myocarditis and myocardial infarction during influenza.
  Wiadomosci Lekarskie 25(14):1249-1253, 1972.

2225
LASSERS, B.W.
  First-year follow-up after recovery from acute myocardial infarction with complete heart-block.
  Lancet 1:1172-1174, 1969.

2226
LASSERS, B.W., AND D.G. JULIAN.
  Artificial pacing management of complete heart block complicating acute myocardial infarction.
  British Medical Journal 2:142-146, 1968.

2227
LASSERS, B.W., M.L. WAHLQUIST, L. KAIJSER, AND L.A. CARLSON.
  Effect of nicotinic acid on myocardial metabolism in man at rest and during exercise.
  Journal Applied Physiology 33(1):72-80, 1972.

2228
LATEGOLA, M.T., AND J. NAUGHTON.
  Restoration of cardiovascular integrity in post myocardially-infarcted aviation personnel.
  Aerospace Medicine 38:1067-1070, 1967.

2229
LATEGOLA, M.T., J. NAUGHTON, C.M. BRAKE, AND P. LYNE.
  Use of simultaneous multilead telecardiography for monitoring cardiovascular rehabilitants during exercise.
  Aerospace Medicine 40:1258, 1969.

2230
LATOSZEK, M.
  The sociologist in rehabilitation of cardiovascular diseases.
  Przeglad Lekarski 25:343-346, 1969.

2231
LAUBINGER, G.
   Early mobilization after myocardial infarction.
   Herz/Kreislauf 5:439, 1973.

2232
LAUFER, A.
   Acute myocardial anoxia. Anatomical changes and their possible relation to immunological pro-
   cesses.
   Cardiologia 56:65-72, 1972.

2233
LAURSEN, B., AND J. GORMSEN.
   Studies on fibrinolytic activity in normal persons and patients with atherosclerotic vascular disease
   after physical activity and injections of nicotinic acid.
   Angiology 21:486, 1970.

2234
LAUTER, C.B., M.R. EL-KHATIB, J.A. RISING, AND E. ROBIN.
   The nitroblue tetrazolium test and acute myocardial infarction.
   Annals Internal Medicine 79:59, 1973.

2235
LAUWERS, P.
   Exercise-electrocardiography diagnosis.
   Lancet 2:47, 1967.

2236
LAUWERS, P., W. AELVOET, R. SNEPPE, AND M. REMION.
   Effect of car driving on the electrocardiogram of patients with myocardial infarction and an
   electrocardiogram at rest devoid of dysrhythmia and repolarization abnormalities. Comparison with
   the electrocardiogram changes obtained during exercise.
   Acta Cardiologica 28(1):27-43, 1973.

2237
LAVIN, M.A.
   Bed exercises for acute cardiac patients.
   American Journal Nursing 73:1226, 1973.

2238
LAVINE, P., D. KIMBIRIS, B.L. SEGAL, AND J.W. LINHART.
   Left main coronary artery disease: clinical, arteriographic and hemodynamic appraisal.
   American Journal Cardiology 30(8):791-796, 1972.

2239
LAWECKI, J., L. CEREMUZYNSKI, J. KUCH, H. ROGALA, AND M. MARKIEWICZ.
   Insulinemia and relationship between catecholamine and glycemia in the course of a recent
   myocardial infarction.
   Acta Diabetologica Latina 9:800, 1972.

2240
LAWECKI, J., J. KUCH, L. CEREMUZYNSKI, AND H. ROGALA.
   The behavior of blood sugar and serum insulin (IRI) after oral administration of glucose in
   different stages of myocardial infarction.
   Acta Diabetologica Latina 9:97-110, 1972.

2241
LAWRENCE, G.H., R.C.R. RIGGINS, R. HIPP, AND R.R. JOHNSTON.
Status of 100 patients after coronary artery bypass surgery.
American Journal Surgery 126:277-285, 1973.

2242
LAWRENCE, T., AND W.S. FRANKL.
Beta-adrenergic receptor blocking drugs.
Medical Clinics North America 57:985, 1973.

2243
LAWRIE, D.M., M.R. HIGGINS, M.J. GODMAN, M.F. OLIVER, D.G. JULIAN, AND K.W. DONALD.
Ventricular fibrillation complicating acute myocardial infarction.
Lancet 2:523-528, 1968.

2244
LAYMAN, W.A.
Psychologic impact of a coronary care unit.
Journal Medical Society New Jersey 69(12):1001-1006, 1972.

2245
LAYTON, C., H. DI NUNZIO, G. GENT, ET AL.
Rate corrected systolic time intervals and Valsalva manoeuvre.
British Heart Journal 35(3):236-244, 1973.

2246
LAZARUS, H.R., AND J.H. HAGENS.
Prevention of psychosis following open-heart surgery.
American Journal Psychiatry 124(9):1190-1195, 1968.

2247
LEACHMAN, R.D., D.V. COKKINOS, O. ZAMALLOA, AND C. DEL RIO.
Intercoronary artery steal. A real entity?
Cardiovascular Research Center Bulletin 10(3):71-83, 1972.

2248
LEAL, R.I., T.N. CARIS, AND M.C. LANCASTER.
Silent and atypical myocardial infarct.
Archivos del Instituto de Cardiologia de Mexico 41(3):249-254, 1971.

2249
LEAVITT, L.A., AND H. WING.
Values of electrodiagnosis in medicine.
Southern Medical Journal 57:960-963, 1964.

2250
LEBOVITS, B.Z., R.B. SCHEKELLE, A.M. OSTFELD, AND O. PAUL.
Prospective and retrospective psychological studies of coronary heart disease.
Psychosomatic Medicine 29:265-272, 1967.

2251
LECEROF, H.
Influence of body position on exercise tolerance, heart rate, blood pressure, and respiration rate in coronary insufficiency.
British Heart Journal 33(1):78-83, 1971.

2252
LECEROF, H. AND R.O. MALMBORG.
Hemodynamic effects of oxprenolol alone and combined with nitroglycerin in patients with ischemic heart disease.
Acta Medica Scandinavica 192(6):499-506, 1972.

2253
LECOMTE, J., J. TROQUET, AND J. BOLAND.
Indications and contraindications of balneotherapy, particularly carbon dioxide baths, in certain cardiovascular affections.
Revue Médicale de Liège 27(5):150-156, 1972.

2254
LEDSOME, J.R., R.J. LINDEN, AND J. NORMAN.
The use of sympathetic beta receptor blocking agents in the investigation of reflex changes in heart rate.
British Journal Pharmacology Chemotherapy 24:781-788, 1965.

2255
LEE, G.B., W. WILSON, K. AMPLATZ, ET AL.
Correlation of vectorcardiogram and electrocardiogram with the coronary arteriogram.
Circulation 38:189-200, 1968.

2256
LEE, K.T., W.M. LEE, J. HAN, J. JARMOLYCH, ET AL.
Experimental model for study of "sudden death" from ventricular fibrillation or asystole.
American Journal Cardiology 32:62, 1973.

2257
LEE, S.J.K., B. JONSSON, S. BEVEGARD, I. KARLÖF, AND H. ASTRÖM.
Hemodynamic changes at rest and during exercise in patients with aortic stenosis of varying severity.
American Heart Journal 79(3):318-331, 1970.

2258
LEE, S.J.K., G. LIESKOVSKY, AND J.C. CALLAGHAN.
Anoxic cardiac arrest and acute myocardial infarction during coronary bypass operations.
Canadian Journal Surgery 16:241, 1973.

2259
LEE, S.J.K., A.R. MCCLELLAND, AND A.J. ZARAGOZA.
The right ventricular function during exercise in patients with and without right ventricular failure.
Acta Cardiologica 25(4):313-325, 1970.

2260
LEES, R.S., AND D.S. FREDRICKSON.
Carbohydrate induction of hyperlipemia in normal man.
Clinical Research 13:327, 1965.

2261
LEETMA, H.E., M.M. GERTLER, E. SALUSTE, AND J. ROSENBERGER.
Carbohydrate, insulin and lipid interrelationship in ischemic heart and cerebrovascular disease.
Circulation 38(Suppl. 6):124, 1968.

2262
LEETMA, H.E., M.M. GERTLER, J.J. WELSH, E. SALUSTE, AND H.H. WHITER.
Insulin response to glucose stress in covert ischemic coronary and cerebrovascular disease.
Circulation 38(Suppl. 6):124, 1968.

2263
LEFEBVRE, L.
Rehabilitation of cardiac patients in factories.
Revue Médicale de Liège 26:102-107, 1971.

2264
LEGATO, M.J.
Ultrastructure of the atrial, ventricular, and Purkinje cell, with special reference to the genesis of arrhythmias.
Circulation 47:178-189, 1973.

2265
LEGORRETA, M.E., E. CALVA, AND F. LOPEZ SORIANO.
Redox potential, excess lactate and pyruvate extraction in experimental myocardial infarction.
Archivos del Instituto de Cardiologia de Mexico 42:766, 1972.

2266
LEHMAN, E.W.
Social class and coronary heart disease: A sociological assessment of the medical literature.
Journal Chronic Diseases 20:381-391, 1967.

2267
LEHR, I., H.B. MESSINGER, AND R.H. ROSENMAN.
A socio biological approach to the study of coronary heart disease.
Journal Chronic Diseases 26:13-30, 1973.

2268
LEIGH, H., M.A. HOFER, J. COOPER, AND M.F. REISER.
A psychological comparison of patients in 'open' and 'closed' coronary care units.
Journal Psychosomatic Research 16(6):449-457, 1972.

2269
LEIJNSE, B., AND C.T. BARTELS.
Methods and standardization of clinico-chemical examination for the detection and prevention of ischemic heart disease.
Heart Bulletin 3:103, 1972.

2270
LEINBACH, R.C., AND C.A. CACERES.
The electrocardiogram in tachycardia. Common errors of interpretation.
American Heart Journal 71(5):611-615, 1966.

2271
LELLOUCH, J., AND J.L. RICHARD.
   A few results on pressure lability.
   Revue du Praticien 22(16):2553-2557, 1972.

2272
LELY, A.H., AND C.H. VAN ENTER.
   Noncardiac symptoms of digitalis intoxication.
   American Heart Journal 83:149, 1972.

2273
LEMAIRE, A.
   Dietetics of atheroma and hypercholesterolemia
   Presse Médicale 71(26):1321-1324, 1963

2274
LEMAITRE, J., AND A. COLEMONT.
   Study of 32 cases of myocardial infarctus occurring before the age of 46.
   Acta Cardiologica 26(1):66-82, 1971.

2275
LEMBERG, L., A.G. ARCEBAL, A. CASTELLANOS, JR., AND D. SLAVIN.
   Use of alprenolol in acute cardiac arrhythmias.
   American Journal Cardiolgy 30(1):77-81, 1972.

2276
LEMBERG, L., A. CASTELLANOS, JR., AND A.G. ARCEBAL.
   The use of propranolol in arrhythmias complicating acute myocardial infarction.
   American Heart Journal 80(4):479-487, 1970.

2277
LEMBRIGHT, K.A.
   Role of the occupational health nurse.
   Journal Rehabilitation 32:80, 1966.

2278
LEMP, A., F. KOENIG, F. TREPEL, K.-L. FROER, AND K.P. BOERGEN.
   The venous pressure load as a criterion of cardiac capacity: II. Report. Simultaneous measurement
   of peripheral and central venous pressure of healthy persons and patients with cardiac insuf-
   ficiency.
   Zeitschrift für Kreislaufforschung 57(4):366-379, 1968.

2279
LEMMENS, M., AND A. DECORTIS.
   Coronary insufficiency and working capacity.
   Revue de Readaptation 13:170, 1971.

2280
LENKEI, S.C., S.M. FOX, III, AND T.N. LYNN.
   Accurate technique for the volumetric calibration of dye dilution curves.
   Circulation 20:727, 1959.

2281
LENKOVA, R.I., S.V. USIK, AND N.N. IAKOVLEV.
Urea content variations in blood and tissues during muscular activity in relation to the adaptation level of the organism.
Fiziologicheskii Zhurnal SSSR 59:1097-1101, 1973.

2282
LEON, A.S.
Comparative cardiovascular adaptation to exercise in animals and man and its relevance to coronary heart disease.
In: Bloor, C.M., Ed. Comparative pathophysiology of circulatory disturbances, pp. 143-174. New York, Plenum, 1972.

2283
LEONARD, F.
A rationale for the preparation of nonthrombogenic materials.
Transactions American Society Artificial Internal Organs 15:15, 1969.

2284
LEONARD, F.
Rapidly polymerizing adhesives and hemostatic agents.
In: Bement, A.L. Jr., Ed. Biomaterials, pp. 129-131. Seattle, Batelle Seattle Research Center and University of Washington Press, 1971.

2285
LEONARD, F., J.W. BOKE, R.J. RUDERMAN, AND A.F. HEGYELI.
Initiation and inhibition of subcutaneous calcification.
Calcified Tissue Research 10:269-279, 1972.

2286
LEONARD, F., R.K. KULHARNI, J. NELSON, ET AL.
Tissue adhesives and hemostasis-inducing compounds: The alkyl cyanoacrylates.
Journal Biomedical Materials Research 1:3-9, 1967.

2287
LEONARD, F., C.A. NIELSON, A.M. FADALI, ET AL.
Thromboresistant polymers by emulsion polymerization with anionic surfactants. I.
Journal Biomedical Materials Research 3:455-464, 1969.

2288
LEONARD, F., AND R.I. SCULLIN.
New mechanism for calcification of skeletal tissues.
Nature 224:1113-1114, 1969.

2289
LEONARD, F., C.W.R. WADE, AND A.F. HEGYELI.
Mechanism of calcification.
Clinical Orthopaedics 78:168-172, 1971.

2290
LEONE, A.
Post mortem coronary angiography in the pathological study of the heart.
Giornale Italiano di Cardiologia 2(5):688-692, 1972.

2291
LENNARD, H.L., AND C.Y. BLOCK.
Studies in hypertension. IV. Differences in the distribution of hypertension in negroes and whites: An appraisal.
Journal Chronic Diseases 5(2):186-196, 1957.

2292
LENZNER, A.S., AND A.L. ARONSON.
Psychiatric vignettes from a coronary care unit.
Psychosomatics 13:179-184, 1972.

2293
LEPESCHKIN, E.
Evaluation of S-T elevation and T wave inversion after exercise.
Journal Electrocardiology 4:84-85, 1971.

2294
LEPESCHKIN, E., AND B. SURAWICZ.
Characteristics of true-positive and false-positive results of electrocardiographic Master two-step exercise tests.
New England Journal Medicine 258:511-520, 1958.

2295
LEREN, P.
The effect of plasma cholesterol lowering diet in male survivors of myocardial infarction.
Acta Medica Scandinavica (Suppl.):466:1, 1966.

2296
LEREN, P.
The effect of plasma lowering cholesterol diet in male survivors of myocardial infarction. A controlled clinical trial.
In: Aarhus, C., Ed. Norwegian Monographs on Medical Science, Oslo, Norway. Universitets Forlaget, 1967.

2297
LEREN, P.
The effect of cholesterol lowering diet in male survivors of myocardial infarction.
Nordisk Medicin 77:658-661, 1967.

2298
LEREN, P.
Plasma cholesterol lowering diet. The effect in male survivors of myocardial infarction.
Minnesota Medicine 52(8):1231-1235, 1969.

2299
LEREN, P.
The Oslo diet-heart study: Eleven-year report.
Circulation 42(5):935-942, 1970.

2300
LEREN, P.
The Oslo diet-heart study—an 11 year report.
Arbeitsmedizin, Sozialmedizin, Arbeitshygiene 7:221-226, 1972.

2301
LEREN, P.
  Cardiac infarcts.
  Tidsskrift for den Norske Laegeforening 92(26):1672-1674, 1723, 1972.

2302
LESCHINSKII, L.A., AND V.V. KHARITONOVA.
  Combined therapy with metadienone and potassium salts in ischemic heart disease.
  Terapevticheskii Arkhiv 44:40, 1972.

2303
LESHIN, S.J., L.D. HORWITZ, R.R. ECKER, G. BLOMQVIST, ET AL.
  Exercise testing in patients with occluded aortocoronary saphenous vein bypass grafts.
  Journal Clinical Investigation 51:55A, 1972.

2304
LESSIN, L.S., W.N. JENSEN, G.A. KELSER, T. MOTOMIYA, AND G. NACHNANI.
  Vascular catheters and thrombogenesis.
  New England Journal Medicine 287:468, 1972.

2305
LESSIN, L.S., W.N. JENSEN, AND P. KLUG.
  Ultrastructure of the normal and hemoglobinopathic red blood cell membrane.
  Freeze-etching and stereoscan electron microscopic studies.
  Archives Internal Medicine 129:306-319, 1972.

2306
LESSIN, L.S., AND P. KLUG.
  Hemolytic anemias associated with hemoglobinopathies.
  Modern Treatment 8:352-378, 1971.

2307
LESSIN, L.S., AND W.F. ROSSE.
  Diagnostic approach to hemolytic anemias.
  Modern Treatment 8:321-328, 1971.

2308
LESTER, B.K., R. BLOCK, AND C.G. GUNN.
  The relation of cardiac arrhythmias to phases of sleep.
  Clinical Research 17(2):456, 1969.

2309
LESTER, F.M., L.T. SHEFFIELD, AND T.J. REEVES.
  Maximum exercise in elderly males.
  Clinical Research 14(1):42, 1966.

2310
LESTER, F.M., L.T. SHEFFIELD, AND T.J. REEVES.
  Electrocardiographic changes in clinically normal older men following near minimal and maximal
  exercise.
  Circulation 36:5-14, 1967.

2311
LEVANDER-LINDGREN, M.
   Studies in neurocirculatory asthenia.
   Acta Medica Scandinavica 172:665-676, 1962.

2312
LEVANDER-LINDGREN, M.
   Studies in neurocirculatory asthenia. 4. Course during common treatment and physical training and relations between symptoms and signs.
   Acta Medica Scandinavica 175:791-799, 1964.

2313
LEVENKOV, N.V.
   Differential diagnosis of angina pectoris and cardialgic neurosis.
   Terapevticheskii Arkhiv 43(9):70-79, 1971.

2314
LEVENSON, R.M.
   Work evaluation units as a resource in exercise programs.
   Journal South Carolina Medical Association 65(Suppl.1):69-70, 1969.

2315
LEVENSON, R.M., R.H. ROSENMAN, AND J.J. SCHWAB.
   A summary of a symposium on counseling the cardiac on work and sex.
   Ohio State Medical Journal 66(10):1003-1007, 1970.

2316
LEVENSON, R.M., AND D.R. SPARKMAN.
   Exercise testing of cardiac patients in evaluating work potential.
   American Journal Cardiology 7(3):330-334, 1961.

2317
LEVEY, G.S.
   Phospholipids, adenylate cyclase, and the heart.
   Journal Molecular Cellular Cardiology 4(3):283-285, 1972.

2318
LEVIN, B.S.
   Comparative analysis of the therapeutic effect of hydrogen sulfide baths in relation to a therapeutic diet.
   Voprosy Kurortologii, Fizioterapii i Lechebnoi Fizicheskoi Kul'tury 34(4):335-340, 1969.

2319
LEVIN, D.C., AND H.A. BALTAXE.
   Angiographic demonstration of important anatomic variations of the posterior descending coronary artery.
   American Journal Roentgenology 116(1):41-49, 1972.

2320
LEVIN, D.C., R.G. CARLSON, AND H.A. BALTAXE.
   Angiographic determination of operability in candidates for aorto coronary bypass.
   American Journal Roentgenology 116(1):66-73, 1972.

2321
LEVIN, P.M., N.M. RICH, AND J.E. HUTTON, JR.
Patency of venous grafts in the venous system.
Journal Cardiovascular Surgery 13(5):421-427, 1972.

2322
LEVINE, H.J., W.A. NEILL, R.J. WAGMAN, N. KRASNOW, AND R. GORLIN.
The effect of exercise on mean left ventricular ejection rate in man.
Journal Clinical Investigation 41:1050, 1962.

2323
LEVINE, S., AND N.A. SCOTCH.
Social stress and cardiac disease. Workshop summary. Toward the development of theoretical models: II.
Milbank Memorial Fund Quarterly 45(Suppl.):163-174, 1967.

2324
LEVINE, S.A., AND B. LOWN.
"Armchair" treatment of acute coronary thrombosis.
Journal American Medical Association 148:1365, 1952.

2325
LEVINSON, G.E., J.F. MARTIN, AND C.J. SCHWARTZ.
The effect of rest and physical effort on the left ventricular burden in mitral and aortic regurgitation.
American Heart Journal 80(6):791-801, 1970.

2326
LEVINSON, H.
Emotional toxicity of the work environment.
Archives Environmental Health 19(2):239-243, 1969.

2327
LEVITAS, I.M., AND J.J. KRISTAL.
Stress exercise testing of the young diabetic for the detection of unknown coronary artery disease.
In: Shafrier, P., Ed. Impact of insulin on metabolic pathways. International Symposium, Jerusalem, Israel, 1971, pp. 491-493. New York, Academic Press, 1972.

2328
LEVITT, B., A. RAINES, Y.J. SOHN, AND F.G. STANDAERT.
Sleep regimen for myocardial infarction.
Lancet 1:1308-1309, 1968.

2329
LEVY, A.M., B.S. TABAKIN, AND J.S. HANSON.
Hemodynamic responses to graded treadmill exercise in young untreated labile hypertensive patients.
Circulation 35(6):1063-1072, 1967.

2330
LEVY, J.V.
Positive inotropic effects of papaverine and aminophylline on isolated human atrial preparations.
Research Communications Chemical Pathology Pharmacology 4(2):261-266, 1972.

2331
LEVY, M.J., B. VIDNE, J. SALOMON, AND D. ESHKOL.
Long-term follow-up (one to four years) of heart valve prostheses (102 consecutive patients).
Diseases Chest 56(5):440-446, 1969.

2332
LEVY, M.N., T. IANO, AND H. ZIESKE.
Effects of repetitive bursts of vagal activity on heart rate.
Circulation Research 30:186, 1972.

2333
LEVY, R.I.
Classification and etiology of hyperlipoproteinemias.
Federation Proceedings 30:829-834, 1971.

2334
LEVY, R.I., AND D.S. FREDRICKSON.
The current status of hypolipidemic drugs.
Postgraduate Medicine 47:130-136, 1970.

2335
LEVY, R.I., D.S. FREDRICKSON, N.J. STONE, D.W. BILHEIMER, W.V. BROWN, C.J. GLUECK, A.M. GOTTO, P.N. HERBERT, P.O. KWITEROVICH, T. LANGER, J. LaROSA, S.E. LUX, A.K. RIDER, R.S. SHULMAN, AND H.R. SLOAN.
Cholestyramine in type II hyperlipoproteinemia.
Annals Internal Medicine 79:51, 1973.

2336
LEVY, R.I., R.S. LEES, AND D.S. FREDRICKSON.
The nature of pre-beta (very low density) lipoproteins.
Journal Clinical Investigation 45: 63-77, 1966.

2337
LEW, E.A.
Survivorship after myocardial infarction.
American Journal Public Health 57:118-127, 1967.

2338
LEWES, D., AND D.W. HILL.
Application of multipoint electrodes to telemetry in patient-monitoring and during physical exercise.
British Heart Journal 29:689-699, 1967.

2339
LEWIS, A.J., G. AILSHIE, AND J.M. CRILEY.
Pre-hospital cardiac care in a paramedical mobile intensive care unit.
California Medicine 117(4):1-8, 1972.

2340
LEWIS, B.S., A. BAKST, D. KITCHINER, AND M.S. GOTSMAN.
Effectiveness of sectral (M & B 17803A) as a beta-blocking agent in man.
South African Medical Journal 47: 1181, 1973.

2341

LEWIS, B.S., AND M.S. GOTSMAN.
  Left ventricular function in systole and diastole in constructive pericarditis.
  American Heart Journal 86: 23, 1973.

2342

LEWIS, C.E.
  Factors influencing the return to work of men with congestive heart failure.
  Journal Chronic Diseases 19(11/12):1193-1209, 1966.

2343

LEWIS, C.M.
  Studies in exercise tolerance as an aid to cardiological diagnosis and assessment.
  South African Medical Journal 38(1): 2-9, 1964.

2344

LEWIS, F.J., S. DELLER, M. QUINN, ET AL.
  Continuous patient monitoring with a small digital computer.
  Computers Biomedical Research 5(4):411-428, 1972.

2345

LEWIS, L.
  Convalescence: a positive approach.
  Journal Rehabilitation 32:35, 1966.

2346

LEWIS, R.P., H. BOUDOULAS, W.F. FORESTER, AND A.M. WEISSLER.
  Shortening of electromechanical systole as a manifestation of excessive adrenergic stimulation in
  acute myocardial infarction.
  Circulation 46(5):856-862, 1972.

2347

LEWIS, R.P., J.D. BRISTOW, AND H.E. GRISWOLD.
  Exercise hemodynamics in aortic regurgitation.
  American Heart Journal 80(2):171-176, 1970.

2348

LEWIS, W.H.
  Iatrogenic psychotic depressive reaction in hypertensive patients.
  American Journal Psychiatry 127(10):1416-1417, 1971.

2349

LI, Y.-B., TING NONG, CHIANG BI-NIN, E.R. ALEXANDER, R.A. BRUCE, AND J.T. GRAYSTON.
  Electrocardiographic response to maximal exercise treadmill and double Master exercise tests in
  middle-aged Chinese men.
  American Journal Cardiology 20(4):541-548, 1967.

2350

LICHSTEIN, E., K.D. CHADDA, AND P.K. GUPTA.
  Complete right bundle branch block with left axis deviation: significance of vectorcardiographic
  morphology.
  American Heart Journal 86:13, 1973.

2351
LICHTIG, C., S. GLAGOV, S. FELDMAN, AND R.W. WISSLER.
Myocardial ischemia and coronary artery atherosclerosis. A comprehensive approach to post-mortem studies.
Medical Clinics North America 57(1):79-91, 1973.

2352
LICHTLEN, P.
The hemodynamics of clinical ischemic heart disease.
Annals Clinical Research 3(6):333-343, 1971.

2353
LICHTLEN, P., H. ALBERT, AND M. SPIEGEL.
On the effect of beta-receptor blockade in coronary insufficiency: II. Left ventricular dynamics during exercises before and after administration of propranolol and the combination of propranolol and nitroglycerin.
Zeitschrift für Kreislaufforschung 59(3):207-218, 1970.

2354
LICHTLEN, P., P.C. BAUMANN, AND H. ALBERT.
The role of left ventricular abnormalities in exercise induced performance in patients with severe coronary artery disease.
Cardiologia 54(5):295-319, 1969.

2355
LICHTMAN, J., R.A. O'ROURKE, A. KLEIN, AND J.S. KARLINER.
Electrocardiogram of the athlete.
Archives Internal Medicine 132: 763, 1973.

2356
LIEB, S.
Compensable heart disease.
Bulletin Academy Medicine New Jersey 11(2):121-126, 1965.

2357
LIEBOLD, F., T. LUTHER, G. SCHLEUSING, AND J. SCHAUER.
Influence of remedial exercises on the cardiopulmonary system in postinfarction conditions.
Medizin und Sport 12(5):158-160, 1972.

2358
LIFSHITS, R.I., V.B. SLOBODIN, V.S. YAKUSHEV. ET AL.
Isoenzymes of lactic dehydrogenase of the heart, liver, and kidneys in experimentally induced ischemic conditions.
Byulleten Eksperimental'noi Biologii i Meditsiny 74(12):49-51, 1972.

2359
LIKOFF, W.
The acute coronary attack.
Journal Rehabilitation 32:25, 1966.

2360
LIKOFF, W.
Office management of patients after heart surgery.
In: Bailey, C., A.G. Shapiro, and S. Gollub, Eds. Therapeutic advances in the practice of cardiology, pp 427-432. New York, Grune and Stratton, 1970.

2361
LIKOFF, W.
  Medical management of angina pectoris.
  Geriatrics 27(5):91-98, 1972.

2362
LIKOFF, W., S. BENDER, AND L. DREIFUS.
  The fate of a patient with so-called mild coronary.
  Journal American Medical Association 177: 579, 1961.

2363
LIKOFF, W., B. SEGAL, AND B. INSULL.
  Atherosclerosis and coronary heart disease.
  New York, Grune and Stratton, 1972.

2364
LILJEFORS, I.
  Coronary heart disease in male twins: Hereditary and environmental factors in concordant and
  discordant pairs.
  Acta Medica Scandinavica (Suppl.)511:9-90, 1970.

2365
LILJEFORS, I., AND R.H. RAHE.
  An identical twin study of psychosocial factors in coronary heart disease in Sweden.
  Psychosomatic Medicine 32(5):523-538, 1970.

2366
LILJEFORS, I., AND R.H. RAHE.
  Hereditary and environmental factors in coronary heart disease: A study on twins.
  Opuscula Medica 16(7):243-246, 1971.

2367
LILJESTRAND, G., E. LYSHOLM, AND G. NYLIN.
  The immediate effects of muscular work on stroke and heart volume in man.
  Scandinavian Archives Physiology 80:265, 1938.

2368
LIM, C.H., AND C.C.S. TOH.
  Cardiogenic shock following acute myocardial infarction and the role of ethyl adrianol in its
  treatment.
  Singapore Medical Journal 13(4):172-177, 1972.

2369
LIN, W.L.
  Circulatory effects of peridural anesthesia in aged men.
  Japanese Journal Anesthesiology 21(9):823-839, 1972.

2370
LINARES CASAS, J.C., R. ARCAS MECA, A. OCHOTECO, AND J. ESPINO VELA.
  Postoperative arrhythmias in auricular septal defect.
  Archivos del Instituto de Cardiologia de Mexico 42:614, 1972.

2371
LIND, A.R. Cardiovascular responses to static exercise. (Isometrics, Anyone?)
Circulation 41:173, 1970.

2372
LIND, A.R., AND G.W. McNICOL.
Muscular factors which determine the cardiovascular responses to sustained and rhythmic exercise.
Canadian Medical Association Journal 96:706-713, 1967.

2373
LIND, E., AND T. THEORELL.
Sociological characteristics and myocardial infarctions.
Journal Psychosomatic Research 17:59-73, 1973.

2374
LINDE, L.M., S.W. TURNER, AND S. AWA.
Present status and treatment of paroxysmal supraventricular tachycardia.
Pediatrics 50(1):127-130, 1972.

2375
LINDEN, V.
Myocardial infarction and urolithiasis. A preliminary communication.
Journal Kansas Medical Society 73(12):503-505, 1972.

2376
LINDERHOLM, H., R. MÜLLER, T. RINGQVIST, AND R. SÖRNÄS.
Hereditary abnormal muscle metabolism with hyperkinetic circulation during exercise.
Acta Medica Scandinavica 185(3):153-166, 1969.

2377
LINDNER, E.
Pharmacologic and clinical effects of Segontin (Prenylamin). II. Distribution and degradation of Prenylamin in the body.
Herz Kreislauf 5(7):288-291, 1973.

2378
LINDQUIST, V.A.Y., R.D. SPANGLER, AND S.G. BLOUNT, JR.
A comparison between the effects of dynamic and isometric exercise as evaluated by the systolic time intervals in normal man.
American Heart Journal 85(2):227-236, 1973.

2379
LINDSAY, C.J.E., AND W.H. PHILLIPS.
Structural changes in exercising middle-aged males during a 2-year period.
Journal Applied Physiology 27(6):787-794, 1969.

2380
LINFORS, O.
Reconstructive vascular surgery of the lower extremities.
Finska Lakaresallskapets Handligar 116:106, 1972.

2381
LINHART, J.W.
Atrial pacing in coronary artery disease, including preinfarction angina and postoperative studies.
American Journal Cardiology 30(6):603-610, 1972.

2382
LINHART, J.W., B.M. BELLER, AND R.C. TALLEY.
Coronary artery disease evaluation by the multi-stage treadmill exercise test and right atrial pacing.
Chest 63:505, 1973.

2383
LINN, J.E., JR.
It takes an all-out effort to keep your patient alive in this classic crisis—if you can get there in time.
Emergency Medicine 5:24, 1973.

2384
LINSCHOTEN, H., N.G. MEIJNE, H.M. MELLINK, AND A.D. OVERDIJK.
Pacemaker implanatation and infection.
Journal Cardiovascular Surgery 14:126, 1973.

2385
LINZBACH, C., R. FELIX, P. THURN, ET AL.
The coronary circulation following vascular occlusion. III: Contractile inadequacy of ventricular myocardium after acute coronary occlusion.
Fortschritte auf dem Gebiete der Roentgenstrahlen und der Nuklearmedizin 116(5):599-606, 1972.

2386
LIPMAN, R.L., P. RASKIN, T. LOVE, J. TRIEBWASSER, ET AL.
Glucose intolerance during decreased physical activity in man.
Diabetes 21(2):101-107, 1972.

2387
LIPP, H., M. GAMBETTA, J. SCHWARTZ, ET AL.
Intermittent pansystolic murmur and presumed mitral regurgitation after acute myocardial infarction.
American Journal Cardiology 30(6):690-694, 1972.

2388
LIPSETT, D., B.K. MADRAS, R.J. WURTMAN, AND H.N. MUNRO.
Serum tryptophan level after carbohydrate ingestion. Selective decline in nonalbumin-bound tryptophan coincident with reduction in serum free fatty acids.
Life Sciences, Part II. Biochemistry, General and Molecular Biology 12(2):57-64, 1973.

2389
LISAK, R.P., J. LEBEAU, S.H. TUCKER, AND L.P. ROWLAND.
Hyperkalemic periodic paralysis and cardiac arrhythmia.
Neurology 22(8):810-815, 1972.

2390
LISKER, S.A., AND D. FINKELSTEIN.
The cardio-auditory syndrome of Jervell and Lange-Nielson: Report of an additional case with radioelectrocardiographic monitoring during exercise.
American Journal Medical Sciences 252(4):458-464, 1966.

2391
LISS, J.P., JR., R.M. JERESATY, AND J. NAKHOUL.
Lidocaine in ventricular arrhythmia.
American Heart Journal 86:143, 1973.

2392
LISTER, J.W., A.N. DAMATO, J.A. RICCI, L.S. SCHWARTZ, AND E. STEIN.
Effect of exercise on atrioventricular transmission in patients with atrioventricular conduction distrubances.
New York State Journal Medicine 68(12):1736-1740, 1968.

2393
LISTER, J.W., E. STEIN, B.D. KOSOWSKY, S.H. LAU, AND A.N. DAMATO.
Atrioventricular conduction in man. Effect of rate, exercise, isoproterenol and atropine on the P-R interval.
American Journal Cardiology 16:516-523, 1965.

2394
LISTER, J.W., F.X. WORTHINGTON, JR., T.O. GENTSCH, ET AL.
Preexcitation and tachycardias in Wolf-Parkinson-White syndrome, type B. A case report.
Circulation 45(4):1081-1090, 1972.

2395
LITTLE, J.A.
Some comments on exercise and changes in blood chemistry.
Canadian Medical Association Journal 96:786, 1967.

2396
LITTLE, J.A.
Fats in adult nutrition.
Canadian Journal Public Health 62(1):27-35, 1971.

2397
LITTLE, J.A., ET AL.
Studies of male survivors of myocardial infarction. IV. Serum lipids and five-year survival.
Circulation 31:854-862, 1965.

2398
LIXI, M., G. PORRAZZO, A. CHERCHI, M.P. ESU, AND P. SASSU.
Metabolic and hemodynamic response to progressive muscular exercise in a sitting position in coronary patients (triangular test 10 watts/min.).
Bollettino della Società Italiana di Cardiologia 14(6):821-836, 1969.

2399
LIXI, M., G. PORRAZZO, P. SASSU, M.P. ESU, P. MONTALDO, AND A. CHERCHI.
The metabolic and hemodynamic response of patients affected by mitral stenosis to progressive orthostatic muscular exercise: II. Systemic arterial pressure, peripheral resistances and tension time index.
Bollettino della Societa Italiana di Cardiologia 14(4):480-483, 1969.

2400
LLOYD, A.M., AND P. JOYCE.
The diagnosis and treatment of anxiety in acute coronary heart disease.
Australian New Zealand Journal Medicine 1(3):274, 1971.

2401
LLOYD-THOMAS, H.G.
The exercise electrocardiogram in patients with cardiac pain.
British Heart Journal 23(5):561-577, 1961.

2402
LOBSTEIN, H.P., L.D. HORWITZ, G.C. CURRY, AND C.B. MULLINS.
Mitral click-murmur syndrome: ECG abnormalities and coronary arteriograms.
New England Journal Medicine 289:127, 1973.

2403
LODIN, A., AND S. ZETTERQUIST.
Metabolic evaluation of the crural blood flow during standing and during sitting leg exercise in patients with congenital absence of venous valves in the legs.
Acta Dermato-Venereologica 45(1):26-33, 1965.

2404
LOELIGER, E.A.
On treatment with oral anticoagulants.
Therapie der Gegenwart 112:1159, 1973.

2405
LOELIGER, E.A., A. HENSEN, F. KROES, L.M. VAN DIJK, ET AL.
A double-blind trial of long-term anticoagulant treatment after myocardial infarction.
Acta Medica Scandinavica 182(5):549-566, 1967.

2406
LOGEAIS, Y., J. FEUILLU, Y. KERDILES, ET AL.
A case of chylopericardium. Diagnostic and therapeutic problems.
Annales de Chirurgie 11(2):231-238, 1972.

2407
LOGIC, J.R., D.H. MORROW, AND R.N. GATZ.
Idioventricular tachycardia complicating experimental myocardial infarction.
Diseases Chest 56:477-480, 1969.

2408
LOMBARDO, T.A., L. ROSE, M. TAESCHLER, S. TULLY, AND R.J. BING.
The effect of exercise on coronary blood flow, myocardial oxygen consumption and cardiac efficiency in man.
Circulation 7:71, 1953.

2409
LONG, R.H.
The physician and the law (third edition).
New York, Appleton-Century-Crofts, 1968.

2410
LONGHURST, J., R.J. CAPONE, E.A. AMSTERDAM, D.T. MASON, AND R. ZELIS.
A microcirculatory defect in congestive heart failure—etiology of depressed oxygen consumption during exercise.
Clinical Research 20(2):208, 1972.

2411
LOOS, A., AND M. KALTENBACH.
The effect of Nifedipine (Bay A 1040) on the work of ECG of angina pectoris patients.
Arzneimittel-Forschung 22:358-362, 1972.

2412
LORENTE, P., A. BOURTHOUMIEUX, P. SKOUFAS, G. MOTTE, AND P.G. PERNOT.
Influence of the inotropic effect of Lanatoside C on the cardiac function and mechanism of valve closure in patients with synus rhythm.
Archives des Maladies du Coeur et des Vaisseaux 63:720-739, 1970.

2413
LORENTE, P., R. SLAMA, AND Y. BOUVRAIN.
The techniques for the determination of cardiac output and their critical study.
Poumon et Coeur 28(5):217-221, 1972.

2414
LOTTENBACH, K.
Vasomotor tone and local vasoconstrictor responses induced by cold.
Angiologica 5:377-385, 1968.

2415
LOTTO, A., B. LOMANTO, AND M. BOSSI.
First experience in the clinical use of a new antiarrhythmic agent, bunaftide.
Cardiologia Pratica 23(2):123-133, 1972.

2416
LOUP, R.J.
Shorter hospitalization for myocardial infarcts.
New England Journal Medicine 289:805, 1973.

2417
LOVELL, R.R.H.
Lessons about myocardial infarction from studies of long-term anticoagulation.
Circulation 40(5 Suppl. 4):119-123, 1969.

2418
LOVELL, R.R.H.
Long-term prognosis after myocardial infarction.
In: Meltzer, L.E. and A.J. Dunning, Eds. Textbook of coronary care, pp. 173-187. Amsterdam, Excerpta Medica, 1972.

2419
LOVELL, R.R.H., M.A. DENBOROUGH, P.J. NESTEL, AND A.J. GOBLE.
A controlled trial of long-term treatment with anticoagulants after myocardial infarction in male patients.
Medical Journal Australia 54(11 Suppl. 3):97-104, 1967.

2420
LOVELL, R.R.H., AND A. VERGHESE.
Personality traits associated with different chest pains after myocardial infarction.
British Medical Journal 3:327-330, 1967.

2421
LOWENTHAL, M.
Exercise programs for health maintenance. An opportunity for rehabilitation medicine.
Archives Physical Medicine Rehabilitation 54:36-38, 1973.

2422
LOWN, B.
   Electrical reversion of cardiac arrhythmias.
   British Heart Journal 29:469, 1967.

2423
LOWN, B., AND P. AXELROD.
   Implanted standby defibrillators.
   Circulation 46(4):637-639, 1972.

2424
LOWN, B., L. EHRLICH, B. LIPSCHULTZ, AND J. BLAKE.
   Effect of digitalis in patients receiving reserpine.
   Circulation 24:1185, 1961.

2425
LOWN, B., A.M. FAKHRO, W.B. HOOD, JR., AND G.W. THORN.
   The coronary care unit: New perspectives and directions.
   Journal American Medical Association 199:188, 1967.

2426
LOWN, B., M.D. KLEIN, I. BARR, ET AL.
   Sensitivity to digitalis drugs in acute myocardial infarction.
   American Journal Cardiology 30(4):388-395, 1972.

2427
LOWN, B., M.D. KLEIN, AND P.I. HERSHBERG.
   Coronary and precoronary care.
   American Journal Medicine 46:705-724, 1969.

2428
LOWN, B., B. KOSOWSKY, AND R. WHITING.
   Exposure of electrical instability in coronary artery disease by exercise stress.
   Circulation 39-40(Suppl. 3):136, 1969.

2429
LOWN, B., AND V.W. SIDEL.
   Duration of hospital stay following acute myocardial infarction.
   American Journal Cardiology 23(1):1-3, 1969.

2430
LOWN, B., AND C. VASSAUX.
   Lidocaine in acute myocardial infarction.
   American Heart Journal 76:586, 1968.

2431
LOWN, B., C. VASSAUX, W.B. HOOD, JR., A.M. FAKHRO, ET AL.
   Unresolved problems in coronary care.
   American Journal Cardiology 20:494, 1967.

2432
LU, H.H., AND C. MCBROOKS.
   An analysis of factors operating at the cellular level to cause arrhythmias.
   Circulation 37-38(Suppl. 6):130, 1968.

2433
LUBBERS, P.
Atrial dissociation (atrial double rhythm) and pseudo atrial double rhythm (the Deitz-Marques phenomenon).
Zeitschrift für Kreislaufforschung 61(7):604-613, 1972.

2434
LUBKE, P., AND H. DANNEMANN.
Circulatory effects of benzoctamine in patients under halothane anesthesia.
Zeitschrift für Praktische Anaesthesie und Wiederbelebung 7(5):270-276, 1972.

2435
LUCAS BERGSTRA, H.J.
Medicosocial work with heart patients.
Metamedica 51(5):107-118, 1972.

2436
LUCE, R.S., AND J.M. LAGERWERFF.
High performance exercise cardiotachometer.
Aerospace Medicine 43(5):537-540, 1972.

2437
LUCIA, W., AND L.B. McGUIRE.
Rehabilitation and functional status after surgery for valvular heart disease.
Archives Internal Medicine 126(6):995-999, 1970.

2438
LUCZAK, J.
Clinical evaluation of fentanyl and droperidol in acute myocardial infarction.
Kardiologia Polska 15:299-306, 1972.

2439
LUDWIG, E.G., AND J. WYSONG.
Work, heart disease and mental health.
Journal Chronic Diseases 21:687-689, 1969.

2440
LUEKER, R.D., J.H.K. VOGEL, AND S.G. BLOUNT, JR.
Cardiovascular abnormalities following surgery for left-to-right shunts. Observations in atrial septal defects, ventricular septal defects, and patent ductus arteriousus.
Circulation 40:785-801, 1969.

2441
LUEKER, R.D., J.H.K. VOGEL, R. PRIOR, AND S.G. BLOUNT, JR.
Unreliable electrocardiographic assessment of hemodynamic changes after correction of ventricular septal defect with pulmonary hypertension.
American Journal Cardiology 28(3):303-308, 1971.

2442
LUEPKER, R.V., S. HOLMBERG, AND E. VARNAUSKAS.
Left atrial pressure during exercise in hemodynamic normals.
American Heart Journal 41(4):494-497, 1971.

2443
LUEPKER, R.V., B. LIANDER, M. KORSGREN, AND E. VARNAUSKAS.
Pulmonary intravascular and extravascular fluid volumes in exercising cardiac patients.
Circulation 44(4):626-637, 1971.

2444
LUISADA, A.A.
The second heart sound in normal and abnormal conditions.
American Journal Cardiology 28:150-161, 1971.

2445
LUISADA, A.A., AND B. ARGANO.
The sound of the heart. The initial component of the first heart sound.
Chest 60(1):79-81, 1971.

2446
LUISADA, A.A., AND B. CORTIS.
The dynamic events of the normal heart in man.
Acta Cardiologica 25:203-212, 1970.

2447
LUISADA, A.A., AND L.P. FEIGEN.
Technical progress in phonocardiography and pulse tracings.
Acta Cardiologica 28(4):392-414, 1973.

2448
LUISADA, A.A., S. KUMAR, AND M.J. POUGET.
On the causes of the changes of the second heart sound in left bundle branch block.
Japanese Heart Journal 13(4):281-294, 1972.

2449
LUKASIK, S., K. WRABEC, K. STANKOWSKA, AND K. JANICKA.
Beta-blocking agents in treatment of angina pectoris: attempt at a critical evaluation.
Polski Tygodnik Lekarski 28(1):17-20, 1973.

2450
LUKOMSKY, P.E.
Cardiac output in patients with disturbed cardiac rhythm.
Cor et Vasa 12(2):97-105, 1970.

2451
LUKOMSKY, P.E., ET AL.
Cardiac output in patients with arrhythmias.
Kardiologiya 9:53-59, 1969.

2452
LUMINET, D., T. FEFER, AND P.C. VAN REETH.
The coronary disease patient and his occupation: Psychosomatic survey, preliminary report.
Acta Neurologica et Psychiatrica Belgica 69:69-77, 1969.

2453
LUND-JOHANSEN, P.
Long term anticoagulant therapy of coronary disease. A retrospective study from an out-patient clinic, 1951-1963.
Acta Medica Scandinavica 177:47-58, 1965.

2454
LUND-JOHANSEN, P.
The work and rehabilitation of patients with coronary heart disease from an urban and rural population of Norway.
Acta Medica Scandinavica 177(1):59-62, 1965.

2455
LUNDBERG, A., AND B. PERNOW.
The effect of physical training on oxygen utilization and lactate formation in the exercising muscle of adolescents with motor handicaps.
Scandinavian Journal Clinical Laboratory Investigation 26:89-96, 1970.

2456
LUNKENHEIMER, P.P.
The possibilities for direct intramural myocardial infusion.
Thoraxchirurgie Vaskuläre Chirurgie 21:211, 1973.

2457
LURIA, M.H.
Selected clinical features of paroxysmal tachycardia. A prospective study in 120 patients.
British Heart Journal 33:351-357, 1971.

2458
LUTHER, T., F. LIEBOLD, AND W. HELBIG.
Affecting hemodynamics and serum lipids by exercise, oxyfedrin and lipostabil in patients after myocardial infarction.
Zeitschrift für die Gesamte Innere Medizin und Ihre Grenzgebiete 26(16):508-515, 1971.

2459
LVOFF, R., AND D.E.L. WILCKEN.
Glucagon in heart failure and in cardiogenic shock, Experience in 50 patients.
Circulation 45(3):534-542, 1972.

2460
LYNCH, J.T., AND G.O. BARNETT.
EKG arrhythmia detection and classification using a digital computer.
Engineering Medicine Biology, Proceedings of the 18th Annual Conference, p. 136, 1965.

2461
LYNGBORG, K., AND J.G. JACOBSEN.
Intractable paroxysmal tachycardia in thyrotoxicosis simulating myocardial infarction.
Acta Medica Scandinavica 192:427-431, 1972.

2462
LYNN, T.N., R. DUNCAN, J.P. NAUGHTON, E.N. BRANDT, J. WULFF, AND S. WOLF.
Prevalence of evidence of prior myocardial infarction, hypertension, diabetes and obesity in three neighboring communities in Pennsylvania.
American Journal Medical Sciences 254:385-391, 1967.

2463
MCARDLE, W.D., F.I. KATCH, G.S. PECHAR, L. JACOBSON, AND S. RUCK.
Reliability and interrelationships between maximal oxygen intake, physical work capacity and step-test scores in college women.
Medicine Science Sports 4:182, 1972.

2464
MCARTHUR, J.D., J.D. HENDERSON, M.M. MANI, AND G. CHERIAN.
Induction cardiac pacing: A new approach.
British Medical Journal 3:328, 1973.

2465
MCBROOM, W.H., AND E.G. LUDWIG.
Clinical evaluations and self-perceptions of employment prospects among cardiovascular disease victims.
Industrial Medicine Surgery 38:309-313, 1969.

2466
MCCALLISTER, B.D., T. YIPINTSOI, F.J. HALLERMANN, R.B. WALLACE, AND R.L. FRYE.
Left ventricular performance during mild supine leg exercise in coronary artery disease.
Circulation 37(6):922-931, 1968.

2467
MCCANN, W.D., N.B. HARBOLD, JR., AND E.R. GIULIANI.
The echocardiogram in right ventricular overload.
Journal American Medical Association 221(11):1243-1245, 1972.

2468
MCCLELLAN, J.T., AND E. JOKL.
Congenital anomalies of coronary arteries as cause of sudden death associated with physical exertion.
In: Jokl, E.E. and J.T. McClellan, Eds. Medicine and Sport 6:91-98. Basel, Switzerland. Karger, 1971.

2469
MCCLOSKEY, D.I., AND J.H. MITCHELL.
Reflex cardiovascular and respiratory responses originating in exercising muscle.
Journal Physiology 224(1):173-186, 1972.

2470
MCCONAHAY, D.R., C.M. MARTIN, AND M.D. CHEITLIN.
Resting and exercise systolic time intervals: Correlations with ventricular performance in patients with coronary artery disease.
Circulation 45(3):592-601, 1972.

2471
MCCONAHAY, D.R., B.D., MCCALLISTER, AND R.E. SMITH.
Postexercise electrocardiography: Correlations with coronary arteriography and left ventricular hemodynamics.
American Journal Cardiology 28(1):1-9, 1971.

2472
MCCREDIE, R.M., D.V. CODY, A.M. MACKIE, K.K. NG, ET AL.
Digoxin preparations: variation in biological availability.
Medical Journal Australia 2:922, 1973.

2473
MCDONALD, I.G.
The shape and movements of the human left ventricle during systole.
American Journal Cardiology 26(3):221-230, 1970.

2474
McDONALD, I.G.
  Contraction of the hypertrophied left ventricle in man studied by cineradiography of epicardial
  markers.
  American Journal Cardiology 30(6):587-594, 1972.

2475
McDONALD, I.G., H. FEIGENBAUM, AND S. CHANG.
  Analysis of left ventricular wall motion by reflected ultrasound. Application to assessment of
  myocardial function.
  Circulation 46(1):14-25, 1972.

2476
McDONALD, L., AND M. EDGILL.
  Coagulability of blood in ischemic heart disease.
  Lancet 2:457,1957.

2477
McDONOUGH, J.R., AND R.A. BRUCE.
  Maximal exercise testing in assessing cardiovascular function.
  Journal South Carolina Medical Association (Suppl.) 65(12):26-33, 1969.

2478
McDONOUGH, J.R., R.A. DANIELSON, R.E. WILLS, AND D.L. VINE.
  Restricted maximal cardiac output and oxygen transport in coronary disease.
  Japanese Circulation Journal 37:971, 1973.

2479
McDONOUGH, J.R., G.E. GARRISON, AND C.G. HAMES.
  Blood pressure and hypertensive disease among negroes and whites. A study in Evans County,
  Georgia.
  Annals Internal Medicine 61(2):208-228, 1964.

2480
McDONOUGH, J.R., C.G. HAMES, S.C. STULB, AND G.E. GARRISON.
  Coronary heart disease among negroes and whites in Evans County, Georgia.
  Journal Chronic Diseases 18:443, 1965.

2481
McDONOUGH, J.R., F. KUSUMI, AND R.A. BRUCE.
  Variation in maximal oxygen intake with physical activity in middle-aged men.
  Circulation 41:743-751, 1970.

2482
McFEE, R., AND S. RUSH.
  Qualitative effects of thoracic resistivity variations on the interpretation of electrocardiograms:
  The low resistance surface layer.
  American Heart Journal 76(1):48-61, 1968.

2483
McGANDY, R.B., AND J. MAYER.
  Improving the nutrition of those most vulnerable to hunger and malnutrition, atherosclerotic
  disease, diabetes, and hypertension: Background considerations.
  In: Mayer, J., Ed. U.S. Nutrition Policies in the Seventies, pp. 37-43. San Francisco, California.
  Freeman, 1973.

2484
MCGILL, F., AND U.C. LUFT.
  Physical performance in relation to fat free weight in women.
  In: Balke B., Ed. Physiological aspects of sports and physical fitness, p. 82. The Athletic
  Institute, 1968.

2485
MCGILL, H.C., JR.
  Geographic pathology of atherosclerosis.
  Baltimore, Williams and Wilkins, 1968.

2486
MCGOON, D.C.
  Surgery for complications of myocardial infarction.
  Medical Journal Australia (Special Suppl.)2:13-14, 1972.

2487
MCGREGOR, M., AND G.A. KLASSEN.
  Observations on the effect of heart rate on cardiac output in patients with complete heart block
  at rest and during exercise.
  Circulation Research 14(Suppl. II):215, 1964.

2488
MCGUINNESS, W.B., AND A.W. SLOAN.
  Dynamic fitness of young adults and its relation to physical training and body fat.
  Journal Sport Medicine 11:179, 1971.

2489
MCGUIRE, L.B., AND M.S. KROLL.
  Evaluation of cardiac care units and myocardial infarction.
  Archives Internal Medicine 130(5):677-681, 1972.

2490
MCHENRY, P.L., O.J. COGAN, W.C. ELLIOT, AND S.B. KNOEBEL.
  False positive ECG response to exercise secondary to hyperventilation: cineangiographic
  correlation.
  American Heart Journal 79:683-698, 1970.

2491
MCHENRY, P.L., C. FISCH, J.W. JORDAN, AND B.R. CORYA.
  Cardiac arrhythmias observed during maximal treadmill exercise testing in clinically normal men.
  American Journal Cardiology 29(3):331-336, 1972.

2492
MCHENRY, P.L., C.P. LISA, AND S.B. KNOEBEL.
  Correlation of treadmill exercise electrocardiogram with arteriographic location of coronary
  disease.
  American Journal Cardiology 26:649, 1970.

2493
MCHENRY, P.L., J.F. PHILLIPS, AND J.J. JACOBS.
  Correlation of the computer quantitated S-T response to exercise with the arteriographic location
  of coronary artery disease.
  American Journal Cardiology 29:276, 1971.

2494
MCHENRY, P.L., J.F. PHILLIPS, AND S.B. KNOEBEL.
Correlation of computer-quantitated treadmill exercise electrocardiogram with arteriographic location of coronary artery disease.
American Journal Cardiology 30:747-752, 1972.

2495
MCHENRY, P.L., D.E. STOWE, AND M.C. LANCASTER
Computer quantitation of the ST-segment response during maximal treadmill exercise.
Circulation 38:691-701, 1968.

2496
MCINERNY, T.K., D.P. GILMOUR, AND J.R. BLINKS.
Comparison of effects of propranolol and other cardiac adrenergic blocking agents on inotropic and chronotropic actions of catecholamines.
Federation Proceedings 24(No. 2 Part 1):712, 1965.

2497
MCINTOSH, H.D., Y. KONG, AND J.J. MORRIS, JR.
Haemodynamic effects of supraventricular arrhythmias.
American Journal Medicine 37:712, 1964.

2498
MCINTOSH, H.D., AND J.J. MORRIS, JR.
The hemodynamic consequences of arrhythmias.
Progress Cardiovascular Diseases 8(4):330, 1966.

2499
MCKECHNIE, J.K., J.V.O. REID, AND S.M. JOUBERT.
The effect of dietary sucrose on the performance of marathon runners.
South African Journal Nutrition 6(2):42-45, 1970.

2500
MCNABB, M.E., ET AL.
The management of angina pectoris.
Journal Arkansas Medical Society 61:331-336, 1965.

2501
MCNAMARA, J.J.
Issues in youth fitness.
Journal School Health 42:621, 1972.

2502
MCNEILL, R.S., J.R. NAIRN, J.S. MILLER, AND C.G. INGRAM.
Exercise-induced asthma.
Quarterly Journal Medicine 35:55-67, 1966.

2503
MCNEILLY, R.H., AND J. PENBERTON.
Duration of last attack in 998 fatal cases of coronary artery disease and its relation to possible cardiac resuscitation.
British Medical Journal 3:139, 1968.

2504
MCNIECE, H.
   Heart disease and the law. The legal basis for awards in cardiac cases.
   Englewood Cliffs, N.J. Prentice-Hall, 1961.

2505
MCNIECE, H.F.
   Essentials of the legal issues in workmen's compensation.
   Journal Rehabilitation 32:82, 1966.

2506
MCNIECE, H.F.
   Legal aspects of exercise testing.
   New York State Journal Medicine 72:1822-1824, 1972.

2507
MCPHERSON, B.D., ET AL.
   Psychological effects of an exercise program for post-infarct and normal adult men.
   Journal Sports Medicine Physical Fitness 7:95-102, 1967.

2508
MCQUEEN, M.F., I.W. GARLAND, AND H.G. MORGAN.
   "Glycerate dehydrogenase" activity in acute myocardial infarction and myocardial ischemia.
   Clinical Chemistry 18(3):275-279, 1972.

2509
MACALPIN, R.N., A. ALVARO AND A.A. KATTUS.
   Effect of propranolol and nitroglycerin on exercise tolerance in angina pectoris.
   In: Kattus, A.A., G. Ross and V.E. Hall, Eds. Cardiovascular beta-adrenergic responses, pp.
   191-202. Los Angeles, University of California Press, 1970.

2510
MACALPIN, R.N., AND A.A. KATTUS.
   Adaptation to exercise in angina pectoris. The electrocardiogram during treadmill walking and
   coronary angiographic findings.
   Circulation 33:183-201, 1966.

2511
MACALPIN, R.N., A.A. KATTUS, AND A.B. ALVARO.
   Angina pectoris at rest with preservation of exercise capacity: Prinzmetal's variant angina.
   Circulation 47:946, 1973.

2512
MACALPIN, R.N., A.A. KATTUS, AND M.E. WINFIELD.
   Evidence for adaptive mechanisms in angina pectoris leading to improvement in exercise capacity.
   Circulation 30(4 Suppl. 3):119-120, 1964.

2513
MACALPIN, R.N., A.A. KATTUS, AND M.E. WINFIELD.
   The effect of a β-adrenergic-blocking agent (nethalide) and nitroglycerin on exercise tolerance in
   angina pectoris.
   Circulation 31(6):869-875, 1965.

2514
MACFADYEN, B.V., JR., S.J. DUDRICK, E.P. TAGUDAR, A.T. MAYNARD, ET AL.
Triglyceride and free fatty acid clearances in patients receiving complete parenteral nutrition using a ten percent soybean oil emulsion.
Surgery Gynecology Obstetrics 137:813, 1973.

2515
MACGREGOR, A.G.
Supraventricular Tachycardia-II.
British Medical Journal 4:419-422, 1971.

2516
MACKENZIE, G.J., S.H. TAYLOR, D.C. FLENLEY, A.H. MCDONALD, ET AL.
Circulatory and respiratory studies in myocardial infarction and cardiogenic shock.
Lancet 2:825, 1964.

2517
MACLEOD, C.A., E.Z. HIRSCH, AND H. SCHWARTZ.
Cardiac response to physical training in coronary heart disease.
Circulation 39-40(Suppl. 3):137, 1969.

2518
MACMILLAN, R., F.D. ROSE, AND W.S. FRANKL.
The His bundle electrocardiogram.
Medical Clinics North America 57:975, 1973.

2519
MACMILLAN, R.L., ET AL.
Changing perspectives in coronary care. A five year study.
American Journal Cardiology 20:451-456, 1967.

2520
MACHIDA, K.
The changes of left and right ventricular volumes induced by propranolol and subsequent carotid occlusion.
Japanese Heart Journal 13(5):445-456, 1972.

2521
MACKAY, R.S.
Non invasive cardiac output measurement.
Microvascular Research 4(4):438-452, 1972.

2522
MAGGI, U., P. PIETROBONO, R. ZATELLI, AND G.A. VENCHI.
Clinical experience with pancuronium bromide, a new muscle relaxing drug, in 72 chest, abdominal and vascular surgery cases.
Minerva Anestesiologica 38:565, 1972.

2523
MAGLIO, A., AND A. VENERANDO.
On evaluation of cardiocirculatory efficiency of a sport rehabilitated paraplegic.
Gazzetta Internazionale de Medicina e Chirugia 70:1007-1013, 1965.

2524
MAGRINI, F., C. FIORENTINI, A. POLESE, ET AL.
Cardiovascular features in a case of Ehlers Danlos syndrome.
Japanese Heart Journal 13(3):272-279, 1972.

2525
MAHON, W.A., J.E. MORCH, AND S.W. KLEIN.
Cardiovascular effects of intravenous glucagon in man.
Circulation 37-38(Suppl. 6):132, 1968.

2526
MAKARTSEV, V.I.
Comparative characteristics of the ECG in various cardiovascular tests.
Gigiena Truda i Professional'nye zabolevaniia 10:57-58, 1966.

2527
MAKOUS, N.
The diagnosis of coronary heart disease.
Industrial Medicine Surgery 39(9):398-401, 1970.

2528
MAKSUD, M.G., K.D. COUTTS, F.E. TRISTANI, J.R. DORCHAK, J.J. BARBORIAK, AND L.H.
HAMILTON.
The effects of physical conditioning and propranolol of physical work capacity.
Medicine Science Sports 4:225-229, 1972.

2529
MALAYA, L.T., AND S.A. LAZAREVA.
Activity of kininogenase and kininase in myocardial infarction.
Vrachebnoe Delo 11:11, 1972.

2530
MALHOTRA, S.L.
Dietary factors causing hypertension in India.
American Journal Clinical Nutrition 23(10):1353-1363, 1970.

2531
MALINOVSKY, N.N., R.P. ZUBAREV, AND A.I. GUSEV.
Continuous myocardial electrostimulation of the heart in complete bundle branch block.
Grudnaia Khirurgiia 14:41, 1972.

2532
MALLAGHAN, M.
Behavioral changes in coronary patients.
British Journal Preventive Social Medicine 26:58, 1972.

2533
MALMBERG, P.
Heart lymph enzyme activity in myocardial cell injury.
Acta Universitatis Uppsala 135, 1972.

2534
MALMCRONA, R., G. CRAMER, AND E. VARNAUSKAS.
Hemodynamic data during rest and exercise for patients who have or have not been able to retain their occupation after myocardial infarction.
Acta Medica Scandinavica 174:557, 1963.

2535
MALMCRONA, R., AND E. VARNAUSKAS.
Haemodynamics during rest and exercise at the end of convalescence from myocardial infarction. Comparison with earlier and later stages of the disease.
Acta Medica Scandinavica 175(1):19-30, 1964.

2536
MALMROS, H.
Dietary prevention of atherosclerosis.
Lancet 2:479, 1969.

2537
MALMSTROM, C., AND B. NORDGREN.
Registration of ECG during bicycle ergometry at health survey studies.
Forsvarsmedicin 8(4):158-160, 1972.

2538
MALSKY, S.J., J. HAFT, D. HAYT, ET AL.
Radiation exposure of staff cardiologist vs. senior resident cardiologist and patients during cardiac catheterization.
Radiation Data Reports 13:387, 1972.

2539
MANDEL, W.J., H. HAYAKAWA, H.N. ALLEN, ET AL.
Assessment of sinus node function in patients with the sick sinus syndrome.
Circulation 46(4):761-769, 1972.

2540
MANDEL, W.J., H. HAYAKAWA, J.K. VYDEN, ET AL.
Diphenidol: a new agent for the treatment of digitalis induced arrhythmias. Electrophysiologic and hemodynamic studies.
American Journal Cardiology 30(1):67-73, 1972.

2541
MANDEL, W.J., J. LOZANO, AND H. HAYAKAWA.
Atrial ectopic tachycardia.
American Heart Journal 86:285, 1973.

2542
MANDUCA, A.
Thermal treatment and rehabilitation.
Giornale di Gerontologia 20(2):201-208, 1972.

2543
MANGIOLA, S.
Intermittent left anterior hemiblock with Wenckebach phenomenon.
American Journal Cardiology 30(8):892-895, 1972.

2544
MANN, G.V., H.L. GARRETT, A. FARHI, ET AL.
Exercise to prevent coronary heart disease: an experimental study of the effects of training on risk factors for coronary disease in men.
American Journal Medicine 46:12-27, 1969.

2545
MANN, G.V., A. SPOERRY, M. GRAY, AND D. JARASHOW.
Atherosclerosis in the Masai.
American Journal Epidemiology 95(1):26-37, 1972.

2546
MANN, R.H., AND H.B. BURCHELL.
Premature ventricular contractions and exercise.
Mayo Clinic Proceedings 27:383-389, 1952.

2547
MANT, A.K.
Sudden and unexpected death.
Practitioner 209:273-278, 1972.

2548
MANVI, K.N., AND M.H. ELLESTAD.
Elevated ST segments with exercise in ventricular aneurysm.
Journal Electrocardiology 5(4):317-323, 1972.

2549
MARCEC-SEIDEL, V.
A case of myocardial infarction following severe emotional stress.
Lijecnicki Vjesnik 86:471-475, 1964.

2550
MARCHIONNI, R., AND R. CLEMENTE.
Resumption of work after myocardial infarct.
Giornale di Igiene e Medicina Preventiva 9:339-348, 1968.

2551
MARETIC, Z., AND J. MIHOVILOVIC MAZUR.
Electrocardiographic changes in influenza.
Zeitschrift für Kreislaufforschung 61(8):700-708, 1972.

2552
MARGARIA, R.
Anaerobic metabolism in muscle.
Canadian Medical Association Journal 96:770-774, 1967.

2553
MARGARIA, R.
Energy sources for anaerobic work.
In: Balke, B., Ed. Physiological aspects of sports and physical fitness, pp. 20-25. The Athletic Institute, 1968.

2554
MARGARIA, R., P. AGHEMO, AND G. SASSI.
  Lactic acid production in supramaximal exercise.
  Pfluegers Archiv European Journal Physiology 326:152, 1971.

2555
MARGARIA, R., P. CERRETELLI, AND F. MANGILI.
  Balance and kinetics of anerobic energy release during strenuous exercise in man.
  Journal Applied Physiology 19:623, 1964.

2556
MARGARIA, R., P. CERRETELLI, P.E. DI PRAMPERO, C. MASSARI, AND G. TORELLI.
  Kinetics and mechanism of oxygen debt contraction in man.
  Journal Applied Physiology 18:371, 1963.

2557
MARGOLIS, J.R., W.B. KANNEL, M. FEINLEIB, T.R. DAWBER, AND P.M. McNAMARA.
  Clinical features of unrecognized myocardial infarction—silent and symptomatic. Eighteen year
  follow-up: The Framingham Study.
  American Journal Cardiology 32:1, 1973.

2558
MARK, H., AND L.S. LUNA.
  Treatment of Wolff-Parkinson-White syndrome.
  American Heart Journal 83(4):565-569, 1972.

2559
MARK, R.J., E.L. LANSDOWN, D. MYMIN, AND D. JACKSON.
  Second look at coronary angiography.
  Journal American Medical Association 225:979, 1973.

2560
MARKIEWICZ, M.
  P wave in patients with myocardial infarction.
  Polski Tygodnik Lekarski 27(33):1263-1265, 1972.

2561
MARKS, A.D.
  The cardiovascular manifestations of systemic Lupus Erythematosus.
  American Journal Medical Sciences 264(4):254-265, 1972.

2562
MARMO, E., A.P. CAPUTI, AND S. CATALDI.
  Review of the literature and report of experiments relating to a coronaroactive drug (hexo-
  bendine).
  Minerva Cardioangiologica 20:571, 1972.

2563
MAROKO, P.R., P. LIBBY, C.M. BLOOR, ET AL.
  Reduction by hyaluronidase of myocardial necrosis following coronary artery occlusion.
  Circulation 46(3):430-437, 1972.

2564
MAROKO, P.R., P. LIBBY, B.E. SOBEL, ET AL.
  Effect of glucose insulin potassium infusion on myocardial infarction following experimental coronary artery occlusion.
  Circulation 45(6):1160-1175, 1972.

2565
MARON, B.J., B.B. BELL, AND M. MIROWSKI.
  Coexistence of passive and active junctional rhythms with rates up to 300 per minute in a child with atrial parasystole.
  Chest 64:276, 1973.

2566
MARRIOTT, H.J.L.
  Arrhythmias in myocardial infarction. Diagnosis and treatment (No. 4).
  Chest 57:180-181, 1970.

2567
MARRIOTT, H.J.L., AND E. FOGG.
  Constant monitoring for cardiac dysrhythmias.
  Modern Concepts Cardiovascular Disease 39:103, 1970.

2568
MARSHALL, W.L., H. STRAWBRIDGE, AND A. KELTNER.
  The role of mental relaxation in experimental desensitization.
  Behavioral Research Therapy 10:355-366, 1972.

2569
MARTIN, A.M., JR., D.B. HACKEL, M.L. ENTMAN, M.P. CAPP, AND M.S. SPACH.
  Mechanisms in the development of myocardial lesions in hemorrhagic shock.
  Annals New York Academy Sciences 156:79-90, 1969.

2570
MARTIN, C.M., AND D.R. McCONAHAY.
  Maximal treadmill exercise electrocardiography. Correlations with coronary arteriography and cardiac hemodynamics.
  Circulation 46:956-962, 1972.

2571
MARTIN, C.M., E.G. SOUTHWICK, AND H.I. MAIBACH.
  Propranolol induced alopecia.
  American Heart Journal 86:236, 1973.

2572
MARTIN, H.L.
  The relationship between premonitory distress state and rehabilitation in patients with coronary occlusion.
  Medical Journal Australia 1:480-483, 1967.

2573
MARTIN, H.L.
  The significance of discussion with patients about their diagnosis and its implications.
  British Journal Medical Psychology 40:233-242, 1967.

2574
MARTIN, H.L.
   Social correlates of rehabilitation following a first coronary occlusion.
   Rehabilitation (London) 68:67-70, 1969.

2575
MARTINI, G., AND C. SARACCO.
   Point of views in rehabilitation of elderly people.
   Giornale di Gerontologia 20(1):70-74, 1972.

2576
MARTINI, U., M. IANNETTI, C. PASTORINI, AND S. CAPONNETTO.
   Effect of muscular work on the time of cardiac revolution in normal subjects and in some
   pathologic conditions.
   Archivio E. Maragliano di Patologia e Clinica 23(1):55-67, 1967.

2577
MARTYNOV, I.F.
   Function of the apparatus of external respiration with physical exercise in patients with mitral
   stenosis following mitral commissurotomy.
   Kardiologiya 5(4):69-72, 1965.

2578
MARTZ, R., D.J. BROWN, R.B. FORNEY, ET AL.
   Propranolol antagonism of marihuana induced tachycardia.
   Life Sciences 111(21):999-1005, 1972.

2579
MASICA, D.N., B.J. MARON, AND L.J. KROVETZ.
   Racial variations in the childhood electrocardiogram: preliminary observations.
   American Heart Journal 84(2):153-160, 1972.

2580
MASLOVA, K.K. AND IU. IA. VYSHNEPOL'SKIY.
   Preliminary results of treated patients having hypertension with reserpine and hydrochlorothiazide
   at industrial establishments in Moscow.
   Kardiologiya 6:79-80, 1966.

2581
MASON, B., N. OAKLEY, AND V. WYNN.
   Studies of carbohydrate and lipid metabolism in women developing hypertension on oral contra-
   ceptives.
   British Medical Journal 3:317, 1973.

2582
MASON, D.T.
   Usefulness and limitations of the rate of rise of intraventricular pressure (dp/dt) in the evaluation
   of myocardial contractility in man.
   American Journal Cardiology 23:516, 1969.

2583
MASON, D.T.
   Digitalis and angina-pectoris.
   Chest 64(4):415-416, 1973.

2584

MASON, D.T., ET AL.
Medical management of chronic ischemic heart disease.
Geriatrics 28(4):126, 1973.

2585

MASON, J.K., F.M. TOWNSEND, AND J.R. JACKSON.
Death from coronary disease while at the controls of an aircraft.
Aerospace Medicine 34:858, 1963.

2586

MASON, R.E., AND I. LIKAR.
A new system of multiple-lead exercise electrocardiography.
American Heart Journal 71:196-205, 1966.

2587

MASON, R.E., I. LIKAR, R.O. BIERN, AND R.S. ROSS.
Multiple-lead exercise electrography. Experience in 107 normal subjects and 67 patients with angina pectoris, and comparison with coronary cinearteriography in 84 patients.
Circulation 36:517, 1967.

2588

MASON, R.E., I. LIKAR, R.O. BIERN, AND R.S. ROSS.
Correlation of graded exercise electrocardiographic response with clinical and coronary cinearteriographic finding.
In: Blackburn, H., Ed. Measurement in exercise electrocardiography. The Ernst Simonson Conference. Springfield, Ill. Thomas, 1969.

2589

MASON, R.E., I.N. LIKAR, AND R.S. ROSS.
New system of multiple leads in exercise electrocardiography. Comparison with coronary arteriography.
Circulation 30(Suppl. 3):123, 1964.

2590

MASSIE, J., A. RODE, T. SKRIEN, AND R.J. SHEPHARD.
A critical review of the "aerobics" points system.
Medicine Science Sports 2:1, 1970.

2591

MASSIE, J.F., AND R.J. SHEPHARD.
Physiological and psychological effects of training—a comparison of individual and gymnasium programs, with a characterization of the exercise "drop-out."
Medicine Science Sports 3:110, 1971.

2592

MASSONI, G.
The use of ajmaline in the therapy of cardiac arrhythmias in old age.
Giornale di Gerontologia 19:510, 1971.

2593

MASSUMI, R.A., N. ALI, R. SARIN, M. POOYA, H. SCHEFFEL, AND J.C. RIOS.
The mechanism of pulsus paradoxua in pericardial effusion.
Circulation 39-40(Suppl. 3):142, 1969.

2594

MASSUMI, R.A., N. ALI, M. POOYA, R. SARIN, J.C. RIOS, AND H. SCHEFFEL.
   Accelerated idioventricular rhythm.
   Circulation 39-40(Suppl. 3):142, 1969.

2595

MASSUMI, R.A., J.C. RIOS, A.S. GOOCH, V.T. DE VITA, AND D. NUTTER.
   Hemodynamic studies in acute phases of primary myocardial disease.
   Circulation 28:764, 1963.

2596

MASSUMI, R.A., J.C. RIOS, A.S. GOOCH, D. NUTTER, V.T. DE VITA, AND D.W. DATLOW.
   Primary myocardial disease. Report of 50 cases and review of the subject.
   Circulation 31:19-41, 1965.

2597

MASSUMI, R.A., R. SARIN, A. TAWAKKOL, AND J.C. RIOS.
   Time sequence of right and left atrial depolarization as a guide to the origin of the P waves.
   American Journal Cardiology 24:28, 1969.

2598
MASTER, A.M.
   The two-step test of myocardial function.
   American Heart Journal 10:495-510, 1935.

2599
MASTER, A.M.
   The two-step exercise electrocardiogram: a test for coronary insufficiency.
   Annals Internal Medicine 32:842-863, 1950.

2600
MASTER, A.M.
   Iproniazid (Marsilid) in angina pectoris.
   American Heart Journal 56:570-582, 1958.

2601
MASTER, A.M.
   Survival and rehabilitation in coronary occlusion.
   American Journal Cardiology 7(3):340-349, 1961.

2602
MASTER, A.M.
   "Silent" coronary artery disease.
   Medical Tribune 5:15, 1964.

2603
MASTER, A.M.
   The Master two-step test.
   American Heart Journal 75:809-837, 1968.

2604
MASTER, A.M.
   Clofibrate and the Master two-step test.
   Circulation 39-40(Suppl. 3):17, 1969.

2605
MASTER, A.M.
    The natural history of angina pectoris.
    Circulation 39-40(Suppl. 3):17, 1969.

2606
MASTER, A.M.
    The Master two-step test. Some historical highlights and current concepts.
    Journal South Carolina Medical Association (Suppl.) 65(12):12-17, 1969.

2607
MASTER, A.M.
    Is the highest rate attained in the Master "two-step" test sufficient?
    Circulation 41(Suppl. 3):19, 1970.

2608
MASTER, A.M.
    "Augmented" two-step test.
    Transactions Association Life Insurance Medical Directors of America 54:42-59, 1970.

2609
MASTER, A.M.
    Reminiscences of fifty years in cardiology at Mount Sinai with special reference to the two step test.
    Mount Sinai Journal Medicine 39(5):486-505, 1972.

2610
MASTER, A.M.
    Exercise testing for evaluation of cardiac performance.
    American Journal Cardiology 30(7):718, 1972.

2611
MASTER, A.M.
    Cardiac arrhythmias elicited by the two-step exercise test.
    American Journal Cardiology 32:766, 1973.

2612
MASTER, A.M., AND C.W. ADAMS.
    The exercise tolerance test.
    Journal American Medical Association 204(1):80, 1968.

2613
MASTER, A.M., S. DACK, AND H.L. JAFFE.
    Premonitory symptoms of acute coronary occlusion. A study of 260 cases.
    Annals Internal Medicine 14:1155-1165, 1941.

2614
MASTER, A.M., L.E. FIELD, AND E. DONOSO.
    Coronary artery disease and the "two-step exercise test."
    New York State Journal Medicine 57:1051-1061, 1957.

2615
MASTER, A.M., R. FRIEDMAN, AND S. DACK.
  The electrocardiogram after standard exercise as a functional test of the heart.
  American Heart Journal 24:777-793, 1942.

2616
MASTER, A.M., AND A.J. GELLER.
  Magnitude of silent coronary disease.
  New York State Journal Medicine 64:2865-2869, 1964.

2617
MASTER, A.M., AND A.J. GELLER.
  The extent of completely asymptomatic coronary artery disease.
  American Journal Cardiology 23:173-179, 1969.

2618
MASTER, A.M., AND H.L. JAFFE.
  Electrocardiography changes after exercise in angina pectoris.
  Journal Mount Sinai Hospital 7:629-632, 1941.

2619
MASTER, A.M., AND E.T. OPPENHEIMER.
  A simple tolerance test for circulatory efficiency with standard tables for normal individuals.
  American Journal Medical Sciences 177:223-242, 1929.

2620
MASTER, A.M., AND I. ROSENFELD.
  The "two-step" exercise test brought up to date.
  New York State Journal Medicine 61:1850, 1961.

2621
MASTER, A.M., AND I. ROSENFELD.
  Criteria for the clinical application of the two-step exercise test.
  Journal American Medical Association 178:283-289, 1961.

2622
MASTER, A.M., AND I. ROSENFELD.
  The Master two-step test. Use in diagnosis of "incipient" coronary artery disease.
  Ohio State Medical Journal 58:1011-1017, 1962.

2623
MASTER, A.M., AND I. ROSENFELD.
  The Master 2-step tests: evaluation of clinical usefulness in 650 persons subjected to extended follow-up studies.
  American Journal Cardiology 13(1):122-123, 1964.

2624
MASTER, A.M., AND I. ROSENFELD.
  Monitored and post-exercise two-step test.
  Journal American Medical Association 190:494-500, 1964.

2625
MASTER, A.M., AND I. ROSENFELD.
  Silent coronary heart disease.
  Modern Medicine 33:78-79, 1965.

2626
MASTER, A.M., AND I. ROSENFELD.
  Arrhythmias in the two-step test.
  Circulation 34(Suppl. 3):22, 1966.

2627
MASTER, A.M., AND I. ROSENFELD.
  Criterion of positive two-step exercise test.
  New York State Journal Medicine 66(20):2641-2645, 1966.

2628
MASTER, A.M., AND I. ROSENFELD.
  Two-step exercise test. Current status after 25 years.
  Modern Concepts Cardiovascular Disease 36:19-24, 1967.

2629
MASTER, A.M., AND I. ROSENFELD.
  Exercise electrocardiography as an estimation of cardiac function.
  Diseases Chest 51:347-383, 1967.

2630
MASTER, A.M., AND I. ROSENFELD.
  Arrhythmias in two-step test-monitored and after exercise.
  Circulation 36:(Suppl. 2):26, 1967.

2631
MASTROPAOLO, J.A., J. STAMLER, D.M. BERKSON, AND W.E. JACKSON.
  Physical activity of work, physical fitness and coronary heart disease in middle-aged Chicago men.
  In: Karvonen, M.J. and A.J. Barry, Eds. Physical activity and the heart, pp. 266-300. Springfield,
  Ill. Thomas, 1967.

2632
MATARAZZO, R.G., D. BRISTOW, AND R. REAUME.
  Medical factors relevant to psychological reactions in mitral valve disease.
  Journal Nervous Mental Disease 137(4):380-388, 1963.

2633
MATE, K., G. BIRTALAN, I. HORVATH, V. NEMES, ET AL.
  Clinical experiences in the application of electrolytes in cardiopathies.
  In: Bajusz, E., Ed. Electrolytes and cardiovascular disease: 2. Clinical aspects, pp. 260-276. Basel,
  Switzerland. S. Karger, 1966.

2634
MATEEF, D.
  The new in the theory of exercise and its influence on growth, development and aging.
  XVI Weltcongress für Sportmedizin, pp. 379-383. Hanover, 1966.

2635

MATESHVILI, G.G., AND G.A. TROFIMOV.
Detection of the cardiac antigen in patients with myocardial infarction.
Kardiologiya 12(11):56-60, 1972.

2636

MATHER, H.G., N.G. PEARSON, K.L.Q. READ, D.B. SHAW, ET AL.
Acute myocardial infarction: Home and hospital treatment.
British Medical Journal 3:334, 1971.

2637

MATHISEN, H., H. LÖKEN, D. BROX, AND O. STENBAEK.
The prognosis in long term treated and "untreated" essential hypertension.
Acta Medica Scandinavica 185(4):253-258, 1969.

2638

MATHIVAT, A., J.-P. BOURDARIAS, J. BARDET, J.-P. NORMAND, ET AL.
Prolonged circulatory assistance by intra-aortic unidirectional counterpulsation in a state of shock following myocardial infarction.
Nouvelle Presse Médicale 2:2663, 1973.

2639

MATHUR, P.P.
Cardiovascular effects of a newer antiarrhythmic agent, diisopyramide phosphate.
American Heart Journal 84(6):764-770, 1972.

2640

MATSUBARA, H.
Long-term prognosis of myocardial infarction, with emphasis on recurrence.
Japanese Circulation Journal 31:1579-1584, 1967.

2641

MATSUDA, T.
Effects of long-term anticoagulant therapy on the prognosis of myocardial infarction.
Japanese Circulation Journal 31(11):1602-1606, 1967.

2642

MATSUDA, T.
Fibrinogen fibrin degradation products in patients with various diseases.
Acta Haematologica Japan 35:52-60, 1972.

2643

MATSUMOTO, M., AND T. KUMAGAI.
A case of variant form of angina pectoris presenting transient ST-segment elevation without anginal pain on exercise tests.
Akita Central Hospital Medical Journal 6(1):32-37, 1969.

2644

MATSUMOTO, T., K.C. PANI, R.M. HARDWAY, III, F. LEONARD, AND C.A. HEISTERKAMP.
Cyanoacrylate tissue adhesive in surgery in anticoagulated subjects.
Archives Surgery 94:187, 1967.

2645
MATSUO, S., AND A. BENCHIMOL.
   Phasic aortic flow velocity during ventricular tachycardia in man.
   American Journal Medical Sciences 262(5):291-300, 1971.

2646
MATSUURA, T., AND A.V.N. GOODYER.
   Effects of a pressure load on left ventricular systolic time intervals.
   American Journal Physiology 224(1):80-85, 1973.

2647
MATTEO, J. DI, A. VACHERON, C. KELLERSHOHN, AND P. DE VERNEJOUL.
   Measurement of coronary blood flow by radiocardiography.
   In: Halonen, P., and A. Louhija, Eds. Early diagnosis of coronary heart disease, pp. 203-13. Basel,
   Switzerland. S. Karger, 1973.

2648
MATTEO, J., DI, A. VACHERON, A. HEULIN, P. DE VERNEJOUL, AND L. BARRITAULT.
   Changes of the coronary artery blood flow in the course of myocardial infarction.
   Archives des Maladies du Coeur et des Vaisseaux 66:1233, 1973.

2649
MATTINGLY, T.W.
   The post-exercise electrocardiogram. Its value in the diagnosis and prognosis of coronary arterial
   disease.
   American Journal Cardiology 9:395-409, 1962.

2650
MATTIOLI, G., AND G. DOMENICHINI.
   Serum iron changes during myocardial infarction.
   Gazzetta Italiana di Cardiologia 2:1024, 1972.

2651
MATUSOVA, A.P., AND M.S. BUBEL.
   Principles and methods of the rehabilitation of patients who sustained myocardial infarction.
   Kardiologiya 10(2):14-18, 1970.

2652
MATZDORFF, F.
   The exertion electrocardiogram—indication, methods, significance.
   Deutsches Medizinisches Journal 22:480-485, 1971.

2653
MATZDORFF, F.
   Seminar in cardiology—life after myocardial infarction. Introduction to rehabilitation of patients
   with myocardial infarction.
   Herz Kreislauf 5(10):437-438, 1973.

2654
MATZDORFF, F., E. LIPPERT, A. SCHMIDT, AND K. SCHMIDT.
   Risk factors of re-infarction.
   Deutsche Medizinische Wochenschrift 98:2183, 1973.

2655
MAUGH, T.H., II.
  Coffee and heart disease: Is there a link?
  Science 181:534-535, 1973.

2656
MAUTNER, B., AND A.L. GIROTTI.
  Premature ventricular beats. Experimental study.
  American Heart Journal 85(3):389-396, 1973.

2657
MAYER, J.
  Obesity, cardiovascular disease, and the dietitian.
  Journal American Dietetic Association 52(1):13-20, 1968.

2658
MAYER, J.
  Improving the nutrition of those most vulnerable to hunger and malnutrition, and heart disease:
  Plans of action.
  In: Mayer, J., Ed. U.S. Nutrition Policies in the Seventies, pp. 44-52. San Francisco, California.
  Freeman, 1973.

2659
MAYOU, R.
  The patient with angina symptoms and disability.
  Postgraduate Medicine Journal 49:250, 1973.

2660
MAYRON, B., M. POUGET, W.S. HARRIS, AND J.P. NAUGHTON.
  Exercise-induced prolongation of left ventricular ejection in angina.
  Circulation 39-40(Suppl. 3):143, 1969.

2661
MEADE, T.W., AND R. CHAKRABARTI.
  Arterial disease research: observation or intervention?
  Lancet 2:913-916, 1972.

2662
MECL, A.
  Rehabilitation in cardiology and its reflection on the assessment of work capacity.
  Ceskoslovenske Zdravotnictvi 13:294-298, 1965.

2663
MEDALIE, J.H., ET AL.
  Angina pectoris among 10,000 men. Five year incidence and univariate analysis.
  American Journal Medicine 55:583, 1973.

2664
MEDALIE, J.H., H.A. KAHN, H.N. NEUFELD, E. RISS, ET AL.
  Myocardial infarction over a five-year period. Part I. Prevalence, incidence and mortality experience.
  Journal Chronic Diseases 26:63-84, 1973.

2665
MEDRANO, G.A., C. BRENES, A. DE MICHELI, AND D. SODI PALLARES.
Clinical electrocardiographic and vectorcardiographic diagnosis of left posterior subdivision block, isolated or associated with RBBB.
American Heart Journal 84:727, 1972.

2666
MEERKAMM, F., AND F.H. HERTLE.
Electrocardiographic observations of healthy persons and cardiac infarct patients under standardized submaximal ergometer stress.
Archiv für Kreislaufforschung; Beihefte zur Zeitschrift für Kreislaufforschung 57(3/4):240-256, 1968.

2667
MEERSON, F.Z.
Possible mechanisms of cardiac hypertrophy.
Acta Biologica et Medica Germanica 29(2):271-280, 1972.

2668
MEHMEL, H.C., H.P. KRAYENBUEHL, AND P. WIRZ.
Isovolumic contraction dynamics in man according to two different muscle models.
Journal Applied Physiology 33(4):409-414, 1972.

2669
MEIER, F., H.P. WEISFLOG, AND N. GANZONI.
Circulatory arrest following suxamethonium administration in accident victims.
Schweizerische Medizinische Wochenschrift 102:1653, 1972.

2670
MEIGS, J.W.
Epidemiology of coronary disease in industrial workers. III. Absentee rates and parental disease histories.
Archives Environmental Health 13:655-661, 1966.

2671
MEIGS, J.W., T.B. CALDWELL, AND M.J. ALBRINK.
Epidemiology of coronary disease in industrial workers.
Archives Environmental Health 10(3):467-474, 1965.

2672
MELAMED, S.B., AND V.M. PAVLOV.
Capacity for work of patients with rheumatic cardiac failures after elimination of auriculur fibrillation with an electropulse discharge.
Terapevticheskii Arkhiv 43(1):44-47, 1971.

2673
MELICOW, M.M.
Coitus, impotence and angina pectoris.
New York State Journal Medicine 45:1325-1328, 1945.

2674
MELLEROWICZ, H.
Ergometric electrocardiography. Method and interpretation.
Malattie Cardiovascolari 10:107-108, 1969.

2675
MELLEROWICZ, H., AND H. SCHMUTZLER.
Blood pressure during ergometric work in middle-aged healthy men and its use in diagnosis and rehabilitation.
Malattie Cardiovascolari 10:263-256, 1969.

2676
MELLINGER, G.D., M.B. BALTER, AND D.I. MANHEIMER.
Patterns of psychotherapeutic drug use among adults in San Francisco.
Archives General Psychiatry 25:385, 1971.

2677
MELLON, L.J., W.D. JENSEN, E. MCLAIN, AND F.J. SAMBUCO.
Experience with computerized electrocardiograms.
Industrial Medicine 40(7):7-9, 1971.

2678
MELTZER, L.E.
Concept of system for intensive coronary care.
Bulletin Academy Medicine New Jersey 10(4):304-311, 1964.

2679
MELTZER, L.E.
Coronary care units: current policies and results.
In: Julian, D.G. and M.F. Oliver, Eds. Acute myocardial infarction, pp. 3-8.
Baltimore, Williams and Wilkins, 1968.

2680
MELTZER, L., H.E. COHEN, AND S.L. WOLFGANG.
Sleep regimen for myocardial infarction.
Lancet 1:1308-1309, 1968.

2681
MELTZER, L.E., AND J.R. KITCHELL, EDS.
The current status of intensive coronary care.
New York. Charles Press, 1966.

2682
MELTZER, L.E., AND J.R. KITCHELL.
The development and current status of coronary care.
In: Meltzer, L.E. and A.J. Dunning, Eds. Textbook of coronary care, pp. 3-25.
Amsterdam, Netherlands. Excerpta Medica, 1972.

2683
MÉNARD, J. AND J. PESLERBE.
Practical value of plasmatic renin activity determination in the investigation of arterial hypertension.
Coeur et Médecine Interne 10(1):93-98, 1971.

2684
MENDEZ, L.
Prevention in cardiology.
Archivos del Instituto de Cardiologia de Mexico 43:373, 1973.

2685
MENON, I.S.
Chest pain as the presenting complaint: A clinicians' dilemma.
Clinician 37(4):157-158, 1973.

2686
MENON, I.S., F. BURKE, AND H.A. DEWAR.
Effects of strenuous and graded exercise on fibrinolytic activity.
Lancet 1:700, 1967.

2687
MENOTTI, A.
Current trends in the reading and interpretation of electrocardiograms.
Policlinico: Sezione Pratica 73:1206-1210, 1966.

2688
MENOTTI, A., AND V. PUDDU.
Epidemiology of coronary heart disease: a ten years study in two Italian rural population groups.
Acta Cardiologica 28(1):66-88, 1973.

2689
MENOTTI, A., V. PUDDU, M. MONTI, AND F. FIDANZA.
Habitual physical activity and myocardial infarction.
Cardiologia 54:119-128, 1969.

2690
MENSEN, H.
Problems of rehabilitation and prevention.
Hippokrates 35:879-889, 1964.

2691
MERCERON, R., Y. WEISS, M. SAFAR, AND P. MILLIEZ.
Comparison between the haemodynamic effects of clonidine, alpha-methyldopa, guanethidine and reserpine. Preliminary study.
Coeur et Médecine Interne 12:425, 1973.

2692
MERLI, M., C. CATTANI, A. PELLEGRINI, AND E.M. PRATELLI.
The role of prophylactic antibiotic therapy in cardiac surgery.
Journal Cardiovascular Surgery 14:131, 1973.

2693
MERRIMAN, J.E.
Exercise tolerance tests in cardiac patients and the use of the computer in such studies.
Malattie Cardiovascolari 10(1-2):373-379, 1969.

2694
MERRIMAN, J.E.
Long-term activity programs for coronary patients.
In: Naughton, J., H.K. Hellerstein and I.C. Mohler, Eds. Exercise testing and exercise training in coronary heart disease, pp. 347-354. New York, Academic Press, 1973.

2695
MERRIMAN, J.E., AND M.E. DONEGAN.
  The coronary risk factors and exercise tolerance of participants.
  In: Naughton, J., H.K. Hellerstein, and I.C. Mohler, Eds. Exercise testing and exercise training in coronary heart disease, pp. 421-426. New York, Academic Press, 1973.

2696
MERRIMAN, J.E., AND S.M. FATTAH.
  Hospital-based exercise training program in the rehabilitation of patients with ischemic heart disease.
  Circulation 43-44(Suppl. 2):201, 1971.

2697
MERSHON, J.C., AND R.J. CUNNINGHAM.
  Continuous ECG monitoring. To evaluate unexplained dizziness, syncope and chest pain.
  Journal Kansas Medical Society 73(11):458-465, 1972.

2698
MERSHON, J.C., J.R. MEDINA, R.W. EVANS, J.W. EDGETT, ET AL.
  Use of the vectorcardiogram to recognize right ventricular hypertrophy in mitral stenosis.
  Chest 64:173, 1973.

2699
MERTENS, C.
  Psychological factors in the etiology of cardiovascular diseases.
  Acta Psychiatrica Belgica 72:26-28, 1972.

2700
MERTENS, C., AND G. MEULEMANS.
  Specificity of psychosomatic relationships in coronary ailments.
  Acta Psychiatrica Belgica 72:65-79, 1972.

2701
MESHULAM, N., AND D. BRUNNER.
  Reconditioning of coronary patients by physical exercises.
  Circulation 40:18, 1969.

2702
MESSENBOURG, B.A.P., ET AL.
  Occupational therapy in coronary rehabilitation.
  American Journal Occupational Therapy 24:428-431, 1970.

2703
MESSER, J.V., R. J. WAGMAN, H.J. LEVINE, W.A. NEILL, ET AL.
  Patterns of human myocardial oxygen extraction during rest and exercise.
  Journal Clinical Investigation 41(4):725-742, 1962.

2704
MESSER, J.V., H.J. LEVINE, R.J. WAGMAN, AND R. GORLIN.
  Effect of exercise on cardiac performance of human subjects with coronary artery disease.
  Circulation 28(3):404-414, 1963.

2705
METELITSA, V.I.
  Prevalence and prevention of ischemic heart disease (epidemiological studies).
  Sovetskaya Meditsina 36(9):53-58, 1973.

2706
METELITSA, V.I., ET AL.
  Factors predisposing 50 to 59 year-old men to ischemic heart disease.
  Kardiologiya 9:130-132, 1969.

2707
METIVIER, J.
  Clinical and anatomic study of cardiopathies in the elderly (subjects over age 70 years).
  Annales de Médecine Interne 122(3):367-372, 1971.

2708
MEUWISSEN, O.J.A.T., A.C. VERVOORN, O. COHEN, F.L.J. JORDAN, AND F.A. NELEMANS.
  Double blind trial of long-term anticoagulant treatment after myocardial infarction.
  Acta Medica Scandinavica 186(5):361-368, 1969.

2709
MEYER, A.-E., GOLLE, R., AND W. WEITEMEYER.
  Duration of illness and elevation of neuroticism scores.
  Journal Psychosomatic Research 11(4):347-355, 1968.

2710
MEYER, J.
  Comparative investigations on various computer programs in the analysis of electrocardiograms.
  Deutsche Medizinische Wochenschrift 97:552-559, 1972.

2711
MEZEY, K.C.
  Pharmacology of compounds used in the treatment of arterial hypertension.
  Chimie Therapeutique 6:477-482, 1968.

2712
MGELADZE, N.V., AND O.A. DZHAGASHVILI.
  Clinical physiological study of patients with hypotension during adaptation to a mountain climate
  and during readaptation.
  Voprosy Kurortologii Fizioterapii Lechebnoi Fizicheskoi Kul'tury 37:101-105, 1972.

2713
MICHAEL, E., AND L. ECKARDT.
  The selection of hard work by trained and non-trained subjects.
  Medicine Science Sports 4:107, 1972.

2714
MICHAELIS, L.L., H.A. WELLONS, JR., W.L. LOVETT, AND S.P. NOLAN.
  Transvenous cardiac pacing as an adjunct to the medical management of dissecting aortic hema-
  toma.
  Journal Thoracic Cardiovascular Surgery 64(2):322-323, 1972.

2715
MICHAELS, L.
  Heparin administration in acute coronary insufficiency. Its value in the initial stages of treatment.
  Journal American Medical Association 221(11):1235-1239, 1972.

2716
MICHAELS, L., AND J.E. KLOVAN.
  Wave amplitude relationships in the normal electrocardiogram.
  British Heart Journal 30:412-418, 1968.

2717
MICHIE, I.
  Electrocardiographic changes in the elderly.
  Gerontologia Clinica 12:193-202, 1970.

2718
MIETTINEN, O.S., AND R.K. NEFF.
  Computer processing of epidemiologic data.
  Hart Bulletin 2(4):98-103, 1971.

2719
MIETTINEN, T.A.
  Mechanisms of hyperlipidaemias in different clinical conditions.
  In: Early diagnosis of coronary heart disease. Proceedings of the second Paavo Nurmi Symposium,
  Porvoo, Finland, 1971. Basel, S. Karger, 1973.

2720
MIHAIL, A., P. POPESCU, X. PETRESCU, AND N. POPA.
  The treatment of angina pectoris with pindolol (β-blocking agents).
  Medicina Internă 24:925, 1972.

2721
MILHAUD, A., J. CHANARD, R. LEVY, G. FONTAINE, ET AL.
  Observations on the use of lignocaine in the treatment of the hyperexcitation syndrome in recent
  myocardial infarction.
  Archives des Maladies du Coeur et des Vaisseaux 62:1474-1484, 1969.

2722
MILLER, A.B., J. NAUGHTON, AND P. GORMAN.
  Left axis deviation: diagnostic contribution of exercise stress testing.
  Chest 63:159, 1973.

2723
MILLER, C.K.
  Psychological correlates of coronary artery disease.
  Psychosomatic Medicine 27(3):257-265, 1965.

2724
MILLER, D.T., AND J.P. GILMORE.
  Excitation contraction correlates in true ischemia.
  Journal Electrocardiology 5(3):257-264, 1972.

2725
MILLER, G.J., AND M.T. ASHCROFT.
The use of submaximal exercise tests for the investigation of heart disease in Jamaica.
Clinical Science 42(4):200, 1972.

2726
MILLER, G.J., AND M.T. ASHCROFT.
Reappraisal of cardiovascular surveys in Jamaica. Use of submaximal exercise tests for clinical investigation.
British Heart Journal 34(11):1113, 1120, 1972.

2727
MILLER, M.G.
The capacity of the cardiac pensioner to resume employment.
Medical Journal Australia 2:335-340, 1969.

2728
MILLER, P.B., R.L. JOHNSON, AND L.E. LAMB.
Effects of four weeks of absolute bed rest on circulatory functions in man.
Aerospace Medicine 35:1194, 1964.

2729
MILLER, P.B., AND L.W. POLLARD.
Paroxysmal tachycardia after exercise.
Circulation 26(3):363-372, 1962.

2730
MILLIKEN, J.A., J. WARTAK, D.W. LYWOOD, ET AL.
Validity of computer interpretation of the electrocardiogram.
Canadian Medical Association Journal 105(11):1147-1150, 1971.

2731
MILLS, I.H.
The cardiovascular system and renal control of sodium excretion.
Canadian Journal Physiology Pharmacology 46:297-303, 1968.

2732
MILZ, H.P.
Exercise therapy as structural principles of a modern cardiovascular hospital.
Archiv für Physikalische Therapie 22:93-104, 1970.

2733
MINC, S.
Psychological factors in coronary heart disease.
Geriatrics 20:747-755, 1965.

2734
MINC, S.
Emotions and ischaemic heart disease.
Medical Journal Australia 1:856-858, 1966.

2735
MINC, S., G. SINCLAIR, AND R. TAFT.
Some psychological factors in coronary heart disease.
Psychosomatic Medicine 25(2):133-139, 1963.

2736
MINOGUE, W.F., A.A. SMESSART, AND W.J. GRACE.
External cardiac massage for cardiac arrest due to myocardial infarction: a changing concept.
American Journal Cardiology 13:25, 1964.

2737
MIR, G.C., AND F.L. SHAPIRO.
The heart in kwashiorkor.
Medicina Clinica 61:11-14, 1973.

2738
MIR, M.A.
M complex: the electrocardiographic sign of impending cardiac rupture following myocardial infarction.
Scottish Medical Journal 17(10):319-325, 1972.

2739
MIRAKYAN, V.O., AND I.D. SHPERLING.
Myogenic cellular elements in the granulated tissue of the affected myocardium.
Arkhiv Patologii 34:29, 1972.

2740
MIROWSKI, M., M.M. MOWER, V.L. GOTT, AND R.K. BRAWLEY.
Feasibility and effectiveness of low energy catheter defibrillation in man.
Circulation 47(1):79-85, 1973.

2741
MIRSKY, I., R.C. ELLISON, AND P.G. HUGENHOLTZ.
Assessment of myocardial contractility in children and young adults from ventricular pressure recordings.
American Journal Cardiology 27:359-367, 1971.

2742
MIRSKY, I., A. PASTERNAC, AND R.C. ELLISON.
General index for the assessment of cardiac function.
American Journal Cardiology 30(5):483-491, 1972.

2743
MISNER, J.E., B.H. MASSEY, AND B.T. WILLIAMS.
The effect of physical training on the response of serum enzymes to exercise stress.
Medicine Science Sports 5(2):86, 1973.

2744
MITCHELL, J.H., L.L. HEFNER, AND R.G. MONROE.
Performance of the left ventricle.
American Journal Medicine 53(4):481-494, 1972.

2745
MITCHELL, J.H., B.J. SPROULE, AND C.B. CHAMPMAN.
   The physiological meaning of the maximal oxygen intake test.
   Journal Clinical Investigation 37:538, 1958.

2746
MITCHELL, J.H., AND K. WILDENTHAL.
   Left ventricular function during exercise.
   In: Larsen, O.A. and R.O. Malmborg, Eds. Coronary heart disease and physical fitness, pp. 93-96.
   Baltimore, University Park Press, 1971.

2747
MIYAHARA, A., ET AL.
   Cardiac arrhythmia diagnosis by digital computer. Considerations related to the temporal distri-
   bution of P and R waves.
   Computers Biomedical Research 1:277-300, 1968.

2748
MIZUNO, Y.
   Vectorcardiographic diagnosis of congenital heart diseases.
   Japanese Circulation Journal 30:1562-1564, 1966.

2749
MIZUNO, Y., AND S. YASUI.
   The relation of the conventional electrocardiogram to orthogonal leads with special reference to
   ventricular hypertrophy.
   Japanese Circulation Journal 31:1634-1639, 1967.

2750
MIZUTANI, K., A. TAKAHASHI, Y. MIYAGISHIMA, AND O. MINAMIKAWA.
   A clinical study on the hemodynamic response to exercise in patients with ischemic heart disease
   and with heart failure.
   Japanese Circulation Journal 31(12):1920, 1967.

2751
MIZUTANI, T.
   A study of coronary circulation in experimental aortic insufficiency with special reference to
   phasic coronary flow pattern.
   Japanese Circulation Journal 37:123, 1973.

2752
MÖBIUS, R., S. SCHÖNER, AND M. WUNDERLICH.
   Early rehabilitation after cardiac infarction at the health spa.
   Zeitschrift für Physiotherapie 23:137-144, 1971.

2753
MOELLER, J.
   Epidemiology of essential hypertension.
   Therapie der Gegenwart 109(11):1594-1608, 1970.

2754
MOENE, R.J., AND J.P. ROOS.
   Preventive effect of practolol on episodes of tachycardia in the Wolff-Parkinson-White syndrome.
   Nederlands Tijdschrift voor Geneeskunde 116(21):877-880, 1972.

2755
MOHLER, S.R.
   Functional aging: present status of assessments regarding airline pilot retirement.
   Aerospace Medicine 44:1062-1066, 1973.

2756
MOIR, T.W., AND D.W. DEBRA.
   Effect of left ventricular hypertension, ischemia and vasoactive drugs on the myocardial distribution of coronary flow.
   Circulation Research 21:65-74, 1967.

2757
MOLENDA, R.
   Investigation on the usefulness of histochemical examination of succinic dehydrogenase in the diagnosis of myocardial damage.
   Archiwum Medycyny Sadowej i Kryminologii 22:39, 1972.

2758
MOLNAR, S., J.E. WILEY, AND T.K. CURETON.
   Prediction of endurance performance and oxygen consumption from cardiac time components.
   Research Quarterly 44:278, 1973.

2759
MOLZAHN, M., T. DISSMANN, S. HALIM, F.W. LOHMANN, AND W. OELKERS.
   Orthostatic changes of haemodynamics, renal function, plasma catecholamines and plasma renin concentration in normal and hypertensive man.
   Clinical Science 42(2):209-222, 1972.

2760
MOND, H., R. TWENTYMAN, D. SMITH, AND G. SLOMAN.
   The pacemaker clinic.
   Cardiology 57(5):262-276, 1972.

2761
MONE, L.C.
   Short-term group psychotherapy with postcardiac patients.
   International Journal Group Psychotherapy 20:99-108, 1970.

2762
MONROE, R.G., AND G. FRENCH.
   Ventricular pressure-volume relationship and oxygen consumption in fibrillation and arrest.
   Circulation Research 8:260, 1960.

2763
MONSALLIER, J.F., J.C. HAYAT, A. CARLI, AND C. ST. MAURICE.
   Posttraumatic myocardial necrosis.
   Cahiers d'Anesthésiologie 20(5):545-556, 1972.

2764
MONTBELLI, M.L.
   Mental deterioration in the sequelae of myocardial infarct.
   Giornale di Psichiatria e di Neuropatologia 92:435-445, 1964.

2765
MONTEIRO, L.A.
  Lay views on activity after myocardial infarction. Sample of Rhode Island residents expect rehabilitated cardiac to return to work.
  Rhode Island Medical Journal 55:77-81, 1972.

2766
MONTEIRO, L.A.
  After heart attack: behavioral expectations for the cardiac.
  Social Science Medicine 7(7):555, 1973.

2767
MONTERO, A.C., W.G. SMITH, H. TAKEZAWA, J.M. LEWIS, AND J.K. ALEXANDER.
  Hemodynamic responses to exercise in constrictive periocarditis.
  Circulation 33-34(Suppl. 3):172, 1966.

2768
MONTOYE, H.J.
  Summary of research on the relationship of exercise to heart disease.
  Journal Sports Medicine 2:35, 1962.

2769
MONTOYE, H.J.
  Participation in athletics.
  Canadian Medical Association Journal 96:813-820, 1967.

2770
MONTOYO, J.V., J. ANGEL, V. VALLE, AND C. GAUSI.
  Cardioversion of tachycardias by transesophageal atrial pacing.
  American Journal Cardiology 32:85, 1973.

2771
MOOKERJEE, S.
  Prediction of ischemic heart diseases and their preventive rehabilitation.
  In: Plavšić, C. and M.M. Gertler, Eds. The first international biennial conference on cardiac rehabilitation, Dubrovnik, Yugoslavia, 1969.

2772
MOOLTEN, S.E., P.B. JENNINGS, AND A. SOLDEN.
  Dietary fat and platelet adhesiveness in arteriosclerosis and diabetes.
  American Journal Cardiology 11(3):290-300, 1963.

2773
MOORE, G.E., AND J.R. PARRATT.
  Effect of noradrenaline and isoprenaline on blood flow in the acutely ischaemic myocardium.
  Cardiovascular Research 7:446-457, 1973.

2774
MOORE, T.O., Y.C. LIN, D.A. LALLY, AND S.K. HONG.
  Effects of temperature, immersion, and ambient pressure on human apneic bradycardia.
  Journal Applied Physiology 33(1):36-41, 1972.

2775
MOOSA, N., D.M. GRIGGS, JR., H. KASPARIAN, AND P. NOVACK.
Effects of nitroglycerin on hemodynamics during rest and exercise in patients with coronary insufficiency.
Circulation 35(1):46-54, 1967.

2776
MOOSMAN, D.A.
The anatomy of infraclavicular subclavian vein catheterization and its complications.
Surgery Gynecology Obstetrics 136(1):71-74, 1973.

2777
MORBELLI, E., AND L. MASCARETTI.
Cardiac output at rest and during graded exercise in normals and in patients with heart disease.
Cardiologia 43:317-336, 1963.

2778
MORDKOFF, A.M., AND M.A. RAND.
Personality and adaptation to coronary artery disease.
Journal Consulting Clinical Psychology 32:648-653, 1968.

2779
MORDKOFF, A.M., AND R.M. GOLAS.
Coronary artery disease and response to the Rosenzweig Picture-Frustration Study.
Journal Abnormal Psychology 73(4):381-386, 1968.

2780
MOREIRA, A.C., O.C. FREITAS, A. RUFFINO NETTO, AND F.L. VICHI.
An electrocardiographic study of the site of origin of ventricular premature beats in chronic Chagas' heart disease.
Arquivos Brasileiros de Cardiologia 25(2):141-145, 1972.

2781
MORET, P., E. COVARRUBIAS, J. COUDERT, AND F. DUCHOSAL.
Cardiocirculatory adaptation to chronic hypoxia. II. Comparative study of myocardial metabolism of glucose, lactate, pyruvate and free fatty acids between sea level and high altitude residents.
Acta Cardiologica 27(4):483-503, 1972.

2782
MOREYRA, E., L.E. ALDAY, L.M. AMUCHASTEGUI, ET AL.
Myocardial infarction and ventricular aneurysms with normal data of coronary arteriography.
Revista Medica de Cordoba 60(7):198-206, 1972.

2783
MORGAN, W.P.
Psychological effect of weight reduction in the college wrestler.
Medicine Science Sports 2:24, 1970.

2784
MORGANS, C.M.
Supervised physical training after myocardial infarction.
British Heart Journal 34:203, 1972.

2785
MORGANS, C.M., AND W.M. BUSTON.
  Supervised circuit training after myocardial infarction.
  Physiotherapy 58(10):340-343, 1972.

2786
MORI, H., T. NAGAYAMA, T. ODA, K. OSHITA, ET AL.
  Analog computer analysis of spatial vectorcardiogram: spatial magnitude, velocity and acceleration electrocardiograph and its clinical applications. Japanese Circulation Journal 32:149-160, 1968.
  Japanese Circulation Journal 32:149-160, 1968.

2787
MORI, H., AND K. OHSHITA.
  Diagnosis of myocardial infarction: Electrocardiograms, vectorcardiograms and its analog computer analysis.
  Japanese Circulation Journal 31:1644-1649, 1967.

2788
MORI, H., T. SHIBATA, K. OSHITA, AND H. KAWAMURA.
  Spatial analytico-geometrical analysis of the vectorcardiogram by electronic computer.
  Japanese Circulation Journal 30:1017-1029, 1966.

2789
MORI, K.
  The effect of exercise on myocardial metabolism of inorganic phosphorus and creatine in patients with circulatory diseases.
  Japanese Circulation Journal 36:1123-1135, 1972.

2790
MORO, C.O., S. MATARESE, B. GALLO, D. IARUSSI, AND A. JACONO.
  Epidemiologic study on ischemic cardiopathy and some metabolic changes in the workers of a steel industry of southern Italy. Preliminary report on 294 subjects.
  Gazzetta Italiana di Cardiologia 2:807-812, 1972.

2791
MORRA, C.A.
  Some aspects of the cardiac patient's personality and conflictual derivations with respect to his disease and his familiar and social enclosure values.
  Revista de la Facultad de Ciencias Medicas de la Universidad Nacional de Cordoba 25(3):267-277, 1967.

2792
MORRIS, E.
  Cardiac rehabilitation. Community service to older cardiac patients.
  New York State Journal Medicine 64(21):2678-2683, 1964.

2793
MORRIS, J.N.
  Four cheers for prevention.
  Proceedings Royal Society Medicine 63:225-232, 1973.

2794
MORRIS, J.N., S.P.W. CHAVE, C. ADAM, ET AL.
  Vigorous exercise in leisure time and the incidence of coronary heart disease.
  Lancet 1:333-339, 1973.

2795
MORRIS, J.N., AND M.D. CRAWFORD
Coronary heart disease and physical activity of work. Evidence of a National Necropsy Survey.
British Medical Journal 2:1485-1496, 1958.

2796
MORRIS, J.N., AND M.J. GARDNER.
Epidemiology of ischemic heart disease.
American Journal Medicine 46:674, 1969.

2797
MORRIS, J.N., J.A. HEADY, AND P.A.B. RAFFLE.
Physique of London busmen: Epidemiology of uniforms.
Lancet 2:569-570, 1956.

2798
MORRIS, J.N., J.A. HEADY, P.A.B. RAFFLE, C.G. ROBERTS, AND J.W. PARKS.
Coronary heart disease and physical activity of work.
Lancet 2:1053, 1111, 1953.

2799
MORRIS, J.N., A. KAGAN, D.C. PATTISON, M.J. GARDNER, AND P.A.B. RAFFLE.
Incidence and prediction of ischemic heart disease in London busmen.
Lancet 2:553-559, 1966.

2800
MORRIS, J.T.
Supraventricular tachycardia of Wolff-Parkinson-White syndrome converted to sinus rhythm by intravenous lidocaine.
Journal Medical Association Alabama 42(4):271-273, 1972.

2801
MORRIS, W.H.M.
The coronary farmer.
Journal Rehabilitation 32:76, 1966.

2802
MORRIS, W.H.M.
Heart disease in farm workers.
Canadian Medical Association Journal 96:821-824, 1967.

2803
MORRISON, J., AND T. KILLIP.
Serum digitalis and arrhythmia in patients undergoing cardiopulmonary bypass.
Circulation 47:341-352, 1973.

2804
MORROW, A.G., D.T. MASON, J. ROSS, JR., AND E. BRAUNWALD.
Combined prosthetic replacement of the mitral and aortic valves: preoperative and postoperative hemodynamic studies including left ventricular response to muscular exercise.
Circulation 33-34(4 Suppl. 3):175, 1966.

2805
MORSE, R.L., ED.
  Exercise and the Heart: Guidelines for Exercise Programs.
  Springfield, Ill. Thomas, 1972.

2806
MORTON, E.V.B.
  Ischaemic heart disease in the elderly.
  Practitioner 209:794-799, 1972.

2807
MORWOOD, J.
  Sleep and ischaemic heart disease.
  Practitioner 209:696-697, 1972.

2808
MOSCATELLO, B., A. MALARBI, L. PIERANGELI, M. GIOFFRE, ET AL.
  Pharmacodynamic study of stenocardia of effort: V. Effect of theophylline ethylenediamine.
  Bollettino della Società Italiana di Cardiologia 15(3):258-266, 1970.

2809
MOSCHOS, C.B., K. LAHIRI, M. LYONS, A.B. WEISSE, ET AL.
  Relation of microcirculatory thrombosis to thrombus in the proximal coronary artery: Effect of aspirin, dipyridamole, and thrombolysis.
  American Heart Journal 86:61, 1973.

2810
MOSCHOS, C.B., K. LAHIRI, A. PETER, ET AL.
  Effect of aspirin upon experimental coronary and noncoronary thrombosis and arrhythmia.
  American Heart Journal 84(4):525-530, 1972.

2811
MOSES, C.
  Heart attack; changing habits, reducing risks.
  Postgraduate Medicine 53(2):104-108, 1973.

2812
MOSHKOV, Y.N., AND A.I. ZHURAVLEVA.
  New data in the use of therapeutic exercise in diseases of the peripheral vessels.
  Translation into English from "Novyye Dannyye v Primenenii Lechebnoy Fizkultury pri Zabolevaniyakh Pifericheskikh Sosudov" pp. 18-22. Washington, D.C. Scripta Technica, 1973.

2813
MOSS, A.J., J. DEWEESE, E. LIPCHICK, AND E. OLSAN.
  Combined septal rupture repair and infarctectomy in acute myocardial infarction.
  Journal American Medical Association 213(3):460-462, 1970.

2814
MOSINGER, M., G. DEBISSCHOP, AND R. LUCCIONI.
  Occupational rehabilitation of patients who had suffered from myocardial infarct, regarding 35 observations.
  Archives des Maladies Professionelles de Médecine du Travail et de Sécurité Sociale 30:518, 1969.

2815
MOSINGER, M., AND R. LUCCIONI.
  Vocational rehabilitation of patients with myocardial infarct. A propos of 33 cases.
  Archives des Maladies Professionelles, de Médecine du Travail et de Sécurité Sociale 29:573-576, 1968.

2816
MOSSARD, J.M., G. JOSSOT, L.S. WOLFE, ET AL.
  The heart in Fabry's disease.
  Archives des Maladies du Coeur et des Vaisseaux 65(4):495-503, 1972.

2817
MOST, A.S., T.R. HORNSTEN, V. HOFER, AND R.A. BRUCE.
  Exercise ST changes in healthy men.
  Archives Internal Medicine 121(3):225-229, 1968.

2818
MOST, A.S., H.G. KEMP, AND R. GORLIN.
  Postexercise electrocardiography in patients with arteriographically documented coronary artery disease.
  Annals Internal Medicine 71(6):1043-1050, 1969.

2819
MOST, A.S., AND D.R. PETERSON.
  Myocardial infarction surveillance in a metropolitan community.
  Journal American Medical Association 208:2433-2438, 1969.

2820
MOTA, E., AND M.H. PIRES DE CARVALHO.
  Auricular fibrillation in the Wolff-Parkinson-White syndrome.
  Boletim da Sociedade Portugesa de Cardiologia 9:75, 1971.

2821
MÖTTÖNEN, M.
  Myocardial infarction and coronary atherosclerosis among and comparison between intellectual and manual workers in Finland.
  Beiträge zur Pathologischen Anatomie und zur Allgemeinen Pathologie 141(2):148-154, 1970.

2822
MOULOPOULOS, S.D., AND L.P. ANTHOPOULOS.
  Reversible A-V conduction changes during exercise.
  Acta Cardiologica 23:352-366, 1968.

2823
MOULOPOULOS, S.D., J. DARSINOS, AND D.A. SIDERIS.
  Atrioventricular block response to exercise and intraventricular conduction at rest.
  British Heart Journal 34(10):998-1004, 1972.

2824
MOWE, G.
  Rehabilitation in patients with prior myocardial infarct. Medical and sociomedical problems in the light of a follow-up study.
  Tidsskrift for den Norske Laegeforening 86:527-532, 1966.

2825
MOWE, G.
Work capacity and sick leave among industrial workers with prior myocardial infarct. Five-year case material from the Borregaard Factories, Sarpsborg.
Tiddsskrift for den Norske Laegeforening 86:532-534, 1966.

2826
MOXLEY, R.T., P. BRAKMAN, AND T. ASTRUP.
Resting levels of fibrinolysis in blood in inactive and exercising men.
Journal Applied Physiology 28:549, 1970.

2827
MOYANO, A., L.E. ALDAY, E. MOREYRA, ET AL.
Termination of paroxysmal auricular flutter by stimulation of the right ventricle.
Revista Argentina de Cardiologia 40(5):361-365, 1972.

2828
MOYER, J.H., ET AL.
The changing outlook for the patient with hypertension.
American Journal Cardiology 17:673-681, 1966.

2829
MUELLER, M.
Estimating the limitation of performance in congenital and acquired heart defects.
Zeitschrift für Kreislaufforschung 52(7):623-640, 1968.

2830
MUHLBERG, H., AND G. SCHLEUSING.
Stress electrocardiogram and spiroergometry in the diagnosis of coronary diseases.
Zeitschrift für die Gesamte Innere Medizin und Ihre Grenzgebiete 23:121-125, 1968.

2831
MUHLBERG, H., AND G. SCHLEUSING.
Modern method of electrocardiogram after work.
Zeitschrift für die Gesamte Innere Medizin und Ihre Grenzgebiete 23(20):626-633, 1968.

2832
MUIR, J.R.
Excitation contraction coupling in normal and failing hearts.
Annales de Cardiologie et d'Angéiologie 21(6):535-543, 1972.

2833
MUKERJEE, A.B., AND S. DASGUPTA.
Idiopathic paroxysmal ventricular tachycardia.
Journal Indian Medical Association 58(7):247-249, 1972.

2834
MUKHERJEE, S.K.
The electrocardiogram in left ventricular hypertrophy.
Indian Heart Journal 23(1):45-54, 1971.

2835
MULCAHY, R., AND N.J. HICKEY.
The long-term management of patients with coronary heart disease.
Irish Journal Medical Science Series 6:9-16, 1965.

2836
MULCAHY, R., AND N. HICKEY.
The rehabilitation of patients with coronary heart disease.
Scandinavian Journal Rehabilitation Medicine 2-3:108, 1970.

2837
MULCAHY, R., AND N. HICKEY.
The rehabilitation of patients with coronary heart disease: A comparison of the return to work experience of National Health Insurance patients with coronary heart disease and of a group of coronary patients subjected to a spccific rehabilitation programme.
Journal Irish Medical Association 60:541-545, 1971.

2838
MULCAHY, R., N. HICKEY, AND N. COGHLAN.
Rehabilitation of patients with coronary heart disease.
Geriatrics 27:120-121 passim, 1972.

2839
MULLER, E.A.
Physiologic methods of increasing human physical work capacity.
Ergonomics 8:409, 1965.

2840
MULLER, E.A.
Influence of training and of inactivity on muscle strength.
Archives Physical Medicine Rehabilitation 51:449-462, 1970.

2841
MUNDY, G.R., R. CUTFORTH, AND P.M. BROOKS.
Serum lipid abnormalities and the atrial pacing test.
Medical Journal Australia 2(10):535-537, 1972.

2842
MURAKI, H., K. NAKAGAWA, Y. HASHIMOTO, ET AL.
The Frank vectorcardiogram in mitral stenosis and its postoperative changes.
Japanese Circulation Journal 36(6):529-538, 1972.

2843
MURATA, K., F. TERASAWA, M. KURAMOCHI, ET AL.
The relation of blood pressure and degree of coronary atherosclerosis to myocardial lesions and cardiac hypertrophy.
Japanese Heart Journal 13(1):34-42, 1972.

2844
MURAYAMA, M., K. HARUMI, M. YAMAMOTO, K. IGUCHI, AND C.M. CHEN.
Further study on exercise vectorcardiogram with Frank's lead: Spatial ST, T changes produced by exercise in health and disease.
Japanese Heart Journal 11(4):400-416, 1970.

2845
MURAYAMA, M., K. HARUMI, C.M. CHEN, AND S. MURAO.
Postextrasystolic ST, T changes in the exercise vectorcardiogram with Frank's lead.
Japanese Heart Journal 12(2):185-190, 1971.

2846
MURPHY, G.W., B.F. SCHREINER, JR., P.L. BLEAKEY, AND P.N. YU.
Left ventricular performance after digitalization in patients with and without heart failure.
Circulation 28:775, 1963.

2847
MURRAY, J.A., I.S. KASSER, L.B. ROWELL, AND R.A. BRUCE.
Aortic pressure and oxygen transport responses to upright exercise in angina pectoris.
Circulation 37-38(Suppl. 6): 145, 1968.

2848
MURRAY, M.J.
Reflex constriction of coronary arteries.
American Journal Cardiology 15:141, 1965.

2849
MUTI, R., AND V. TAVORMINA.
New research on the vascularisation of the atrioventricular cardiac valves in adult man.
Anatomischer Anzeiger 131(3):298-310, 1972.

2850
MIYAKE, K.
Studies on rehabilitation of cardiac patients: evaluation of cardiac function by step test.
Japanese Circulation Journal 36:1005, 1972.

2851
MYBURGH, D.P.
Post extrasystolic T and U wave changes in diseased and normal hearts.
South African Medical Journal 46(43):1615-1617, 1972.

2852
MYERBURG, R.J., H. GELBAND, AND B.F. HOFFMAN.
Confinement of premature impulses in functional compartments of regions of the A-V conducting system.
Cardiovascular Research 7(1):69-81, 1973.

2853
MYMIN, D., T.E. CUDDY, S.N. SINHA, AND D.A. WINTER.
Inhibition of demand pacemakers by skeletal muscle potentials.
Journal American Medical Association 223(5):527-529, 1973.

2854
MYRSTEN, A.-L., B. POST, M. FRANKENHAEUSER, AND G. JOHANSSON.
Changes in behavioral and physiological activation induced by cigarette smoking in habitual smokers.
Psychopharmacologia 27:305-312, 1972.

2855
MYSLIWIEC, M., A. PERZANOWSKI, AND M. BIELAWIEC.
   Platelet adhesiveness in patients with a history of former myocardial infarction.
   Polski Tygodnik Lekarski 27:1034, 1972.

2856
NACHNANI, G.H., L.S. LESSIN, T. MOTOMIYA, ET AL.
   Scanning electron microscopy of thrombogenesis on vascular catheter surfaces.
   New England Journal Medicine 286: 139-140, 1972.

2857
NADAL-GINARD, B., G. SANZ, AND J. FROUFE.
   Total dextroposition of the great vessels with obstruction of the left ventricular outlet.
   Chest 64: 270, 1973.

2858
NAGASAKA, T., S. ANDO, T. TAKAI, M. HARA, ET AL.
   An analysis of EKG recorded by radiotelemetry on Mt. Aconcagua and in a low pressure chamber
   at sea level.
   Nagoya Journal Medicine 29: 377-384, 1967.

2859
NAGEL, M.R., J.A. RONAN, JR., AND W.C. ROBERTS.
   Left-to-right shunt at atrial level after rupture of papillary muscle from acute myocardial infarc-
   tion.
   American Heart Journal 86: 112, 1973.

2860
NAGER, F., F. BURKART, M. FRIEDEMANN, ET AL.
   Prevention and treatment of arrhythmias due to myocardial infarction.
   Schweizerische Medizinische Wochenschrift 102(50): 1836-1851, 1972.

2861
NAGLE, F., B. BALKE, G. BAPTISTA, J. ALLEYIA, ET AL.
   Compatibility of progressive treadmill, bicycle and step tests based on oxygen uptake responses.
   Medicine Science Sports 3(4): 149-154, 1971.

2862
NAGLE, F.J., B. BALKE, AND J.P. NAUGHTON.
   Gradational step tests for assessing work capacity.
   Journal Applied Physiology 20:745-748, 1965.

2863
NAGLE, F.J., J. NAUGHTON, AND B. BALKE.
   Comparisons of direct and indirect blood pressure with pressure-flow dynamics during exercise.
   Journal Applied Physiology 21: 317, 1966.

2864
NAGLE, R., R. GANGOLA, AND I. PICTON-ROBINSON.
   Factors influencing return to work after myocardial infarction.
   Lancet 2:454-456, 1971.

2865
NAGLE, R., AND I. PICTON-ROBINSON.
  Rehabilitation after myocardial infarction.
  Proceedings Royal Society Medicine 65(4):327-328, 1972.

2866
NAGLE, R.E., B. SMITH, AND D. O. WILLIAMS.
  Familial atrial cardiomyopathy with heart block.
  British Heart Journal 34: 205, 1972.

2867
NAHUN, L.H.
  The rest dogma.
  Connecticut Medical Journal 27: 134, 1963.

2868
NAHUN, L.H.
  Returning the cardiac to work.
  Connecticut Medicine 29:169-172, 1965.

2869
NAIMARK A., K. WASSERMAN, AND M.B. McILROY.
  Continuous measurement of ventilatory exchange ratio during exercise.
  Journal Applied Physiology 19(4):644-652, 1964.

2870
NAIR, K.G., T. UMALI, AND J. POTTS.
  Ribonucleic acid (RNA) polymerase and adenyl cyclase in cardiac hypertrophy and cardio-
  myopathy.
  American Journal Cardiology 32:423, 1973.

2871
NAJAFI, H., W.S. DYE, H. JAVID, ET AL.
  Acute aortic regurgitation secondary to aortic dissection. Surgical management without valve
  replacement.
  Annals Thoracic Surgery 14(5):474-482, 1972.

2872
NAJMI, M., H. KASPARIAN, D.M. GRIGGS, JR., AND W. LIKOFF.
  Correlation of selective cinecoronary arteriography with clinical findings and resting and exercise
  hemodynamics in normal subjects and patients with coronary heart disease.
  Circulation 33-34 (Suppl. III):179, 1966.

2873
NAKAMURA, T., AND N. SUZUKI.
  Organ characteristics of the vascular system in man. V. Vascular characteristics of the heart.
  Tohoku 83(4):145-314, 1971.

2874
NAKANO, J., AND T. KUSAKARI.
  Effects of propranolol on the cardiovascular performance.
  Federation Proceedings 24(2 Part 1):712, 1965.

2875
NAKAYAMA, M.
  Exercise phonocardiogram: With special reference to Q-II$_A$ interval on exercise.
  Japanese Circulation Journal 35(12):1551-1557, 1971.

2876
NAKAYAMA, R., T. KOBAYASHI, K. KIMURA, AND T. AZUMA.
  A theoretical approach to the volume pulse wave.
  American Heart Journal 86: 96, 1973.

2877
NAKHJAVAN, F.K., M.R. KATZ, V. MARANHAO, AND H. GOLDBERG.
  Analysis of influence of catecholamine and tachycardia during supine exercise in patients with mitral stenosis and sinus rhythm.
  British Heart Journal 31(6): 753-761, 1969.

2878
NAKHJAVAN, F.K., V. MARANHAO, H. SHEDROVILZKY, M. KATZ, AND H. GOLDBERG.
  Hemodynamic effects of exercise, catecholamine stimulation and tachycardia at comparable heart rates in mitral stenosis.
  Federation Proceedings 27(2):326, 1968.

2879
NAPOLITANO, D., A. CUOMO, AND M. IMPROTA.
  Protease inhibitors in cardiogenic shock due to infarction.
  Rassegna Internazionale di Clinica e Terapia 52(19):1186-1193, 1972.

2880
NARULA, O.S., M. RUNGE, AND P. SAMET.
  Second degree Wenckebach type AV block due to block within the atrium.
  British Heart Journal 34(11):1127-1136, 1972.

2881
NASH, F.A.
  The growing heart.
  Preventive Techniques for the Modern Community. The Chest and Heart Association, London, England, 1971.

2882
NATARAJAN, G., AND A.S. GOOCH.
  Arrthythmia behavior during exercise in digitoxic patients.
  Clinical Research 29(3):390, 1972.

2883
NATHAN, M.J., W.Z. YAHR, AND J.J. GREENBERG.
  Temporary permanent pacemaker lead for cardiac surgery.
  Journal Thoracic Cardiovascular Surgery 64:957, 1972.

2884
NAUGHTON, J.
  The myocardiopathies—some electrocardiographic features.
  Journal Oklahoma State Medical Association 58:50, 1965.

2885
NAUGHTON, J.
Clinical considerations in the diagnosis of atrial septal defects.
Journal Oklahoma State Medical Association 59:52, 1966.

2886
NAUGHTON, J.
Cardiopulmonary responses during physical training in patients who have recovered from myocardial infarction.
In: Raab, W., Ed. Prevention of ischemic heart disease, pp. 332-337. Springfield, Ill. Thomas, 1966.

2887
NAUGHTON, J.
Assessment of the physical performance of middle-aged American men.
Medical Times 95:220-227, 1967.

2888
NAUGHTON, J.
Cardiorespiratory endurance. Before and after regular physical activity.
Minnesota Medicine 51:619-623, 1968.

2889
NAUGHTON, J.
The hemodynamic appraisal of the patient with cardiac disease.
Journal Oklahoma State Medical Association 61:72-76, 1968.

2890
NAUGHTON, J.
Examples of graded exercise tests.
Journal South Carolina Medical Association 65(Suppl. 1, No 12):96, 1969.

2891
NAUGHTON, J.
Active pre-season evaluation of prospective athletes.
In: American Academy of Orthopediatric Surgeons Symposium on Sports Medicine, pp. 30-36. St. Louis, Mo. Mosby, 1969.

2892
NAUGHTON, J.
Games that cardiacs can play.
Internal Medicine Digest 5(12):26-34, 1970.

2893
NAUGHTON, J.
Can myocardial infarction be prevented?
Medical Digest 17:30-39, 1971.

2894
NAUGHTON, J.
Heart patients and sex.
Sexual Behavior 1:45-47, 1971.

2895
NAUGHTON, J.
Sex for cardiac patients. Answers to questions.
Journal Human Sexuality 6:80, 1972.

2896
NAUGHTON, J.
Sex in patients with neck, back and radicular pain syndromes.
Medical Aspects Human Sexuality 6(12):25-27, 1972.

2897
NAUGHTON, J.
Infarcts and exercise.
Consultant; Journal Medical Consultations, p. 154, September, 1972.

2898
NAUGHTON, J.
Coronary heart disease.
In: Levine, E. and J. Garrett, Eds. Rehabilitation practices with the physically disabled, pp. 209-239. New York, Columbia University Press, 1973.

2899
NAUGHTON, J.
Preferred coital position after coronary.
Medical Aspects Human Sexuality 7:177-181, 1973.

2900
NAUGHTON, J.
The effects of acute and chronic exercise on cardiac patients.
In: Naughton, J.P. , H.K. Hellerstein, and I.C. Mohler, Eds. Exercise testing and exercise training in coronary heart disease, pp. 337-346. New York, Academic Press, 1973.

2901
NAUGHTON, J., AND B. BALKE.
Physical working capacity in medical personnel and the response of serum cholesterol to acute exercise and to training.
American Journal Medical Sciences 247:286, 1964.

2902
NAUGHTON, J., B. BALKE, AND F. NAGLE.
Refinements in method of evaluation and physical conditioning before and after myocardial infarction.
American Journal Cardiology 14(6):837-843, 1964.

2903
NAUGHTON, J., B. BALKE, AND F. NAGLE.
The effect of physical conditioning on an individual before and after suffering a myocardial infarction.
U.S. Civil Aeromedical Research Institute 1-10, 1964.

2904
NAUGHTON, J., B. BALKE, AND A. POARCH.
Modified work capacity studies in individuals with and without coronary artery disease.
Journal Sports Medicine 4:208, 1964.

2905
NAUGHTON, J., R. BLOCK, AND M. WELCH.
  Central alveolar hypoventilation.
  American Review Respiratory Disease 103(4):557-565, 1971.

2906
NAUGHTON, J., AND J. BRUHN.
  Emotional stress, physical activity and ischemic heart disease.
  Disease-a-Month 3:1-34, 1970.

2907
NAUGHTON, J., J.G. BRUHN, AND M.T. LATEGOLA.
  Regular physical activity and the cardiac patient.
  Geriatrics 23:157-164, 1968.

2908
NAUGHTON, J., J.G. BRUHN, AND M.T. LATEGOLA.
  Effects of physical training on physiologic and behavioral characteristics of cardiac patients.
  Archives Physical Medicine Rehabilitation 49:131, 1968.

2909
NAUGHTON, J., J.G. BRUHN, M.T. LATEGOLA, AND T. WHITSETT.
  Rehabilitation following myocardial infarction.
  American Journal Medicine 46(5):725-734, 1969.

2910
NAUGHTON, J., AND R. HAIDER.
  Methods of exercise testing.
  In: Naughton, J.P., H.K. Hellerstein, and I.C. Mohler, Eds. Exercise testing and exercise training in coronary heart disease pp. 79-91. New York, Academic Press, 1973.

2911
NAUGHTON, J.P., H.K. HELLERSTEIN, AND I.C. MOHLER, EDS.
  Exercise testing and exercise training in coronary heart disease.
  New York, Academic Press, 1973.

2912
NAUGHTON, J., AND M.T. LATEGOLA.
  Physical activity and coronary atherosclerosis.
  Journal Oklahoma State Medical Association 60:76-81, 1967.

2913
NAUGHTON, J., AND M.T. LATEGOLA.
  Cardiorespiratory adjustments during exercise in patients with healed myocardial infarction.
  Journal Arkansas Medical Society 65:241-244, 1968.

2914
NAUGHTON, J., AND M.T. LATEGOLA.
  The evaluation of physical performance in cardiac patients.
  Medicine Sport 4:156-166, 1970.

2915
NAUGHTON, J. AND M.T. LATEGOLA.
  Medical rehabilitation.
  Encyclopedia Sports Science Medicine, pp. 1505-1508. New York, MacMillan, 1971.

2916
NAUGHTON, J., M.T. LATEGOLA, C.M. BRAKE, AND P. LYNE.
Electrocardiographic monitoring during physical activity.
Cardiology Digest 3:31, 1968.

2917
NAUGHTON, J., M. LATEGOLA, J. BRUHN, AND S. WOLF.
Rehabilitation for patients after myocardial infarction.
Southern Medical Bulletin 55(1):29-35, 1967.

2918
NAUGHTON, J., M.T. LATEGOLA, AND K. SHANBOUR.
A physical rehabilitation program for cardiac patients: A progress report.
American Journal Medical Sciences 252(5):545-553, 1966.

2919
NAUGHTON, J., AND W. LEACH.
The effect of a simulated warm-up on ventricular performance.
Medicine Science Sports 3(4):169-171, 1971.

2920
NAUGHTON, J., AND J.F. McCOY.
Observations on the relationship of physical activity to the serum cholesterol concentration of healthy men and cardiac patients.
Journal Chronic Diseases 19:727-733, 1966.

2921
NAUGHTON, J., AND F. NAGLE.
Peak oxygen intake during physical fitness program for middle-aged men.
Journal American Medical Association 191:899, 1965.

2922
NAUGHTON, J., W. O'NEILL, AND J. PATTERSON.
Characterization of heart rate response to graded exercise before and after vasodilators.
Medicine Science Sports 4(1):33-36, 1972.

2923
NAUGHTON, J., J. PATTERSON, AND S.M. FOX, III.
Exercise tests on patients with chronic diseases.
Journal Chronic Diseases 9:519, 1971.

2924
NAUGHTON, J., G. SEVELIUS, AND B. BALKE.
Physiological responses of normal and pathological subjects to a modified work capacity test.
Journal Sports Medicine 3:201, 1963.

2925
NAUGHTON, J., K. SHANBOUR, R. ARMSTRONG, J. Mc COY, AND M. T. LATEGOLA.
Cardiovascular responses to exercise following myocardial infarction.
Archives Internal Medicine 117:541, 1966.

2926
NAUGHTON, J., AND J. WULFF.
Effect of physical activity on carbohydrate metabolism.
Journal Laboratory Clinical Medicine 70:996, 1967.

2927
NAYLER, W.G., AND V. CARSON.
Effect of stellate ganglion stimulation on myocardial blood flow, oxygen consumption, and cardiac efficiency during beta-adrenoceptor blockade.
Cardiovascular Research 7(1):22-29, 1973.

2928
NAYLER, W.G., AND I. McINNES.
Salbutamol and orciprenaline induced changes in myocardial function.
Cardiovascular Research 6(6):725-733, 1972.

2929
NEAL, C., C. SMITH, K. DUBOWSKI, AND J. NAUGHTON.
3-methoxy-4-hydroxymandelic acid excretion during physical exercise.
Journal Applied Physiology 24:619, 1968.

2930
NEBLETT, C.R., D.P. McNEEL, T.A. WALTZ, JR., AND G.M. HARRISON.
Effect of cardiac glycosides on human cerebrospinal fluid production.
Lancet 2:1008-1009, 1972.

2931
NEDELJKOVIC, S.
Electrocardiogram following exercise loading .I.
Medicinski Glasnik 21:40-41, 1967.

2932
NEDOSTUPOV, S.P., K.M. ALEKSANDROVA, E. YU. MERKULOVA, O.I. VAKHNOVASKAYA, ET AL.
Experience in the use of hexonium electrophoresis in health-resort treatment of patients with hypertension.
Vrachebnoe Delo 4:73-75, 1970.

2933
NELSON, A.M.
Diet therapy in coronary disease. Effect on mortality of high protein, high seafood, fat controlled diet.
Geriatrics 27(12):103-116, 1972.

2934
NERDRUM, H.J., AND S. NORDOY.
Changes of serum glutamic oxaloacetic transaminase following exercise in patients with and without coronary disease.
Scandinavian Journal Clinical Laboratory Investigation 16:617-623, 1964.

2935
NEREM, R.M., AND W.A. SEED.
An in vivo study of aortic flow disturbances.
Cardiovascular Research 6(1):1, 1972.

2936
NEUFELD, H.N.
   Proceedings of the 4th Asian Pacific Congress of Cardiology of the Israel Heart Society session on ischemic heart disease, prevention, and rehabilitation. Jerusalem and Tel Aviv, Israel, September 1-7, 1968.
   Israel Journal Medical Sciences 5:783-793, 1969.

2937
NEUMAN, A.
   Intermittent regional delay of left ventricular activation: The influence of such a delay on the standard electrocardiogram, report of 33 cases.
   Chest 61(7): 633-639, 1972.

2938
NEUMAN, M.P. DE, S. TALMASKY, L.P. DE LIPPENHOLTZ, ET AL.
   Free fatty acids in acute myocardial infarction.
   Prensa Mèdica Argentina 59(35):1323-1326, 1972.

2939
NEUMANN, E.H., AND A. PIERACH.
   Convalescence of the heart patient.
   Internist 6:373-385, 1965.

2940
NEW, P.K.M., ET AL.
   The support structure of heart and stroke patients: A study of the role of significant others in patient rehabilitation.
   Social Science Medicine 2:185-200, 1968.

2941
NEWHOUSE, M.T., ET AL.
   Long-term dipyridamole therapy of angina pectoris.
   American Journal Cardiology 16: 234-237, 1965.

2942
NEWMAN, L.B., R.R. WASSERMAN, AND C. BORDEN.
   Productive living for those with heart disease: The role of physical medicine and rehabilitation.
   Archives Physical Medicine Rehabilitation 37:137-149, 1956.

2943
NIARCHOS, A.P.
   Propranolol induced bradycardia and syncope. A report of three cases.
   Acta Cardiologica 27(4):504-510, 1972.

2944
NICHAMAN, M.Z., E. BOYLE, JR., T.P. LESESNE, AND H.I. SAUER.
   Cardiovascular disease mortality by race.
   Geriatrics 17:724-737, 1962.

2945
NICHOLS, J.R.
   Vocational rehabilitation of the cardiac patient.
   Maryland State Medical Journal 15:93-94, 1966.

2946
NICOLAS, F.
    Cardiac glucosides and drugs used in anesthesia and in resuscitation.
    Minerva Anestesiologica 38:127, 1972.

2947
NIEUWENHUIZEN, C.L., C. VAN.
    On the rehabilitation of cardiac patients.
    Tidjdschrift voor Sociale Geneeskunde 42:913-918, 1964.

2948
NIITANI, H., S. IINO, T. NARUSAWA, S. NISHINOIRI, ET AL.
    Limitations in the diagnosis of the exercise electrocardiogram.
    Japanese Circulation Journal 30:1564-1565, 1966.

2949
NIITANI, H., S. IINO, T. NARUSAWA, S. NISHINOIRI, ET AL.
    Clinical application of telemetering (the second report). (1) Strenuous two-step exercise test with
    the 3-channel radioelectrocardiograph. (2) Radioelectrocardiography during bathing of cardio-
    vascular patients.
    Japanese Journal Medicine 6(1):24-26, 1967.

2950
NIITANI, H., AND K. MIYAKE.
    Clinical application of exercise tolerance test with emphasis on the physical fitness index.
    Japanese Circulation Journal 35(1):71-75, 1971.

2951
NIKITINE, S., C. SCHWAB, C. CARABATOS, ET AL.
    Frequency spectrum of the heart using Fourier's transformation method.
    Archives des Maladies du Coeur et des Vaisseaux 65(6):729-734, 1972.

2952
NIKKILÄ, E.A.
    Serum lipids and lipoproteins as related to coronary heart disease.
    Duodecim 88(21):1271-1282, 1972.

2953
NIKKILÄ, E.A., AND P. TORSTI.
    Adjustment of fat metabolism to exercise as studied in vitro.
    In: Karvonen, M.J., and A.J. Barry, Eds. Physical activity and the heart, pp. 216-227. Springfield,
    Ill. Thomas, 1967.

2954
NISHIMOTO, S., Y. NAWADA, Y. FUYUNO, AND H. YAMAMOTO.
    Rehabilitation of geriatric circulatory diseases.
    Japanese Circulation Journal 35(6):704, 1971.

2955
NISHINO, K., M. ITO, H. YAGI, A. KOIKE, ET AL.
    Studies on lipids and fibrinolytic activity in blood during hemodialysis.
    Japanese Circulation Journal, 37(8):889, 1973.

2956
NITTER-HAUGE, S., K. KIRKEBY, J.O. ALVSAKER, AND A. AAKVAAG.
Plasma 11-hydroxycorticosteroids in acute myocardial infarction.
Acta Medica Scandinavica 192(6):535-538, 1972.

2957
NITTER-HAUGE, S., O. MULLER, G. SEMB, K.V. HALL, ET AL.
Myocardial infarctectomy.
Acta Medica Scandinavica 191:405-408, 1972.

2958
NIXON, P.G.F.
Recovery from coronary illness.
Rehabilitation 81:23-25, 1972.

2959
NIXON, P.G.F., H. IKRAM, AND S. MORTON.
Cardiogenic shock treated with infusion of dextrose solution.
American Heart Journal 73:843, 1967.

2960
NIXON, P.G.F., D.J.E. TAYLOR, S.D. MORTON, AND M. BROMFIELD.
A sleep regimen for acute myocardial infarction.
Lancet 1:726-728, 1968.

2961
NOGUEIRA, J.B., J. SAAVEDRA, V. KASPRZYKOWSKI, R. RANCHHOD, ET AL.
The cardiac profile in arterial hypertension.
Münchner Medizinische Wochenschrift 113:1259-1264, 1971.

2962
NOLAN, J.C.
Vocational assessment.
Journal Rehabilitation 32:61, 1966.

2963
NOMURA, Y., Y. TAKAKI, AND S. TOYAMA.
A method for computer diagnosis of the electrocardiogram.
Japanese circulation Journal 30:499-508, 1966.

2964
NOMURA, Y., Y. TAKAKI, AND S. TOYAMA.
Computer analysis of the spatial vectorcardiogram with Frank's lead system.
Japanese Circulation Journal 31:1441-1451, 1967.

2965
NOMURA, Y., Y. TAKAKI, AND S. TOYAMA.
Logics for computer diagnosis of the electrocardiogram.
Journal Electrocardiology 2(2):117-126, 1969.

2966
NORDAN, R., K. OSTENDORF, AND J.P. NAUGHTON.
Return to the land of the living: An approach to the problem of chronic hemodialysis.
Pediatrics 48(6):939-945, 1971.

2967
NORDELL, K., L. MOGENSEN, O. NYQUIST, AND E. ORINIUS.
Thrombophlebitis following intravenous lignocaine infusion.
Acta Medica Scandinavica 192(4):263-265, 1972.

2968
NORRIS, R.M.
Long-term survival after cardiac arrest.
New Zealand Medical Journal 69(6):144-146, 1969.

2969
NORRIS, R.M.
Factors affecting long-term prognosis after myocardial infarction.
Medical Journal Australia 2(1):26-27, 1973.

2970
NORRIS, R.M., P.W.T. BRANDT, AND A.J. LEE.
Mortality in a coronary-care unit analysed by a new coronary prognostic index.
Lancet 1:278-281, 1969.

2971
NORRIS, R.M., ET AL.
A new coronary prognostic index.
Lancet 1:274-278, 1969.

2972
NORRIS, R.M., C.J. MERCER, AND M.S. CROXSON.
Conduction disturbances due to anteroseptal myocardial infarction and their treatment by endo-cardial pacing.
American Heart Journal 84(4):560-566, 1972.

2973
NORRIS, R.M., C.J. MERCER, AND S.E. YEATES.
Idioventricular rhythm complicating acute myocardial infarction.
British Heart Journal 32:617-621, 1970.

2974
NORRIS, R.M., C.J. MERCER, AND S.E. YEATES.
Sinus rate in acute myocardial infarction.
British Heart Journal 34(9):901-904, 1972.

2975
NOUZHA, E., O. BEUGNET, C. HUET, ET AL.
Congenital total absence of pericardium discovered at thoracotomy.
Annales de Chirurgie 26:137-142, 1972.

2976
NOVACK, P., D. POMERANTZ, H. KASPARIAN, A. KASPAR, AND B. SEGAL.
Response of the coronary heart disease patient to exercise.
Circulation 28(4 Part 2):779-780, 1963.

2977
NOVACK, P.
Haemodynamics of ventricular tachycardia.
In: Dreifus, L.S. and W. Likoff, Eds. Mechanisms and therapy of cardiac arrhythmias, pp. 265-273. New York, Grune and Stratton, 1966.

2978
NOWLIN, J.B., W.G. TROYER, W.S. COLLINS, G. SILVERMAN, ET AL.
The association of nocturnal angina pectoris with dreaming.
Annals Internal Medicine 63:1040, 1965.

2979
NOWOSIELECKA, DERUS E., K. DOBOSIEWICZ, AND G. KLUSZCZYK.
The results of rehabilitation of patients after acute myocardial infarction.
Wiadomosci Lekarskie 24(21):1981-1985, 1971.

2980
NULAND, W.
The use of hypnotherapy in the treatment of the postmyocardial infarction.
International Journal Clinical Experimental Hypnosis 16(3):139-150, 1968.

2981
NUNNELEY, S.A., S. FINKELSTEIN, AND U.C. LUFT.
Longitudinal study on physical performance of ten pilots over a ten-year period.
Aerospace Medicine 43:541-544, 1972.

2982
NÜSSEL, E., AND F.J. HEHL.
Morbidity and mortality of myocardial infarction.
In: Schlegel, B., Ed. Verhandlungen der Deutschen Gesselschaft für Innere Medizin. Wiesbaden, West Germany, April 9-13, 1972, pp. 104-117. München, Bergmann, 1972.

2983
NÜSSEL, E., H. JAHN, AND A. ATANASOV.
Comparative sociomedical study of myocardial infarct and liver patients of the regional insurance agency of Baden.
Archiv für Kreislaufforschung 57:113-127, 1968.

2984
NUSSER, E., AND H. DONATH.
Cardiac arrhythmias.
Stuttgart, German Federal Republic. Schattauer Verlag, 1972.

2985
NUTTER, D.O., R.C. SCHLANT, AND J.W. HURST.
Isometric exercise and the cardiovascular system.
Modern Concepts Cardiovascular Disease 41:11-15, 1972.

2986
NYBERG, G.
Drugs for angina pectoris.
British Medical Journal 3:47, 1973.

2987
NYE, E.R.
   Exercise in the treatment of coronary artery disease.
   Journal Royal College Physicians (London) 6(1):69, 1971.

2988
NYE, E.R., AND P.G. WOOD.
   Exercise and the patient with ischaemic heart disease.
   New Zealand Medical Journal 70(446):31-34, 1969.

2989
NYQUIST, O.
   Shock complicating acute myocardial infarction. A clinical, hemodynamic and therapeutic study.
   Acta Medica Scandinavica (Suppl.) 536:1-72, 1972.

2990
OBEL, I.W.P., P. MARCHAND, AND R.N. SCOTT MILLAR.
   Cardiac pacemaking. Experience with the first 120 patients treated in Johannesburg.
   South African Medical Journal 46:2002, 1972.

2991
OBEREMCHENKO, Y.V., N.L. PROSHCHENKO, V.Z. MIKHALSKY, AND G.I. LIVSHITS.
   Treatment of acute disorders of atrio ventricular conduction.
   Vrabchebnoe Delo, 10:28-34, 1972.

2992
OBERWITTLER, W.
   Occupational analysis of workers with myocardial infarction.
   Medizinische Welt 21:1180, 1966.

2993
OBERWITTLER, W.
   Framingham study, anti-coronary club, heart prophylaxis.
   Therapiewoche 21(5):299-301, 1971.

2994
OBEYESEKERE, I., AND G.U. DeSILVA.
   Emotional stress and ischaemic heart disease in Ceylon.
   Ceylon Medical Journal 9:154-159, 1964.

2995
OBEYESEKERE, I. AND Y. HERMON.
   Myocarditis and cardiomyopathy after arbovirus infections (dengue and chikungunya fever).
   British Heart Journal 34(8):821-827, 1972.

2996
O'BRIEN, G.S., D.H. MCKENNA, C.V. JARAMILLO, AND G.G. ROWE.
   Systemic and coronary hemodynamic effects of beta-adrenergic blockade with Hethalide.
   Federation Proceedings 24(2 Part 1):713, 1965.

2997
O'BRIEN, J.R., AND W.J.H. BUTTERFIELD.
   Aspirin in the prevention of thrombosis.
   American Heart Journal 86:711, 1973.

2998

O'BRIEN, K.P., L.M. HIGGS, D.L. CLANCY, AND S.E. EPSTEIN.
Hemodynamic accompaniments of angina. A comparison during angina induced by exercise and by atrial pacing.
Circulation 39(6):735-743, 1969.

2999

O'CONNELL. D.D., AND R.M. LUNDY.
Level of aspiration in hypertensive cardiac patients compared with nonhypertensive cardiac patients with arteriosclerotic heart disease.
Journal Consulting Psychology 25:353, 1961.

3000

OGILVIE, R.I., AND J. RUEDY.
An educational program in digitalis therapy.
Journal American Medical Association 222(1):50-55, 1972.

3001

OGSTON, D.
Fibrinolytic activity and anxiety and its relation to coronary artery disease.
Journal Psychosomatic Research 8:219-222, 1964.

3002

OHM, O.J.
Displacement and fracture of pacemaker electrode during physical exertion. Report on three cases.
Acta Medica Scandinavica 192(1-2):33-35, 1972.

3003

OKADA, K., S. SHIBATA, T. CHIBA, ET AL.
Case reports of cardiac arrest during hypothermia supposedly caused by the temperature difference between the rectum and the esophagus.
Japanese Journal Anesthesiology 21(4):389-394, 1972.

3004

OKAMOTO, N., AND E. SIMONSON.
Separation of normal and abnormal vectorcardiograms. Use of spatial orientation of initial, central and terminal segmental planes of QRS loop.
American Journal Cardiology 18:682-689, 1966.

3005

OKUBO, Y., K. OKUBO, Y. ONUMA, AND Y. ISAWA.
A psychosomatic study of circulatory diseases: second report.
Journal Japanese Psychosomatic Society 12:297-298, 1972.

3006

OKUDA, M., T. YAMADA, AND K. HOSONO.
Characterization of a myocardial depressant factor isolated from cardiogenic shock.
Japanese Circulation Journal 37:982, 1973.

3007

OLAGUE DE ROS, J., J. COSIN AGUILAR, M. BELTRAN CARRASCOSA, F.J. ALGARRA VIDAL AND J.M. CAFFARENA RAGGIO.
Disturbances in intraventricular conduction through open heart surgery in congenital and acquired cardiopathies. Our experience.
Medicina Española 69:176, 1973.

3008
OLAZABAL, F., JR., J. OMS, AND R. RODRIGUEZ.
Quantitative vectorcardiography in the coronary care unit.
Boletin de la Asociacion Medica de Puerto Rico 64(8):206-210, 1972.

3009
O'LEARY, J.P., R.L. COLUMBARO, J.J. SCHWAB, AND W.H. McGINNIS.
Anxiety in cardiac patients.
Diseases Nervous System 29(7):443-448, 1968.

3010
OLENEVA, V.A., N.S. TAITS, AND T.A. KUZ'MINOVA.
Effect of diet reduction on the condition of the cardiovascular system in obese patients.
Voprosy Pitaniya 26(4):35-40, 1967.

3011
OLEWINE, D., M. SIMPSON, D. JENKINS, F. RAMSAY, S. ZYZANSKI, AND C.G. HAMES.
Catecholamines platelet aggregation and the coronary prone behavior pattern.
Psychosomatic Medicine 34:473, 1972.

3012
OLIN, H.S. AND T.P. HACKETT.
The denial of chest pain in 32 patients with acute myocardial infarction.
Journal American Medical Association 190(11):977-981, 1964.

3013
OLINGER, G.N., F.W. RIO, AND J.V. MALONEY, JR.
Closed valvulotomy for calcific mitral stenosis.
Journal Thoracic Cardiovascular Surgery 62(3):357-365, 1971.

3014
OLIVA, P.B., M.L. JOHNSON, M. POMERANTZ, AND A. LEVENE.
Dysfunction of the Beall mitral prosthesis and its detection by cinefluoroscopy and echocardio-
graphy.
American Journal Cardiology 31(3):393-396, 1973.

3015
OLIVER, M.F.
The place of the coronary care unit.
Royal College Physicians 3:47, 1968.

3016
OLIVER, M.F.
Glucose, insulin, potassium in acute myocardial infarction.
Acta Cardiologica Suppl. 17:257, 1973.

3017
OLIVER, M.F., AND P.A. YATES.
Induction of ventricular arrhythmias by elevation of arterial free fatty acids in experimental
myocardial infarction.
Cardiologia 56(1):359, 1972.

3018
OLIVER, R.M.
Physique and serum lipids of young London busmen in relation to ischemic heart disease.
British Journal Industrial Medicine 24:181-188, 1967.

3019
OLSEN, E.G.J.
Pathology of primary cardiomyopathies.
Postgraduate Medical Journal 48:732-737, 1972.

3020
OLSON, R.E.
"Excess lactate" and anaerobiosis.
Annals Internal Medicine 59:960, 1963.

3021
OLSON, R.E.
Basic relationships: Diet and heart disease.
Academy Medicine New Jersey Bulletin 10(4):250-261, 1964.

3022
OLSSON, L.G., AND A. REDFORS.
A simple system for displaying ECG and heart rate, recorded by portable tape recorders.
Scandinavian Journal Clinical Laboratory Investigation 30(2):159-162, 1972.

3023
OLSSON, S.B.
Recording of monophasic action potentials in the study of atrial dysrhythmias.
Gazzetta Italiana di Cardiologia 2(4):536-541, 1972.

3024
OLSSON, S.B. AND E. VARNAUSKAS.
A preliminary report on the duration of beta blockade after oral intake of LB 46.
Indian Heart Journal 24(Suppl. 1):167-171, 1972.

3025
ONO, K.
Influence of β-blocking agent on hemodynamics and myocardial metabolism: Supplement. A consideration of angina pectoris due to exercise.
Nippon University Medical Journal 27(2):109-127, 1968.

3026
ONO, N.
Studies of the easy exercise test and the coronary vasodilator injection test in the electrocardiogram.
Japanese Journal Medicine 6(1):26-27, 1967.

3027
OOSTENBRINK, A.A.
Study on the prognosis of myocardial infarction and angina pectoris in insurance medicine.
Tijdscrift voor Sociale Geneeskunde 49(24):894-901, 1971.

3028
OPIE, L.H.
  Exercise and myocardial factor in ischemic heart disease.
  Lancet 1:1067-1068, 1973.

3029
OPPENHEIMER, E.H. AND J.R. ESTERLY.
  Myocardial lesions in patients with cystic fibrosis of the pancreas.
  Johns Hopkins Medical Journal 133:252, 1973.

3030
ORANSKII, I.E., AND V.S. VOLKOV.
  The effect of physical exertion on the systolic structure of the left and right ventricles of healthy
  persons and patients with postinfarction cardiosclerosis.
  Kardiologiya 11(3):126-130, 1971.

3031
ORAVETZ, J., AND H.A. ZIMMERMAN.
  The fallacious T-wave and the second sound.
  Angiology 20:496-501, 1969.

3032
ORESKOVIC, A.
  Walking exercise in the rehabilitation of patients with coronary artery disease.
  In: Plavšić, C. and M.M. Gertler, Eds. The first international biennial conference on cardiac
  rehabilitation, Dubrovnik, Yogoslavia, 1969.

3033
ORHA, I., AND A. MOGA.
  Aspects of the relationship between physical work and homeostasis of lipid metabolism under
  physiologic conditions and in atherosclerosis patients.
  Fiziologia Normală și Patologică 16(5):417-426, 1970.

3034
ORINIUS, E., AND U. SÄWE.
  Fluoroscopic screening for left ventricular aneurysm following acute myocardial infarction.
  Acta Medica Scandinavica 192(3):197-199, 1972.

3035
ORLOVA, N.P.
  Changes in blood coagulation activity in patients with ischemic heart disease under the effect of
  physical exertion.
  Kardiologiya 11(11):117-119, 1971.

3036
OSCAI, L.B., J.A. PATTERSON, D.L. BOGARD, R.J. BECK AND B.L. ROTHERMEL.
  Normalization of serum triglycerides and lipoprotein electrophoretic patterns by exercise.
  American Journal Cardiology 30(7):775, 1972.

3037
OSHIMA, H.
  Study on the cardiopulmonary function in chronic pulmonary disease with special reference to
  exercise load test.
  Journal Osaka City Medical Center 16(9/10):573-593, 1967.

3038
OSNESS, W.H., B. BALKE, E.S. GORDON AND J. RANKIN.
   The metabolic role of lipids in the production of energy during exercise.
   In: Balke, B., Ed. Physiological aspects of sports and physical fitness, pp. 91-99. The Athletic
   Institute, 1968.

3039
OSTFELD. A.M.
   Heart disease and stroke in an elderly welfare population.
   Bulletin New York Academy Medicine 49(6):458-466, 1973.

3040
OSTFELD, A.M., ET AL.
   A propsective study of the relationship between personality and coronary heart disease.
   Journal Chronic Diseases 17:265, 1964.

3041
OSTRAND, I.
   Exercise electrocardiograms recorded twice with an 8-year interval in a group of 204 women and
   men 48-63 years old.
   Acta Medica Scandinavica 178:27-39, 1965.

3042
OSTRANDER, L.D., JR.
   Identification and management of the precursors of coronary heart disease.
   University Michigan Medical Center Journal 38(3):93-97, 1972.

3043
OSTRANDER, L.D., JR., W.D. BLOCK, D.E. LAMPHIEAR, AND F.H. EPSTEIN.
   Altered carbohydrate and lipid metabolism and coronary heart disease among men in Tecumseh,
   Michigan.
   In: Camerini-Davalos, R.A. and H.S. Cole, Eds. Advances in metabolic disorders. Supplement 2.
   Vascular and neurological changes in early diabetes. Proceedings of the Second International
   Diabetes Symposium, Curacao, Netherlands Antilles, Dec. 1971, pp. 73-81. New York, Academic
   Press, 1973.

3044
OSTRANDER, L.D., T. FRANCIS, JR., N.S. HAYNER, M.O. KJELSBERG, AND F.H. EPSTEIN.
   The relationship of cardiovascular disease to hyperglycemia.
   Annals Internal Medicine 62:1188, 1965.

3045
OSTRANDER, L.D., AND B.J. WEINSTEIN.
   Electrocardiographic changes after glucose ingestion.
   Circulation 30:67, 1964.

3046
OSTWALD, R., ET AL.
   Changes in tissue lipids in response to diet. I. Fatty acids of subcutaneous, mesenteric and
   scapular fat.
   Journal Nutrition 76:341, 1962.

3047
OWEN, C.A., E.F. BEARD, P.C. THOMAS, AND H.A. WALLACE.
An exercise prescription intervention program with periodic ergometric grading.
Journal Occupational Medicine 13(6):271-276, 1971.

3048
PAASIKIVI, J.
Long term tolbutamide treatment of survivors from myocardial infarction.
Acta Diabetologica Latina 8(1):437-443, 1971.

3049
PACIARONI, E., AND E.G. RASPA.
The rehabilitation of the aged cardiac patient.
Rassegna Geriatria 6(3):119-126, 1970.

3050
PAFFENBARGER, R.S., JR., AND M.E. LAUGHLIN.
Physical activity of work as related to death from coronary heart disease and stroke.
Circulation 39-40(Suppl. III):158, 1969.

3051
PAFFENBARGER, R.S., JR., M.E. LAUGHLIN, A.S. GIMA, AND R.A. BLACK.
Work activity of longshoremen as related to death from coronary heart disease and stroke.
New England Journal Medicine 282:1109-1114, 1970.

3052
PAFFENBARGER, R.S., JR., J. NOTKIN, D.E. KRUEGER, P.A. WOLF, ET AL.
Chronic disease in former college students. II. Methods of study and observations on mortality from coronary heart disease.
American Journal Public Health 56:962, 1966.

3053
PAFNOTE, M., I. VAIDA, AND M. DUMITRIU.
Correlations between the heart rate, body temperature and that of the environment during work performance.
Fiziologia Normala și Patologică 18(5):425-432, 1972.

3054
PAGE, I.H., J.N. BERRETTONI, A. BUTKUS, AND F.M. SONES.
Prediction of coronary heart disease based on clinical suspicion, age, total cholesterol and triglyceride.
Circulation 42:625, 1970.

3055
PALMA, A., ET AL.
Social and rehabilitation problems in myocardial infarct.
Rassegna Internazionale di Clinica e Terapia 48:1278-1283, 1968.

3056
PALMER, J., J. WOODHILL, AND R. BLACKET.
Strict modified fat diet in coronary heart disease.
Israel Journal Medical Sciences 5:754-759, 1969.

3057
PANTRIDGE, J.F.
   Flying squad services.
   In: Julian, D.G. and M.F. Oliver, Eds. Acute myocardial infarction. Edinburgh, Livingstone, 1968.

3058
PANTRIDGE, J.F., AND A.A.J. ADGEY.
   Pre-hospital coronary care. The mobile coronary care unit.
   American Journal Cardiology 24:666-673, 1969.

3059
PAPADOPOULOS, N.M., AND J.L. BEDYNEK.
   Serum lipoprotein patterns in liver and heart disease.
   Annals Clinical Laboratory Science 2:343, 1972.

3060
PAPE, J.
   On the significance of intracellular potassium and magnesium ions in the etiology of myocardial infarction.
   Medizin Ernährung 6:143, 1963.

3061
PAPP, O.A., L. PADILLA, AND A.L. JOHNSON.
   Dietary intake in patients with and without myocardial infarction.
   Lancet 2:259-261, 1965.

3062
PARAMONOVA, E.G.
   Dietary cure in coronary atherosclerosis. (From the findings of the Cardiovascular Division, Clinic of Therapeutic Nutrition, Institute of Nutrition, Academy of Medical Sciences of the USSR.)
   Vestnik Akademii Meditsinskikh Nauk SSSR 19:69-75, 1964.

3063
PARAMANOVA, E.G., G.S. KOROBKINA, A.N. SYCHEVA, E.P. CHUNAKOVA, ET AL.
   The curative effect of a diet including sea products in patients with coronary atherosclerosis.
   Sovetskaya Meditsina 29:(2):11-15, 1966.

3064
PARAMONOVA, E.G., AND V.A. SHATERNIKOV.
   Some aspects of lipid metabolism in patients with coronary atherosclerosis and influence exerted thereupon by dietetic treatment.
   Terapevticheskii Arkhiv 38(12):46-50, 1966.

3065
PARKER, G.W., AND R. GORLIN.
   Immediate post-exercise vital capacity: A measure of increased pulmonary capillary pressure.
   American Journal Medical Sciences 257:365-369, 1969.

3066
PARKER, J.O.
   Hemodynamic and metabolic changes during myocardial ischemia.
   Archives Internal Medicine 129(5):790-798, 1972.

3067
PARKER, J.O., S. DI GIORGI, AND R.O. WEST.
  A hemodynamic study of acute coronary insufficiency precipitated by exercise.
  American Journal Cardiology 17(4):470-483, 1966.

3068
PARKER, J.O., R.W. WEST, AND S. DI GIORGI.
  The hemodynamic response to exercise in patients with healed myocardial infarction without angina. With observations on the effects of nitroglycerin.
  Circulation 36(5):734-751, 1967.

3069
PARKER, J.O., R.O. WEST, AND S. DI GIORGI.
  Hemodynamics in coronary heart disease.
  Canadian Medical Association Journal 98(2):111, 1968.

3070
PARKER, J.O., R.O. West, R.B. CASE, AND M.A. CHIONG.
  Relation of metabolic, hemodynamic and electrocardiographic changes during myocardial ischemia produced by atrial pacing or exercise.
  Circulation 37-38(Suppl. 6):153, 1968.

3071
PARKER, J.O., R.O. WEST, R.B. CASE, AND M.A. CHIONG.
  Temporal relationships of myocardial lactate metabolism, left ventricular function, and S-T segment depression during angina precipitated by exercise.
  Circulation 40(1):7, 1969.

3072
PARKER, J.O., R.O. WEST, AND S. DI GIORGI.
  The effect of nitroglycerin on coronary blood flow and the hemodynamic response to exercise in coronary artery disease.
  American Journal Cardiology 27(1):59-65, 1971.

3073
PARKER, J.O., R.O. WEST, R.J. LEDWICH, AND S. DI GIORGI.
  The effect of acute digitalization on the hemodynamic response to exercise in coronary artery disease.
  Circulation 40(4):453-462, 1969.

3074
PARLEY, K.
  How to balance your tensions.
  American Journal Nursing 67(10):2099-2101, 1967.

3075
PARMLEY, W.W., AND E.H. SONNENBLICK.
  Series elasticity in heart muscle. Its relation to contractile element velocity and proposed muscle models.
  Circulation Research 20:112, 1967.

3076
PARMLEY, W.W., J.F. SPANN, R.R. TAYLOR, AND E.H. SONNENBLICK.
 The series elasticity of cardiac muscle in hyperthyroidism, ventricular hypertrophy, and heart failure.
 Proceedings Society Experimental Biology Medicine 127:606, 1968.

3077
PARMLEY, W.W., H. TOMODA, S. FUJIMURA, AND J.M. MATLOFF.
 Relation between pulsus alternans and transient occlusion of the left anterior descending coronary artery.
 Cardiovascular Research 6(6):709-715, 1972.

3078
PARRATT, J.R., I.M. LEDINGHA, AND C.S. McARDLE.
 Effect of a coronary vasodilator drug (Carbochromen) on blood flow and oxygen extraction in acute myocardial infarction.
 Cardiovascular Research 7(3):401-407, 1973.

3079
PARSONNET, V.
 A stretch fabric pouch for implanted pacemakers.
 Archives Surgery 105(4):654-656, 1972.

3080
PARSONNET, V., L. GILBERT, AND I.R. ZUCKER.
 The natural history of pacemaker wires.
 Journal Thoracic Cardiovascular Surgery 65:315, 1973.

3081
PASCH, T., R.D. BAUER, AND J. VON DER EMDE.
 Comparative measurements of blood flow with the electromagnetic and the ultrasonic Doppler procedures.
 Zeitschrift für Kreislaufforschung 61(6):485-491, 1972.

3082
PASSA, P., AND J. CANIVET.
 Electrocardiographic changes after glucose loading.
 Nouvelle Presse Médicale 1:1831-1834, 1972.

3083
PASSOWICZ, L.
 The effect of clofibrat isopharm on fat tolerance in atherosclerotic patients.
 Polski Tygodnik Lekarski 27(30):1163-1166, 1972.

3084
PASSOWICZ, L., AND K. WRABEC.
 Fat tolerance test in patients with past myocardial infarction undergoing long-term treatment with physical exercises.
 Polski Tygodnik Lekarski 27(34):1306-1307, 1972.

3085
PASSMORE, R., AND J.V.G.A. DURNIN.
 Human energy expenditure.
 Physiological Reviews 35:801-840, 1955.

3086
PATHAK, C.L.
Intrinsic autoregulatory control of heart rate and its applied and clinical implications.
Acta Cardiologica 27(5):630-647, 1972.

3087
PATRUSHEV, V.I.
On the effect of hypochloride diet on the arterial pressure and mineral metabolism in hypertensive disease.
Voprosy Pitaniya 22(1):22-28, 1963.

3088
PATTERSON, J.A., J. NAUGHTON, R.J. PIETRAS, AND R.M. GUNNAR.
Treadmill exercise in the assessment of functional capacity of cardiac patients.
Circulation 43-44(Suppl. II):209, 1971.

3089
PATTERSON, J.A., J. NAUGHTON, R.J. PIETRAS, AND R.M. GUNNAR.
Treadmill exercise in assessment of functional capacity of patients with cardiac disease.
American Journal Cardiology 30(7):757-762, 1972.

3090
PAUL, L.T.
The effect of epinephrine on myocardial synchronization and diastolic filling time.
Proceedings Society Experimental Biology Medicine 140(4):1197-1202, 1972.

3091
PAUL, O.
Risks of mild hypertension: a ten-year report.
British Heart Journal 33(Suppl.):116-121, 1971.

3092
PAUL, O.
Factors in mortality from coronary disease.
In: American Clinical Climatological Association, Ed. Transactions of the American Clinical and Climatological Association 84:132-143. Richmond, Va. American Clinical and Climatological Association, 1973.

3093
PAUL, O.
Epidemiological and clinical aspects of sudden cardiac death.
Triangle 12(1):17-20, 1973.

3094
PAUL, O., M.H. LEPPER, W.H. PHELAN, G.W. DUPERTUIS, ET AL.
A longitudinal study of coronary heart disease.
Circulation 28:20, 1963.

3095
PAULAY, K.L., P.J. VARGHESE, AND A.N. DAMATO.
Atrial rhythms in response to an early atrial premature depolarization in man.
American Heart Journal 85(3):323-331, 1973.

3096
PAULEV, P.E.
    Respiratory and cardiac responses to exercise in man.
    Journal Applied Physiology 30:165-172, 1971.

3097
PĂUNESCOU-PODEANU, A.
    Respiration, oxygen, and atherosclerosis.
    Revue Roumaine de Médicine Interne 8(4):297-308, 1971.

3098
PAVLIK, L. AND S. KEPIC.
    Experience with precoronary care for career soldiers.
    Vojenske Zdravotnicke Listy 41:182, 1972.

3099
PAYNE, P.R., E.F. WHEELER, AND C.B. SALVOSA.
    Prediction of daily energy expenditure from average pulse rate.
    American Journal Clinical Nutrition 24:1164-1170, 1971.

3100
PAYNE, R.M., L.D. HORWITZ, AND C.B. MULLINS.
    Comparison of isometric exercise and angiotension infusion as stress test for evaluation of left
    ventricular function.
    American Journal Cardiology 31:428-433, 1973.

3101
PAZZANESE, D., V. BERTOLAMI, AND O.P. PORTUGAL.
    The role of the departments of public health in the prevention of myocardial infarction.
    Anais Paulistas de Medicina e Cirurgia 96(6):376-389, 1969.

3102
PCHELINTSEV, V.P., AND P.I. FILONENKO.
    Excretion of catecholamines and vanillyl-amygdalic acid in patients with ischemic disease of the
    heart and the effect of physical effort on it.
    Terapevticheskii Arkhiv 42(11):40-43, 1970.

3103
PEAL, S.
    Some psychological observations of patients with myocardial infarction, a pilot study.
    Psychiatric Communications 10:1-12, 1968.

3104
PEARSON, H.E.S.
    Stress and occlusive coronary artery disease.
    American Heart Journal 66(6):836-838, 1963.

3105
PEARSON, J.S., AND R.M. STEINHILBER.
    Psychological assessment of therapy in coronary artery disease.
    Journal American Medical Association 217(1):72-74, 1971.

3106
PEDERSEN, A.
Electrocardiography in extremity, precordial and Frank leads, recorded continuously on magnetic tape during a graded exercise. Experiences from a population study of about 400 not admitted 70-year old persons.
Scandinavian Journal Clinical Laboratory Investigation 19(Suppl. 100):52, 1967.

3107
PEDERSEN-BJERGAARD, O.
The effect of physical training in myocardial infarction.
In: Larsen, O., and R.O. Malmborg, Eds. Coronary heart diseases and physical fitness, pp. 115-116. Baltimore, University Park Press, 1971.

3108
PEDERSEN, O.F., AND E.S. STAFFELDT.
The relationship between four tests of back muscle strength in untrained subjects.
Scandinavian Journal Rehabilitation Medicine 4:175-181, 1972.

3109
PEDRAZA, N.M., L.H. HARTLEY, W.C. DAY, AND W.H. ABELMANN.
Abnormal response to exercise conditioning after myocardial infarction.
Circulation 48(4):203, 1973.

3110
PEDROTE GUINEA, J.A., J. BURGOS CORNEJO, A. CORREDOR MORALES, ET AL.
Cardiac rupture in myocardial infarction.
Revista Española de Cardiologia 25(3):261-264, 1972.

3111
PELIDES, L.J., D.S. REID, M. THOMAS, AND J.P. SHILLINGFORD.
Inhibition by beta-blockade of the ST segment elevation after acute myocardial infarction in man.
Cardiovascular Research 6(3):295-301, 1972.

3112
PELL, S. AND C.A. D'ALONZO.
Immediate mortality and five-year survival of employed men with a first myocardial infarction.
New England Journal Medicine 270(18):915-922, 1964.

3113
PELL, S., AND C.A. D'ALONZO.
Three-year study of myocardial infarction in a large employed population.
Journal American Medical Association 175:463-469, 1961.

3114
PELLEGRINO, L., A. DI MICHELE, AND D. PRENCIPE.
Disopyramide in cardiac arrhythmia.
Bolletino della Società Italiana di Cardiologia 17(8):617-625, 1972.

3115
PELSER, H.E.
Psychological aspects of the treatment of patients with coronary infarct.
Journal Psychosomatic Research 11:47-49, 1967.

3116
PENNEY, J.P.M.
   Return to work after myocardial infarction.
   Lancet 2:711-712, 1971.

3117
PENSE, G., E. BANZHAF, AND G. PANZRAM.
   Physiologic glycosuria in healthy subjects and patients with arteriosclerosis.
   Zeitschrift für Gesamte und Innere Medizin 26(7):230-233, 1971.

3118
PENTECOST, B.L.
   Prophylactic lignocaine after myocardial infarction.
   Lancet 1:1073, 1971.

3119
PEPINE, C.J., AND L. WIENER.
   Relationship of anginal symptoms to lung mechanics during myocardial ischemia.
   Circulation 46(5):863-869, 1972.

3120
PEREIRA-MIGUEL, M.J., M. HALPERN, J.M. PEREIRA-MIGUEL, M.G. AMADOR, ET AL.
   Hyperlipemias in the rural Portuguese population.
   Annales de Biologie Clinique 31(Special Number):147-148, 1973.

3121
PEREZ, C.F.
   Psychogenesis and psychological problems of coronary disease.
   Revista Española de Cardiologia 19:239-244, 1966.

3122
PEREZ, F.F., J.A. VELASCO RAMI, AND V. TORMO ALFONSO.
   Intracardial phonocardiography in the diagnosis of tricuspid insufficiency.
   Revista Española de Cardiologia 25(5):437-442, 1972.

3123
PERLMAN, L.V., S. FERGUSON, K. BERGUM, E.L. ISENBERG, AND J.F. HAMMARSTEN.
   Precipitation of congestive heart failure: Social and emotional factors.
   Annals Internal Medicine 75(1):1-7, 1971.

3124
PERNOD, J., J.G. BERNARD, AND J. KERMAREC.
   Myocardial infarction in the young adult. The role of emotional stress and dangerous occupations.
   Agressologie 7(4):27, 1966.

3125
PERNOD, J., J.G. BERNARD, AND J. KERMAREC.
   Myocardial infarction in the young adult. The role of emotional stress and dangerous occupations.
   Anesthesie Analgesie Reanimation 23(4):CLXIX-CLXXI, 1966.

3126
PERNOD, J., B. COBLENCE, R. CARRE, N. VASILE, AND J. BARAGAN.
   Study of the normal carotidogram (apropos of 1000 traces taken in 500 subjects).
   Archives des Maladies du Coeur et des Vaisseaux 60(9):1241-1249, 1967.

3127
PERNOT, C.
  Work adjustment of cardiacs.
  Archives des Maladies Professionelles 26:496-501, 1965.

3128
PERNOT, C.
  Myocardial infarction in railway environment. Medico-professional aspects concerning 100 cases.
  Archives des Maladies Professionnelles de Médecine du Travail et de Sécurité Sociale 34(3):165,
  1973.

3129
PEROSIO, A.M., L.D. SUAREZ, AND J.J. LLERA.
  Atrial dissociation.
  American Heart Journal 85(3):401-404, 1973.

3130
PERRET, C., J.F. ENRICO, S. POLI, AND J.J. AMACKER.
  Myocardial infarction: potential and limits of intensive care.
  Schweizerische Medizinische Wochenschrift 102(50):1830-1836, 1972.

3131
PERSIC, T., R. IVANCIC, V. RUKAVINA, E. KOREN, AND F. CUSTOVIC.
  Heart infarction in younger age.
  Medicina (Rijeka) 9:295-301, 1972.

3132
PETERSON, C.R.
  Clinical and invasive studies of coronary artery disease—one-year follow-up of 505 patients.
  Minnesota Medicine 56:944, 1973.

3133
PETERSON, D.R., D.J. THOMPSON, AND N. CHINN.
  Ischemic heart disease prognosis: A community-wide assessment (1966-1969).
  Journal American Medical Association 219(11):1423-1427, 1972.

3134
PETITIER, H., J.M. POLU, B. DODINOT, P. SOMMELET, P. MATHIEU, AND G. FAIVRE.
  Irreducible ventribular tachycardia: treatment by electrocoagulation of the ectopic nucleus.
  Presse Médical 79(2):54, 1971.

3135
PETITIER, H., J.M. POLU, B. DODINOT, P. SOMMELET, P. MATHIEU, AND G. FAIVRE.
  Irreducible ventricular tachycardia: treatment by electrocoagulation.
  Archives des Maladies du Coeur et des Vaisseaux 64:331-351, 1971.

3136
PFLANZ, M., AND L. LAMBELET.
  "Civilizational diseases" and psychosomatic problems in agricultural India.
  Münchener Medizinische Wochenschrift 107:1493-1502, 1965.

3137
PHILLIPS, J.H., JR., AND G.E. BURCH.
  A review of cardiovascular diseases in the white and negro races.
  Medicine 39:241-288, 1960.

3138
PHILLIPS, J., AND H. ICHINOSE.
  Clinical and pathologic studies in the hereditary syndrome of a long QT interval, syncopal spells
  and sudden death.
  Chest 58(3):236-243, 1970.

3139
PHILLIPS, W.J., H.B. HIGGINBOTHAM, H. FRERKING, ET AL.
  Evaluation of myocardial state by synchronized radiography and exercise.
  New England Journal Medicine 274(15):826-829, 1966.

3140
PHLIPPEN, R., H. HECK, AND B. GRÜNEWALD.
  Long-term ECG investigations on the question of heart strain of the aged during skiing.
  Medizinische Welt 46:1985-1990, 1970.

3141
PIARNAT, I.A.P., A.A. VIRU, AND A.P. PISUKE.
  Interrelations of the indices of work capacity of the cardiovascular and respiratory systems and
  the blood compositon of runners during muscular work of increasing magnitude.
  Fiziologicheskii Zhurnal SSSR Imeni I.M. Sechenova 56:1427-1432, 1970.

3142
PICK, A.
  Mechanisms of cardiac arrhythmias: From hypothesis to physiologic fact.
  American Heart Journal 86:249, 1973.

3143
PICKERING, J.E.
  Lidocaine blood levels in patient with acute myocardial infarction.
  Pennsylvania Medicine 76(3):57-60, 1973.

3144
PIDRMAN, V., AND A. HAMET.
  Conversion of atrial fibrillation and flutter by a combination of antiarrhythmic drugs.
  Vnitrni Lekarstvi 18(9):845-848, 1972.

3145
PIESSENS, J., W. VAN MIEGHEN, H. KESTELOOT, AND H. DE GEEST.
  Value of the effort electrocardiogram and of atrial pacing in the diagnosis of coronary atheromat-
  osis.
  Archives des Maladies du Coeur et des Vaisseaux 66:1351, 1973.

3146
PIGOTT, V.M., R. RYAN PLATT, E. ELBER, AND D.H. SPODICK.
  The influence of recording speed on apexcardiographic timing. A multi observer study of precision
  and performance utilizing randomized tracings in multiple subjects.
  Cardiology 57(4):232-239, 1972.

3147
PILCHER, J., AND M.K. HEALY.
The Birmingham (Lucas) pacemaker: A follow up with particular reference to dependence and parasystole.
British Heart Journal 34(10):1052-1056, 1972.

3148
PILEGGI, F., E. SOSA, G. BELLOTTI, ET AL.
Electrogram of the His bundle in atrial fibrillation. A study of atrioventricular conduction.
Arquivos Brasileiros de Cardiologia 25(2):125-133, 1972.

3149
PILOWSKY, I., D. SPALDING, J. SHAW, AND P.J. KORNER.
Hypertension and personality.
Psychosomatic Medicine 35:50-56, 1973.

3150
PINCHERLE, G.
Factors affecting the mean serum cholesterol.
Journal Chronic Diseases 24(5):289-297, 1971.

3151
PINNER, J.I., AND A.H. ALTMAN.
Selective placement in industry.
Journal Rehabilitation 32:71-73, 1966.

3152
PIPBERGER, H.V.
Computer analysis of the electrocardiogram.
In: Stacy, R.W. and B.D. Waxman, Eds. Computers in biomedical research p. 377. New York, Academic Press. 1965.

3153
PIPBERGER, H.V., AND F.W. STALLMANN.
Computation of differential diagnosis in electrocardiography.
Annals New York Academy Sciences 115:1115-1128, 1964.

3154
PIPBERGER, H.V., F.W. STALLMAN, K. YANO, AND H.W. DRAPER.
Digital computer analysis of the normal and abnormal electrocardiogram.
Progress Cardiovascular Diseases 5(4):378-392, 1963.

3155
PISTOLESE, M., G. RICHICHI, V. CATALANO, AND A. MORABITO.
Permanent atrial pacing: indications and method.
Gazzetta Italiana di Cardiologia 2(4):519-526, 1972.

3156
PITT, A., AND S.T. ANDERSON.
A comparison of the effects of "Trasicor" (oxprenolol) and "Inderal" (propranolol) on left ventricular myocardial function.
Medical Journal Australia 1:1089-1093, 1970.

3157
PITT, B., AND G.S. KURLAND.
Use of edrophonium chloride (Tensilon) to detect early digitalis toxicity.
American Journal Cardiology 18:557, 1966.

3158
PITTELOUD, J.J.
Total hemoglobin and the control of tolerance to muscular efforts in cardiovascular diseases.
Malattie Cardiovascolari 10(1-2):359-367, 1969.

3159
PIXBERG, H.U., W. ECKHARDT, AND M. CACHOVAN.
Determination of blood volume in defined regions of the body, using 113m In (III) chloride.
Nuclear Medizin 11(2):132-137, 1972.

3160
PLAGNE, A., AND M. BARACHET.
Use of propanidid during correction of cardiac arrhythmias by external electric shock. (258 cases).
Anesthesie Analgesie Réanimation 29(3):347-354, 1972.

3161
PLAS, F.
Myocardial infarction and sport.
Anesthésie Analgesie Réanimation 23(4):218, 1966.

3162
PLAS, R.
The electrocardiogram of sportsmen.
Annales de Cardiologie et d'Angéiologie 20(6):729-731, 1971.

3163
PLASS, R., K.H. SCHMIDT, AND K.H. GUNTHER.
Parameters of contractility of the left ventricle under physical stresses.
Cor Vasa 13(1):43-49, 1971.

3164
PLATT, R.
Heredity in hypertension.
Lancet 1:899-904, 1963.

3165
PLAVŠIĆ, C., AND V. BAKASUN.
Some parameters and the successful rehabilitation of patients with myocardial infarction.
Bollettino della Società Italiana di Cardiologia 16(9):553-557, 1971.

3166
PLAVŠIĆ, C., AND M.M. GERTLER, EDS.
The first international biennial conference on cardiac rehabilitation.
Dubrovnik, Yugoslavia, 1969.

3167
POCOCK, W.A., AND J.B. BARLOW.
Postexercise arrhythmias in the billowing posterior mitral leaflet syndrome.
American Heart Journal 80(6):740-745, 1970.

3168
POCOCK, W.A., AND J.B. BARLOW.
Etiology and electrocardiographic features of the billowing posterior mitral leaflet syndrome. Analysis of a further 130 patients with a late systolic murmur or nonejection systolic click.
American Journal Medicine 51:731-739, 1971.

3169
POHLMANN, K.E.
Labor and the coronary worker.
Journal Rehabilitation 32(2):79, 1966.

3170
POKROVSKY, A.V., L.T. NADZHIMITDINOV, AND M.A. GLADKOVA.
Rehabilitation of patients at remote periods after resection of a coarctation of the aorta with prosthesis implantation.
Klinicheskaya Meditsina 50(8):51-54, 1972.

3171
POLAND, J.L., AND D.H. BLOUNT.
The effects of training on myocardial metabolism.
Proceedings Society Experimental Biology Medicine 129:177, 1968.

3172
POLANI, P.E., AND E.J. MOYNAHAN.
Progressive cardiomyopathic lentiginosis.
Quarterly Journal Medicine 41(162):205-225, 1972.

3173
POLE, D.J.
Myocardial infarction in Perth.
Medical Journal Australia 2(1):23-26, 1973.

3174
POLEDNAK, A.P.
Longevity and cardiovascular mortality among former college athletes.
Circulation 46(4):649-654, 1972.

3175
POLEDNAK, A.P., AND A. DAMON.
College athletics, longevity and cause of death.
Human Biology 42:28, 1970.

3176
POLIC-TADEJEVIC, A., AND T. MATIC.
Heart infarction: Ten years material.
Medicina (Rijeka) 9:283-294, 1972.

3177
POLIS, O., E. GHUYS, P. SMETS, J.W. DE KEYSER, ET AL.
Study of left ventricular ejection time during physical effort and during recovery.
Acta Cardiologica 26(1):38-65, 1971.

3178
POLLOCK, M.L., J. BROIDA, Z. KENDRICK, H.S. MILLER, JR., ET AL.
Effects of training two days per week at different intensities on middle-aged men.
Medicine Science Sports 4:192-197, 1972.

3179
POLLOCK, M.L., H.S. MILLER, JR., R. JANEWAY, A.C. LINNERUD, ET AL.
Effects of walking on body composition and cardiovascular function of middle-aged men.
Journal Applied Physiology 30:126-130, 1971.

3180
POLTORANOV, V.V.
Efficiency of health resort treatment of patients with cardiovascular diseases.
Vrachebnoe Delo 6:5-9, 1970.

3181
POLU, J.M., and J.M. GILGENKRANTZ.
The vectorcardiogram of the Wolff-Parkinson-White syndrome.
Annales de Cardiologie et d'Angéiologie 21(4):335-346, 1972.

3182
POMEROY, W.C., AND P.D. WHITE.
Coronary heart disease in former football players.
Journal American Medical Association 167:711, 1958.

3183
POOL, J., H.W.H. WEEDA, AND L.L.M. THOMAS.
Physical training of patients after myocardial infarction.
British Heart Journal 30(3):462, 1968.

3184
POOLE, P.E.
Implementing behavior in male patients with coronary artery disease.
Nursing Research 15:172-175, 1966.

3185
POORTMANS, J.R., AND R.W. JEANLOZ.
Urinary excretion of high-weight substances during physical exercises.
In: Balke, B., Ed. Physiological aspects of sports and physical fitness, pp. 83-86. The Athletic Institute, 1968.

3186
POOYA, M., N. KHOI, R. SARIN, J.C. RIOS, AND R.A. MASSUMI.
Clinical and hemodynamic features of idiopathic hypertrophic subaortic stenosis (IHSS).
Medical Annals District of Columbia 37:594, 1968.

3187
POPE, B., AND W. H. SCOTT.
Psychological diagnosis in clinical practice with applications in medicine, law, education, nursing, and social work.
New York, Oxford University Press, 1967.

3188
POPOV, V.G., A.L. SYRKIN, I.N. IVANITSKAYA, A.I. SHATIKHIN, ET AL.
   Regimen for a patient with myocardial infarction.
   Terapevticheskii Arkhiv 43(5):39-44, 1971.

3189
PORJÉ, I.G.
   Coronary diseases and physical activity.
   Nordisk Medicin 82(33):1019-1020, 1969.

3190
PORTE, D., JR., D.W. CRAWFORD, D.B. JENNINGS, C. ABER, AND M.B. MCILROY.
   Cardiovascular and metabolic responses to exercise in a patient with McArdle's syndrome.
   New England Journal Medicine 275(8):406-412, 1966.

3191
PORTER, A.L., C.D. MCCARTHY, AND H.E. PEARMAN.
   Effect of stressful physical illness on future time perspective.
   Journal Clinical Psychology 27(4):447-448, 1971.

3192
PORTER, G.A., AND N.A. DAVID.
   Bendroflumethiazide diuresis in congestive heart failure.
   Journal New Drugs 1(4):150-156, 1961.

3193
PORTNOY, B., K. ENGLEMAN, AND R. WYATT.
   Plasma catecholamines in hypertensive and psychiatric disorders.
   Clinical Research 17:258, 1969.

3194
POSCHL, M.
   Tasks of the sport medicine physician.
   Münchener Medizinische Wochenschrift 114:1321-1324, 1972.

3195
POSTMA, J.U.
   The importance of ballistocardiographic examination for patients with intermittent cerebrovascular insufficiency.
   Geneeskundige Gids 2(9):334-339, 1971.

3196
POUGET, J.M., W.S. HARRIS, B.R. MAYRON, AND J.P. NAUGHTON.
   Abnormal responses of the systolic time intervals to exercise in patients with angina pectoris.
   Circulation 43:289-298, 1971.

3197
POUGET, J.M., W.S. HARRIS, B.R. MAYRON, AND J.P. NAUGHTON.
   Abnormal responses of systolic time intervals to exercise in patients with angina pectoris.
   Cardiology Digest 7(4):10, 1972.

3198
POWELL, W.J., JR., R.B. WHITING, R.D. DINSMORE, AND C.A. SANDERS.
Symptomatic prognosis in patients with idiopathic hypertrophic subaortic stenosis (IHSS).
American Journal Medicine 55:45, 1973.

3199
PRAGLOWSKI, T., A. MISIEWICZ, AND J. SZCZEPANSKI.
Infarctions of the heart muscle in young people in the autopsy material.
Archiwum Medycyny Sadoweji Kryminologii 22:31, 1972.

3200
PRAKASH, R., W.W. PARMLEY, H.N. ALLEN, AND J.M. MATLOFF.
Effect of sotalol on clinical arrhythmias.
American Journal Cardiology 29:397-400, 1972.

3201
PRAKASH, R., W.W. PARMLEY, K. DIKSHIT, J. FORRESTER, AND H.J.C. SWAN.
The effects of isometric handgrip stress in patients with acute myocardial infarction.
Clinical Research 20(2):209, 1972.

3202
PRAKASH, R., W.W. PARMLEY, K. DIKSHIT, J. FORRESTER, AND H.J.C. SWAN.
Hemodynamic effects of posture change in acute myocardial infarction.
Clinical Research 20(3):392, 1972.

3203
PRASAD, K.
Transmembrane potential, contraction and ATPase activity of human heart in relation to ouabain.
Japanese Heart Journal 13(1):59-72, 1972.

3204
PRASAD, K., AND K.K. MIDHA.
Effect of rubidium on cardiac function.
Japanese Heart Journal 13(4):317-324, 1972.

3205
PRASAD, K., AND K.K. MIDHA.
Effect of cesium on the properties of cardiac muscle.
Japanese Heart Journal 14:454, 1973.

3206
PREIMATE, E.Y.
Frequency of ischemic heart disease in Riga according to epidemiological studies.
Latvijas PSR Zinatnu Akademijas Vestis 4:119-125, 1971.

3207
PREIMATE, E.Y.
Incidence of ischemic heart disease and certain factors of risk in the male population of Riga.
Kardiologiya 12:48-53, 1972.

3208
PREIMATE, E.Y.
Spread of some risk factors and their combination in ischemic disease of the heart in the city of
Riga: Epidemiological study.
Terapevticheskii Arkhiv 44:35-38, 1972.

3209

PREIMATE, E.Y.
   Clinical and morphological study of heart ischemia and arterial hypertension.
   Latvijas PSR Zinatnu Akademijas Vestis 11:112-116, 1972.

3210

PRESBER, W., AND K.H. SCHULZE.
   Participation of persons with cardiovascular diseases in special vocational rehabilitation.
   Zeitschrift für die Gesamte Hygiene und Ihre Grenzgebiete 17:71-77, 1971.

3211

PRIKAZCHIKOV, A.I.
   Some problems of etiology and pathogenesis of repeated myocardial infarction.
   Terapevticheskii Arkhiv 43(7):43-46, 1971.

3212

PRIMEAU, R.
   Peaked symmetrical T waves, an early sign of myocardial infarct.
   Union Médicale du Canada 98:104-105, 1969.

3213

PRINCE, R.A.
   An assessment of short and long term anticoagulant therapy in myocardial infarction.
   Drug Intelligence Clinical Pharmacy 7(5):202, 1973.

3214

PRIOR, I.A.M., J.G. EVANS, R.B.I. MORRISON, AND B.S. ROSE.
   The Carterton Study: 6. Patterns of vascular, respiratory, rheumatic and related abnormalities in
   a sample of New Zealand European adults.
   New Zealand Medical Journal 71:169-177, 1970.

3215

PRYS-ROBERTS, C., R. MELOCHE, AND P. FOËX.
   Studies of anaesthesia in relation to hypertension. I. Cardiovascular responses of treated and
   untreated patients.
   British Journal Anaesthesiology 43:122-137, 1971.

3216

PUGH, L.G.C.E.
   Deaths from exposure on Four Inns walking competition, March 14-15, 1964.
   In: Jokl, E. and J.T. McClellan, Eds. Medicine and Sport 5:112-120. Basel, Karger, 1971.

3217

PUNSAR, S., AND M.J. KARVONEN.
   Angina pectoris and ECG abnormalities in relation to prognosis of coronary heart disease in
   population studies in Finland.
   In: Early diagnosis of coronary heart disease. Proceedings of the second Paavo Nurmi Symposium,
   Porvoo, Finland, 1971. Basel, S. Karger, 1973.

3218
PYE, O.F., C.G. BROOKS, AND M.M. WINSTON.
Developing a program of learning on the fat-controlled diet.
Journal American Dietetic Association 57:428-431, 1970.

3219
PYFER, H.R., AND B.L. DOANE.
Cardiac arrest during exercise training. Report of a successfully treated case attributed to preparedness.
Journal American Medical Association 210(1):101-102, 1969.

3220
PYFER, H.R., AND B.L. DOANE.
Exercise for the cardio-pulmonary patient. A feasibility study.
Northwest Medicine 68(2):129-134, 1969.

3221
PYFER, H.R., AND B.L. DOANE.
Economic aspects of cardiac rehabilitation programs.
In: Naughton, J., H.K. Hellerstein, and I.C. Mohler, Eds. Exercise testing and exercise training in coronary heart disease, pp. 365-369. New York, Academic Press, 1973.

3222
PYÖRÄLÄ, K., R. KÄRÄVÄ, S. PUNSAR, P. OJA, ET AL.
A controlled study of the effects of 18 months physical training in sedentary middle-aged men with high indexes of risk relative to coronary heart disease.
In: Larsen, O.A., and R.O. Malmborg, Eds. Coronary heart diseases and physical fitness. pp. 261-265. Baltimore, University Park Press, 1971.

3223
PYÖRÄLÄ, K., M.J. KARVONEN, P. TASKINEN, J. TAKKUNEN, ET AL.
Cardiovascular studies on former endurance athletes. Report 19 Institute Occupational Health, Helsinki, 1965.
In: Noro, L., Ed. Annual Report, Occupational Medical Foundation and Institute of Occupational Health, Helsinki, Finland, 1966.

3224
PYÖRÄLÄ, K., M.J. KARVONEN, P. TASKINEN, J. TAKKUNEN, ET AL.
Cardiovascular studies on former endurance athletes.
In: Karvonen, M.J. and A.J. Barry, Eds. Physical activity and the heart, pp. 301-310. Springfield, Ill. Thomas, 1967.

3225
QUIRET, J.C., J. LIENARD, V. BAIL, J. PH. LESBRE, ET AL.
ECG during exercise in a "healthy" high risk population for coronary heart disease.
Nouvelle Presse Médicale 2:2749, 1973.

3226
QIZILBASH, A.H., AND C.J. SCHWARTZ.
False aneurysm of left ventricle due to perforation of mitral-aortic intervalvular fibrosa with rupture and cardiac tamponade. Rare complication of infective endocarditis.
American Journal Cardiology 32:110, 1973.

3227
RAAB, W.
   Civilization-induced neurogenic degenerative heart disease. Origin and prevention.
   Cardiologia 41(3):129-143, 1962.

3228
RAAB, W.
   The sympathogenic biochemical trigger mechanism of angina pectoris. Its therapeutic
   suppression and long-range prevention.
   American Journal Cardiology 9:576-590, 1962.

3229
RAAB, W.
   The nonvascular metabolic myocardial vulnerability factor in "coronary heart disease".
   American Heart Journal 66(5):685-706, 1963.

3230
RAAB, W.
   Rehabilitation in cardiovascular diseases.
   Verhandlungen der Deutschen Gesellschaft für Kreislaufforschung 30:325-334, 1964.

3231
RAAB, W.
   Rehabilitation of patients with cardiovascular diseases.
   Klinische Wochenschrift 42:767-768, 1964.

3232
RAAB, W.
   Exercise and ischemic heart disease.
   National Conference Cardiovascular Diseases 2:356, 1964.

3233
RAAB, W.
   Emotional and sensory stress factors in myocardial pathology.
   American Heart Journal 72(4):538-564, 1966.

3234
RAAB, W.
   Pluricausal pathogenesis and preventability of ischemic heart disease.
   Diseases Chest 53:629, 1968.

3235
RAAB, W.
   Exercise habits and emotional patterns in myocardial pathophysiology.
   In: Brunner, D. and E. Jokl, Eds. Physical activity and aging, pp. 132-135.
   Baltimore, University Park Press, 1970.

3236
RAAB, W., P. DE PAULA, E. SILVA, H. MARCHET, ET AL.
   Cardiac adrenergic preponderance due to lack of physical exercise and its pathogenic implications.
   American Journal Cardiology 5:300, 1960.

3237
RAAB, W., AND L.B. GILMAN.
Report on study tour of German reconditioning centers. Insurance-sponsored, preventive, cardiac reconditioning centers in West Germany.
American Journal Cardiology 13:670-673, 1964.

3238
RAAB, W., AND H.J. KRZYWANEK.
Cardiovascular sympathetic tone and stress response related to personality patterns and exercise habits: a potential cardiac risk and screening test.
American Journal Cardiology 16(1):42-53, 1965.

3239
RADFORD, M.D., AND D.W. EVANS.
Long-term results of DC reversion of atrial fibrillation.
British Heart Journal 30(1):91-96, 1968.

3240
RADKE, J.D., H.K. HELLERSTEIN, S.H. SALZMAN, H.M. MAISTELMAN, AND R. RICKLIN.
The quantitative effects of physical conditioning on the exercise electrocardiogram of subjects with arteriosclerotic heart disease and normal subjects.
Medicine Sport 4:168-194, 1970.

3241
RAFFO, M., C. BIDDAU, M. BINA, R. FONZA, ET AL.
Study on the effect of orally given potassium on the electrocardiogram taken during effort of normal people, neurodistonics, pericardiacs, and coronary patients.
Bolletino della Società Italiana di Cardiologia 14:839, 1969.

3242
RAHE, R.H., D.J. MCKEAN, AND R.J. ARTHUR.
A longitudinal study of life-change and illness patterns.
Journal Psychosomatic Research 10:355-366, 1967.

3243
RAHE, R.H., AND J. PAASIKIVI.
Psychosocial factors and myocardial infarction. II. An outpatient study in Sweden.
Journal Psychosomatic Research 15:33-39, 1971.

3244
RAHE, R.H., C.F. TUFFLI, JR., R.J. SUCHOR, JR., AND R.J. ARTHUR.
Group therapy in the outpatient management of post-myocardial infarction patients.
Psychiatry Medicine 4:77-88, 1973.

3245
RAHIMTOOLA, S.H., H.S. LOEB, A. EHSANI, ET AL.
Relationship of pulmonary artery to left ventricular diastolic pressures in acute myocardial infarction.
Circulation 46(2):283-290, 1972.

3246
RAHIMTOOLA, S.H., M. ZIAD SINNO, R. CHUQUIMIA, ET AL.
Effects of ouabain on impaired left ventricular function in acute myocardial infarction.
New England Journal Medicine 287(11):527-531, 1972.

3247
RAINE, J., AND J.M. BISHOP.
   The distribution of alveolar ventilation in mitral stenosis at rest and after exercise.
   Clinical Science (London) 24(1):63-68, 1963.

3248
RAIZNER, A.E., M.E. SILVERMAN, AND W.C. WATERS.
   Conduction disturbances and pacemaker failure in Loffler's endomyocarditis.
   American Journal Medicine 53(3):343-347, 1972.

3249
RAJ, D.V., AND K. VENKATA REDDY.
   A simple pacemaker.
   Indian Journal Medical Science 26(10):644-646, 1972.

3250
RAJAGOPALAN, R.S., T.G. JAGANNADHAN, K.S.C. APPU, ET AL.
   Acute cardiac infarction treated in an intensive coronary care unit.
   Indian Heart Journal 24(2):92-100, 1972.

3251
RALSTON, H.J., AND L. LUKIN.
   Energy levels of human body segments during level walking.
   Ergonomics 12(1):39-46, 1969.

3252
RAMIREZ, E.A., P.H. GARCIA PONT, AND F. ALVARADO NORAT.
   A five-year double blind controlled clinical trial of D-thyroxine on euthyroid coronary subjects.
   Final report.
   Boletin de la Asociacion Medica de Puerto Rico 64(4):64-73, 1972.

3253
RAMOS, O.L., H. AJZEN, AND M.C. LIMA.
   Effect of diet, posture, and guanethidine, on $T^C H_2 O$ in hypertensive subjects.
   Journal Applied Physiology 19(6):1175-1178, 1964.

3254
RAO, B.S., J.J. KELLY, JR., K.E. COHN, AND A. SELZER.
   Hemodynamic response to exercise and isoproterenol (IP) in normal individuals and in congestive
   failure (CHF) during beta-adrenergic blockade with MJ1999.
   Circulation 37-38(Suppl. 6):161, 1968.

3255
RAPAPORT, E.
   Exercise responses in patients with heart failure or valvular or congenital heart disease.
   Journal South Carolina Medical Association (Suppl.) 65(12):61-64, 1969.

3256
RAPOPORT, M.Y.
   Functional cardiac troubles and the sexual sphere.
   Sovetskaya Meditsina 34(7):69-73, 1971.

3257

RASTAN, H., B. HEISIG, D. RASTAN, C. BAUMGARTEN, AND D. REGENSBURGER.
Improved method of atrioseptectomy.
Thoraxchirurgie Vaskuläre Chirurgie 21:226, 1973.

3258

RATER, D., D. PUGH, AND W. GRAY.
Practical significance of systolic time intervals in coronary heart disease.
Chest 64:186, 1973.

3259

RAUSCH DE TRAUBENBERG, N.
Vocational guidance of professional cardiopaths.
Revue de Neuropsychiatrie Infantile et d'Hygiene Mentale de l'Enfance 11:173-177, 1963.

3260

RAUTAHARJU, P.M.
Deterministic type waveform analysis in electrocardiography.
Annals New York Academy Sciences 128:939-945, 1966.

3261

RAUTAHARJU, P., AND H. BLACKBURN.
The exercise electrocardiogram. Experience in analysis of "noisy" cardiograms with a small computer.
American Heart Journal 69(4):515-520, 1965.

3262

RAUTAHARJU, P.M., S. PUNSAR, H. BLACKBURN, J. WARREN, AND A. MENOTTI.
Waveform patterns in Frank-lead rest and exercise electrocardiograms of healthy elderly men.
Circulation 48:541-548, 1973.

3263

RAWLINS, M.D., D. MENDEL, AND M.V. BRAIMBRIDGE.
Ventricular septal defect and mitral regurgitation secondary to myocardial infarction.
British Heart Journal 34:322-324, 1972.

3264

RAYMAN, R.B.
Sudden incapacitation in flight, 1 January 1966- 30 November 1971.
Aerospace Medicine 44:953-955, 1973.

3265

RAYNAUD, J., H. BERNAL, J.P. BOURDARIAS, P. DAVID, AND J. DURAND.
Oxygen delivery and oxygen return to the lungs at onset of exercise in man.
Journal Applied Physiology 35:259-262, 1973.

3266

RAYNAUD, R., J.M. BOIVIN, M. BROCHIER, P. MORAND, ET AL.
Myocardial infarction in young adults.
Semaine des Hôpitaux de Paris 49:1809-1814, 1973.

3267
RAYNAUD, R., M. BROCHIER, J.P. FAUCHIER, AND P. RAYNAUD.
Arrhythmias of the atrioventricular node.
Annales de Cardiologie et d' Angéiologie 21(5):417-431, 1972.

3268
RAYNAUD, R., M. BROCHIER, J.L. NEEL, J.P. FAUCHIER, AND P. RAYNAUD.
Ventricular tachycardia with variable pattern and loss of potassium.
Archives des Maladies du Coeur et des Vaisseaux 62:1578-1598, 1969.

3269
RAYNAUD, R., M. BROCHIER, P. RAYNAUD, AND J.P. FAUCHIER.
Potassium deficit and severe troubles of cardiac rhythm.
Coeur et Médecine Interne 9:13, 1970.

3270
RECHNITZER, P.A.
Rehabilitation of the coronary patient.
Manitoba Medical Review 47:94-95, 1967.

3271
RECHNITZER, P.A., H.A. PICKARD, A.U. PAIVIO, M.S. YUHASZ, ET AL.
Long-term follow-up study of survival and recurrence rates following myocardial infarction in exercising and control subjects.
Circulation 45(4):853-857, 1972.

3272
RECHNITZER, P.A., ET AL.
The effects of a graduated exercise program on patients with previous myocardial infarction.
Canadian Medical Association Journal 92:858-860, 1965.

3273
RECHNITZER, P.A., M.S. YUHASZ, A. PAIVIO, H.A. PICKARD, ET AL.
Effects of a 24-week exercise programme on normal adults and patients with previous myocardial infarction.
British Medical Journal 1:734, 1967.

3274
REDDY, M.V., L.L. KASTENSCHMIDT, R.G. CASSENS, AND E.J. BRISKEY.
Studies on stress susceptibility: The relationship between serum enzyme changes and the degree of stress susceptibility.
Life Sciences 10(II/24):1381-1391, 1971.

3275
REDWOOD, D.R., D.R. ROSING, R.E. GOLDSTEIN, G.D. BEISER, AND S.E. EPSTEIN.
Importance of the design of an exercise protocol in the evaluation of patients with angina pectoris.
Circulation 43(5):618-628, 1971.

3276
REDWOOD, D.R., D.R. ROSING, AND S.E. EPSTEIN.
Circulatory and symptomatic effects of physical training in patients with coronary-artery disease and angina pectoris.
New England Journal Medicine 286(18):959-965, 1972.

3277
REEDER, L.G., J.M. CHAPMAN, AND A.H. COULSON.
Socioenvironmental stress, tranquilizers and cardiovascular disease.
In: Pletscher, A., and A. Marino, Eds. Psychotropic drugs in internal medicine. Excerpta Medica International Congress Series No. 182, pp. 226-238. Amsterdam, Netherlands. Excerpta Medica Foundation, 1970.

3278
REEDER. L.G., P.G.M. SCHRAMA, AND J.M. DIRKEN.
Stress and cardiovascular health: An international cooperative study. I.
Social Science Medicine 7:573, 1973.

3279
REES, W.D.
The distress of dying.
American Heart Journal 86:141, 1973.

3280
REEVES, T.J., AND L.T. SHEFFIELD.
The influence of age and athletic training on maximal heart rate during exercise.
In: Larsen, O.A., and R.O. Malmborg, Eds. Coronary heart disease and physical fitness, pp. 209-216. Baltimore, University Park Press, 1971.

3281
REICH, T., J. TUCKMAN, M.C.H. WANG, AND J.H. JACOBSON, II.
Effect of normobaric and hyperbaric oxygen tensions on resting and postexercise calf blood flow in normal man and in patients with arterial insufficiency.
Circulation 33-34(Suppl. III):196, 1966.

3282
REICHERT, P.
Does heart disease end sex activity?
Sexulogy 29:76-81, 1962.

3283
REICHLE, F.A., AND R.R. TYSON.
Revascularization of severely ischemic lower extremities in the elderly by femorotibial bypass.
Journal American Geriatric Society 20(10):497-499, 1972.

3284
REID, D.D.
Smoking and ischemic heart disease prevention; problems and potential.
Preventive Medicine 1:84-91, 1972.

3285
REID, D.D., AND J.V. WARREN.
Collaborative analysis of long-term anticoagulant administration after acute myocardial infarction.
Lancet 1:203-209, 1970.

3286
REIDEMEISTER, J.C., E. MARX, H.D. SCHULTE, ET AL.
Preliminary experiences with isotope pacemakers.
Thoraxchirurgie Vaskuläre Chirurgie 20(6):435-440, 1972.

3287
REIFF, G.G., H.J. MONTOYE, R.D. REMINGTON, J.A. NAPIER, ET AL.
Assessment of physical activity by questionnaire and interview.
In: Karvonen, M.J. and A.J. Barry, Eds. Physical activity and the heart, pp. 336-377. Springfield, Ill. Thomas, 1967.

3288
REINDELL, H., K. KÖNIG, AND H. ROSKAMM.
Functional diagnosis of the healthy and sick heart.
Stuttgart, West Germany. G. Thieme, 1967.

3289
REINHOLD, D.
Rehabilitation and physical therapy in patients with ischemic heart diseases.
Archiv für Physikalische Therapie 22(6):329-337, 1970.

3290
REINHOLD, D.
The significance of therapeutic functional training in the rehabilitation of coronary patients.
Medizin und Sport 12(5):155-157, 1972.

3291
REINHOLD, D., AND U. REINHOLD.
Effects of the complex spa treatment on myocardial oxygen consumption in coronary patients.
Zeitschrift für Physiotherapie 23(2):129-136, 1971.

3292
REITERER, W., AND H. CZITOBER.
The behavior of the systolic and diastolic blood pressure and of the heart rate in graduated exercise tests in subjects 50 to 80 years old under iodosol therapy.
Zeitschrift für Angewandte Bäder-und Klimaheilkunde 19(1):27, 1972.

3293
REMINGTON, R.D., AND M.A. SCHORK.
Determination of number of subjects needed for experimental epidemiologic studies of the effect of increased physical activity on incidence of coronary heart disease-preliminary considerations.
In: Karvonen, M.J. and A.J. Barry, Eds. Physical activity and the heart, pp. 311-319. Springfield, Ill. Thomas, 1967.

3294
REMMLINGER, H.
Balneological factors in the rehabilitation of cardiovascular disease.
Medizinische Welt 43:2428-2432, 1965.

3295
RENGGLI, L., R. BUCHER, F. BURKART, W. SCHWEIZER, ET AL.
Angina pectoris and abnormal electrocardiographic response to exercise in 3,000 professional people: The Basel Study II.
Medizinische Welt 19:1194, 1967.

3296
RENKER, U.
On the occupational reinstatement of patients with heart and circulatory diseases.
Zeitschrift für Aerztliche Fortbildung (Jena) 59:823-824, 1965.

3297
RESNEKOV, L.
Circulatory effects of cardiac dysrhythmias.
Cardiovascular Clinics 2(2):23-48, 1970.

3298
REYNELL, P.C., AND M.C. REYNELL.
The cost benefit analysis of a coronary care unit.
British Heart Journal 34(9):897-900, 1972.

3299
REYNOLDS, J.L.
Modification of atherosclerotic disease risk factors in children.
Journal Louisiana Medical Society 124(10):353-360, 1972.

3300
RICCI, B.
Measurement of oxygen debt and of blood lactate and pyruvate.
In: Balke B., Ed. Physiological aspects of sports and physical fitness, p. 12.
The Athletic Institute, 1968.

3301
RICCIUTTI, M.A.
Myocardial lysosome stability in the early stages of acute ischemic injury.
American Journal Cardiology 30(5):492-497, 1972.

3302
RICCIUTTI, M.A.
Lysosomes and myocardial cellular injury.
American Journal Cardiology 30(5):498-502, 1972.

3303
RICE, H., AND R.B. CONNERS.
A simple technique for identifying waveforms in a multiple display.
Medical Biological Engineering 10:113-114, 1972.

3304
RICHARDS, R.L., AND T.B. BEGG.
Long-term anticoagulant therapy in atherosclerotic peripheral arterial disease.
Vascular Disease 4(1):27-35, 1967.

3305
RICHARDSON, J.F.
The sugar intake of businessmen and its inverse relationship with relative weight.
British Journal Nutrition 27(3):449-460, 1972.

3306
RICHTER, K., AND G. BÖCK.
Determination of cardiovascular diseases by x-ray surveys and their methodical problems.
Zeitschrift für Erkrankungen der Atmungsorgane 133(1-3):188-194, 1970.

3307
RIEGER, P.
   The phonocardiogram after exercise.
   Zeitschrift für Kreislaufforschung 59(8):699-708, 1970.

3308
RIEVET, M., AND D. WASSERMANN.
   Role of sympathetic vasomotor tonus in the renal vasoconstrictive action of angiotensin.
   Comptes Rendus Société Biologique (Paris) 164:247-251, 1970.

3309
RIFKIN, B.G.
   The treatment of cardiac neurosis using systematic desensitization.
   Behavior Research Therapy 6(2):239-241, 1968.

3310
RILEY, C.P., A. OBERMAN, AND L.T. SHEFFIELD.
   Electrocardiographic effects of glucose ingestion.
   Archives Internal Medicine 130:703, 1972.

3311
RILEY, C.P., R.O. RUSSELL, JR., AND C.E. RACKLEY.
   Left ventricular gallop sound and acute myocardial infarction.
   American Heart Journal 86:598, 1973.

3312
RIME, B., AND M. BONAMI.
   Psychological approach to coronary disease: Comparative analysis of interviews with 20 myocardial infarct patients.
   Acta Psychiatrica Belgica 72:29-45, 1972.

3313
RINZLER, S.H., H. BAKST, AND J. ROSENFELD.
   Comparison of the usefulness of the Dock electromagnetic ballistocardiograph and the exercise tolerance test in the detection of coronary insufficiency.
   New York State Journal Medicine 52:1277, 1952.

3314
RIOS, J.C., AND N. ALI.
   Normal electrocardiographic variants.
   Medical Times, 98(2):81-94, 1970.

3315
RIOS, J.C., C.A. DZIOK, AND N. A. ALI.
   Digitalis-induced arrhythmias: Recognition and management.
   Cardiovascular Clinics 2(2):262-279, 1971.

3316
RIOS, J.C., G.A. EWY, AND R.A. MASSUMI.
   Lateral displacement of the head: A sign of decreased right ventricular performance.
   Chest 64:313, 1973.

3317

RIOS, J.C., AND R.A. MASSUMI.
Correlation between the apexcardiogram and the left ventricular pressure.
American Journal Cardiology 15:647, 1965.

3318

RIOS, J.C., R.A. MASSUMI, AND W.T. BREESMEN.
Auscultatory features of acute tricuspid regurgitation.
American Journal Cardiology 23:41, 1969.

3319

RIOS, J.C., R.A. MASSUMI, R. FLETCHER, AND G.A. EWY.
Electrocardiographic features of trifascicular block.
Circulation 39(Suppl. III):170, 1969.

3320

RIOS, J.C., R.A. MASSUMI, A. TAWAKKOL, AND A. ROSS.
Technique for insertion of an intrapericardial catheter for physiologic studies of pericardial effusion.
British Heart Journal 30:333, 1968.

3321

RIOS, J.C., A. TRIESTER, J. SCHATZ, AND H. KASPARIAN.
Left atrial enlargement in coronary artery disease.
Circulation 45-46(Suppl. II):211, 1972.

3322

RISSANEN, V.
Aortic and coronary atherosclerosis in a Finnish autopsy series of violent deaths.
Annales Academiae Scientiarum Fennicae, Series A V, Medica 155, 1972.

3323

RITTENHOUSE, E.A., H.M. RADKE, AND D.S. SUMNER.
Carotid artery aneurysm. Review of the literature and report of a case with rupture into the oropharynx.
Archives Surgery 105(5):786-789, 1972.

3324

RIZK, G., R. GOODALE, AND K. AMPLATZ.
Vascular endoscopy.
Radiology 106(1):33-35, 1973.

3325

ROBB, G.P., AND H.H. MARKS.
Evaluation of type and degree of changes in post-exercise electrocardiography in detecting coronary artery disease.
Proceedings Society Experimental Biology Medicine 103:450-452, 1960.

3326

ROBB, G.P., AND H.H. MARKS.
Latent coronary artery disease: Determination of its presence and severity by the exercise electrocardiogram.
American Journal Cardiology 13:603, 1964.

3327
ROBB, G.P., AND H.H. MARKS.
Postexercise electrocardiogram in arteriosclerotic heart disease: Its value in diagnosis and prognosis.
Journal American Medical Association 200(11):918-926, 1967.

3328
ROBBINS, A.F.
Exercise prescription.
Obesity Bariatric Medicine 2:26, 1973.

3329
ROBBINS, P.R.
Personality and psychosomatic illness: A selective review of research.
Genetic Psychology Monographs 80:51-90, 1969.

3330
ROBERTS, J.A., AND J.W. ALSPAUGH.
Specificity of training effects resulting from programs of treadmill running and bicycle ergometer riding.
Medicine Science Sports 4:6-10, 1972.

3331
ROBERTS, L.
Hemorrhagic myocardial infarction during long term anticoagulant therapy.
Canadian Medical Association Journel 89(26):1325-1327, 1963.

3332
ROBERTS, W.C., AND S.M. FOX, III.
Mumps of the heart: clinical and pathologic features.
Circulation 32:342-345, 1965.

3333
ROBERTS, W.C.
Does thrombosis play a major role in the development of symptom-producing a therosclerotic plaque?
Circulation 48:1161, 1973.

3334
ROBINSON, B.F.
Relation of heart rate and systolic blood pressure to the onset of pain in angina pectoris.
Circulation 35(6):1073-1083, 1967.

3335
ROBINSON, J.S., G. SLOMAN, T.H. MATHEW, AND A.J. GABLE.
Survival after resuscitation from cardiac arrest in acute myocardial infarction.
American Heart Journal 69:740, 1965.

3336
ROBINSON, N., R. SUTTON, AND E. CRAIGE.
Implanted bipolar pacemakers. Analysis of function.
Journal American Medical Association 223(5):505-511, 1973.

3337
ROBINSON, S.
   Experimental studies of physical fitness in relation to age.
   Arbeitsphysiologie 10:251, 1938.

3338
ROBINSON, S., ET AL.
   Mental disorders following open heart surgery.
   Harefuah Journal Israel Medical Association 77(7):294-296, 1969.

3339
ROCACHE, M., A. CABROL, G. GUIRAUDON, ET AL.
   Long term results of aortic valve annuloplasty.
   Archives des Maladies du Coeur et des Vaisseaux 65(9):1123-1128, 1972.

3340
ROCHELLE, R.
   Blood plasma cholesterol changes during a physical training program.
   Research Quarterly; American Association Health, Physical Education, Recreation 32:538, 1961.

3341
ROCHMIS, P., AND H. BLACKBURN.
   Exercise tests. A survey of procedures, safety, and litigation experience in approximately 170,000 tests.
   Journal American Medical Association 217:1061-1066, 1971.

3342
RODBARD, S., AND M. FARBSTEIN.
   Improved exercise tolerance during venous congestion.
   Journal Applied Physiology 33:704, 1972.

3343
RODDA, B.E., M. CLINTON MILLER, III, AND J.G. BRUHN.
   Prediction of anxiety and depression patterns among coronary patients using a Markov process analysis.
   Behavioral Science 16(5):482-489, 1971.

3344
RODE, A., AND R.J. SHEPHARD.
   Cardiac output, blood volume, and total hemoglobin of the Canadian Eskimo.
   Journal Applied Physiology 34(1):91-96, 1973.

3345
RODRIGUEZ, M., ET AL.
   Dietary interviews in an epidemiological study of coronary artery disease in Puerto Rico.
   Boletin Asociacion Medica de Puerto Rico 61:202, 1969.

3346
ROELANDT, J., L. SCHAMROTH, AND P.G. HUGENHOLTZ.
   Effects of new beta-blocking agent (DL-tiprenolol) on conduction within normal and anomalous atrioventricular pathways in Wolff-Parkinson-White syndrome.
   British Heart Journal 34(12):1272-1282, 1972.

3347
ROGERS, W.R., AND W.D. HURST.
   Moderate exercise testing in ischemic heart disease.
   Northwest Medicine 63(10):702-706, 1964.

3348
ROGGE, J.D., J.F. MEYER, AND W. K. BROWN.
   Comparison of the incidence of cardiac arrhythmias during $+G_x$ acceleration, treadmill exercise
   and tilt table testing.
   Aerospace Medicine 40(1):1-5, 1969.

3349
ROHL, D., AND D. SUMMERS.
   Treatment of cardiogenic shock after myocardial infarction.
   Deutsche Medizinische Wochenschrift 98:1537, 1973.

3350
ROITMAN, D., W.B. JONES, AND L.T. SHEFFIELD.
   Comparison of submaximal exercise ECG test with coronary cineangiocardiogram.
   Annals Internal Medicine 72(5):641-647, 1970.

3351
ROKSETH, R., AND L. HATLE.
   Sinus arrest in acute myocardial infarction.
   British Heart Journal 33:639-642, 1971.

3352
ROLETT, E.L., W.P. HOOD, JR., C.E. RACKLEY, AND D.T. YOUNG.
   Ejection fraction, stroke volume, and exercise cardiac output in man.
   Clinical Research 15(3):31, 1967.

3353
ROMAN, L., AND S. BELLET.
   Significance of the QX/QT ratio and the QT ratio (QT_r) in the exercise electrocardiogram.
   Circulation 32:435, 1965.

3354
ROMAN, O., E. MOTLES, AND L. KOCH.
   The physical working capacity in healthy subjects and in cardio-respiratory patients.
   Revista Medica de Chile 93:646, 1965.

3355
ROMANOVA, D., AND P. BARIN.
   The influence of physical exercise on the content of serum protein, lipoprotein and total
   cholesterol in persons of middle and elderly age with symptoms of atherosclerosis.
   Kardiologia Polska 1:36, 1961.

3356
ROMERO, T., J. COVELL, AND W.F. FRIEDMAN.
   A comparison of pressure volume relations of the fetal, newborn, and adult heart.
   American Journal Physiology 222(5):1285-1290, 1972.

3357
ROMHILT, D.W., AND E.H. ESTES, JR.
A point-score system for the ECG diagnosis of left ventricular hypertrophy.
American Heart Journal 75:752-758, 1968.

3358
ROMO, M.
Factors related to sudden death in acute ischemic heart disease: Community study in Helsinki.
Acta Medica Scandinavica Suppl. 547:1, 1973.

3359
ROMSLO, I.
Distribution of serum lipids in Norwegian recruits.
Acta Medica Scandinavica 190(5):401-406, 1971.

3360
RONZITTI, M.
Evaluation of a new association cardiokinetic drug by means of the polygraphic survey.
Giornale di Gerontologia 21:339, 1973.

3361
ROSAI, J., AND E.F. LASCANO.
On the chemical nature of basophilic (mucoid) degeneration of myocardium.
American Heart Journal 84(3):419-420, 1972.

3362
ROSE, G.
A study of blood pressure among negro school children.
Journal Chronic Diseases 15:373-380, 1962.

3363
ROSE, G.
Physical activity and coronary heart disease.
Proceedings Royal Society Medicine 62:1183, 1969.

3364
ROSE, G.
Current developements in Europe, changing incidence of disease.
In: Jones, R.J., Ed. "Atherosclerosis: Proceedings, second international symposium," pp. 310-314.
New York, Springer, 1970.

3365
ROSE, G.
Predicting coronary heart disease from minor symptoms and electrocardiographic findings.
British Journal Preventive Social Medicine 25:94, 1971.

3366
ROSE, G.
Screening for early heart disease.
Preventive Techniques for the Modern Community. The Chest and Heart Association. London, England, 1971.

3367
ROSE, G., R.J. PRINEAS, AND J.R.A. MITCHELL.
   Myocardial infarction and the intrinsic calibre of coronary arteries.
   British Heart Journal 29:548, 1967.

3368
ROSE, G.A., AND H. BLACKBURN.
   Cardiovascular survey methods.
   Geneva, Switzerland. World Health Organization, Monograph Series, No. 56, p. 29, 1968.

3369
ROSE, K.D., F. STONE, S.I. FUENNING, AND J. WILLIAMS.
   Cardiac contusion resulting from "spearing" in football.
   Archives Internal Medicine 118:129-131, 1966.

3370
ROSE, L.I., H.S. FRIEDMAN, S.C. BEERING, AND K.H. COOPER.
   Plasma cortisol changes following a mile run in conditioned subjects.
   Journal Clinical Endocrinology 31:339-341, 1970.

3371
ROSEN, A.J., AND R.G. DePALMA.
   Risk factors in peripheral atherosclerosis.
   Archives Surgery 107:303-308, 1973.

3372
ROSEN, K.M., A. BARWOLF, A. EHSANI, AND S.H. RAHIMTOOLA.
   Effects of lidocaine and propranolol on the normal and anomalous pathways in patients with preexcitation.
   American Journal Cardiology 30(8):801-809, 1972.

3373
ROSEN, K.M., A. EHSANI, AND S.H. RAHIMTOOLA.
   H-V intervals in left bundle branch block. Clinical and electrocardiographic correlations.
   Circulation 46(4):717-723, 1972.

3374
ROSEN, M.R., H. GELBAND, C. MERKER, AND B.F. HOFFMAN.
   Mechanisms of digitalis toxicity. Effects of ouabain on phase four of canine Purkinje fiber transmembrane potentials.
   Circulation 47:681-689, 1973.

3375
ROSEN, M.R., AND B.F. HOFFMAN.
   Mechanisms of action of antiarrhythmic drugs.
   Circulation Research 32(1):1-8, 1973.

3376
ROSENBAUM, F.F., AND E.L. BELKNAP, EDS.
   Work and the heart.
   New York, Hoeber, 1959.

3377
ROSENBLUM, R., A.R. TAI, AND D. LAWSON.
Dopamine in man: Cardiorenal hemodynamics in normotensive patients with heart disease.
Journal Pharmacology Experimental Therapeutics 183(2):256-263, 1972.

3378
ROSENBLUM, W.I.
Report on symposium on atherosclerosis.
Stroke 3:683-685, 1972.

3379
ROSENKRANZ, K.A.
The treatment of sympatheticotonic dysregulations with pindolol.
Münchener Medizinische Wochenschrift 114:1154, 1972.

3380
ROSENMAN, R.H.
The role of personality and behavior patterns in the genesis of coronary heart disease.
Journal American Medical Women's Association 20:161-167, 1965.

3381
ROSENMAN, R.H.
Emotional patterns in the development of cardiovascular disease.
Journal American College Health Association 15:211-214, 1967.

3382
ROSENMAN, R.H.
Emotional factors in coronary heart disease.
Postgraduate Medicine 42:165-171, 1967.

3383
ROSENMAN, R.H.
Prospective epidemiological recognition of the candidate for ischemic heart disease.
Psychotherapy Psychosomatics 16:193-201, 1968.

3384
ROSENMAN, R.H.
The influence of different exercise patterns on the incidence of coronary heart disease in the Western Collaborative Group Study.
In: Brunner, D., And E. Jokl, Eds. Physical activity and aging, p. 272. Baltimore, University Park Press, 1970.

3385
ROSENMAN, R.H., AND M. FRIEDMAN.
Association of specific behavior pattern in women with blood and cardiovascular findings.
Circulation 24:1173-1184, 1961.

3386
ROSENMAN, R.H., AND M. FRIEDMAN.
Behavior patterns, blood lipids, and coronary heart disease.
Journal American Medical Association 184:934-938, 1963.

3387
ROSENMAN, R.H., M. FRIEDMAN, AND S.O. BYERS.
   Glucose metabolism in subjects with behavior pattern A and hyperlipemia.
   Circulation 33:704-707, 1966.

3388
ROSENMAN, R.H., M. FRIEDMAN, AND A. CARROLL.
   Study of the possible effect of gainful employment on serum cholesterol, and incidence of
   hypertension, arcus senilis, and clinical coronary heart disease in urban American females.
   Circulation 24(4 Part 2):1101-1102, 1961.

3389
ROSENMAN, R.H., M. FRIEDMAN, D. JENKINS, R. STRAUS, ET AL.
   The prediction of immunity to coronary heart disease.
   Journal American Medical Association 198:1159, 1956.

3390
ROSENMAN, R.H., M. FRIEDMAN, C.D. JENKINS, R. STRAUS, ET AL.
   The relationship of behavior Pattern A to the state of the coronary vasculature.
   American Journal Medicine 44:525, 1968.

3391
ROSENMAN, R.H., M. FRIEDMAN, R. STRAUS, M. WURM, ET AL.
   A predictive study of coronary heart disease: The Western Collaborative Group Study.
   Journal American Medical Association 189:15, 1964.

3392
ROSENMAN, R.H., M. FRIEDMAN, R. STRAUS, C.D. JENKINS, ET AL.
   Coronary heart disease in the Western Collaborative Group Study. A follow-up experience of 4½
   years.
   Journal Chronic Diseases 23(3):173-190, 1970.

3393
ROSENSTIEL, H.C.
   Recording Master's two-step test electrocardiograms.
   Journal American Medical Association 203(11):990, 1968.

3394
ROSENTRETER, E.
   Results of investigations into the problem of early invalidism and its rehabilitation.
   Zeitschrift für die Gesamte Hygiene 18(1):32-42, 1972.

3395
ROSING, D.R., P. BRAKMAN, D.R. REDWOOD, R.E. GOLDSTEIN, C.D. BEISER, T. ASTRUP, AND
   S.E. EPSTEIN.
   Blood fibrinolytic activity in man. Diurnal variation and the response to varying intensities of
   exercise.
   Circulation Research 27:171, 1970.

3396
ROSKAMM, H.
   Optimum patterns of exercise for healty adults.
   Canadian Medical Association Journal 96:895-898, 1967.

3397
ROSKAMM, H.
  Comparison between ECG during exercise and ECG during hypoxia in patients with angina pectoris.
  Malattie Cardiovascolari 10(1-2):73-77, 1969.

3398
ROSKAMM, H.
  General circulatory adjustment to exercise in well-trained subjects.
  In: Larsen, O.A., and R.O. Malmborg, Eds. Coronary heart disease and physical fitness, pp. 17-20. Baltimore, University Park Press, 1971.

3399
ROSKAMM, H., F. LANDRY, L. SAMEK, N. SCHLAGER, ET AL.
  Effects of a standardized ergometer training program at three different altitudes.
  Journal Applied Physiology 27:840-847, 1969.

3400
ROSKAMM, H., AND H. REINDELL.
  Physical training for the normal and diseased heart.
  Medizinische Monatsschrift 19:2-10, 1965.

3401
ROSKAMM, H., AND H. REINDELL.
  Optimum patterns of exercise for healthy adults.
  In: Brunner, D. and E. Jokl, Eds. Physical activity and aging. Baltimore, University Park Press, 1970.

3402
ROSKAMM, H., H. REINDELL, J. EMMRICH, J. BARMEYER, ET AL.
  Relation of electrocardiogram during graded exercise to heart size and physical ability of normal persons and infarct patients.
  Deutsche Archiv für Klinische Medizin 209(4):331-359, 1964.

3403
ROSKAMM, H., G. SCHULTZE-WERNINGHAUS, F. LANDRY, L. SAMEK, ET AL.
  Oxygen uptake capacity during four weeks of physcial training.
  Internationale Zeitschrift für Angewandte Physiologie 28:197-208, 1970.

3404
ROSKAMM, H., J. SKINNER, A. LESCH, ET AL.
  The contractility reserve of the healthy left ventricle during physical stress after blocking of beta-receptors.
  Zeitschrift für Krieslaufforschung 61(9):802-811, 1972.

3405
ROSKAMM, H., H. WEIDEMANN, B. MEINECKE, J. PETERSEN, AND H. REINDELL.
  Diagnosis of beginning cardiac insufficiency by means of a floating catheter system. Studies on 15 patients with myocardial infarction 3 to 6 weeks after infarction and 10 patients after more than 4 months after the acute stage.
  Zeitschrift für Kreislaufforschung 59(2):119-138, 1970.

3406
ROSKAMM, H., H. WEIDEMANN, K. SCHNELLBACHER, D. SUPLIE, ET AL.
The effect of propranolol and nitroglycerin on the electrocardiogram and intra-pulmonary pressure during physical exercise of patients with angina pectoris.
Deutsche Medizinische Wochenschrift 95(52):2593-2599, 1970.

3407
ROSNER, S.W., R.C. LEINBACH, A.J. PRESTO, L.K. JACKSON, ET AL.
Computer analysis of the exercise electrocardiogram.
American Journal Cardiology 20:356-362, 1967.

3408
ROSS, J., JR., AND E. BRAUNWALD.
The study of left ventricular function in man by increasing resistance to ventricular ejection with angiotensin.
Circulation 29:739, 1964.

3409
ROSS, J., JR., J.H. GAULT, D.T. MASON, J.W. LINHART, AND E. BRAUNWALD.
Left ventricular performance during muscular exercise in patients with and without cardiac dysfunction.
Circulation 34(4):597-608, 1966.

3410
ROSS, R.S., AND G.C. FRIESINGER.
Coronary arteriography.
In: Symposium on coronary artery disease. American Heart Association Monograph 2, second edition, pp.59-66. New York, American Heart Association, 1968.

3411
ROSSI, F., L. DEAMBROGGI, AND C. GALBIATI.
Use of orthogonal leads in electrocardiographic exercise test.
Giornale Italiano di Cardiologia 2(5):693-701, 1972.

3412
ROSSI, L.
Histopathologic features of cardiac arrhythmias.
Milan, Italy. Casa Editrice Ambrosiana, 1969.

3413
ROSSI, L.
Histopathology of the conducting system.
Gazzetta Italiana di Cardiologia 2(4):484-491, 1972.

3414
ROSSI, P.
Selective angiography in the endoperitoneal organs.
Radiologica Medica 58(7):578-587, 1972.

3415
ROSTAFINSKA, J., L. KLIMIUK, Z. KARCZEWSKA, ET AL.
The application of apex cardiography for examination of the work of the left ventricle in patients with hyperthyroidism.
Polski Tygodnik Lekarski 28(4):123-125, 1973.

3416
ROSTON, S.
   The energy output of the left ventricle and the mechanism of congestive heart failure.
   Bulletin Mathematical Biophysics 33(2):195-201, 1971.

3417
ROTH, O., A. BERKI, AND G.D. WOLFF.
   Long range observations in fifty-three young patients with myocardial infarction.
   American Journal Cardiology 19(3):331-338, 1967.

3418
ROTHAN, A.
   Occupational reclassification of cardiacs.
   Gazette Médicale de France 72:2937-3044, 1965.

3419
ROTHFELD, E.L., I.R. ZUCKER, AND V. PARSONNET.
   Postinfarction ventricular septal defect and the Eisenmenger syndrome.
   Chest 62(2):224-226, 1972.

3420
ROTMAN, M., G.S. WAGNER, AND R.A. WAUGH.
   Significance of high degree atrioventricular block in acute posterior myocardial infarction. The
   importance of clinical setting and mechanism of block.
   Circulation 47:257-262, 1973.

3421
ROUBELAK, G., AND G. MICHAELI.
   Hospital mortality at acute stage of myocardial infarction—statistical study of 600 cases.
   Annales de Cardiologie et d'Angéiologie 22(4):303-309, 1973.

3422
ROUGIER, G., P. BLANCHOT, AND P. FONTANILLE.
   Cardiac volume of former sportsmen.
   Coeur et Médecine Interne 11(1):63-68, 1972.

3423
ROUSSEAU, M.F., L.A. BRASSEUR, AND J-M. R. DETRY.
   Hemodynamic determinants of maximal oxygen intake in patients with healed myocardial in-
   farction. Influence of physical training.
   Circulation 48(5):943-949, 1973.

3424
ROUSSEAU, M.F., L.A. BRASSEUR, AND J-M. R. DETRY.
   Hemodynamic and electrocardiographic effects of practolol during upright exercise in coronary
   heart disease.
   Cardiovascular Research 7:306-312, 1973.

3425
ROWE, G.G.
   Coronary vasodilator therapy for angina pectoris.
   American Heart Journal 68:691, 1964.

3426
ROWE, G.G., C.A. CASTILLO, S. AFONSO, AND C.W. CRUMPTON.
   Coronary flow measured by the nitrous-oxide method.
   American Heart Journal 67:457, 1964.

3427
ROWE, G.G., C.A. CASTILLO, G.M. MAXWELL, ET AL.
   A hemodynamic study of hypertension including observations on coronary blood flow.
   Annals Internal Medicine 54:405-412, 1961.

3428
ROWELL, L.B.
   The liver as an energy source in man during exercise.
   In: Pernow, B. and B. Saltin, Eds. Muscle metabolism during exercise, pp. 127-141. New York,
   Plenum Press, 1971.

3429
ROWELL, L.B.
   Distribution of cardiac output during exercise and the effect of training.
   In: Larsen, O., and R.O. Malmborg, Eds. Coronary heart disease and physical fitness, pp. 57-61.
   Baltimore, University Park Press, 1971.

3430
ROWELL, L.B., ET AL.
   Reductions in cardiac output, central blood volume, and stroke volume with thermal stress in
   normal men during exercise.
   Journal Clinical Investigation 45:1801-1816, 1966.

3431
ROWELL, L.B., H.L. TAYLOR, E. SIMONSON, AND W.S. CARLSON.
   The physiological fallacy of adjusting for body weight in performance of the Master two-step test.
   American Heart Journal 70:461, 1965.

3432
ROYSTON, G.R.
   Long-term anticoagulant treatment in coronary disease.
   Angiology 18(3):133-149, 1967.

3433
ROYSTON, G.R.
   Short stay hospital treatment and rapid rehabilitation of cases of myocardial infarction in a
   district hospital.
   British Heart Journal 34:526-532, 1972.

3434
ROZENBLIT, Y.A., A.A. KRAMER, AND R.A. GRIGORYANTS.
   The central hemodynamics in patients with coronary atherosclerosis in physical effort.
   Kardiologiya 11(1):77-82, 1971.

3435
ROZHNOVA, Z.I.
   The pressor action of blood in the treatment of essential hypertension with diet and sleep.
   Byulletin Eksperimental 'noi Biologii i Meditsiny 57(1):28-30, 1964.

3436
ROZSAHEGYI, I.
   Occupational rehabilitation of heart and circulatory diseases in rural areas.
   Zeitschrift für die Gesamte Hygiene und Ihre Grenzgebiete 15(10):786-787, 1969.

3437
RUBANOVSKII, B.R.
   Use of hydrochlorothiazide therapy on patients with hypertension and the possibility of its
   long-term use.
   Sovetskaya Meditsina 28(9):26-30, 1964.

3438
RUBENSTEIN, C., R. YATTEAU, AND A. WALSTON.
   Significance of exercise S-T elevation.
   Circulation 44(Suppl. II):219, 1971.

3439
RUBIN, M.I.
   Systemic hypertension.
   Pediatric Clinics North America 11:431-463, 1964.

3440
RUBINS, S., J. LOZANO, H. CARRASCO, T-W. LANG, AND E. CORDAY.
   Tachyarrhythmias. Differential diagnosis and therapy after acute myocardial infarction.
   Geriatrics 27:123-133, 1972.

3441
RUBIO, G.A., AND C.R.M. BACA.
   The sociological aspects of heart disease.
   Revista del Colegio Medico de Guatemala 12(3):137-145, 1961.

3442
RUDD, J.L., AND W.C. DAY.
   A physical fitness program for patients with hypertension.
   Journal American Geriatrics Society 15:373-379, 1967.

3443
RUDNICKI, S., Z. KRASZEWSKA, K. SLIDZIEWSKI, R. J. ZOCHOWSKI, AND J. BARYLAK.
   Value of radioelectrocardiographic examination in following the rehabilitation of patients with
   recent myocardial infarction.
   Polskii Archivum Medycyny Wewnetrznej 41(6):7811-815, 1968.

3444
RUDNICKI, S., K. SLIDZIEWSKI, K. TYMINSKA, ET AL.
   Rehabilitation in hospital of patients with recent myocardial infarction.
   Polski Tygodnik Lekarski 27(34):1313-1315, 1972.

3445
RUDNICKI, S., E. WELC, J. KOSINSKI, AND D. STRZELECKA.
   Evaluation of the effectiveness of the method of physical rehabilitation in the sanatorium of
   patients with recent myocardial infarction.
   Polski Tygodnik Lekarski 27(33):1265-1268, 1972.

3446
RUDOLPH, W.
   Myocardial metabolism in cyanotic congenital heart disease.
   Cardiologia 56(1-2):209, 1972.

3447
RUDUSKY, B.M.
   The fifth dimension of electrocardiography.
   Vascular Disease 4(1):36-41, 1967.

3448
RUIZ, L., M. FIGUEROA, C. HORNA, AND D. PENALOZA.
   Prevalence of arterial hypertension and ischemic heart disease at high altitudes.
   Archivos del Instituto de Cardiologia de Mexico 39(4):476-489, 1969.

3449
RULLI, V.
   Rehabilitation of the coronary patient. II. The psychological aspects.
   Giornale Italiano di Cardiologia 1:371-375, 1971.

3450
RULLI, V.
   Rehabilitation of the patient with coronary disease. III. Socioeconomic aspects.
   Giornale Italiano di Cardiologia 1:591-593, 1971.

3451
RULLI, V., A. NARDELLI, AND P. SIGNORETTI.
   The factors limiting functional capacity after myocardial infarction.
   Gazzetta Italiana de Cardiologia 2(6A):802-806, 1972.

3452
RULLI, V., A. NARDELLI, P. SIGNORETTI, AND A. MENOTTI.
   Preliminary studies of short-term rehabilitation of subjects with myocardial infarct.
   Gazzetta Italiana di Cardiologia 2:676-687, 1972.

3453
RULLI, V., AND A. VENERANDO.
   Rehabilitation of the cardiopathic patient. I.
   Cardiologia Pratica 19:1-16, 1968.

3454
RUMBALL, A., AND E.D. ACHESON.
   Latent coronary heart disease detected by electrocardiogram before and after exercise.
   British Medical Journal 1:423, 1963.

3455
RUMBAUGH, D.M.
   The cardiac adjustment scale.
   San Diego, California. Educational and Industrial Testing Service, 1964.

3456
RUMBAUGH, D.M.
   The psychological aspects.
   Journal Rehabilitation 32:56-58, 1966.

3457
RUNYAN, J.W., JR., W.E. PHILLIPS, O. HERRING, AND L. CAMPBELL.
A program for the care of patients with chronic diseases.
Journal American Medical Association 211(3):476-479, 1970.

3458
RUSH, R.A., AND L.B. GEFFEN.
Radioimmunoassay and clearance of circulating dopamine β-hydroxylase.
Circulation Research 31(3):444-452, 1972.

3459
RUSHMER, R.F.
Structure and function of the cardiovascular system.
Philadelphia, Saunders, 1972.

3460
RUSHMER, R.F. , ET AL.
Mechanisms of cardiac control in exercise.
Circulation Research 7:602, 1959.

3461
RUSK, H.A.
Co-ordination of treatment and aftercare.
In: The disabled in the modern world. Proceedings of the Fifth World Congress International
Society, Welfare Cripples. Stockholm, September 1951.

3462
RUSK, H.A.
The philosphy and need of rehabilitation. Readings in Unemployment. Special Committee on
Unemployment Problems, U.S. Senate, 86th Congress, 1st Session.
U.S. Government Printing Office, Washington, D.C., 1960.

3463
RUSKIN, H.D., L.L. STEIN, I.M. SHELSKY, AND M.L. BAILEY.
MMPI: Comparison between patients with coronary disease and their spouses together with other
demographic data: A preliminary report.
Scandinavian Journal Rehabilitation Medicine 2(2/3):99-104, 1970.

3464
RUSSEK, H.I.
Emotional stress and coronary heart disease in American physicians.
American Journal Medical Sciences 240:711, 1960.

3465
RUSSEK, H.I.
Evaluation of drug therapy in angina pectoris employing the Master two-step test: Vasodilators,
amine and oxidase inhibitors, and hypocholesteremic agents.
Circulation 24(4 Part 2):1028, 1961.

3466
RUSSEK, H.I.
Emotional stress and coronary heart disease in American physicians, dentists, and lawyers.
American Journal Medical Sciences 243:716, 1962.

3467
RUSSEK, H.I.
Tobacco consumption and emotional stress in the etiology of coronary heart disease.
Geriatrics 19:425-433, 1964.

3468
RUSSEK, H.I.
Control of obesity in the cardiac patient.
American Journal Medical Sciences 249:305-308, 1965.

3469
RUSSEK, H.I.
Stress, tobacco and coronary disease in North American professional groups: survey of 12,000 men in 14 occupational groups.
Journal American Medical Association 192: 189-194, 1965.

3470
RUSSEK, H.I.
Combined vasodilator and tranquilizer therapy in angina pectoris: A comparative study with statistical analysis.
American Journal Medical Sciences 249:420-424, 1965.

3471
RUSSEK, H.I.
Emotional stress in the etiology of coronary heart disease.
Geriatrics 22:84-89, 1967.

3472
RUSSEK, H.I.
Propranolol and isosorbide dinitrate in the long-term therapy of angina pectoris.
Diseases Chest 56(3):267, 1969.

3473
RUSSEK, H.I.
Prognosis in severe angina pectoris: Medical versus surgical therapy.
American Heart Journal 83(6):762-768, 1972.

3474
RUSSEK, H.I., AND B.L. ZOHMAN.
Relative significance of heredity, diet, and occupational stress in coronary heart disease of young adults.
American Journal Medical Sciences 235:266, 1958.

3475
RUSSELL, A.S.
Antecedents of myocardial infarction.
Canadian Medical Association Journal 109(7):571, 1973.

3476
RUSSELL, R.O., D. HUNT, C. POTANIN, AND C.E. RACKLEY.
Hemodynamic monitoring in a coronary intensive care unit: Clinical application.
Archives Internal Medicine 130:370-376, 1972.

3477
RUSSELL, R.O., JR., D. HUNT, AND C.E. RACKLEY.
Left ventricular hemodynamics in anterior and inferior myocardial infarction.
American Journal Cardiology 32:8, 1973.

3478
RUSSELL, R.O., JR., AND C.E. RACKLEY.
You've got a lot of remedies for this complication but for every rhythm there's a particular combination.
Emergency Medicine 5:27, 1973.

3479
RUSSELL, R.O., JR., AND C.E. RACKLEY.
Cardiac arrhythmias in acute MI.
Emergency Medicine 5(7):27, 1973.

3480
RUSSELL, W.R.
Yoga and vertebral arteries.
British Medical Journal 4:685, 1972.

3481
RUTENBERG, H.L., AND J.F. SPANN, JR.
Alterations of cardiac sympathetic neurotransmitter activity in congestive heart failure.
Journal Cardiology 32:472, 1973.

3482
RUTISHAUSER, W.
Exercise tests in disorders of coronary circulation.
Deutsche Medizinische Wochenschrift 95(52):2617-2618, 1970.

3483
RUTISHAUSER, W.
Hemodynamics and coronary circulation in coronary heart disease.
Zeitschrift für Kreislaufforschung 60(7):663-664, 1971.

3484
RUTISHAUSER, W., H. HIRZEL, I. AMENDE, ET AL.
Myocardial function and coronary flow in coronary sclerosis.
Schweizerische Medizinische Wochenschrift 102(47):1709-1716, 1972.

3485
RUTISHAUSER, W., G. NOSEDA, P. WIRZ, AND M. GANDER.
Left ventricular performance at rest, during exercise and electrical pacing in conscious man before and after beta-blockade.
Zeitschrift für Kreislaufforschung 59(11):1037-1050, 1970.

3486
RYABOVA, V.V.
Trace elements in the myocardium during experimentally induced severe myocardial ischemia.
Trudy Voronezhskogo Meditsinskogo Instituta 58:94-97, 1967.

3487
RYAN, C.S. W.W. STEWART, AND J.J. KELLY.
  Detection of latent coronary artery disease by exercise tests.
  Industrial Medicine Surgery 37:929-937, 1968.

3488
RYDEN, L., A. WALDENSTROM, L. EHN, S. HOLMBERG, AND M. HUSAINI.
  Comparison between effectiveness of intramuscular and intravenous lignocaine on ventricular
  arrhythmia complicating acute myocardial infarction.
  British Heart Journal 35:1124, 1973.

3489
RYDEN, L., H. WASIR, T.B. CONRADSSON, AND B. OLSSON.
  Blood levels of lignocaine after intramuscular administration to patients with proven or suspected
  acute myocardial infarction.
  British Heart Journal 34(10):1012-1017, 1972.

3490
RYMASZEWSKI, Z., W. POPLAWSKA, J. PREIBISZ, AND W. JANUSZEWICZ.
  Clinical evaluation of practolol in acute arrhythmias.
  British Heart Journal 34:260-262, 1972.

3491
RYNEARSON, R.R.
  Psychological aspects of cardiovascular disease in the aged.
  Postgraduate Medicine 46:177-178, 1969.

3492
RYUMINA, E.N., AND K. AMANNEPESOV.
  Radiocardiography in the study of the remote results of surgical treatment of interatrial septal
  defects.
  Kardiologiya 10:89-93, 1970.

3493
SAAD, E.A., F.J. BARBOSA, P. GINEFRA, ET AL.
  Familial cardiomyopathy.
  Journal Brasileiro de Doencas Toracicas 1:147-160, 1965.

3494
SACHERO, A.
  The contribution of cardiological instrumental methods in the early diagnosis of coronary insuf-
  ficiency, with particular regard to effort electrocardiogram and to vectorcardiography.
  Rivista Istituto Vaccinogeno Consorzi Provincia Antituberculosi, Milano 19(3):421-454, 1969.

3495
SADOKOVA, Z.M.
  Cardiac rupture in myocardial infarction.
  Terapevticheskii Arkhiv 43(8):70-72, 1971.

3496
SADOUGHI, W., ET AL.
  Sexual adjustment of the chronically ill and physically disabled population: A pilot study.
  Archives Physical Medicine Rehabilitation 52:311-317, 1971.

3497
SADOYAN, V.S., G.A. MINASYAN, AND D.L. ASTVATS-ATRYAN.
The effect of exercise on the function of the cardiovascular system of patients with myocardial infarct.
Zhurnal Eksperimental'noi i Teoreticheskoi Fizikii 5(1):78-82, 1965.

3498
SAFAR, M., Y. WEISS, A. SOBEL, G. LAGRUE, AND P. MILLIEZ.
Anti-hypertensive effects of a beta-blocker: pindolol.
Nouvelle Presse Médicale 2:2685, 1973.

3499
SAIMYOJI, H., Y. YAMANE, S. KUBO, N. SAITO, ET AL.
Clinical studies on the "water-electrolyte regulation mechanism" in chronic congestive heart failure.
In: Proceedings of the 3rd Asian-Pacific Congress of Cardiology in association with the 28th annual meeting of the Japanese Circulation Society, Kyoto, 10-14 May 1964, pp. 1386-1391. Kyoto, Kawakita Printing Co., 1964.

3500
SAINANI, G.S., AND A.K. MUKHERJEE.
A double blind drug trial of LB 46 (Visken) in angina pectoris.
Indian Heart Journal 24(Suppl. 1):192-196, 1972.

3501
SAINT PIERRE, A., AND A. PERRIN.
Spontaneous, delayed and paradoxical conversions of permanent atrial fibrillations.
Archives des Maladies du Coeur et des Vaisseaux 66(1):71-83, 1973.

3502
SAITTA, G., I. DI BLASI, F. GALLI, ET AL.
The L/R ratio precordial leads from footballers.
Medicina dello Sport 25:81, 1972.

3503
SAKSENA, F.B., AND H.E. ALDRIDGE.
Atrial septal defect in the older patient. A clinical and hemodynamic study in patients operated on after age 35.
Circulation 42:1009-1020, 1970.

3504
SALAZAR, E., A. GARCIA ALFAGEME, AND R. DAVILA.
Interatrial communication. Analysis of 462 cases studied in the National Institute of Cardiology.
Archivos del Instituto de Cardiologia de Mexico 42(1):4-32, 1972.

3505
SALEL, A.F., E.A. AMSTERDAM, D.T. MASON, AND R. ZELIS.
The importance of type IV hyperlipoproteinemia as a major predisposing metabolic factor in coronary artery disease.
Circulation 44(Suppl. II):II-47, 1971.

3506
SALERNI, R., AND D.F. LEON.
  Current status of cardiac pacing.
  Disease-a-Month 10:1, 1972.

3507
SALES, S.M., AND J. HOUSE.
  Job dissatisfaction as a possible risk factor in coronary heart disease.
  Journal Chronic Diseases 23(12):861-873, 1971.

3508
SALGADO, J.A., C. VELOSO, J. GALIZZI, JR., ET AL.
  Electrocardiographic studies in patients with schistosomiasis mansoni treated with hycanthone.
  Revista da Sociedade Brasileira de Medicina Tropical 6(3):129-133, 1972.

3509
SALTIN, B.
  Physiological effects of physical conditioning.
  Medicine Science Sports 1:50-56, 1969.

3510
SALTIN, B.
  Central circulation after physical conditioning in young and middle-aged men.
  In: Larsen, O.A. and R.O. Malmborg, Eds. Coronary heart disease and physical fitness, pp. 21-26.
  Baltimore, University Park Press, 1971.

3511
SALTIN, B., G. BLOMQVIST, J.H. MITCHELL, R.L. JOHNSON, ET AL.
  Response to exercise after bed rest and after training.
  Circulation 38 (Suppl.7):1-78, 1968.

3512
SALTIN, B., L.H. HARTLEY, A. KILBOM, AND I. ÅSTRAND.
  Physical training in sedentary middle-aged and older men. II. Oxygen uptake, heart rate, and
  blood lactate concentration at submaximal and maximal exercise.
  Scandinavian Journal Clinical Laboratory Investigation 24:323-334, 1969.

3513
SALTUPS, B., B.D. McCALLISTER, F.J. HALLERMANN, R.B. WALLACE, ET AL.
  Left ventricular hemodynamics in patients with coronary artery disease and in normal subjects:
  Correlations with the extent of coronary artery lesions and the electrocardiogram.
  American Journal Medicine 50(1):8-19, 1971.

3514
SALUSTE, E., M.M. GERTLER, H.E. LEETMA, AND J.L. ROSENBERGER.
  Uric acid as a homeostatic factor in glucose-insulin-free fatty acid (FFA) metabolism in ischemic
  heart (IHD) and thrombotic cerebrovascular disease (ITCVD).
  Circulation 41 (Suppl. 3):22, 1970.

3515
SALVADOR, M., C. THOMAS, M. MAZENQ, J. CONTE, ET AL.
  Rhythm troubles directly caused or favored by potassium depletion.
  Archives des Maladies du Coeur et des Vaisseaux 63:230, 1970.

3516
SALVINI, M.
Rehabilitation of the heart patient to industrial work.
Minerva Medica 58:1659, 1967.

3517
SAMEK, L., H. ROSKAMM, H. WEIDEMANN, T. MEIER-LIEHL, ET AL.
The effect of four weeks training in the low pressure chamber (2250 and 3450 m) on the erythrocytes during rest and during maximal ergometer stress.
Blut 20:156-164, 1970.

3518
SAMET, P.
Hemodynamic sequelae of cardiac arrhythmias.
Circulation 47:399-407, 1973.

3519
SAMET, P., AND W.H. BERNSTEIN.
Hemodynamic alterations due to A-V block.
In: Dreifus, L.S., W. Likoff and J.H. Moyer, Eds. Mechanisms and therapy of cardiac arrhythmias New York, Grune and Stratton, pp. 498-509, 1966.

3520
SAMSONOVA, M.A., AND B.Z. AKKERMAN.
Psychophysiological phase of therapeutic exercise in the acute period of myocardial infarction.
Kazanskii Meditsinkii Zhurnal, 6:23-24, 1972.

3521
SAMUEL, P., AND J. GOLDSTEIN.
Long-term reduction of serum cholesterol levels of patients with atherosclerosis by small doses of Neomycin.
Circulation 35(5):938-945, 1967.

3522
SAMUELS, B.M.
Exercise program after myocardial infarction.
British Medical Journal, 4:493, 1973.

3523
SANDBERG, L.
Electrocardiographic studies of cases where bundle-branch block develops during exercise tests.
Acta Medica Scandinavica 169 (Suppl.):78-87, 1961.

3524
SANDERS, C.A.
The coronary care unit: necessity or luxury?
New England Journal Medicine 288(2):101-102, 1973.

3525
SANDLER, G.
Nitrites and nitrates in ischemic heart disease.
British Medical Journal 1:108, 1967.

3526
SANDLER, G.
Comparison of radiocardiography and conventional electrocardiography in the exercise tolerance test.
British Heart Journal 29(5):719-724, 1967.

3527
SANDLER, G., AND A. PISTEVOS.
Clinical evaluation of oxprenolol in angina pectoris.
British Heart Journal 34(8):847-850, 1972.

3528
SANDLER, G., AND A. PISTEVOS.
Mobile coronary care. The coronary ambulance.
British Heart Journal 34(12):1283-1291, 1972.

3529
SANDOE, E., AND K. OLESEN.
Hypokalaemia, hypochloraemia, and baseosis in long-term treatment of oedematous heart failure with benzothiadiazine diuretics. I. Incidence and pathophysiology.
Acta Medica Scandinavica 172(6):691-697, 1962.

3530
SANDOE, E., E. FLENSTED-JENSEN, AND B. DUPONT.
Long-term prognosis in patients resuscitated from cardiac arrest.
Israel Journal Medical Sciences 5(4):769-771, 1969.

3531
SANGHVI, V.R., F. KHAJA, A.L. MARK, AND J.O. PARKER.
Effects of blood volume expansion on left ventricular hemodynamics in man.
Circulation 46(4):780-787, 1972.

3532
SANGIORGI, M., AND D. CANNATA.
Interatrial partial block with double atriogram and phases of double atrial heterotopic rhythm with interference.
Gazzetta Italiana di Cardiologia 2(5):655-664, 1972.

3533
SANGIORGI, M., B. MOSCATELLO, A. MALARBI, F. SARDELLA, ET AL.
Pharmacodynamic study of the stenocardia of effort. II. Effect of sodium nitrite.
Bollettino della Società Italiana di Cardiologia 15(3):200-255, 1970.

3534
SANKALE, M., P. KOATE, N. PADONOU, AND O. BAO.
On 600 cases of complete cardiac insufficiency in Black Africans in a hospital in Dakar.
Bulletin de la Société Médicale d'Afrique Noire de Langue Française 18(Suppl.):111-113, 1971.

3535
SANNE, H., D. ELMFELDT, G. GRIMBY, C. RYDIN, AND L. WILHELMS.
Exercise tolerance and physical training of non-selected patients after myocardial infarction.
Acta Medica Scandinavica Suppl. 551-:1, 1973.

3536
SANNE, H., D. ELMFELDT, AND L. WILHELMSEN.
Preventive effect of physical training after a myocardial infarction.
In: Tibblin, G., Ed. Preventive cardiology, pp. 154-160. New York, Wiley, 1972.

3537
SANNE, H., G. GRIMBY, AND L. WILHELMSEN.
Physical training during convalescence after myocardial infarction.
In: Larsen, O.A. and R. O. Malmborg, Eds. Coronary heart diseases and physical fitness, pp. 183-188. Baltimore, University Park Press, 1971.

3538
SANNE, H.M., AND L. WILHEMSEN.
Physical activity as prevention and therapy in coronary heart disease.
Scandinavian Journal Rehabilitation Medicine 3(1/2):47-56, 1971.

3539
SANNERSTEDT, R.
Hemodynamic response to exercise in patients with arterial hypertension.
Acta Medica Scandinavica 180(Suppl. 458):7-83, 1966.

3540
SANNERSTEDT, R.
Hemodynamic effects of pargyline hydrochloride at rest and during exercise in hypertension.
Acta Medica Scandinavica 181(6):699-706, 1967.

3541
SANNERSTEDT, R.
Hemodynamic findings at rest and during exercise in mild arterial hypertension.
American Journal Medical Sciences 258(2):70-79, 1969.

3542
SANNERSTEDT, R., J. BJURE, AND E. VARNAUSKAS.
Correlation between electrocardiographic changes and systemic hemodynamics in human arterial hypertension.
American Journal Cardiology 26(2): 117-122, 1970.

3543
SANNERSTEDT, R., S. PAULIN, AND E. VARNAUSKAS.
Correlation between radiological chest findings and systemic haemodynamics in human arterial hypertension.
British Heart Journal 32(4):477-482, 1970.

3544
SANTORO, G., D. BERNARDI, AND C. GIUSTI.
Instrumental classification of patients with previous myocardial infarction in the phase of so-called electrocardiographic recovery.
Bollettino della Società Italiana di Cardiologia 17(8):539-543, 1972.

3545
SAPIRA, J.D., E.T. SCHEIB, R. MORIARTY, AND A.P. SHAPIRO.
Differences in perception between hypertensive and normotensive populations.
Psychosomatic Medicine 33(3):239-250, 1971.

3546
SARACHEK, N.S., J. ROBERTS, AND J.J. LEONARD.
A new method to measure nonuniformity in the intact heart.
Journal Electrocardiology 5(4):341-438, 1972.

3547
SARDELLA, F., G. RECINE, R. CALABRÒ, ET AL.
Changes in the electrocardiogram, general arterial pressure, heart rate and respiratory rate in coronary disease patients during muscular exertion.
Bollettino della Società Italiana de Cardiologica 12:226-239, 1967.

3548
SASAMOTO, H., K. HOSONO, Y. KASUGA, Y. NAKAMURA, ET AL.
Studies of electrocardiogram during exercise.
Japanese Circulation Journal 28(11):833-839, 1964.

3549
SASLAW, M.S.
Coronary care units: one hundred day evaluation.
Angiology 23(6):372-376, 1972.

3550
SASLOW, G., AND P.H. BLACHLY.
Timberline conference on psychophysiologic aspects of cardiovascular disease.
Psychosomatic Medicine 26(4):490-411, 1964.

3551
SASSA, H., K. MINAKUCH, A. FUTENMA, T. ITO, ET AL.
Fibrinolysis in patients with ischemic heart disease in relation to etiologic factor of myocardial infarction.
Japanese Circulation Journal 37(8):909, 1973.

3552
SAVAGNONE, E., AND E. MURATORE.
Neurological and psychiatric complications in cardiovascular pathology.
Acta Neurologica 25(1):83-115, 1970.

3553
SÄWE, U.
Early diagnosis of acute myocardial infarction with special reference to the diagnosis of the Intermediate Coronary Syndrome. A clinical study.
Acta Medica Scandinavica 193(Suppl. 545):1, 1973.

3554
SCHACHENMAYR, W., AND O. HAFERKAMP.
Hemorrhagic myocardial infarction.
Deutsche Medizinische Wochenschrift 97(32):1172-1174, 1972.

3555
SCHACKE, G., C.D. BLOEDNER, H. VALENTIN, AND O. ELLNER.
Preventive long term investigations of ECG and heart rate performed by means of radiotelemetry, during sympatholysis.
Arzneimittel-Forschung 26(11):394-401, 1972.

3556
SCHALLER, K.
  Causes of the change in Falithrom requirement after myocardial infarction.
  Zeitschrift für Gesamte Innere Medizin 27(17):756-758, 1972.

3557
SCHAMROTH, L.
  The disorders of cardiac rhythm.
  Philadelphia, Pa. F.A. Davis, 1971.

3558
SCHAMROTH, L.
  Potassium and the electrocardiogram.
  South African Medical Journal 46(30):15-18, 1972.

3559
SCHAMROTH, L.
  How to approach an arrhythmia.
  Circulation 47(2):420-426, 1973.

3560
SCHAMROTH, L., AND G.B. LAPINSKY.
  The Wolff-Parkinson-White syndrome associated with myocardial infarction and right bundle
  branch block.
  Journal Electrocardiology 5(3):299-305, 1972.

3561
SCHANE, W.P.
  Continuous ECG recording of helicopter instructor pilots.
  Aerospace Medicine 43:560-536, 1972.

3562
SCHAPER, W., W. FLAMENG, A. JAGENEAU, AND L. SNOECKX.
  Physical exercise and collateral development.
  Zeitschrift für Kreislaufforschung 60(7):667, 1971.

3563
SCHAR, M.
  The significance for social medicine of rehabilitation.
  Bulletin der Schweizerischen Akademie der Medizinischen Wissenschaften 28(1/2):6-11, 1972.

3564
SCHAR, M.
  Risk factors in coronary disease.
  Schweizerische Medizinische Wochenschrift 102(47):1702-1704, 1972.

3565
SCHAR, M., L.G. REEDER, AND J.M. DIRKEN.
  Stress and cardiovascular health: An international cooperative study. II. The male population of a
  factory at Zurich.
  Social Science Medicine 7:585, 1973.

3566
SCHATZ, J.W., L. WIENER, H.S. GALLAGHER, AND R.J. EBERLY.
Salmonella pericarditis: An unusual complication of myocardial infarction.
Chest 64:267, 1973.

3567
SCHAUDIG, A.
Rehabilitation after pacemaker implantation.
Fortschritte der Medizin 90:1118, 1972.

3568
SCHAUF, G.E.
Etiology of obesity—the QQF theory.
Journal American Geriatric Society 21(8):346, 1973.

3569
SCHECTER, N.
Psychological aspects of chronic cardiac disease.
Psychosomatics 8:166-169, 1967.

3570
SCHEIER, I.H., AND R.B. CATTELL.
Handbook for the IPAT 8-parallel form anxiety battery.
Champaign, Ill. IPAT, 1960.

3571
SCHEIFFARTH, F.
Immunopathogenesis from myocardiopathies.
Medizinische Welt 23:1638-1639, 1972.

3572
SCHEINMAN, M., AND B. BRENMAN.
Clinical and anatomic implications of intraventricular conduction blocks in acute myocardial infarction.
Circulation 46(4):753-760, 1972.

3573
SCHEINMAN, M.M.
Retrograde ventriculoatrial conduction in patients with acute myocardial infarction.
Chest 59(2):165-168, 1971.

3574
SCHEINMAN, M.M., AND J.A. ABBOTT.
Clinical significance of transmural versus nontransmural electrocardiographic changes in patients with acute myocardial infarction.
American Journal Medicine 55:602, 1973.

3575
SCHERF, D.
The electrocardiographic exercise test.
Journal Electrocardiology 1(2):141-144, 1968.

3576
SCHERF, D.
  Concerning paroxysmal tachycardia.
  Diseases Chest 56(6):465-466, 1969.

3577
SCHERF, D.
  Atropine in acute myocardial infarction.
  American Heart Journal 86:284, 1973.

3578
SCHERF, D., AND J. COHEN.
  The atrioventricular node and selected cardiac arrhythmias.
  New York, Grune and Stratton, 1964.

3579
SCHERF, D., AND A.I. SCHAFFER.
  The electrocardiographic exercise test.
  American Heart Journal 43:927, 1952.

3580
SCHERF, D., AND A. SCHOTT.
  Extrasystoles and allied arrhythmias.
  New York, Grune and Stratton, 1953.

3581
SCHERLAG, B.J., P. SAMET, AND R.H. HELFANT.
  His bundle electrogram: A critical appraisal of its uses and limitations.
  Circulation 46(3):601-613, 1972.

3582
SCHEUER, J.
  Physical training, and intrinsic cardiac adaptations.
  Circulation 47:677, 1973.

3583
SCHICK, K.
  Differential diagnosis of Q in section 3.
  Medizinische Klinik 62(6):225-229, 1967.

3584
SCHIEBLER, T.H., R. GOSSRAU, AND H. VON MOHRENSCHILD.
  On the histochemistry and capillary supply of the sinatrial node.
  Histochemie 30(3):181-200, 1972.

3585
SCHIEFFER, H., N. STERNITZKE, AND L. BETTE.
  Affecting the temporal dynamics of the heart and contractility of the right ventricle by physical
  stress in healthy persons and heart patients.
  Zeitschrift für Kreislaufforschung 60(7):668, 1971.

3586
SCHILLER, E.
   Cardiac rehabilitation. Its potential in the early prevention of disability after myocardial infarction.
   Medical Journal Australia 2(14):751-757, 1972.

3587
SCHILLER, E., AND G. MORRIS.
   Coronary disease and return to work. A practical rating scale for early identification of the problem case.
   Medical Journal Australia 58-1(17):889-892, 1971.

3588
SCHILLING, W.
   Medical rehabilitation by athletic activities in patients with pulmonary cardiopathy.
   Medizin und Sport 12(8):225-229, 1972.

3589
SCHIMMLER, W., AND G. WEGNER.
   Aortic pulse rate in young sportsmen as compared to untrained persons.
   Zeitschrift für Kreislaufforschung 61:648-652, 1972.

3590
SCHIRMER, E.
   What a leading economic official ought to know about rehabilitation.
   Zeitschrift für die Gesamte Hygiene 18(1):27-29, 1972.

3591
SCHJONSBY, H.P.
   Coronary disease in Etnedal. A cross sectional investigation.
   Tidsskrift for den Norske Laegeforening 92(33):2269-2274,2276, 1972.

3592
SCHLANT, R.C., AND J.W. HURST.
   Advances in electrocardiography.
   New York, Grune and Stratton, 1972.

3593
SCHLARB, K.
   Subclavian puncture. Technique, indication, contraindication, complication and clinical experiences.
   Anaesthesist 21(11):477-481, 1972.

3594
SCHLESINGER, P., AND A.B. BENCHIMOL.
   Lidoflazine in angina pectoris.
   Arquivos Brasileiros de Cardiologia 25(5):397-403, 1972.

3595
SCHLESINGER, Z., Y. LIEBERMAN, A. LANDESBERG, AND H.N. NEUFELD.
   Repair of ventricular septal defect and left ventricular aneurysm following myocardial infarction.
   Thorax 26:615-618, 1971.

3596
SCHLEY, G., W. MEESMANN, F.W. SCHULZ, ET AL.
Studies on the effect of spontaneous collateral vessels of the heart on cardiac dysrhythmias following acute experimental coronary artery occlusion.
Archiv für Kreislaufforschung 67(4):305-325, 1972.

3597
SCHLUGER, J., J.H. TRAVERS, R.E. WOLF, AND J.M. GREEN.
Sinus arrest induced by swallowing and propranolol.
Chest 64:651, 1973.

3598
SCHLUSSEL, H.
Therapy of cardiovascular diseases with dietetic measures.
Medizin und Ernährung 3(1):1-4, 1962.

3599
SCHMIDT, F.L.
Kinetotherapy in patients with coronary disease. Criteria for an individual dosage.
Medizinische Klinik 64(46):2135-2139, 1969.

3600
SCHMIDT, G.B., M.A. MEIER, AND M.S. SADOVE.
Sudden appearance of cardiac arrhythmias after dexamethasone.
Journal American Medical Association 221(12):1402-1404, 1972.

3601
SCHMUTZLER, H.
The value of the exercise tolerance test for the functional diagnosis of acquired heart disease.
Anglo-German Medical Review 4:209-223, 1967.

3602
SCHMUTZLER, H., G.A. NEUHAUS, AND H. PAEPRER.
The pressure curve of the left auricle in steady state body work of patients with mitral stenosis.
Verhandlungen der Deutschen Gesellschaft für Kreislaufforschung 35:251, 1967.

3603
SCHNEIDER, B.
Computer application on ECG and VCG analysis in Hannover. Report on the IFIPTC-4 Working conference.
Methods Information Medicine 11:257, 1972.

3604
SCHNEIDER, H., H. BURRMANN, H.W. WACHE, AND H. BARTELS.
Investigations on the correlation of postprandial glucose tolerance changes to age, body weight, blood pressure, cholesterol as well as to asymptomatic and manifest diabetes mellitus in a closed rural population in the second half of life.
Zeitschrift für die Gesamte Innere Medizin und Ihre Grenzgebiete 18:592-596, 1971.

3605
SCHNEIDER, K.W.
On the question of digitalization in case of danger of infarction.
Therapie der Gegenwart 111(1):41-45, 1972.

3606
SCHNEIDER, R.A., AND J.P. COSTILOE.
Level and variability of serial resting blood pressures in subjects with and without ischemic heart disease.
Angiology 17(3):201-211, 1966.

3607
SCHNEIDER, R.A., J.P. COSTILOE, AND S. WOLF.
Arterial pressures recorded in hospital and during ordinary daily activities: Contrasting data in subjects with and without ischemic heart disease.
Journal Chronic Diseases 23(9):674-657, 1971.

3608
SCHNELLBACHER, K., H. ROSKAMM, H. WEIDEMANN, ET AL.
Effects of prolonged physical training on the course of coronary heart diasease.
Münchener Medizinische Wochenschrift 114(31):1343-1348, 1972.

3609
SCHOLLMEYER, P.
Cardiac rhythm disturbances. Part I. Pathogenesis and clinical meaning.
Medizinische Klinik 66(16):613-619, 1971.

3610
SCHOLLMEYER, P.
Cardiac rhythm disturbance.
Medizinische Klinik 66:644-649, 1971.

3611
SCHOPL, S.R.M., K. DIRNAGL, H. DREXEL, AND M.J. HALHUBER.
Ergometric control studies of infarction and hypertension in patients treated in a rehabilitation clinic.
Zeitschrift für Physikalische Medizin 1(5):426-442, 1970.

3612
SCHOUTEN, J. AND J.T.R. SCHREUDER.
Exercise after infarction.
British Medical Journal 1:640, 1968.

3613
SCHOWENGERDT, C.G., AND M.P. MASANGKAY.
Implantation of cardiac pacemakers. A review of complications.
Ohio State Medical Journal 68(11):1015-1018, 1972.

3614
SCHREUDER, H.B.
Influence of age on insulin secretion and lipid mobilization after glucose stimulation.
Israel Journal Medical Science 8:832-834, 1972.

3615
SCHRIEFERS, K.H.
Portal surgery in portal hypertension following liver cirrhosis.
Revista Brasileira Cardiovascular 8(2):163-170, 1972.

3616
SCHRIER, R.W., H.S. HENDERSON, C.C. TISHER, AND R.L. TANNEN.
Nephropathy associated with heat stress and exercise.
In: Jokl, E., and J.T. McClellan, Eds. Medicine and Sport 5:121-147. Basel, Karger, 1971.

3617
SCHRIRE, V., W. BECK, R.P. HEWITSON, AND C.N. BARNARD.
Immediate and long-term results of aortic valve replacement with University of Cape Town aortic valve prosthesis.
British Heart Journal 32(2):255-269, 1970.

3618
SCHRODER, R.
Dicoumarol therapy following cardiac infarction.
Deutsche Medizinische Wochenschrift 98:2220, 1973.

3619
SCHRYVER, C. DE, AND J. MERTENS-STRYTHAGEN.
Intensity of exercise and heart tissue catecholamine content.
Pflügers Archiv (European Journal Physiology) 336(4):345, 1972.

3620
SCHUITEMAKER, H.G.
Toward larger scales.
Tijdschrift voor Aangepaste Werkvoorziening 7(2):36-40, 1972.

3621
SCHULTE, W.
The hazards of extreme pharmacotherapy and extreme psychotherapy in psychiatry.
Landarzt 42:1514-1519, 1966.

3622
SCHULTE, W.
Psychotherapy in old age with utilization of autoprotective mechanisms in involution.
Zeitschrift für Alternsforschung 20(2):129-133, 1967.

3623
SCHULTZ, K.T., AND H.E. LEBOVITZ.
Exaggerated insulin secretion in experimental myocardial infarction.
Circulation 39-40(Suppl. 3):187, 1969.

3624
SCHUMACHER, R.R., A.D. LIEBERSON, R.H. CHILDRESS, AND J.F. WILLIAMS.
Hemodynamic effects of lidocaine in patients with heart disease.
Circulation 37:965, 1968.

3625
SCHUREN, K.P., AND U. HÜTTEMANN.
Chronic obstructive lung disease: Pulmonary circulation, right ventricular function, and oxygen transport in different clinical types.
Klinische Wochenschrift 51:605, 1973.

3626
SCHUTZ, E., AND A. LEHMENKUHLER.
  On the local movements of the heart muscle.
  Zeitschrift für Kardiologie 62:925, 1973.

3627
SCHWAB, J.J., L. MARDER, R.S. CLEMMONS, AND N.H. McGINNIS.
  Anxiety, severity of illness and other medical variables.
  Journal Psychosomatic Research 10(6):297-303, 1966.

3628
SCHWARTZ, A., L.A. SORDAHL, M.L. ENTMAN, J.C. ALLEN, ET AL.
  Abnormal biochemistry in myocardial failure.
  American Journal Cardiology 32:407-422, 1973.

3629
SCHWARTZ, A., J.M. WOOD, J.C. ALLEN, E.P. BORNET, ET AL.
  Biochemical and morphologic correlates of cardiac ischemia.
  American Journal Cardiology 32:46, 1973.

3630
SCHWARTZ, M.K., AND P. HILL.
  Problems in the interpretation of serum cholesterol values.
  Preventive Medicine 1:167-177, 1972.

3631
SCHWARTZKOPFF, W., S. THONIG, F. SORGE, ET AL.
  Hyperlipoproteinemia, a risk factor in peripheral arterial and coronary occlusive diseases.
  Arzneimittel-Forschung 22(10a):1811-1815, 1972.

3632
SCHWARZ, F., AND H. BRAUN.
  Biatrial myxoma masquerading as generalized inflammatory vascular disease.
  Deutsche Medizinische Wochenschrift 97(41):1550-1553, 1972.

3633
SCHWEIZER, W.
  Early diagnosis of coronary heart disease.
  Deutsche Medizinische Wochenschrift 98:1543, 1973.

3634
SCIORTINO, G.
  Data on cardiovascular diseases as a cause of civilian disability.
  Minerva Medica 60:2777-2778, 1969.

3635
SCOTT, J.C.
  Physical activity and the coronary cirulation.
  Canadian Medical Association Journal 96:853-859, 1967,

3636
SCOTT, M.L., D.R. WEBRE, J.F. ARENS, AND J.L. OCHSNER.
  Clinical application of a flow directed balloon tipped cardiac catheter.
  American Surgeon 38:690, 1972.

3637
SCOTT, R.F., AND T.S. BRIGGS.
Pathologic findings in prehospital deaths due to coronary atherosclerosis.
American Journal Cardiology 29(6):782-787, 1972.

3638
SCRIPCARU, G., AND M. COVIC.
Study of the dynamics of left ventricular systole in myocardial infarction.
Archives des Maladies du Coeur et des Vaisseaux 65(10):1243-1250, 1972.

3639
SEALEY, B.J., J. LILJEDAL, B. ABLAD, AND G. NYBERG.
The effects of intravenous alprenolol on exerise tolerance in patients with angina pectoris. A preliminary report.
Pharmacologia Clinica 2(1):46-50, 1969.

3640
SEGAL, B.L.
Efficacy of tranquilizers as antianginal agents.
In: Brest, A.N. and J.H. Meyer, Eds. Cardiovascular Drug Therapy: The eleventh Hahnemann symposium, pp. 304-308. New York, Grune and Stratton, 1965.

3641
SEGALL, H.N.
Rehabilitation of the aged with coronary heart disease.
Journal American Geriatrics Society 11:964-967, 1963.

3642
SEGALL, H.N.
Return older patients to work after a heart attack—or not?
Consultant 8(2):41-44, 1968.

3643
SEGARRA, A.S.
Disease among leaders and managers: Causes, symptoms, prevention and treatment.
Revista de Sanidad e Higiene Pública 42(11/12):811-829, 1968.

3644
SEGEL, N., W.A. HUDSON, P. HARRIS, AND J.M. BISHOP.
The circulatory effect of electrically induced changes in ventricular rate at rest and during exercise in complete heart block.
Journal Clinical Investigation 43:1541, 1964.

3645
SEGERS, M.J., AND C. MERTENS.
Anxiety depression and the risk of coronary atherosclerosis.
Acta Psychiatrica Belgica 72:46, 1972.

3646
SEGERS, M.J., C. MERTENS, AND R. HOGENRAAD.
Self evaluation of anxiety depression and coronary predisposition. Part 2. Modalities of expression and bioclinical risk.
Journal Psychosomatic Research 17:207-214, 1973.

3647
SEGERS, M.J., C. MERTENS, AND M. VASTESAEGER.
Self evaluation of anxiety depression and coronary predisposition. Part 1. Psycho-bioclinical relationships.
Journal Psychosomatic Research 17:197-206, 1973.

3648
SEGNI, E. DI, G. CURZI, V. DI LUZIO, ET AL.
Effects of dopamine on the contractile state of the left ventricle in man.
Bolletino della Società Italiana di Cardiologia 17(2):113-119, 1972.

3649
SEIDEN, G.E., AND C. STAHL.
A new method for diagnosing myocardial damage in patients with normal electrocardiograms and vector cardiograms.
Transactions New York Academy Sciences 35(4):283, 1973.

3650
SEIGEL, D.G., ET AL.
A critique of studies of long-term survivorship of patients with a myocardial infarction.
American Journal Public Health 58:1348-1354, 1968.

3651
SEIPEL, L. AND F. LOOGEN.
On the question of working capacity of patients after surgery for mitral stenosis.
Zeitschrift für Kreislaufforschung 60(2):122-129, 1971.

3652
SELDEN, R., AND T.W. SMITH.
Ouabain pharmacokinetics in dog and man. Determination by radioimmunoassay.
Circulation 45(6):1176-1182, 1972.

3653
SELDON, W.A.
Cardiac disorders.
British Medical Journal 3:548, 1968.

3654
SELDON, W.A., D.E. ANDERSON, AND A.M. LLOYD.
Cardiac rehabilitation—experience with 1,000 cases.
New Zealand Medical Journal 66:66-68, 1967.

3655
SELLER, R.H., O. RAMIREZ, A.N. BREST, AND J.H. MOYER.
Refractory heart failure. Differential diagnosis and management.
Postgraduate Medicine 40(5):599-607, 1966.

3656
SELTZER, C.C., AND J. MAYER.
A simple criterion of obesity.
Postgraduate Medicine 38:101-107, 1965.

3657
SELVESTER, R.H., R. KALABA, C.R. COLLIER, R. BELLMAN, AND H. KAGIWADA.
A digital computer model of the vectorcardiogram with distance and boundary effects: Simulated myocardial infarction.
American Heart Journal 74(6):792-808, 1967.

3658
SELVINI, A.
Psychological aspects of angina patients.
Minerva Medica 57:289-292, 1966.

3659
SELYE, H.
The evolution of the stress-concept—Stress and cardiovascular disease.
American Journal Cardiology 26:289-299, 1970.

3660
SELYUMINOVA, N. YA.
Effect of therapeutic exercises on patients with chronic coronary insufficiency.
Voprosy Kurortologii Fizioterapii i Lechebnoi Kultury 35(1):71-72, 1970.

3661
SEMOVA, N.
Peculiarities of the electrocardiogram at the age of 7-17 years.
Higiena i Zdraveopazvane 15(3):273-281, 1972.

3662
SEMPLE, T.
Rehabilitation of the coronary patient.
Transactions Society Occupational Medicine 18:135-141, 1968.

3663
SEMPLE, T.
The after care of heart attacks.
Rehabilitation 81:21-23, 1972.

3664
SEMRAD, B., AND B. FISER.
The relation between the PR interval and height of pulse pressure in patients with artifical pacemakers.
Vnitrni Lekarstir 19(1):35-40, 1973.

3665
SENGUPTA, A.N., AND M. SENGUPTA.
Psychological reaction after myocardial infarction.
Journal Indian Medical Association 58:241-242, 1972.

3666
SERRADIMIGNI, A., M. BORY, P. DJIANE, ET AL.
The ECG effort test in the diagnosis of cornonary heart disease. Comparative study with coronarography.
Nouvelle Presse Médicale 1(14):939-944, 1972.

3667
SERRADIMIGNI, A., M. BORY, L. POGGI, M. GAUDY, ET AL.
Correlations between effort electrocardiogram and coronarography.
Archives des Maladies du Coeur et des Vaisseaux 64(11):1669-1680, 1971.

3668
SETTEL, E.
Further experience with spironolactone-hydrochlorothiazide (Aldactazide-A) in long-term treatment of refractory cardiac edema.
Journal American Geriatrics Society 13(7):655-662, 1965.

3669
SEXTON, U.A.G., AND R.L. WICK.
15-Year survey of pilots returned to flying status following a myocardial infarction.
Aerospace Medicine 44:1287, 1973.

3670
SHABETAI, R.
Systolic time intervals: a non-invasive method to determine left ventricular function—current status, advantages and limitations.
Journal Maine Medical Association 64:134, 1973.

3671
SHADAKSHARAPPA, K.S., AND J. NAUGHTON.
An unusual triad of congenital cardiac defects.
Journal Oklahoma State Medical Association 61:225-228, 1968.

3672
SHAFTEL, N., H.E. SHAFTEL, AND A. HALPERN.
Work stressor tests and coronary disease.
Angiology 13(10):488-493, 1962.

3673
SHAH, P., AND L. KIDD.
Hemodynamic responses to exercise and to isoproterenol following total correction of Fallot's tetralogy.
Journal Thoracic Cardiovascular Surgery 52(1):138-145, 1966.

3674
SHAH, V.V., V.N. PANSE, S.A. KAMATH, P.L. GOODLUCK, AND C.M. BALCHANDANN.
A study of physical, nutritional and psychosocial characteristics in coronary heart disease.
In: Proceedings of the third Asian Pacific Congress of Cardiology in association with the 28th annual meeting of the Japanese Circulation Society, Kyoto, 10-14, May 1964, pp. 19-25. Kyoto, Kawakita Printing Company, 1964.

3675
SHANOFF, H.M., ET AL.
Studies of male survivors of myocardial infarction due to "essential" atherosclerosis. III. Corneal arcus: Incidence and relation to serum lipids and lipoproteins.
Canadian Medical Association Journal 91:835-839, 1964.

3676
SHANOFF, H.M., AND J.A. LITTLE.
Studies of male survivors of myocardial infarction. VIII. The electrocardiogram and ten-year survival.
American Journal Cardiology 18:535-539, 1966.

3677
SHAPER, A.G.
Diet and the risk of coronary heart disease.
Diagnostica 27:12, 1973.

3678
SHAPER, A.G., J.N. MORRIS, AND T.W. MEADE.
The London busmen.
In: Larsen, O.A. and R.O. Malmborg, Eds. Coronary heart disease and physical training, pp. 240-243. Baltimore, University Park Press, 1971.

3679
SHAPIRA, J., D.R. YOUNG, B. DATNOW, AND R. PELLIGRA.
Development of a standard prolonged work test for the evaluation of fatigue and stress in man.
Aerospace Medicine 38(3):268-272, 1967.

3680
SHAPIRO, A., H.D. COHEN, AND E. MELKONIAN.
Psychophysiology and sinus arrhythmia.
Bibliotheca Cardiologica 26:235-242, 1970.

3681
SHAPIRO, S.
Angina pectoris—an effective therapeutic approach.
Clinical Medicine 70(9):1627-1636, 1963.

3682
SHAPIRO, S., E. WEINBLATT, AND C.W. FRANK.
Return to work after first myocardial infarction.
Archives Environmental Health 24(1):17-26, 1971.

3683
SHAPIRO, S., E. WEINBLATT, C.W. FRANK, AND R.V. SAGER
The H.I.P. study of incidence and prognosis of coronary heart disease. Preliminary findings on incidence of myocardial infarction and angina.
Journal Chronic Diseases 18:527-558, 1965.

3684
SHAPIRO, S., E. WEINBLATT, C.W. FRANK, AND R.V. SAGER.
Incidence of coronary heart disease in a population insured for medical care (HIP).
American Journal Public Health 59(6 Part II, Suppl.):40, 1969.

3685
SHAPIRO, W., AND K. TAUBERT.
Effects of diuretics and exercise on serum digoxin levels.
Clinical Research 20(1):71, 1972.

3686

SHAPPELL, S.D., J.A. MURRAY, A.J. BELLINGHAM, R.D. WOODSON, ET AL.
Adaptation to exercise: role of hemoglobin affinity for oxygen and 2,3-diphosphoglycerate.
Journal Applied Physiology 30:827-832, 1971.

3687

SHARKEY, B.J.
Intensity and duration of training and the development of cardiorespiratory endurance.
Medicine Science Sports 2:197-202, 1970.

3688

SHARLAND, D.E.
Ability of men to return to work after cardiac infarction.
British Medical Journal 2:718-720, 1964.

3689

SHARMA, B., AND S.H. TAYLOR.
Reversible left-ventricular failure in angina pectoris.
Lancet 2:902-906, 1970.

3690

SHARROCK, N.E., AND E.R. NYE.
Patients with coronary heart disease: effect of recreational activities on heart rate, blood lactate and free fatty acids.
New Zealand Medical Journal 74:78-83, 1971.

3691

SHARROCK, N., H.L. GARRETT, AND G.V. MANN.
Practical exercise test for physical fitness and cardiac performance.
American Journal Cardiology 30(7):727, 1972.

3692

SHATALOV, N.N., AND M.A. MUROV.
The influence of intensive noise and neuropsychic tension of the level of the arterial pressure and incidence of hypertensive vascular disease.
Klinicheskaya Meditsina 48(3):70-73, 1970.

3693

SHAVER, L.G.
Smoking and selected physical fitness measures.
Journal American College Health Association 21:489, 1973.

3694

SHAW, T.R.D., M.R. HOWARD, AND J. HAMER.
Variation in the biological availability of digoxin.
Lancet 2:303-307, 1972.

3695

SHAY, J.
Does calcium influx into ischaemic cells stop A.D.P. phosphorylation?
Lancet II:1392, 1973.

3696
SHEFFIELD, L.T., J.H. HOLT, F.M. LESTER, D.V. CONROY, AND T.J. REEVES.
   On-line analysis of the exercise electrocardiogram.
   Circulation 40(6):935-944, 1969.

3697
SHEFFIELD, L.T., J.H. HOLT, AND T.J. REEVES.
   Exercise graded by heart rate in exercise electrocardiographic testing of angina pectoris.
   Circulation 32:622-629, 1965.

3698
SHEFFIELD, L.T., L.N. LARKIN, M.D. PERRY, J.A. BURDESHAW, AND D.V. CONROY.
   Application of computer techniques to the graded exercise EKG test for ischemic heart disease.
   In: Digest of the seventh international conference on medical and biological engineering, 1967,
   Stockholm, Sweden. Stockholm, Royal Academy of Engineering, 1967.

3699
SHEFFIELD, L.T., AND T.J. REEVES.
   Graded exercise in the diagnosis of angina pectoris.
   Modern Concepts Cardiovascular Disease 34:1-6, 1965.

3700
SHEFFIELD, L.T., D. ROITMAN, AND T.J. REEVES.
   Submaximal exercise testing.
   Journal South Carolina Medical Association 65(12)(Suppl. I):18-25, 1969.

3701
SHEKELLE, R.B., ET AL.
   Social status and incidence of coronary heart disease.
   Journal Chronic Diseases 22(6/7):381-394, 1969.

3702
SHEKELLE, R.B., AND A.M. OSTFELD.
   Psychometric evaluations in cardiovascular epidemiology.
   Annals New York Academy Science 126:696-705, 1965.

3703
SHEKELLE, R.B., A.M. OSTFELD, B.Z. LEBOVITS, AND P. OGLESBY.
   Personality traits and coronary heart disease: A re-examination of Ibrahim's hypothesis using
   longitudinal data.
   Journal Chronic Diseases 23(1):33-38, 1970.

3704
SHELL, W.E.
   Assessment of myocardial infarction with serum enzyme determinations.
   California Medicine 119(5):87-88, 1973.

3705
SHEN, A.C., AND R.B. JENNINGS.
   Myocardial calcium and magnesium in acute ischemic injury.
   American Journal Pathology 67(3):417-440, 1972.

3706
SHEPHARD, R.J.
   Intensity, duration and frequencey of exercise as determinants of the response to a training regime.
   Internationale Zeitschrift für Angewandte Physiologie Einschliess Arbeitzphysiologie 26:272-278, 1968.

3707
SHEPHARD, R.J.
   Methodology of exercise tests in healthy subjects and in cardiac patients.
   Canadian Medical Association Journal 99(8):354-359, 1968.

3708
SHEPHARD, R.J.
   Learning, habituation and training.
   Internationale Zeitschrift für Angewandte Physiologie 28:38-48, 1969.

3709
SHEPHARD, R.J.
   For exercise testing please. A review of procedures available to the clinician.
   Bulletin de Physio-Pathology Respiratoire (Nancy) 6:425-474, 1970.

3710
SHIKAWA, H., ET AL.
   Three cases of emotional angina.
   Journal Japanese Psychosomatic Society 8(4):248-252, 1968.

3711
SHINEBOURNE, E.
   Evidence that the effect of beta-adrenergic blockade on the haemodynamic response of hypertenisve patients to exercise is not solely rate-dependent.
   Cardiovascular Research 3(1):52-55, 1969.

3712
SHINEBOURNE, E., J. FLEMING, AND J. HAMER
   Effects of beta-adrenergic blockade during exercise in hypertension and ischaemic heart disease.
   British Heart Journal 30(3):424, 1968.

3713
SHINEBOURNE, E., J. FLEMING, AND J. HAMER.
   Haemodynamic responses to exercise in hypertension: Place of the sympathetic nervous system evaluated by a new selective cardiac beta-adrenergic blocking agent 1C1 50, 172 [4-(2-hydroxy-3-isopropylaminopropoxy)acetanilide].
   Cardiovascular Research 2(4):379-383, 1968.

3714
SHINODA, T., AND S. HINOHARA.
   A psychosomatic study on the increase of female patients with myocardial infarction.
   Journal Japanese Psychosomatic Society 12:300-301, 1972.

3715
SHIROKOV, V.S.
   Error in the lead-in of phonocardiograms in digital computers.
   Novosti Meditsinskogo Priborostroeniia 2:40-43, 1971.

3716
SHISHMAREV, Y.N.
   Analysis of the cardiac electric field by means of quantitative spatial vectorelectrocardiography.
   Kardiologiya 11(9):121-128, 1971.

3717
SHOCK, N.W.
   Physical activity and the "rate of aging".
   Canadian Medical Association Journal 96:836-840, 1967.

3718
SHORT, D., AND M. STOWERS.
   Earliest symptoms of coronary heart disease and their recognition.
   British Medical Journal 2:387-391, 1972.

3719
SHKHVATSABAYA, I.K., N.M. MUKHARLYAMOV, S.M. KAMENKER, AND K.A. MEMETOV.
   Effect of physical exertion on hemodynamics, oxygen regime and ways of preventing circulatory disorders.
   Kardiologiya 9(7):40-45, 1969.

3720
SHKHVATSABAYA, I.K., AND V.P. ZAITSEV.
   The problems of evaluation and classification of the psychic changes in patients suffering with myocardial infarction in connection with their rehabilitation.
   Kardiologiya 10:12-18, 1970.

3721
SHKVATSABAYA, I.K., AND V.P. ZAITSEV.
   Psychologic factors in myocardial infarction and problems of rehabilitation.
   Terapevticheskii Arkhiv 44(4):22-27, 1972.

3722
SHRIVASTAVA, S., M.L. BHATIA, AND S.B. ROY.
   Propranolol and cardioversion.
   Indian Heart Journal 24(3):282-285, 1972.

3723
SHUBIN, H., AND A. GLASKIN.
   Psychological aspects of coronary heart disease.
   Psychosomatics 5:305-310, 1964.

3724
SHUBIN, H., A.A. ABDELMONEM, N.M. RAND, AND M. H. WEIL.
   Objective index of hemodynamic status for quantitation of severity and prognosis of shock complicating myocardial infarction.
   Cardiovascular Research 2:329, 1968.

3725
SHULTZ, K.T., AND H.E. LEBOVITZ.
   Exaggerated insulin secretion in experimental myocardial infarction.
   Circulation 39-40(Suppl. III):187, 1969.

3726
SHUMWAY, N.D., J.A. JOHNSON, AND R.J. STISH.
The study of ventricular fibrillation by threshold determination.
Journal Thoracic Surgery 34:643, 1957.

3727
SHUSTER, A.
The electrocardiogram in subarachnoid hemmorrhage.
British Heart Journal 22:316-320, 1960.

3728
SHVARTSMAN, Z.D.
Myocardial infarction in senile persons.
Terapevticheskii Arkhiv 43(9):52-55, 1971.

3729
SIBLEY, J.C.
The post-hospital treatment of the patient with cardiac infarction.
Applied Therapeutics 7:300-306, 1965.

3730
SIDERIS, D.A. AND S.F. STAMATELOPOULOS.
Correlation between atrial fibrillation and some hemodynamic factors in mitral stenosis.
Cardiology 55:361-370, 1970.

3731
SIEGEL, G.H.
Legal aspects of informed consent, stress testing, and exercise programs.
In: Naughton, J., H.K. Hellerstein, and I.C. Mohler, Eds. Exercise testing and exercise training in coronary heart disease, pp. 387-391. New York, Academic Press, 1973.

3732
SIEGEL, W., G. BLOMQVIST, AND J. MITCHELL.
Effects of a quantitated physical training program on middle-aged sedentary men.
Circulation 41:19, 1970.

3733
SIEGEL, W., G. BLOMQVIST, J.D. HOUSTON, AND L.S. COHEN.
The apexcardiogram during exercise in coronary heart disease.
Circulation 39-40(suppl. III):187, 1969.

3734
SIGGAARD-ANDERSEN, J., AND F.B. PETERSEN.
Simultaneous venous occlusion plethysmography and Xe^{133} clearance measurements on the calf of the leg after repeated exercise in patients with arteriosclerosis. Concluding remarks on the use of the two methods.
Scandinavian Journal Thoracic Cardiovascular Surgery 3:26-30, 1969.

3735
SIGGAARD-ANDERSEN, J., J. ULRICH, H.C. ENGELL, AND F.B. PETERSEN.
Blood pressure measurements of the lower limb. Arterial occlusions in the calf determined by plethysmographic blood pressure measurements in the thigh and at the ankle.
Angiology 23(6):350-357, 1972.

3736
SIGLER, L.H.
Emotion and atheroslerotic heart disease. I. Electrocardiographic changes observed on the recall of past emotional disturbances.
British Journal Medical Psychology 40:55-64, 1967.

3737
SIGLER, L.H.
Reemployment of the elderly cardiac.
Geriatrics 22:97-105, 1967.

3738
SILBERT, A., P.H. WOLFF, B. MAYER, A. ROSENTHAL, AND A.S. NADAS.
Cyanotic heart disease and psychological development.
Pediatrics 43(2):192-200, 1969.

3739
SILVA, W.N., DA.
Rehabilitation of cardiac patients.
Revista do Hospital das Clinicas da Faculdade de Medicina de Universidade de Sao Paulo 21:96-102, 1966.

3740
SILVIJ, S.
Physiotherapy for cardiac neuroses.
Recenti Progressi in Medicina 52(4):390-391, 1972.

3741
SIMBORG, D.W.
The status of risk factors and coronary heart disease.
Journal Chronic Diseases 22(8/9):515-552, 1970.

3742
SIME, W.E., I.T. WHIPPLE, D.M. BERKSON, ET AL.
Reproducibility of heart rate at rest and in response to submaximal treadmill and bicycle ergometer test in middle-aged men.
Medicine Science Sports 4(1):14-17, 1972.

3743
SIMMONS, R., AND R.J. SHEPHARD.
Effects of physical conditioning upon the central and peripheral circulatory responses to arm work.
Internationale Zeitschrift für Angewandte Physiologie 30:73-84, 1971.

3744
SIMON, A.B., M. FEINLEIB, AND H.K. THOMPSON, JR.
Components of delay in the prehospital phase of acute myocardial infarction.
American Journal Cardiology 30(5):476-482, 1972.

3745
SIMON, A.L.
Angiographic appearance of idiopathic hypertrophic subaortic stenosis.
Circulation 46(3):614-622, 1972.

3746
SIMONSON, E.
   The concept and definition of normality.
   Annals New York Academy Science 134:541-558, 1966.

3747
SIMONSON, E.
   Electrocardiographic stress tolerance tests.
   Progress Cardiovascular Disease 13(3):269-292, 1970.

3748
SIMONSON, E.
   Physiology of work capacity and fatigue, p. 592.
   Springfield, Ill. Thomas, 1971.

3749
SIMONSON, E.
   Evaluation of cardiac performance in exercise.
   American Journal Cardiology 30(7):722, 1972.

3750
SIMONSON, E.
   The effect of age on the electrocardiogram.
   American Journal Cardiology 29(1):64-73, 1972.

3751
SIMONSON, E., C. BAKER, N. BURNS, C. KEIPER, ET AL.
   Cardiovascular stress (electrocardiographic changes) produced by driving an automobile.
   American Heart Journal 75(1):125-135, 1968.

3752
SIMONSON, E., AND R. BERMAN.
   Myocardial infarction in young people. Experience in USSR.
   American Heart Journal 84(6):814, 1972.

3753
SIMONSON, E., AND R. BERMAN.
   New approach in treatment of cardiac decompensation in USSR.
   American Heart Journal 86:117, 1973.

3754
SIMONSSON, B.G., B.E. SKOOGH, AND B. EKSTROM JODAL.
   Exercise induced airways constriction.
   Thorax 27(2):169-180, 1972.

3755
SIMPSON, F.O.
   Beta-blocker?
   Lancet II:1396, 1973.

3756
SIMPSON, F.O., AND H.J. WAAL-MANNING.
   Hypertension and depression: interrelated problems in therapy.
   Journal Royal College Physicians (London) 6(1):14-24, 1971.

3757
SIMPSON, M.T., C.G. HAMES, R. MEIER, D. OLEWINE, AND F. RAMSEY.
   An epidemiological study of platelet aggregation and physical activity.
   Circulation 43-44(Suppl. II):88, 1971.

3758
SINGER, E., A.S. GOOCH, AND D. Morse.
   Exercise induced arrhythmias in patients with pacemakers.
   Journal American Medical Association 224:1515-1518, 1973.

3759
SINGH, I., P.K. KHANNA, M.C. SRIVASTAVA, AND R.S. HOON.
   Extent of possible rehabilitation of service personnel with ischaemic heart disease.
   British Heart Journal 32(5):665-670, 1970.

3760
SINGH, J., ET AL.
   Sex life and psychiatric problems after myocardial infarction.
   Journal Association Physicians India 18:503-507, 1970.

3761
SINNING, W.E.
   Body composition, cardiorespiratory function, and rule changes in women's basketball.
   The Research Quarterly 44:313, 1973.

3762
SIVKOV, I.I., V.G. KUKES, AND N.M. IZMALKOVA.
   Derangements of the acid base balance and their correction in patients with chronically insuf-
   ficient circulation.
   Sovetskaya Meditsina 35(11):15-22, 1972.

3763
SJORGEN, A.
   Left heart failure in acute myocardial infarction: A clinical haemodynamic and therapeutic study.
   Acta Medica Scandinavica (Suppl.) 510:7-87, 1970.

3764
SKAGSETH, E., T. FRÖYSAKER, T. SEMB, G.S. HALL, AND L. EFSKIND.
   Surgical treatment of postinfarctional ventricular septal rupture and aneurysm.
   Scandinavian Journal Thoracic Cardiovascular Surgery 5:239-242, 1971.

3765
SKAVRONSKY, V.I.
   Changes in the level of biogenic amines in patients with ischemic heart disease consuming
   qualitatively differing carbohydrates.
   Voprosy Pitaniya 31(6):38-43, 1972.

3766
SKINNER, J.S.
   The cardiovascular system with aging and exercise.
   In: Brunner, D., and E. Jokl, Eds. Physical activity and aging, pp 100-108. Baltimore, University
   Park Press, 1970.

3767
SKINNER, J.S., H. BENSON, J.R. McDONOUGH, AND C.G. HAMES.
Social status, physical activity, and coronary proneness.
Journal Chronic Diseases 19:773, 1966.

3768
SKINNER, J.S., ET AL.
Effects of a program of endurance exercises on physical work. Capacity and anthropometric
measurements of fifteen middle-aged men.
American Journal Cardiology 14:747-752, 1964.

3769
SKINNER, J.S., J.O. HOLLOSZY, G. TORO, A.J. BARRY, AND T.K. CURETON.
Effects of a six-month program of endurance exercise on work tolerance, serum lipids, and
ULF-ballistocardiograms of fifteen middle-aged men.
In: M. J. Karvonen, and A. J. Barry, Eds. Physical activity and the heart, pp. 79-98, Springfield,
Ill. Thomas, 1967.

3770
SKJAEGGESTAD, O.
The natural history of intermediate coronary syndrome.
Acta Medica Scandinavica 193:533, 1973.

3771
SLACK, J.
Risk of ischemic heart disease in familial hyperlipoproteinemic states.
Lancet 2:1380, 1969.

3772
SLANY, J., H. MOSSLACHER, AND P. BODNER.
Precordial kinetics in coronary disease.
Wiener Klinische Wochenschrift 85:724, 1973.

3773
SLATER, A., S. BELLET, AND D.G. KILPATRICK.
Telemetering of the human electrocardiogram underwater.
Engineering Medicine Biology, Proceedings 18th annual conference p. 143, 1965.

3774
SLEIGHT, P.
What is hypertension? Recent studies on neurogenic hypertension.
British Heart Journal 33(Suppl.):109-112, 1971.

3775
SLOAN, J.M., J.S. MACKAY, AND B. SHERIDAN.
Glucose tolerance and insulin response in atherosclerosis.
British Medical Journal 4:586-599, 1970.

3776
SLODKI, S.J., A.T. HUSSAIN, AND A.A. LUISADA.
The Q-II interval. III. A study of the second heart sound in old age.
Journal American Geriatrics Society 17(7):673-679, 1969.

3777
SLOMAN, G.
  Propranolol in management of muscular subaortic stenosis.
  British Heart Journal 29(5):783-787, 1967.

3778
SLOMAN, G.
  A decade of coronary care in Melbourne, Australia. Part I.
  Heart Lung 2(5):659, 1973.

3779
SLOMAN, G., A. PITT, E.Z. HIRSCH, AND A. DONALDSON.
  The effect of a graded physical training programme on the physical working capacity of patients
  with heart disease.
  Medical Journal Australia 52-1:4-7, 1965.

3780
SLOMAN, G., AND R.J. PRINEAS.
  Major cardiac arrhythmias in acute myocardial infarction, implications for long-term survival.
  Chest 63:513, 1973.

3781
SLOMAN, G., R. J. PRINEAS, AND R.H. STEWART.
  Cardiac arrhythmias in acute myocardial infarction-relation to one-year survival.
  Medical Journal Australia 2(1):52-55, 1973.

3782
SMITH, A.L.,SR., AND A.L. SMITH, JR.
  Evaluation of the vectorcardiogram taken after exercise in 164 cases of angina pectoris.
  Circulation 24(4 Part 2):1044, 1961.

3783
SMITH, J.E., C.R. HARPER, AND G.J. KIDERA.
  Wolff-Parkinson-White syndrome simulating myocardial infarction.
  Aerospace Medicine 41(3):328-330, 1970.

3784
SMITH, J.E., AND G.J. KIDERA.
  Treatment of angina pectoris with exercise stress.
  Aerospace Medicine 38(7):742-745, 1967.

3785
SMITH, G.H., AND K. CHANDRA.
  Haemodynamic effects of glucagon after mitral valve replacement.
  Thorax 27(5):591-593, 1972.

3786
SMITH, H.J., G.A. BOUSVAROS, AND M. McGREGOR.
  Failure of acute digitalization to influence exercise tolerance in angina pectoris.
  British Medical Journal 1:1337-1338, 1966.

3787
SMITH, L.E.
  Facilitatory effects of myotatic stretch training upon leg strength and contralateral transfer.
  American Journal Physical Medicine 49:132-141, 1970.

3788
SMITH, R., L. JOHNSON, D. ROTHFELD, ET AL.
  Sleep and cardiac arrhythmias.
  Archives Internal Medicine 130:751, 1972.

3789
SMITH, R.F.
  Quantitative exercise stress testing in the naval aviator population and in the projected Apollo
  spacecraft experiment MO-IS.
  In: Blackburn, H. Ed. Measurement in exercise electrocardiography, p. 131, Springfield, Ill.
  Thomas, 1969.

3790
SMITH, R.F., AND R.J. WHERRY, JR.
  Quantitative interpretation of the exercise electrocardiogram. Use of computer techniques in the
  cardiac evaluation of aviation personnel.
  Circulation 34:1044-1055, 1966.

3791
SMITH, R.O., W.D. LOVE, P.H. LEHAN, AND H.K. HELLEMS.
  Delayed coronary blood flow detected by computer analysis of serial scans.
  American Heart Journal 84(5):670-677, 1972.

3792
SMITH, T.W.
  Radioimmunoassay for serum digitoxin concentration. Methodology and clinical experience.
  Journal Pharmacology Experimental Therapy 175:352, 1970.

3793
SMITH, T.W., V.P. BUTLER, JR., AND E. HABER.
  Determination of therapeutic and toxic serum digoxin concentrations by radioimmunoassay.
  New England Journal Medicine 281:1212, 1969.

3794
SMITH, T.W., J.G. CURD, AND E. HABER.
  Rapid reversal of digoxin toxicity by Fab fragments from purified digoxin specific antibody.
  Circulation 43:(Suppl. II):41, 1971.

3795
SMITH, T.W., AND E. HABER.
  Digitalis, 2.
  New England Journal Medicine 289(19):1010-1015, 1973.

3796
SMITH, T.W., AND E. HABER.
  Digitalis, 3.
  New England Journal Medicine 289:1063, 1973.

3797
SMITH, W.K., JR., AND W.S. FRANKL.
  Ultrasound cardiography in clinical practice.
  Medical Clinics North America 57:959, 1973.

3798
SMITH, W.M., A.N. DATATO, N.J. GALLUZZI, ET AL.
The evaluation of antihypertensive therapy cooperative clinical trial method. I. Double-blind control comparison of chlorothiazide, rauwolfia serpentina, and hydralazine.
Annals Internal Medicine 61:829-846, 1964.

3799
SMITHEN, C.S., K. BROWN, D. FLUCK, AND E. SOWTON.
Analysis of heart block and dysrhythmias by His bundle electrograms.
Cardiovascular Research 6(2):129-134, 1972.

3800
SMOKLER, P.E., R.N. MACALPIN, A. ALVARO, AND A.A. KATTUS.
Reproducibility of a multi-stage near maximal treadmill test for exercise tolerance in angina pectoris.
Circulation 48:346, 1973.

3801
SMULYAN, H., AND R.H. EICH.
Effect of beta-sympathetic blockade on the initial hemodynamic response to exercise.
Circulation 34(4 Suppl. III):219, 1966.

3802
SMYLLIE, H.C., M.P. TAYLOR, AND R.A. CUNNINGHAME GREEN.
Acute myocardial infarction in Doncaster. I. Estimating size of coronary care unit.
British Medical Journal 1:31-34, 1972.

3803
SNOW, H.M., C.M. FURNIVAL, AND R.J. LINDEN.
Functional distribution of sympathetic and parasympathetic nerves to the heart.
British Heart Journal 21:393, 1969.

3804
SNOW, P.J.D.
Effect of propranolol in myocardial infarction.
Lancet 2:551, 1965.

3805
SO, C.S.
Der Herzinfarkt im Electrokardiogram.
Munich, West Germany. Urban und Schwarzenberg, 1972.

3806
SOARES DA COSTA, J., C. RIBEIRO, T. SOARES DA COSTA, AND J.F. MARTINS CORREIA.
Two cases of Prinzmetal angina.
Boletim da Sociedade Portuguesa de Cardiologia 10:105, 1972.

3807
SOBOLOVA, V., V. SELIGER, D. GRUSSOVA, J. MACHOVCOVA, V. ZELENKA.
The influence of age and sports training in swimming on physical fitness.
Acta Paediatrica Scandinavica (Suppl.) 217:63-67, 1971.

3808
SÖDERHOLM, B., O. THULESIUS, F. HEYMAN, R. MALMCRONA, AND P. BJÖRNTORP.
Myocardial infarction in the younger age groups. III. Follow-up observations with special reference to exercise tolerance tests.
Acta Medica Scandinavica 172(5):585-592, 1962.

3809
SODHI, H.S., AND B.J. KUDCHODKAR.
Synthesis of cholesterol in hypercholesterolemia and its relationship to plasma triglycerides.
Metabolism 22:895, 1973.

3810
SOKOLOV, B.P., K.M. DANILOVA, ET AL.
Clinical importance of some metabolic shifts in myocardial infarction based on the data of a complete biochemical and histoenzymatic investigation.
Sovetskaya Meditsina 35(11):22, 1972.

3811
SOLANKI, S.V., AND V.H. YAJNIK.
Ortner's syndrome.
Indian Heart Journal 24(1):43-46, 1972.

3812
SOLOFF, L.A., AND H. SCHWARTZ.
Relationship between glucose and fatty acid in myocardial infarction.
Lancet 1:449-452, 1966.

3813
SOLOMONOVA, L.N., AND V.V. SOKOLOV.
Changes in the capacity for physical work in patients with atherosclerotic cardiosclerosis during treatment.
Kardiologiya 12:31-35, 1972.

3814
SOLTI, F., AND K. FOLDESY.
Sinoauricular block in carditis patients after exercise.
Zeitschrift für Gesamte Innere Medizin und Ihre Grenzgebiete 17(20):930-933, 1962.

3815
SOLTI, F., Z. SZABO, F. RENYI VAMOS, JR., ET AL.
Treatment of tachyarrhythmias with pacemaker implantation.
Zeitschrift für Kreislaufforschung 61(2):103-114, 1972.

3816
SOMMER, A., R. BENYAMINE, AND A. JOUVE.
Trial of a new antihypertensive drug: Clonidine.
Coeur et Médecine Interne 12:445, 1973.

3817
SOMERVILLE, J., D. ROSS, G. SACHS, ET AL.
Long term results of pulmonary autograft replacement for aortic valve disease.
Lancet 2:730-734, 1972.

3818
SOMERVILLE, W.
Emotions, catecholamines, and coronary heart disease.
In: Halonen, P., and A. Louhija, Eds. Early diagnosis of coronary heart disease. Second Paavo Nurmi symposium, Porvoo, Finland, 1971, pp. 162-173. Basel, Switzerland. S. Karger, 1973.

3819
SOMERVILLE, W., P. TAGGART, AND M. CARRUTHERS.
Addressing a medical meeting: effect on heart rate, electrocardiogram, plasma catecholamines, free fatty acids, and triglycerides.
British Heart Journal 33(4):608, 1971.

3820
SOMOGYI, G., A. KALDOR, AND A. JANKOVICS.
Plasma concentrations of cardiac glycosides in digitalis intoxication.
European Journal Clinical Pharmacology 4(3):158-161, 1972.

3821
SOMOGYI, J.C.
Nutrition and atherosclerosis. Collection on "Nutrition and Diet." No. 12.
Basel, Switzerland. S. Karger, 1969.

3822
SONES, F. M., JR.
Indications and value of coronary arteriography.
In: Halonen, P., and A. Louhija, Eds. Early diagnosis of coronary heart disease. Second Paavo Nurmi Symposium, Porvoo, Finland, 1971, pp. 67-75. Basel, Switzerland. Karger, 1973.

3823
SONG, H., C. YI, Y. NO, S. PAK, ET AL.
An epidemiological study on various cardiac diseases.
Korean Journal Internal Medicine 15:37-38, 1972.

3824
SONNENBLICK, E.H.
Series elastic and contractile elements in heart muscle: changes in muscle length.
American Journal Physiology 207:1330, 1964.

3825
SONNENBLICK, E.H.
Instantaneous force-velocity-length determinants in the contraction of heart muscle.
Circulation Research 16:441, 1965.

3826
SONNENBLICK, E.H., E. BRAUNWALD, AND A.G. MORROW.
The contractile properties of human heart muscle: studies on myocardial mechanics of surgically excised papillary muscles.
Journal Clinical Investigation 44:966, 1965.

3827
SONNENBLICK, E.H., E. BRAUNWALD, J.F. WILLIAMS, JR., AND G. GLICK.
Effects of exercise on myocardial force-velocity relations in intact unanesthetized man. Relative roles of changes in heart rate, sympathetic activity, and ventricular dimensions.
Journal Clinical Investigation 44:2051, 1965.

3828
SONNENBLICK, E.H., AND E.W. GERTZ.
  Mechanisms of heart failure.
  Verhandlungen der Deutschen Gesellschaft für Kreislaufforschung 37:29-42, 1971.

3829
SONNENBLICK, E.H., J. ROSS,JR., J.W. COVELL, G.A. KAISER, AND E. BRAUNWALD.
  Velocity of contraction as a determinant of myocardial oxygen consumption.
  American Journal Physiology 209:919-927, 1965.

3830
SONNENBLICK, E.H., AND C.L. SKELTON.
  Oxygen consumption of the heart: physiological principles and clinical implications.
  Modern Concepts Cardiovascular Disease 40:9-16, 1971.

3831
SOPINA, N.V.
  Effect of exercise therapy on the blood coagulation properties in a combined treatment of
  patients with coronary atherosclerosis.
  Vrachebnoe Delo 5:27-30, 1970.

3832
SORGE, F., H.J. DIEHL, H. HOFFMANN, AND W. SCHWARTZKOPF.
  Insulin response to oral glucose after myocardial infarction and in patients with peripheral vascular
  disease.
  Acta Diabetologica 10(3):658, 1973.

3833
SOROKIN, M.
  Myocardial infarction in Fiji.
  Medical Journal Australia 2(16):764-767, 1973.

3834
SOROUR, A.H., A.M. EL-KEIY, M.S. FAHMY, ET AL.
  Effects of graded exercise on the physical work capacity of patients with coronary heart disease.
  Malattie Cardiovascolari 10(1-2):431-436, 1969.

3835
SOUKUPOVÁ, K., A. HEYROVSKY, E. STUCHLIKOVÁ, AND M. ŠULC.
  Serum lipids, glucose tolerance tests and clinical signs in healthy men with a raised beta/alpha-
  lipoprotein index.
  Gerontologia Clinica 12(1):1-9, 1970.

3836
SOUSA, P.A.
  Topographical localization of the atrial rhythms.
  Boletim da Sociedade Portuguesa de Cardiologia 10:81, 1972.

3837
SOWTON, E.
  Pacemaker treatment of patients without heart block: A new approach to the management of
  intractable arrhythmias.
  British Heart Journal 30(3):420, 1968.

3838
SOWTON, E.
Driving licences for patients with cardiac pacemakers.
British Heart Journal 34(10):977-980, 1972.

3839
SOWTON, E., R. BALCON, T. PRESTON, D. LEAVER, AND M. YACOUB.
Long-term control of intractable supraventricular tachycardia by ventricular pacing.
British Heart Journal 31(6):700-706, 1969.

3840
SOWTON, E., C. SMITHEN, D. LEAVER, AND I. BARR.
Effect of practolol on exercise tolerance in patients with angina pectoris.
American Journal Medicine 51(1):63-70, 1971.

3841
SPAIN, D.M., AND V.A. BRADESS.
Sudden death from coronary atherosclerosis: Age, race, sex, physical activity, and alcohol.
Archives Internal Medicine 100:228, 1957.

3842
SPANGLER, R.D., M.J. HORMAN, S.W. MILLER, D.A. ROTENBERG, J.C. BIRNHOLZ, R.L. SIMMONS, E.E. WESTURA, S.M. FOX, III.
A submaximal exercise electrocardiographic test as a method of detecting occult ischemic heart disease.
American Heart Journal 80(6):752-758, 1970.

3843
SPARKMAN, D.R., AND R.M. LEVENSON.
Employability after cardiac rehabilitation.
Northwest Medicine 64:269-272, 1965.

3844
SPARKS, H.V., H.H. KOPALD, S. CARRIERE, ET AL.
Intrarenal distribution of blood flow with chronic congestive heart failure.
American Journal Physiology 223(4):840-846, 1972.

3845
SPEAR, A., AND W. KLIP.
A digital program for the computation of phase velocity and transmission of waves generated in the arterial system.
Alabama Journal Medical Science 9:57-64, 1972.

3846
SPECHT, D.F.
Vectorcardiographic diagnosis using the polynomia discriminant method of pattern recognition.
IEEE Transactions Bio-Medical Engineering 90-95, 1967.

3847
SPECHT, D.F., J.E. MANGELSDORF, AND J.G. TOOLE.
Classification of electrocardiograms using the polynomial discriminant method of pattern classification.
Biomedical Sciences Instrumentation 4:132-136, 1968.

3848
SPELMAN, M.S. AND P. LEY.
The effect of psycho-social factors on the prognosis of coronary thrombosis.
Medical Journal Australia 2:1189-1193, 1966.

3849
SPENCER, M.E., E.L. YOUMANS, M.J. SHUMEN, AND K. RODHAL.
Effects of rope skipping and physical education classes on physical work capacity of sedentary college women.
In: Balke B., Ed. Physiological aspects of sports and physical fitness, pp. 79-81.
The Athletic Institute, 1968.

3850
SPENCER, W.A.
A new use for the rehabilitation process: Introspection.
Archives Physical Medicine Rehabilitation 51:187-197 1970.

3851
SPENCER, W.A., C. VALLBONA, AND R.E. CARTER, JR.
Physiologic concepts of immobilization.
Archives Physical Medicine Rehabilitation 46:89-100, 1965.

3852
SPERANSKII, G.N., AND IV. M. PRATUSEVICH.
The effect produced by dosed physical exercises eliminating mental fatigue, on induced potentials of the encephalon in children.
Doklady Akademii Nauk SSSR (Moskva) 163:1028-1031, 1965.

3853
SPERANSKY, N.I., E.I. SOROKINA, AND V.E. KRASNIKOV.
Clinical principles of rehabilitation of patients who had sustained myocardial infarction.
Klinicheskaya Meditsina 49(6):24-31, 1971.

3854
SPIEGEL, M., ET AL.
The prehospital phase of acute myocardial infarction in Zurich.
Schweizerische Medizinische Wochenschrift 103:1219, 1973.

3855
SPIEKERMAN, R.E., J.T. BRANDENBERG, R.W.P. ACHOR, AND J.E. EDWARDS.
The spectrum of coronary heart disease in a community of 30,000: a clinicopathologic study.
Circulation 25:57, 1962.

3856
SPITZER, H., AND T. HETTINGER.
Tables for calories conversion (4th edition).
Darmstadt, West Germany. Beuth, 1964.

3857
SPIVACK, A.P., AND R.F. DeBUSK.
Exercise during convalescence from myocardial infarction.
Circulation 40(4 Part 3):192, 1969.

3858
SPODICK, D.H.
   Progress in cardiology (Yu and Goodwin, Eds.)
   Journal American Medical Association 225:317, 1973.

3859
SPOERRI, TH., AND W. TH. WINKLER, EDS.
   Proceedings of the VIIth International Congress of Psychotherapy.
   Basel, Switzerland. S. Karger, 1968.

3860
SPOTNIZ, H.M., AND E.H. SONNENBLICK.
   Structural conditions in the hypertrophied and failing heart.
   American Journal Cardiology 32:398-406, 1973.

3861
SPRAGUE, H.B.
   Environment in relation to coronary artery disease.
   Archives Environmental Health 13:4-12, 1966.

3862
SPRITZER, R.C., L.M. MATTES, C. CARP, A. WEISENSEEL, ET AL.
   Electrocardiographic follow-up of patients with demand pacemakers.
   American Heart Journal 80(3):367-375, 1970.

3863
SPURRELL, R.A.J., D.M. KRIKLER, AND E. SOWTON.
   Study of intraventricular conduction times in patients with left bundle branch block and left axis
   deviation and in patients with left bundle branch block and normal QRS axis using His bundle
   electrocardiograms.
   British Heart Journal 34(12):1244-1249, 1972.

3864
SPURRELL, R.A.J., D. M. KRIKLER, AND E. SOWTON.
   Two or more intra AV nodal pathways in association with either a James or Kent extranodal
   bypass in three patients with paroxysmal supraventricular tachycardia.
   British Heart Journal 35(2):113-122, 1973.

3865
SPYCHER-BRAENDLI, C.B.
   The time parameter of the carotid pulse curve in aortic valvular diseases pre- and postoperatively.
   Archive für Klinische Medizin 213:106-120, 1967.

3866
SRINIVASAN, S.R., P. DOLAN, B. RADHAKRISHNAMURTHY, AND G.S. BERENSON.
   Isolation of lipoprotein acid mucopolysaccharide complexes from fatty streaks of human aortas.
   Atherosclerosis 16(1):95-104, 1972.

3867
SRIVASTAVA, B.N., P.C. JAIN, AND G.P. VYAS.
   A new beta-receptor blocking agent LB 46 in angina pectoris. (A double blind clinical trial).
   Indian Heart Journal 24(Suppl.1):203-204, 1972.

3868
STAEHELIN, B.
  On psychosomatic features of vegetative heart and circulatory disorders.
  Therapeutische Umschau 22:429, 1965.

3869
STAMLER, J.
  Nutrition, metabolism and atherosclerosis. A review of data and theories, and a discussion of
  controversial question.
  In: Ingelfinger, F.J., A.S. Relman, and M. Finland, Eds. Controversy in Internal Medicine, pp.
  27-59. Philadelphia, Saunders, 1966.

3870
STAMLER, J.
  The coronary prone.
  Journal Rehabilitation 32:18, 1966.

3871
STAMLER, J.
  Lectures on preventive cardiology.
  New York, Grune and Stratton, 1967.

3872
STAMLER, J.
  The primary prevention of coronary heart disease.
  Hospital Practice 6:49-59, 1971.

3873
STAMLER, J.
  Acute myocardial infarction—Progress in primary prevention.
  British Heart Journal 33(Supp.):145, 1971.

3874
STAMLER, J., D.M. BERKSON, M. LEVINSON, H.A. LINDBERG, ET AL.
  Coronary artery disease. Status of preventive efforts.
  Archives Environmental Health 13:322-335, 1966.

3875
STAMLER, J., D.M. BERKSON, AND H.A. LINDBERG.
  Risk factors: Their role in the etiology and pathogenesis of the atherosclerotic diseases.
  In: Wissler, R.W., and J.C. Geer, Eds. Pathogenesis of atherosclerosis: Pathology. Baltimore,
  Waverly Press, 1972.

3876
STAMLER, J., D.M. BERKSON, H.A. LINDBERG, I.T. WHIPPLE, ET AL.
  Long-term epidemiologic studies on the possible role of physical activity and physical fitness in
  the prevention of premature clinical coronary heart disease.
  In: Brunner, D., and E. Jokl, Eds. Physical activity and aging, pp. 274-300. Baltimore, University
  Park Press, 1970.

3877
STAMLER, J., ET AL.
  A long term coronary prevention evaluation program.
  Annals New York Academy Science 149:1022-1037, 1968.

3878
STAMLER, J., AND F.H. EPSTEIN.
Coronary heart disease: risk factors as guides to preventive action.
Preventive Medicine 1:27-48, 1972.

3879
STAMLER, J., M. KJELSBERG, AND Y. HALL.
Epidemiologic studies on cardiovascular-renal diseases: I. Analysis of mortality by age-race-sex-occupation.
Journal Chronic Diseases 12(4):440-455, 1960.

3880
STAMLER, J., H.A. LINDBERG, D.M. BERKSON, A. SHAFFER, ET AL.
Prevalence and incidence of coronary heart disease in strata of the labor force of a Chicago industrial corporation.
Journal Chronic Diseases 11:405, 1960.

3881
STAMLER, J., R. STAMLER, AND R.B. SHEKELLE.
Regional differences in prevalence, incidence and mortality from atherosclerotic coronary heart disease.
In: de Haas, J.H., H.C. Hemker, and H.A. Snellen, Eds. Ischaemic heart disease, p. 84. Leiden, The Netherlands. Leiden University Press, 1970.

3882
STANAWAY, R.G., and R.P. HULLIN.
The relationships of exercise response to personality.
Psychological Medicine 3:343, 1973.

3883
STANCARI, V.DI, A. MAZZONI, AND P. ARTUSO.
On some aspects of cardiac neurosis in chauffeurs.
Bollettino della Società Italiana di Cardiologia 9:153-156, 1964.

3884
STANOWSKI, J., AND Z. KORDYL.
Systematic psychotherapy and educational influence as factors enhancing cardiological rehabilitation.
Polski Tygodnik Lekarski 22:94-97, 1967.

3885
STARKEY, P.D.
Sick role retention as a factor in non-rehabilitation.
Dissertation Abstracts 27(12B):4557-B-4558-B, 1967.

3886
STAUFFER, J.J., AND E.B. MOODY.
Cardiac output before and after exercise as indication of functional status in patients with stable heart disease.
Circulation 26(4 Part 2):790, 1962.

3887
STAVRIDIS, I., D. THOMOPOULOS, AND K. GARDIKAS.
The trypsin time as a new method for the determination of blood coagulation in patients under treatment with cumarin derivatives.
Nosokomeiaka Chronika 34(3):225-235, 1972.

3888
STEEL, J.M., J.F. MUNRO, AND L.J.P. DUNCAN.
A comparative trial of different regimens of fenfluramine and phentermine in obesity.
Practitioner 211:232, 1973.

3889
STEEL, R.K., J.K. COOPER, AND S.M. FOX, III.
Mobile coronary services.
Circulation 39:279-281, 1969.

3890
STEENKAMP, W.F.J.
Familial trifascicular block.
American Heart Journal 84/6:758-760, 1972

3891
STEFADOUROS, M.A., M.J. DOUGHERTY, W. GROSSMAN, AND E. CRAIGE.
Determination of systemic vascular resistance by a noninvasive technic.
Circulation 47(1):101-107, 1973.

3892
STEFAN, G., AND R.J. BING.
Echocardiographic findings in experimental myocardial infarction of the posterior left ventricular wall.
American Journal Cardiology 30:629-639, 1972.

3893
STEFFEN, V., AND H. FIEHRING.
Drug prophylaxis and treatment of arrhythmia in acute myocardial infarction.
Zeitschrift für Gesamte Innere Medizin 27(20):875-881, 1972.

3894
STEIGER, B.W., A.J. LIBANOFF, AND E.B. SPRINGER.
Myocardial infarction due to paradoxical embolism.
American Journal Medicine 47:995-998, 1969.

3895
STEIN, E., S.I. COHEN, J.I. HAFT, S.H. LAU, ET AL.
Effect of heart rate of left atrial pressure in mitral stenosis.
Clinical Research 15(2):223, 1967.

3896
STEIN, G.
The stress tolerance of the myocardial infarction patient.
Medizinische Klinik 67(24):836-841, 1972.

3897
STEIN, P.D., H.L. BROOKS, J.L. MATSON, AND J.W. HYLAND.
  Effect of propranolol on coronary blood flow.
  Clinical Research 15(2):223, 1967.

3898
STEIN, S.W., AND G.E. ALTMAN.
  Work experience of cardiac patients following referral to a work evaluation unit.
  Circulation 31:497-505, 1965.

3899
STEINBERG, D., AND H.M. KENNER.
  Community programming for hypertension control.
  Southern Medical Bulletin 55(3):101, 1967.

3900
STEINER, S.H., AND J.L. QUINN, III.
  Cardiovascular hemodynamics.
  Journal American Medical Society 204(8):742, 1968.

3901
STELMASIAK, M., AND J. OSEMLAK.
  Relations of the coronary arteries and areas of the heart supplied by them in man.
  Folia Morphologica 31(4):515-526, 1972.

3902
STENBERG, J., R. SANNERSTEDT, AND L. WERKO.
  Haemodynamic studies on the antihypertensive effect of guancydine.
  European Journal Clinical Pharmacology 3(2):63-67, 1971.

3903
STEPHENS, W.B.
  Post-myocardial infarction pain in a series of male patients in the Albury-Wodonga district.
  Medical Journal Australia 57-2(11):492-494, 1970.

3904
STEPIAN, A., AND E. BUCZYNSKI.
  Comparative studies on content of lipofuscin in the heart.
  Patologia Polska 23(4):451-459, 1972.

3905
STERN, A.
  The molecular mechanism of cardiac glycoside action.
  American Heart Journal 83(5):712-715, 1972.

3906
STERN, M., S. SONNENBERG, AND R.P. LIBERMAN.
  A profile for rating depressive and schizoprenic behavior.
  Comprehensive Psychiatry 13:925, 1972.

3907
STERN, M.J.
  Training nurses to be therapists on a psychiatric inpatient service.
  Hospital Community Psychiatry 23:218, 1972.

3908
STERN, S., AND D. TZIVONI.
Dynamic changes in the ST-T segment during sleep in ischemic heart disease.
American Journal Cardiology 32:17, 1973.

3909
STERNBACH, R.A.
Psychophysiological bases of psychosomatic phenomena.
Psychosomatics 7:81-84, 1966.

3910
STEWART, I. McD. G.
Long-term observations on high blood-pressure presenting in fit young men.
Lancet 1:355-358, 1971.

3911
STICKNEY, J.L.
The effect of reserpine and d,1-propranolol on digitalis-induced arrhythmias.
Archives Internationales de Pharmacodynamie et de Therapie 201(2):368-380, 1973.

3912
STIJNS, H.J.
Some data about physical rehabilitation of 134 patients with uncomplicated acute myocardial infarction.
Tijdschrift voor Geneeskunde 28(4):347-353, 1972.

3913
STILLE, W.
Successful long-term therapy of an enterococci-endocarditis with doxycycline.
Medizinische Welt 15:885-887, 1969.

3914
STOCK, E.
The present status of the exercise electrocardiogram.
Medical Journal Australia 2(19):867, 1967.

3915
STOCK, E.
Myocardial infarction in Fiji.
Medical Journal Australia 2(22):1026-1027, 1973.

3916
STOCKSMEIER, U.
Contributions to the problem of psychosocial stress.
Therapiewoche 23:37-40, 1973.

3917
STOCKSMEIER, U.
Automatic interpretation of rest and exercise ECG.
Munich, West Germany. Urban und Schwarzenberg, 1973.

3918
STOCKSMEIER, U., AND M.J. HALHUBER.
The Höhenried longitudinal cross section study of patients with myocardial infarction. The problem, methods, provisional results. Preliminary communication.
Münchener Medizinische Wochenschrift 114(31):1349-1354, 1972.

3919
STOEDEFALKE, K.G.
The principles of conducting exercise programs.
In: Naughton, J.P., H.K. Hellerstein, and I.C. Mohler, Eds. Exercise testing and exercise training in coronary heart disease, pp. 299-305, New York, Academic Press, 1973.

3920
STOEDEFALKE, K.G.
The physical educator's role in exercise programs.
In: Naughton, J.P., H.K. Hellerstein, and I.C. Mohler, Eds. Exercise testing and exercise training in coronary heart disease, pp. 404-407. New York, Academic Press, 1973.

3921
STONE, J.R., AND R.H. MARTIN.
Bloody pericardial fluid or intracardiac blood? A method for quick and accurate differentiation.
Annals Internal Medicine 77(4):592-594, 1972.

3922
STONE, M.C., AND T.B.S. DICK.
Prevalence of hyperlipoproteinaemias in a random sample of men and in patients with ischaemic heart disease.
British Heart Journal 35:954-961, 1973.

3923
STONE, N., M.D. KLEIN, AND B. LOWN.
Diphenylhydantoin in the prevention of recurring ventricular tachycardia.
Circulation 43:420-427, 1971.

3924
STONE, N.J., AND R.I. LEVY.
The hyperlipidemias and coronary artery disease.
Disease-a-Month 8:1, 1972.

3925
STORSTEIN, L.
LB-46, a new beta-adrenergic receptor blocking agent in cardiac arrhythmias.
Acta Medica Scandinavica 191:423-428, 1972.

3926
STORSTEIN, L., AND H. EIE.
Latent coronary insufficiency in young athletes.
Acta Medica Scandinavica 193:525, 1973.

3927
STOUDENMIRE, J.
Effects of muscle relaxation training on state and trait anxiety in introverts and extraverts.
Journal Personality Social Psychology 24(2):273-275, 1972.

3928
STOVEL, S., G. BAILEY, AND G.R. CUMMING.
   Endurance fitness and a home exercise program in college girls.
   Canadian Medical Association Journal 102:715-717, 1970.

3929
STOWERS, M., AND D. SHORT.
   Warning symptoms before major myocardial infarction.
   British Heart Journal 32(6):833-838, 1970.

3930
STRANDELL, T.
   Electrocardiographic findings at rest, during and after exercise in healthy old men compared with
   young men.
   Acta Medica Scandinavica 174:479-499, 1963.

3931
STRANDELL, T.
   Circulatory studies on healthy old men.
   Acta Medica Scandinavica (Suppl.)414:1, 1964.

3932
STRANDELL, T., AND J. WAHREN.
   Circulation in the calf at rest, after arterial occlusion and after exercise in normal subjects and in
   patients with intermittent claudication.
   Acta Medica Scandinavica 173(1):99-105, 1963.

3933
STRANDNESS, D.E.
   Exercise testing in the evaluation of patients undergoing direct arterial surgery.
   Journal Cardiovascular Surgery 11(3):192-200, 1970.

3934
STRASER, T., AND V. GODIC.
   Overprotection: a negative factor in cardiovascular rehabilitation.
   Srpski Arhiv za Celokupno Lekarstvo 96:517-520, 1968.

3935
STRASSER, T.
   Atherosclerosis and coronary heart disease: The contribution of epidemiology.
   World Health Organization Chronicle 26(11):7-11, 1972.

3936
STRAUBE, K.H.
   On rehabilitation of patients with heart and circulatory diseases.
   Zeitschrift für Aerztliche Fortbildung (Jena) 59:828-832, 1965.

3937
STRAUSS, H.C., A.L. SAROFF, J.T. BIGGER, JR., AND E.G.V. GIARDINA.
   Premature atrial stimulation as a key to the understanding of sinoatrial conduction in man.
   Presentation of data and critical review of the literature.
   Circulation 47(1):86-93, 1973.

3938
STRONG, J.A., AND R.W.D. TURNER.
   Radio-iodine in the management of refractory cardiac pain.
   Quarterly Journal Medicine 31(122): 221-233, 1962.

3939
STRUNGE, P., AND A.F. TROSTMANN.
   The lipoprotein pattern in a Danish family. Children and adolescents.
   Acta Medica Scandinavica 192(4):331-335, 1972.

3940
STUCKE, K., V. FISCHER, H. FELDMEIER, AND L. HENN.
   Promotion of training levels by addition of highly concentrated protein.
   Münchener Medizinische Wochenschrift 114:496-503, 1972.

3941
STUCHLIKOVÁ, E.
   Infarction of the myocardium from the viewpoint of lipid metabolism.
   Protectio Vitae 16(2):68-69, 1971.

3942
STUCKEY, J.G.
   Arrhythmias in prehospital phase of acute myocardial infarction.
   Medical Journal Australia 2(1):29-32, 1973.

3943
SUCK, A.F., ET AL.
   Identification of essential hypertension in patients with labile blood pressures.
   Chest 59:402-406, 1971.

3944
SUGIKI, K., AND J. WADA.
   Studies on three cases of Wolff-Parkinson-White syndrome using the recording technique of His
   bundle electrograms.
   Japanese Circulation Journal 37:181, 1973.

3945
SUGIMOTO, T., AND T. ISHIKAWA.
   Effects of antianginal medication on hemoglobin affinity for oxygen.
   American Heart Journal 84(4):570-571, 1972.

3946
SUGIMOTO, T., S.F. SCHAAL, AND A.G. WALLACE.
   Mechanism of ventricular fibrillation produced by 60 CPS stimulation.
   Clinical Research 15(2):223, 1967.

3947
SUGIURA, M., AND R. OKADA.
   A clinicopathological study on the natural history of myocardial infarction in the aged.
   Japanese Circulation Journal 36(1):2-5, 1972.

3948
SUKHUPRAGARN, S.
   Normal central venous pressure.
   Asian Journal Medicine 8(6):244-246, 1972.

3949
SUMA, K., M. HORI, T. TOYODA, Y. FUJIMORI, ET AL.
The control of heart rate—pacemaker and paired pulse stimulation.
Japanese Circulation Journal 31(1):116-117, 1967.

3950
SUMNER, D.S., AND D.E. STRANDNESS, JR.
The effect of exercise on resistance to blood flow with an occluded superficial femoral artery.
Vascular Surgery 4(4):229-237, 1970.

3951
SUNDSTROM, C.
The relevance of work play theory to human adaptation. The physiological aspects of work and play.
American Journal Occupational Therapy 26(4):173-185, 1972.

3952
SURAWICZ, B.
Clinical management of ventricular arrhythmias.
In: Brest, A.N. and J.H. Moyer, Eds. Cardiovascular Drug Therapy: The eleventh Hahnemann symposium, pp. 512-521. New York, Grune and Stratton, 1965.

3953
SURAWICZ, B.
Evaluation of treatment of acute myocardial infarction with potassium, glucose and insulin.
Progress Cardiovascular Diseases 10:545, 1968.

3954
SURAWICZ, B., AND L.S. GETTES.
Effect of electrolyte abnormalities on the heart and circulation.
In: Conn, H.L., and O. Horwitz, Eds. Cardiac and vascular disease. pp. 539-576. Philadelphia, Lea and Febiger, 1971.

3955
SUREK, C., W. SZIEGOLEIT, AND W. FOERSTER.
Relationships between cardiac infarction morbidity and occupational activity in an industrial city.
Deutsche Gesundheitswesen 27:2212-2215, 1972.

3956
SUTTER, J.M., R. GERARD, H. LUCCIONI, J.C. SCOTTO, AND P. GUIN.
Psychosomatic study of 48 cases of cardiac dysrhythmia.
Presse Médicale 76(33):1639, 1968.

3957
SUTTON, J.R.
Exercise and the treatment of coronary heart disease.
Medical Journal Australia 55(1):98, 1968.

3958
SUY, R., AND J. PIESSENS.
Selective coronary angiography.
Medikon 2:287, 1973.

3959
SUZMAN, M.M.
Diagnostic significance of posture, hyperventilation, exercise and beta-adrenergic blockade in the differentiation of anxiety induced from ischemic cardiac disorders.
Circulation 34(4 Suppl.III):225, 1966.

3960
SUZUKI, N.
Studies on the prognosis and rehabilitation of the myocardial infarction from the viewpoint of collateral circulation.
Japanese Circulation Journal 31:1588-1593, 1967.

3961
SVEDBERG, B.
Group discussion in a rehabilitative workshop. A way to coresponsibility, participation in decision making and increase in job satisfaction.
Social-Medicinsk Tidskrift 49(1):30-34, 1972.

3962
SVEHLA, C.
Fibrinolytic activity in patients with acute myocardial infarction.
American Journal Clinical Pathology 59:120-121, 1973.

3963
SVIRIDOV, A.M., AND V.G. NIKITINA.
Therapeutic and prophylactic domiciliar application of anticoagulants.
Sovetskaya Meditsina 31(6):103-107, 1968.

3964
SWAN, H.J.C., J.S. FORRESTER, R. DANZIG, AND H.N. ALLEN.
Power failure in acute myocardial infarction.
Progress Cardiovascular Diseases 12(6):568-600, 1970.

3965
SWANICK, E.J., F. LaCAMERA. JR., AND H.J.L. MARRIOTT.
Morphologic features of right ventricular ectopic beats.
American Journal Cardiology 39(8):888-891, 1972.

3966
SWANSON, M., L. CACACE, G. CHUN, AND M. ITANO.
Saliva calcium and potassium concentrations in the detection of digitalis toxicity.
Circulation 47:736-743, 1973.

3967
SWEATMAN, T., A. SELZER, M. KAMAGAKI, AND K. COHN.
Echocardiographic diagnosis of mitral regurgitation due to ruptured chordae tendineae.
Circulation 46(3):580-586, 1972.

3968
SWITZER, M.E.
Prospects in vocational rehabilitation.
Journal Rehabilitation 32:104, 1966.

3969
SYCHEVA, A.N.
Dynamics of the indices for the coagulation and anticoagulation systems of the blood in patients with coronary atherosclerosis owing to a diet containing sea products.
Voprosy Pitania 26(1):45-49, 1967.

3970
SYED, S.A., A.S. ABBASI, M.A. BEG, AND M.Z. KHAN.
Accomplishment and method of cardiac evaluation and rehabilitation in Pakistan.
In: Plavšić, C. and M.M. Gertler, Eds. The first international biennial conference on cardiac rehabilitation, Dubrovnik, Yugoslavia, 1969.

3971
SYME, S.L.
Psychological factors and coronary heart disease.
International Journal Psychiatry 5:429-435, 1968.

3972
SYME, S.L.
Stress and coronary heart disease.
Postgraduate Medicine 48(1):123-127, 1970.

3973
SYMES, J.F., I.M.F. ARNOLD, AND P.E. BLUNDELL.
Early revascularization of the acute myocardial infarction: The critical time factor.
Canadian Journal Surgery 16:275, 1973.

3974
SYMES, J.M., AND D.G. EADIE.
Solitary arteriosclerotic aneurysm of the profunda femoris artery.
Journal Cardiovascular Surgery 14:220, 1973.

3975
SYRKIN, A.L., I.N. IVANITSKAYA, V.L. UTKIN, AND A.I. STUKLOV.
A study of cardiodynamics in patients with cardiovascular pathology during physical exercise.
Kardiologiya 13:101-106, 1973.

3976
SZEKERES, L., E. UDVARY, AND J.G. PAPP.
Some cardiac metabolic and haemodynamic alterations due to adrenergic beta receptor blockade.
Acta Biologica et Medica Germanica 28(6):1031-1039, 1972.

3977
SZENT-GYORGYI, N.
Blood pressure studies among American and foreign-born students.
Circulation 14:17-24, 1956.

3978
SZEPLAKI, S.
Stress phonocardiography.
Münchener Medizinische Wochenschrift 110:1420-1429, 1968.

3979
SZEPLAKI, S., E. BOSZORMENYI, AND Z. SZEBLAKI.
ECG model for the evaluation of ST-segment and T-wave changes in Ashman's physiological ECG types.
Cor Vasa 12(3):215-229, 1970.

3980
SZEPLAKI, S., J. SZMANDRA, AND Z. SZEPLAKI.
Lidocaine treatment in coronary ischemia and angina pectoris.
Münchener Medizinische Wochenschrift 114:1997, 1972.

3981
SZMIDT, M., J. ROZNIECKI, AND H. RELIGA.
Hemorrhagic diathesis in a patient with obliterative atherosclerosis during treatment with low molecular dextran.
Polski Tygodnik Lekarski 27(40):1566-1568, 1972.

3982
TABAK, V.Y., AND V.D. ZHUKOVSKY.
The use of electroanaesthesia with interferential currents in electroimpulse treatment of cardiac arrhythmias.
Eksperimetnal'naya Khirurgia i Anesteziologiya 17(6):56-58, 1972.

3983
TABAKIN, B.S., J.S. HANSON, AND A.M. LEVY.
Effects of physical training on the cardiovascular and respiratory response to graded upright exercise in distance runners.
British Heart Journal 27:205-210, 1965.

3984
TACKER, W.A., JR., N.B. HARBOLD, JR., E.R. GIULIANI, AND R.B. WALLACE.
Nocturnal angina pectoris with disease of a single coronary artery.
Journal American Medical Association 221(13):1509-1511,1972.

3985
TAEGERT, J.
Conclusions from a cross-sectional comparison of healthy persons and persons with circulatory diseases for longitudinal epidemiological studies.
Zeitschrift für Kreislaufforschung 59(8):744-756, 1970.

3986
TAGGART, P., M. CARRUTHERS, AND W. SOMERVILLE.
Electrocardiogram, plasma catecholamines and lipids, and their modification by oxprenolol when speaking before an audience.
Lancet 2:341, 1973.

3987
TAJIK, A.J., E.R. GIULIANI, R.L. FRYE, ET AL.
Muscular subaortic stenosis associated with complete heart block.
American Journal Cardiology 31(1):101-104, 1973.

3988
TAKAGI, K.
Clinical study on hemodynamic effects of exercise.
Japanese Circulation Journal 30(9):1213-1236, 1966.

3989
TAKAGI, M., S. ICHINOSE, D. ASHIDA, AND R. TANAKA.
Subthreshold chest wall stimulation in the management of digitalis intoxication in patients wearing ventricular inhibited demand pacemaker.
Japanese Circulation Journal 36(8):779-783, 1972.

3990
TAKAHASHI, H., T. IWATSUKA, I. OHASHI, AND S. HOTTA.
Some observations of the ST depression in the exercise electrocardiogram.
Japanese Heart Journal 4(2):105-117, 1963.

3991
TAKARO, T., H.N. HULTGREN, D. LITTMAN, AND E.C. WRIGHT.
An analysis of deaths occurring in association with coronary arteriography.
American Heart Journal 86:587-597, 1973.

3992
TAKEUCHI, M.
Rehabilitation of patients with myocardial infarction.
Japanese Circulation Journal 31:1594-1598, 1967.

3993
TAKEZAWA, H., AND H. TAKASAKI.
Effect of exercise on hemodynamic parameters in mitral valvular disease: Evaluation and clinical significance.
Israel Journal Medical Sciences 5(4):876-878, 1969.

3994
TAKKUNEN, J., E. HUHTI, O. OILINKI, U. VUOPALA, AND W.J. KAIPAINEN.
Early ambulation in myocardial infarction.
Acta Medica Scandinavica 188(1/2):103-106, 1970.

3995
TAKKUNEN, J., O. OILINKI, E. HUHTI, ET AL.
Medical treatment and mortality in cardiogenic shock. Metaraminol compared with combined phentolamine and norepinephrine. Glucagon therapy.
Acta Medica Scandinavica 192(3):165-170, 1972.

3996
TALBOT, S.A., I. LIKAR, AND W.K. HARRISON, JR.
Exercise escalator for electrocardiographic studies in patients with coronary heart disease.
American Heart Journal 72(1):35-37, 1966.

3997
TALLURY, V.K., N.P. DePASQUALE, M.S. BRUNO, AND A.C. NODY.
Migration of retained transvenous electrode catheter.
Archives Internal Medicine 130(3):390-391, 1972.

3998
TALMON, J.L., G. VAN HERPEN, AND J.H. VAN BEMMEL.
Diagnostic methods.
Progress Report Medicophysical Institute TNO 3:176, 1972.

3999
TANGCHAI, P.
   Atherosclerosis and coronary heart disease in Thailand.
   Journal Medical Association Thailand 55(4):225-227, 1972.

4000
TARJAN, J., M. BROLLY, Z. BALOGH, AND J. CZOPF.
   Ballistocardiographic ice test.
   Magyar Belorvosi Archivum 25(3):150-155, 1972.

4001
TASKAR, P.K., AND N. SENECAL.
   Quebec beer-drinkers' cardiomyopathy: Dietary assesment of patients.
   Canadian Medical Association Journal 97(5):924-925, 1967.

4002
TATSUMI, S.
   Clinical study of cardiac asthma.
   Japanese Circulation Journal 31(8):1211-1226, 1967.

4003
TATTERSFIELD, A.E., M.W. MCNICOL, AND R.W. SILLETT.
   Relationship between haemodynamic and respiratory function in patients with myocardial infarction and left ventricular failure.
   Clinical Science 42(6):751-768, 1972.

4004
TAWAKKOL, A., R.A. MASSUMI, J.C. RIOS, R.K. SARIN, AND A. ROSS.
   True relationship of right and left atrial depolarization in determining the origin of abnormal P waves.
   Circulation 35-36(Suppl. 2):248, 1967.

4005
TAYLOR, A.W., R. LAPPAGE, AND S. RAO.
   Skeletal muscle glycogen stores after submaximal and maximal work.
   Medicine Science Sports 3:75-78, 1971.

4006
TAYLOR, A.W., R. THAYER, AND S. RAO.
   Human skeletal muscle glycogen synthetase activities with exercise and training.
   Canadian Journal Physiology Pharmacology 50:411-415, 1972.

4007
TAYLOR, D.J.E., AND P.G.F. NIXON.
   Assessment of left ventricular function after myocardial infarction.
   British Heart Journal 34(9):905-910, 1972.

4008
TAYLOR, H.L.
   Relationship of physical activity to serum cholesterol concentration.
   In: Rosenbaum, F. and E. Balknap, Eds. Work and the heart, p. 111. New York, Hoeber, 1959.

4009
TAYLOR, H.L.
   Occupational factors in the study of coronary heart disease and physical activity.
   Canadian Medical Association Journal 96:825-831, 1967.

4010
TAYLOR, H.L.
   The effect of rest in bed and of exercise on cardiovascular function.
   Circulation 38:1016, 1968.

4011
TAYLOR, H.L., H. BLACKBURN, AND A. KEYS.
   Coronary heart disease in seven countries. 5 year follow-up of employers of selected U.S. railroad companies.
   Circulation 41(Suppl. 1):20-39, 1970.

4012
TAYLOR, H.L., H. BLACKBURN, T. PUCHNER, C.L. VASQUEZ, R.W. PARLIN, AND A. KEYS.
   Coronary heart disease in selected occupations of American railroads in relation to physical activity.
   Circulation 39-40 (Suppl. 3):202, 1969.

4013
TAYLOR, H.L., E. BUSKIRK, AND A. HENSCHEL.
   Maximal oxygen intake as an objective measure of cardio-respiratory performance.
   Journal Applied Physiology 8:73-80, 1955.

4014
TAYLOR, H.L., ET AL.
   Exercise and cardiovascular disease. A review.
   National Conference Cardiovascular Diseases 2:358, 1964.

4015
TAYLOR, H.L., W.L. HASKELL, S.M. FOX, III, AND H. BLACKBURN.
   Exercise tests: A summary of procedures and concepts of stress testing for cardiovascular diagnostic and function evaluation.
   In: Blackburn, H., Ed. Measurement in exercise electrocardiography, pp. 259-305. Springfield, Ill. Thomas, 1969.

4016
TAYLOR, H.L., E. KLEPETAR, A. KEYS, R.W. PARLIN, ET AL.
   Death rates among physically active and sedentary employees of the railroad industry.
   American Journal Public Health 52:1967, 1962.

4017
TAYLOR, H.L., Y. WANG, L. ROWELL, AND G. BLOMQUIST.
   The standardization and interpretation of submaximal and maximal tests of working capacity.
   Pediatrics 32(Part II):703, 1963.

4018
TAYLOR, J.L.
   Life assurance after myocardial infarction.
   South African Medical Journal 42:890-892, 1968.

4019

TAYLOR, J.O., C.F. LANDERS, D. CHULAY, W.B. HOOD, JR., AND W.H. ABELMANN.
Monitoring high-risk cardiac patients during transportation in hospital.
Lancet 2:1205-1208, 1970.

4020

TAYLOR, R.R., AND B.E. HOPKINS.
Influence of respiration and respiratory sinus arrhythmia on aortic regurgitation.
American Journal Physiology 223(3):668-672, 1972.

4021

TAYLOR, W.J., R. POCELINKO, AND W.B. ABRAMS.
Divergent responses to a chemical and to a thermal challenge both of which presumably mediate catecholamine release.
Clinical Research 15(4):453, 1967.

4022

TECTOR, A.J., C.F. REUBEN, J.F. HOFFMAN, E.T. GELFAND, ET AL.
Coronary artery wounds treated with bypass grafts.
Journal American Medical Association 225:282, 1973.

4023

TEICHMANN, W.
Myocardial infarction in the follow-up course of treatment.
Münchener Medizinishe Wochenschrift 113(11): 374-379, 1971.

4024

TEJERINA, R.M.
Evaluation and importance of continuous monitoring of heart activity with the electrocardiographic system "Avionics" at high altitudes.
Revista Española de Cardiologia 23(4):532-542, 1970.

4025

TEMKIN, L.P., S. WOLFSON, AND L.S. COHEN.
Dynamic (DYN) and isometric handgrip (IHG) exercise effects on systolic time intervals (STI) in normals and patients with coronary artery disease (CAD).
Clinical Research 20(3):400, 1972.

4026

TEMPLER, D.I.
Death anxiety in religiously very involved persons.
Psychological Reports 31:361-362, 1972.

4027

TERASAWA, F., M. KURAMOCHI, H. YAMAGUCHI, ET AL.
Clinical and pathological studies on incomplete left bundle branch block in the aged.
Acta Gerontologica Japonica 52:79-95, 1970.

4028

TERASAWA, F., S. MATSUSHITA, K. KURAMOTO, AND M. SEKI.
An autopsied case of myocardial infarction in the presence of incomplete left bundle branch block diagnosed because of ventricular premature beats.
Acta Gerontologica Japonica 52:73-78, 1970.

4029
TERJUNG, R.T., ET AL.
   Cardiovascular adaptation to 12 minutes of mild daily exercise in middle-aged sedentary men.
   Journal American Geratrics Society 21(4):164, 1973.

4030
TERRY, G., C.W. VELLANI, M.R. HIGGINS, AND A. DOIG.
   Bretylium tosylate in treatment of refractory ventricular arrhythmias complicating myocardial
   infarction.
   British Heart Journal 32:21-25, 1970.

4031
TEUNS, J.P.
   Reactive behavior of heart patients and of their families.
   Nederlands Tijdschrift voor Geneeskunde 109:448-449, 1965.

4032
TEYSSANDIER, M.J.
   Cardiovascular apparatus and physical training.
   Maroc Médical 43:987-994, 1964.

4033
THANABALSUNDRAM, R.S.
   Evaluation of anti-coagulants in myocardial infarction.
   Ceylon Medical Journal 13(2):77-79, 1968.

4034
THEORELL, T.
   Psycho-social factors prior to myocardial infarction.
   Opuscula Medica 16(7):247-250, 1971.

4035
THEORELL, T.
   Psychosocial factors and myocardial infarction. Why and how.
   In: Early diagnosis of coronary heart disease; Proceedings of the second Paavo Nurmi symposium,
   Porvoo, Finland, 1971, pp. 117-131. Basel, Switzerland. S. Karger, 1973.

4036
THEORELL, T., E. LIND, J. FROBERG, ET AL.
   A longitudinal study of 21 subjects with coronary heart disease: Life changes, catecholamine
   excretion and related biochemical reactions.
   Psychosomatic Medicine 34:505-516, 1972.

4037
THEORELL, T., AND R. RAHE.
   Time-relationship of psychosocial factors to myocardial infarction: A principle of systematic
   research.
   Nordisk Medicin 84(27):850-857, 1970.

4038
THEORELL, T., AND R.H. RAHE.
   Psychosocial factors and myocardial infarction. I. An inpatient study in Sweden.
   Journal Psychosomatic Research 15:25-31, 1971.

4039
THEORELL, T., AND R.H. RAHE.
Behavior and life satisfactions characteristics of Swedish subjects with myocardial infarction.
Journal Chronic Diseases 25(3):139-147, 1972.

4040
THEORELL, T., AND P.O. WESTER.
The significance of psychological events in a coronary care unit. Preliminary report.
Acta Medica Scandinavica 193:207-210, 1973.

4041
THIEDE, A., J. SCHAEFER, H. MULLER-WIEFEL, A. KRUG, ET AL.
Surgical therapy of a defect of the ventricular septum and of an aneurysm of the ventricular front wall after myocardial infarction.
Thoraxchirurgie 19:145-149, 1971.

4042
THIEL, H.G., D. PARKER, AND T.A. BRUCE.
Stress factors and the risk of myocardial infarction.
Journal Psychosomatic Research 17(1):43-57, 1973.

4043
THIRLWELL, M.P., AND T.T. ZSOTER.
The effect of propranolol and atropine on venomotor reflexes in man.
Journal Medicine (Basel) 3:65, 1972.

4044
THOCKLOTH, R.Mc., S.C. HO, H. WRIGHT, AND W.A. SELDON.
Is cardiac rehabilitation really necessary?
Medical Journal Australia 2(14):669, 1973.

4045
THOM, A.R., AND G.U. HOWE.
The dental status of cardiac patients.
British Heart Journal 34(12):1302-1307, 1972.

4046
THOMAS, C.
Psychological aspects of blood pressure regulation.
Pyschosomatic Medicine 26:454-480, 1964.

4047
THOMAS, C.B., AND E.A. MURPHY.
Further studies on cholesterol levels in the Johns Hopkins medical students. Effect of stress at examinations.
Journal Chronic Diseases 8:661, 1958.

4048
THOMAS, H.D., B. BOSHELL, C. GAOS, AND T.J. REEVES.
Cardiac output during exercise and anaerobic metabolism in man.
Journal Applied Physiology 19(5):383-848, 1964.

4049
THOMAS, H.V.
Hypertension, millions of Americans don't know they have it.
California Health 30:1-3, 1973.

4050
THOMAS, M.
Haemodynamics after acute myocardial infarction.
Schweizerische Medizinische Wochenschrift 102:1818, 1972.

4051
THOMAS, R.M., E. MYLON, AND M.C. WINTERNITZ.
Myocardial lesions resulting from dietary deficiency.
Yale Journal Biological Medicine 12:345, 1940.

4052
THOMPSON, D.F.J.
The ElectroCardioAnalyzer. Preventive Techniques for the Modern Community.
The Chest and Heart Association. London, England. 1971.

4053
THOMPSON, J.I.
Exercise as treatment in coronary heart disease.
Minnesota Medicine 55(4):381, 1972.

4054
THOMPSON, M.
"Re-creation" for the coronary patient.
Journal Rehabilitation 32:84, 1966.

4055
THOMPSON, P.L., H.R. JENZER, B. LOWN, AND L.A. LOHRBAUE.
Exercise during acute myocardial infarction—experimental study.
Cardiovascular Research 7(5):642-648, 1973.

4056
THOMPSON, W.M., JR., J.R. NIDA, AND H.D. RILEY, JR.
Electrocardiographic findings in adolescents at rest and at maximal exertion.
Pediatrics 43(3):438-442, 1969.

4057
THORPE, P.
Pindolol (Visken) and angina pectoris: A double blind multicentre trial.
New Zealand Medical Journal 76:171-173, 1972.

4058
THORNTON, J.V.
Compensable heart disease.
Journal Occupational Medicine 5:476, 1963.

4059

THUMALA, A., K.E. HAMMERMEISTER, W.B. CAMPBELL, B. POMERANTZ, H. OVERY, AND H. DAVIES.
Hemodynamic studies with sotalol in man, performed at rest, during exercise and during right ventricular pacing.
American Heart Journal 82:439-447, 1971.

4060

TIBBLIN, G.
A population study of 50-year-old men. An analysis of the nonparticipation group.
Acta Medica Scandinavica 178(4):453-459, 1965.

4061

TIBBLIN, G., S.E. BERGENTZ, J. BJURE, AND L. WILHELMSEN.
Hematocrit, plasma protein, plasma volume, and viscosity in early hypertensive disease.
American Heart Journal 72(2):165-176, 1966.

4062

TIBBLIN, G., B. LINDSTROM, AND S. ANDER.
Emotions and heart disease.
In: Porter, R. and J. Knight, Eds. Ciba Foundation Symposium, No. 8 Physiology, emotion and psychosomatic illness, London, England, April 18-20, 1972, pp. 321-336. New York, American Elsevier, 1972.

4063

TIBELL, B.
Peripheral arterial insufficiency. An epidemiological study of 2,243 hospital admissions caused by arteriosclerosis obliterans, diabetes mellitus, thrombangitis obliterans and arterial embolism.
Acta Orthopaedica Scandinavica (Suppl.)139:1, 1971.

4064

TIEDT, N., B. WOHLGEMUTH, AND P. WOHLGEMUTH.
Dynamics of heart rate behavior and appraisal of performance in sinusoid modifications of stress.
Medizin und Sport 12(7):208-213, 1972.

4065

TILIAGOS, M.R.
The influence of cigarette smoking on the coronary vessels.
Nosokomejaka Chronika 34(4):356-364, 1972.

4066

TILLMAN, K.
Relationship between physical fitness and selected personality traits.
Research Quarterly American Association for Health, Physical Education Recreation 36:483-489, 1965.

4067

TILLOTSON, J.L., H. KATO, M.Z. NICHAMAN, D.C. MILLER, M.L. GAY, K.J. JOHNSON, AND G.G. RHOADS.
Epidemiology of coronary heart disease and stroke in Japanese men living in Japan, Hawaii, and California: Methodology for comparison of diet.
American Journal Clinical Nutrition 26:177-184, 1973.

4068
TING, N., Y.B. LI, B.N. CHIANG, E.R. ALEXANDER, AND R.A. BRUCE.
Significance of maximal exercise ST responses in middle-aged Chinese men.
Israel Journal Medical Sciences 5(4):691-695, 1973.

4069
TIPTON, C.M., AND R.J. BARNARD.
Alactacid debt.
In: Balke, B., Ed. Physiological aspects of sports and physical fitness, p. 26. The Athletic Institue, 1968.

4070
TITUS, J.L.
Symposium cardiac arrhythmias, (Part I). Anatomy of the conduction system.
Circulation 47:170-177, 1973.

4071
TIWARI, N.M.
Management of cardiac arrhythmias.
Journal Medical Surgery 18(3):85-88, 1968.

4072
TJOE, S.L., AND M.H. LURIA.
Delays in reaching the cardiac care unit: An analysis.
Chest 61(7):617-621, 1972.

4073
TOBIS, J.S.
Safe exercise after myocardial infarction.
Archives Physical Medicine Rehabilitation 50:663-665, 1969.

4074
TOBIS, J.S.
Programs for cardiac rehabilitation.
In: Russek, H., Ed. Advance in coronary heart disease. Philadelphia, Lippincott, 1971.

4075
TOBIS, J.S., AND L.R. ZOHMAN.
A rehabilitation program for inpatients with recent myocardial infarction.
Archives Physical Medicine Rehabilitation 49(8):443-448, 1968.

4076
TOBIS, J.S., AND L.R. ZOHMAN.
Follow-up study of cardiac patients on a rehabilitation service.
Archives Physical Medicine Rehabilitation 51:286, 1970.

4077
TOBIS, J.S., AND L.R. ZOHMAN.
Rehabilitating the coronary patient.
Postgraduate Medicine 47(2):139-145, 1970.

4078

TODD, J.W.

Psychological hazards of convalescence after myocardial infarction.
Lancet 1:1305, 1971.

4079

TOFLER, O.B., K.A. ROLLO, B.M. SAKER, AND M.J. BURVILL.

A modified oxygen debt test.
In: Eliakim, M., and H.N. Neufeld, Eds. Cardiology, current topics and progress, pp. 157-161. New York, Academic Press, 1969.

4080

TOMASZEWSKI, J., J. MANZLIK, J. LOPATYNSKI, AND B. GILATOWSKA.

Studies on the chemical composition of vascular wall. XI. Glycosaminoglicans of the wall of human aorta in the process of physiological aging.
Polski Archivum Medycyny Wewnetrznej 47(1):51-59, 1971.

4081

TOMLINSON, C.W., AND N.S. DHALLA.

Excitation-contraction coupling in heart: IX. Changes in the intracellular stores of calcium in failing hearts due to lack of substrate and oxygen.
Cardiovascular Research 7:470, 1973.

4082

TOMMASIS, L. DE, O. SALZANO, AND D. CARUSO.

Statistical study on the behaviour of the electrocardiogram in persons over 70 years of age.
Riforma Medica 87(3):102-115, 1973.

4083

TOMODA, H., L. CHUCK, AND W.W. PARMLEY.

Comparative myocardial depressant effects of lidocaine, ajmalin, propranolol and quinidine.
Japanese Circulation Journal 36(5):433-437, 1972.

4084

TOMOMATSU, T., S. YORIFUJI, K. TANEMOTO, K. SERA, ET AL.

The cardiopulmonary effect of exercise in congestive heart failure.
Japanese Circulation Journal 27(10):720, 1963.

4085

TONNESEN, K.H.

Clinical application of Na^{24}-clearance during standard exercise in chronic arterial thrombosis.
Scandinavian Journal Clinical Laboratory Investigation 15(76):64-65, 1963.

4086

TOONE, W.M.

The management of arteriosclerotic occlusive vascular disease with poor distal run-off.
Angiology 18(7):409-413, 1967.

4087

TOOSHI, A.

Effects of three different durations of endurance exercises upon serum cholesterol.
Medicine Sciences Sports 3(1):1, 1971.

4088
TORKELSON, L.O.
Rehabilitation of the patient with acute myocardial infarction.
Journal Chronic Diseases 17:685-704, 1964.

4089
TORRESANI, J., J.L. AMICHOT, J.P. PICARD, AND A. JOUVE.
Recent acquisitions in electrocardiographic exploration technics of the heart cavities.
Archives des Maladies du Coeur 62:193-209, 1969.

4090
TOSHIMA, H.
Collective statistical study on the survival rates of the patients with myocardial infarction.
Japanese Circulation Journal 31(11):1610-1612, 1967.

4091
TOSO, M., G. CASUCCI, G. RENZINI, ET AL.
Changes of the electrical systole after exercise in normal subjects.
Cuore e Circolazione 50:261-268, 1966.

4092
TOUBAS, P., J. LEBLANC, AND J. BENHAIM.
Congenital atrio-ventricular block and pregnancy.
Coeur et Médecine Interne 12:457, 1973.

4093
TOUBOUL, P., AND M. IBRAHIM.
Atrioventricular conduction defects in patients presenting with syncope and normal PR interval.
British Heart Journal 34(10):1005-1011, 1972.

4094
TOUTOUZAS, P., D. GUPTA, R. SAMSON, AND J. SHILLINGFORD.
Q-second sound interval in acute myocardial infarction.
British Heart Journal 31:462-467, 1969.

4095
TOWNE, W.D., W.P. GEISS, H.O. YANES, AND S.H. RAHIMTOOLA.
Intractable ventricular fibrillation associated with profound accidental hypothermia. Successful treatment with partial cardiopulmonary bypass.
New England Journal Medicine 287(22):1135-1136, 1972.

4096
TRACY, R.E.
Sex difference in coronary disease: Two opposing views.
Journal Chronic Diseases 19:1245-1251, 1966.

4097
TRANGEIZER, V.A.
Dynamic changes of some mineral metabolism indices in patients with coronary atherosclerosis occurring under the effect of dietetic treatment.
Voprosy Pitaniya 26:53-55, 1967.

4098
TRANK, J., R. FETTER, AND R.M. LAUER.
  A spray-on electrode for recording the electrocardiogram during exercise.
  Journal Applied Physiology 24(2):267-268, 1968.

4099
TRAP-JENSEN, J., AND J.P. CLAUSEN.
  Effect of training on the relation of heart rate and blood pressure to the onset of pain in effort
  angina pectoris.
  In: Larsen, O.A., and R.O. Malmborg, Eds. Coronary heart disease and physical fitness, pp.
  111-114. Baltimore, University Park Press, 1971.

4100
TRAUTWEIN, H.
  Rehabilitation of cardiac and circulatory patients.
  Medizinische Welt 46:2447-2455, 1964.

4101
TRAUTWEIN, H.
  The rehabilitation of patients after heart surgery.
  Hippokrates 36:378-384, 1965.

4102
TREISTMAN, B., D.A. COOLEY, R. LUFSCHANOWSKI, AND R.D. LEACHMAN.
  Diverticulum or aneurysm of left ventricle.
  American Journal Cardiology 32:119, 1973.

4103
TREMOLIERES, J.
  Food selection in relation to requirement.
  In: Birch, G.G., L.F. Green, and L.G. Plaskett, Eds. Health and food. Symposium, Surrey,
  England, March 27-28, 1972, pp. 170-181. New York, Halsted Press, 1972.

4104
TRENCKMANN, H.
  Outpatient care of patients with infarcts.
  Zeitschrift für Aerztliche Fortbildung 59:824-826, 1965.

4105
TRENHOLM, B.G., D.A. WINTER, D. MYMIN, AND E.L. LANSDOWN.
  Computer determination of left ventricular volume using videodensitometry.
  Medical Biological Engineering 10:163-173, 1972.

4106
TRICOT, R., C. GUEROT, P.E. VALERE, AND A. COSTE.
  Study of atrioventricular conduction by His bundle recording in 60 cases of atrioventricular block.
  Archives des Maladies du Coeur et des Vaisseaux 65(4):441-463, 1972.

4107
TRIGIANO, L.L.
  Move that cardiac early.
  Pennsylvania Medicine 72(1):52-55, 1969.

4108
TRINCAO, M.
   Concepts on the rehabilitation of cardiac patients.
   Coimbra Medica 16(9):1011-1021, 1969.

4109
TRIPATHY, S.R., AND B.C. SINHA.
   Clinical profile of acute myocardial infarction.
   Indian Medical Forum 23(7):233-238, 1972.

4110
TROSHIKHIN, V.A., AND S.I. MOLDAVSKAYA.
   Effect of automobile driving on the cardiovascular system of the driver according to foreign
   literature.
   Gigiena Truda Professional'nye Zabolevaniya 16:43-44, 1972.

4111
TROWELL, H.
   Crude fibre, dietary fibre and atherosclerosis.
   Atherosclerosis 16(1):138-140, 1972.

4112
TROYER, W.G., C.T. TWENTYMAN, R.J. GATCHEL, AND P.J. LANG.
   Age and ischemic heart disease related effects on biofeedback heart rate training.
   Psychosomatic Medicine 35(5):456, 1973.

4113
TRUETT, J.T., H. BENSON, AND B. BALKE.
   On the practicability of submaximal exercise testing.
   Journal Chronic Diseases 19:711-715, 1966.

4114
TRUJILLO, M.H., A. CASTILLO, E. CAVALLIN, ET AL.
   Analysis of intracavitary electrocardiograms through a saline bridge in the diagnosis of cardiac
   arrhythmias.
   American Heart Journal 84(4):451-455, 1972.

4115
TSE, R.L.
   Daily walking exercise in treatment of (human) intermittent claudication: It Works!!: An appeal
   for more frequent use.
   Angiology 22(1):1-3, 1971.

4116
TSFASMAN, A.Z., G.I. KASSIRSKII, AND A.I. MOZEL.
   Hemodynamics under physical stress in patients with auricular fibrillation after mitral commis-
   surotomy and restoration of the sinus rhythm.
   Kardiologiya 13:42-47, 1973.

4117
TULLOCH, J.A., R.B. KANYEREZI, P.G. D'ARBELA, AND N.K. SOOD.
   Prolonged bed rest in the treatment of idiopathic cardiomegaly.
   Transactions Royal Society Tropical Medicine Hygiene 62(3):362-370, 1968.

4118
TULPULE, T.H., H.M. SHAH, S.J. SHAH, AND H.K. HAVELIWALA.
Yogic exercises in the management of ischaemic heart disease.
Indian Heart Journal 23(4):259-264, 1971.

4119
TUNA, N., G.B. LEE, AND K. AMPLATZ.
The value of vectorcardiography, electrocardiography and exercise electrocardiography in the diagnosis of coronary artery disease. Correlation with coronary arteriography.
In: Proceedings XII, international vectorcardiography symposium, p. 368. Amsterdam, The Netherlands. North Holland, 1971.

4120
TURELL, D.J.
Rehabilitation of the post-coronary patient.
Medical Record Annals 54(10):281, 1961.

4121
TURELL, D.J.
Determining a work prescription for the post-coronary patient.
Medical Record Annals 55(2):36, 1962.

4122
TURELL, D.J.
The cardiac patient returns to work.
American Journal Nursing 65(8):115-117, 1965.

4123
TURELL, D.J., AND H.K. HELLERSTEIN.
Evaluation of cardiac function in relation to specific physical activities following recovery from acute myocardial infarction.
Progress Cardiovascular Diseases 1:2, 1958.

4124
TURELL, D.J., AND H.K. HELLERSTEIN.
The feasibility of employing cardiacs.
The Recorder, Columbia Medical Society, Richland County 23(7):15-23, 1959.

4125
TURKULIN, K.
Ergometry tests.
In: Plavšić, C., and M.M. Gertler, Eds. The first international biennial conference on cardiac rehabilitation, Dubrovnik, Yugoslavia, 1969.

4126
TURNER, R., AND K. BALL.
Prevention of coronary heart disease.
Lancet 2:1137, 1973.

4127
TURNER, R.W.D.
Multipoint electrocardiography.
Lancet 1:1158, 1966.

4128
TURPEINEN, O., M. MIETTINEN, M.J. KARVONEN, P. ROINE, M. PEKKARINEN, E.J. LEHTOSUO, AND P. ALIVIRTA.
Dietary prevention of coronary heart disease. Long-term experiment.
American Journal Clinical Nutrition 21:255, 1968.

4129
TURPEINEN, O., M. MIETTINEN, M.J. KARVONEN, P. ROINE, M. PEKKARINEN, E. J. LEHTOSUO, AND P. ALIVIRTA.
Blood lipids and primary coronary events. The effect of diet modification.
Minnesota Medicine 52(8):1247-1252, 1969.

4130
TURTO, H., AND S. LINDY.
Digitoxin treatment and experimental cardiac hypertrophy.
Cardiovascular Research 7:482, 1973.

4131
TYLKA, J.
Peculiarities in adaptation of elderly people following myocardial infarction.
Polski Tygodnik Lekarski 26:2033-2035, 1971.

4132
TZAGOURNIS, M., J.F. SEIDENSTICKER, AND G.J. HAMWI.
Serum insulin, carbohydrate, and lipid abnormalities in patients with premature coronary heart disease.
Annals Internal Medicine 67:42-47, 1967.

4133
TZANKOFF, S.P., S. ROBINSON, F.S. PYKE, AND C.A. BRAWN.
Physiological adjustments to work in older men as affected by physical training.
Journal Applied Physiology 33:346-350, 1972.

4134
UDALOV, Y.F., N.N. BAKHTADZE, AND B.N. GARASHOV.
Prevention of lipid metabolism disorders in persons working under increased neuroemotional stress.
Gigiena Truda Professional'nye Zabolevaniya 17:54-56, 1973.

4135
UEDA, H., T. SAKAMOTO, Z. UOZUMI, N. KAWAI, ET AL.
Clinical aspects of primary myocardial disease. The diagnostic importance of phonocardiography and mechanocardiography.
Japanese Circulation Journal 31:1921, 1967.

4136
UELAND, K., M.J. NOVY, AND J. METCALFE.
Hemodynamic responses of patients with heart disease to pregnancy and exercise.
American Journal Obstetrics Gynecology 113(1):47-59, 1972.

4137
UGOLEVA, G. YA.
The reactivity of tonus of medium sized blood vessels to moderate muscular exercise in arterial hypertension.
Terapevticheskii Arkhiv 36(10):46-52, 1964.

4138
UHLEY, H.N.
A new simple model for the synthesis of the electrocardiogram.
Circulation 40:173-178, 1969.

4139
ULMER, H.V.
A mathematical criterion for the determination of endurance limit.
Internationale Zeitschrift für Angewandte Physiologie 27:299-310, 1969.

4140
ULMER, H.V., U. ROSKE, AND K. LINK.
Validity of E.A. Muller's LPI in determining the physical fitness of trained and untrained subjects.
Internationale Zeitschrift für Angewandte Physiologie 29:343-358, 1971.

4141
UNDT, W., H. KAROBATH, J. BUCHER, ET AL.
Myocardial infarction. Studies on the influence of weather, season, and periodic environmental factors on the moment of onset of the disease.
Zeitschrift für Angewandte Bäder- und Klimaheilkunde 19(2-3):151-169, 1972.

4142
URBACH, J.R., J.J. GRAUMAN, AND S.H. STRAUS.
Quantitative methods for the recognition of atrioventricular junctional rhythms in atrial fibrillation.
Circulation 39:803-817, 1969.

4143
URBAIN, L.S.
Counseling families of cardiac patients. The many faces of direct service.
California's Health 23(10/11):158-160, 1966.

4144
URSCHEL, C.W., AND E.H. SONNENBLICK.
Determinants of cardiac performance.
In: Kenedi, R.M., Ed. Biomechanics and related bioengineering topics. pp. 303-316. London, England. Pergamon, 1965.

4145
URTHALER, F., J.H. ISOBE, K.E. GILMOUR, AND T.N. JAMES.
Morphine and autonomic control of the sinus node.
Chest 64:203, 1973.

4146
URTHALER, F., C.R. KATHCLI, J. MACY, Jr., AND T.N. JAMES.
Mathematical relationship between automaticity of the sinus node and the AV junction.
American Heart Journal 86:189, 1973.

4147
URUTSKOE, S.N., V.B. USMAN, AND E.S. PROKHORO.
Prevalence of ischemic heart disease and its combination with cerebrovascular affections in age category of 50 to 59 years.
Sovetskaya Meditsina (4):3-7, 1973.

4148
USAMI, M., ET AL.
   The diagnostic evaluation of the "cardiac volume function quotient (Reindell)" in the ergometric exercise test.
   Japanese Circulation Journal 31(1):224, 1967.

4149
UUSITALO, A.J.
   The exercise test as a diagnostic tool.
   Duodecim 88(6):443-450, 1972.

4150
VAILLANT, G.E., AND C.C. McARTHUR.
   What kinds of men do not get psychosomatic illness?
   Psychosomatic Medicine 34:476, 1972.

4151
VAJDA, F.J.E., R.J. PRINEAS, R.R.H. LOVELL, AND J.G. SLOMAN.
   The possible effect of long term high plasma levels of phenytoin on mortality after acute myocardial infarction.
   European Journal Clinical Pharmacology 5(3):138-144, 1973.

4152
VALEK, J.
   Stress and the ischemic heart disease.
   Lekarska Veda v Zahranici 10:194-200, 1967.

4153
VALEK, J., E. KUHN, V. BRODAN, AND J. PECHAR.
   Lipid metabolism and emotional stress in patients with ischemic heart disease.
   Acta Diabetologica 10(2):401, 1973.

4154
VALENZUELA, S., AND A.F. BOWYER.
   Left ventricular (LV) response to graded upright exercise in man.
   Circulation 37-38(Suppl. 6):197, 1968.

4155
VALERO, E.M., R. PESCE, S. DRAJER, ET AL.
   Study of complete auriculoventricular block by recording the potentials of the bundle of His.
   Revista Argentina de Cardiologia 40(3):143-161, 1972.

4156
VALGMA, K.A.
   Factors provoking ischemic disease of the heart.
   Terapevticheskii Arkhiv 44(9):38-40, 1972.

4157
VALLBONA, C.
   Computer analysis of the effects of bedrest on cardiac dynamics.
   In: Symposium on the analysis of central nervous system and cardiovascular data using computer methods, Washington, D.C., 1964, pp. 313-331. Washington, D.C. National Aeronautics Space Administration, 1965. (NASA SP-72).

4158
VALLBONA, C., D. CARDUS, W.A. SPENCER, AND H.E. HOFF.
Patterns of sinus arrhytyhmia in patients with lesions of the central nervous system.
American Journal Cardiology 16:379-389, 1965.

4159
VALLBONA, C., J.D. McCRADY, AND H.E. HOFF.
Neuropharmacological factors influencing the central regulation of the respiratory-heart rate (RHR).
Archives Internationales Pharmacodynamie Therapie 153:256-266, 1965.

4160
VALLBONA, C., W.A. SPENCER, L.A. GEDDES, W.F. BLOSE, AND J. CANZONERI, III.
Experience with on-line monitoring in critical illness.
Proceedings National Telemetering Conference, pp. 189-192, 1966.

4161
VALTONEN, E.J.
Psychic and somatic effects of a physical training programme for myocardial infarction convalescents. A preliminary report.
Europa Medicophysica 7(3):158, 1971.

4162
VALTONEN, E.J., AND H.G. LILIUS.
The significance of synchronization in syncardial massage.
Angiologica 10:124, 1973.

4163
VAN BEMMEL, J.H., AND G. VAN HERPEN.
Critical appraisal of quantitative electrocardiology.
Progress Report Medicophysical Institute TNO 3:150, 1972.

4164
VAN CLEVE, R.B.
The rebound phenomenon. Fact or fancy? Experience with discontinuation of long-term anticoagulation therapy after myocardial infarction.
Circulation 32:878-880, 1965.

4165
VAN CLEVE, R.B.
Letting go of the bear's tail. Experience with discontinuation of long-term anticoagulant therapy.
Journal American Medical Association 196(13):1156-1158, 1966.

4166
VANDENBROUCKE, G.
Program of physical readaptation in myocardial infarction.
Revue de Réadaptation 13:86, 1971.

4167
VANDENBROUCKE, G., AND L. BRASSEUR.
A program of physical rehabilitation following myocardial infarction and angina.
Cahiers de Kinesitherapie 42:613-622, 1972.

4168
VAN DER MEER, J.J., AND R.S. RENEMAN.
An improved technique to induce a standardized functional stenosis of a coronary artery.
European Surgical Research 4(6):407-418, 1972.

4169
VANDERMOTEN, P., R. MESSIN, S. DEGRÉ, AND H. DENOLIN.
Interpretation of blood pressure in ergometry.
Malatti Cardiovascolari 10:207-226, 1969.

4170
VAN DER VALK, J.M., AND J.J. GROEN.
Personality structure and conflict situation in patients with myocardial infarction.
Journal Psychosomatic Research 11:41-46, 1967.

4171
VANDERVORT, P.G., AND W.E. PERRIN.
A programmed course in electrocardiography.
Journal American Osteopathic Association 68:255-259, 1968.

4172
VAN DER TWEEL, L.H., F.L. MEIJLER, AND F.J.L. VAN CAPELLE.
Synchronization of the heart.
Journal Applied Physiology 34(2):283-287, 1973.

4173
VAN DIJL, H.
Test behaviour differences between asthmatics and myocardial infarction patients on a self-evaluation test.
Journal Psychosomatic Research 11:51-58, 1967.

4174
VAN DIJL, H., AND F.H. OLTHUIS.
Some test behaviour differences between healthy men and male myocardial infarction patients.
Psychotherapy Psychosomatics 18:286-293, 1970.

4175
VAN DYKE, K., AND E.K. CHUNG.
Serum digoxin determination by radioimmunoassay. Clinical implications.
Postgraduate Medicine 52(5):219-222, 1972.

4176
VAN NOUHUYS, F.
Abnormalities of the ECG during adenotonsillectomy under anaesthesia by the method of Sluder.
Nederlands Tijdschrift voor Geneeskunde 117(4):137-141, 1973.

4177
VANREMOORTERE, E.C.
Vulnerability of premature beats to A.C. Stimuli of long duration.
Acta Cardiologica 26:121-149, 1971.

4178
VAN WINKLE, M., AND L. LEVY.
Further studies on the reversibility of serum sickness cholesterol-induced atherosclerosis.
Journal Experimental Medicine 132(5):858-867, 1970.

4179
VARAT, M.A., N.O. FOWLER, AND R.J. ADOLPH.
  Cardiac output response to exercise in patients with inferior vena caval ligation.
  Circulation 39-40(Suppl. III):207, 1969.

4180
VARNAUSKAS, E.
  The testing of cardiac patients.
  Canadian Medical Association Journal 96(Special Issue):751-758, 1967.

4181
VARNAUSKAS, E., H. BERGMAN, P. HOUK, AND P. BJÖRNTORP.
  Haemodynamic effects of physical training in coronary patients.
  Lancet 2:8-12, 1966.

4182
VARNAUSKAS, E., P. BJÖRNTORP, M. FAHLEN, I. PREROVSKY, AND J. STENBERG.
  Effects of physical training on exercise blood flow and enzymatic activity in skeletal muscle.
  Cardiovascular Research 4:418-422, 1970.

4183
VARNAUSKAS, E., AND S. HOLMBERG.
  Myocardial blood flow during exercise in patients with coronary heart disease. Comments on
  training effects.
  In: Larson, O.A. and R.O. Malmborg, Coronary heart diseases and physical fitness, pp. 102-104.
  Baltimore, University Park Press, 1971.

4184
VARNAUSKAS, E. AND R. WASSEN.
  Continuous monitoring of the heart rate blood pressure product during exercise testing.
  Malatti Cardiovascolari 10(1-2):257-263, 1969.

4185
VASILE, N., A. DELOCHE, AND J.L. GUERMONPREZ.
  Emergency coronary arteriography for impending infarction, Prinzmetal's angina and complicated
  infarction. Report of 25 cases.
  Journal de Radiologie et d'Electrologie 53(8):617-621, 1972.

4186
VASIL'EV, I.T., V.S. FEL'DMAN, AND V.G. STRANIN.
  Properties during the period of the pressure rise in the right ventricle in patients suffering from
  mitral stenosis during physical exercise
  Kardiologiya 9(2):100-107, 1969.

4187
VASSAUX, C. AND B. LOWN.
  Myocardial infarction and the vulnerable period for ventricular tachycardia ($VT_{(vp)}$).
  Clinical Research 15:225, 1967.

4188
VEDIN, J.A., C. WILHELMSSON, D. ELMFELDT, G. TIBBLIN, ET AL.
  Sudden death: identification of high risk groups.
  American Heart Journal 86:124, 1973.

4189
VEDIN, J.A., C.E. WILHELMSSON, L. WILHELMSEN, ET AL.
  Relation of resting and exercise induced ectopic beats to other ischemic manifestations and to coronary risk factors. Men born in 1913.
  American Journal Cardiology 30(1):25-31, 1972.

4190
VENTURA, T., G. NATALI, AND P. MARSILI.
  Cardio pericardiac metastases from pulmonary cancer (with reference to two cases).
  Bolletino della Società Italiana di Cardiologia 17(8):483-491, 1972.

4191
VERA, Z., G. ERTEM, AND T.O. CHENG.
  Left bundle branch block with intermittent right axis deviation. Evidence for left posterior hemiblock accompanying predivisional left bundle branch block.
  American Journal Cardiology 30(8):896-901, 1972.

4192
VERDESCA, A.S.
  The value of the computer as a screening tool for routine electrocardiograms.
  Journal Occupational Medicine 14(4):293-297, 1972.

4193
VERDOUW, P.D., A.V.D. VORM, F. HAGEMEIJ, AND P.G. HUGENHOL.
  Is prognosis of survival following myocardial infarction possible from hemodynamics at time of admission?
  Circulation 48(4):227, 1973.

4194
VERDUN DI CANTOGNO, L., AND L. DUGHERA.
  The importance and distribution of some stress factors in 500 cases of myocardial infarction in the city of Turin.
  Bollettino della Società Italiana di Cardiologia 16(10):609-610, 1971.

4195
VERDUYN LUNEL, A.A.
  Significance of annulus fibrosus of heart in relation to AV conduction and ventricular activation in cases of Wolff-Parkinson-White syndrome.
  British Heart Journal 34(12):1263-1271, 1972.

4196
VERGARA, G.S., F.J. HILDNER, C.B. SCHOENFELD, ET AL.
  Conversion of supraventricular tachycardias with rapid atrial stimulation.
  Circulation 46(4):788-793, 1972.

4197
VERGHESE, A.
  Relationships between the Eysenck Personality Inventory N score, the Cornell Medical Index M-R score, and the psychogalvanic reflex.
  British Journal Psychiatry 116(530):27-32, 1970.

4198
VERGHESE, A.
  Personality traits and coronary heart disease.
  Journal Indian Medical Association 57:9-12, 1971.

4199
VERHEUGEN, P.
  The situation of readaptation in the United States.
  Revue de Réadaptation 13:147, 1971.

4200
VERMAN, G.K.
  Rehabilitation in cardiovascular diseases.
  Indian Medical Journal 61(10):215-216, 1967.

4201
VERNON, P.E.
  Personality assessment.
  London, England. Methuen, 1964.

4202
VERSTRAETE, M.
  The evaluation of the beneficial effects of the new therapy in patients with recent myocardial
  infarction.
  Clinica Terapeutica 65:297, 1973.

4203
VERSTRAETE, M., J. VERMYLEN, R. DeVREKER, A. AMERY, AND C. VERMYLEN.
  Efficacy of thrombolytic therapy with streptokinase using a new administration scheme.
  Scandinavian Journal Clinical Laboratory Investigation (Suppl.) 16(78):15-22, 1964.

4204
VERWOERDT, A., AND R.H. DOVENMUEHLE.
  Heart disease and depression.
  Geriatrics 19:856-864, 1964.

4205
VERWOERDT, A. AND R.H. DOVENMUEHLE.
  Physical illness and depressive symptomatology. III. Aspects of awareness.
  Journal Gerontology 19:330-335, 1964.

4206
VERWOERDT, A., AND R.H. DOVENMUEHLE.
  Physical illness and depressive symptomatology. IV. Personal factors in the grief reaction.
  Journal Gerontology 20(4):470-478, 1965.

4207
VERZA, M.
  Rehabilitation of the cardiovascular geriatric patient.
  Giornale di Gerontologia 20(2):194-200, 1972.

4208
VESSEY, M.P.
  Coffee drinking and acute myocardial infarction.
  Lancet 2:1278-1281, 1972.

4209
VIDEBAEK, J., N.J. CHRISTENSEN, AND B. STERNDORFF.
  Serial determination of plasma catecholamines in myocardial infarction.
  Circulation 46:846-855, 1972.

4210
VIDNE, B., D. ESHKOL, AND M.J. LEVY.
Carotid sinus nerve stimulator for relief of anginal syndrome.
Harefuah 83(5):199-201;221, 1972.

4211
VIEWEG, W.V.R., M.E. THOMPSON, J.J. MCHALE, JR., AND D.A. LEE.
Ventricular tachyarrhythmias controlled by ventricular aneurysmectomy and aortocoronary saphenous vein bypass grafts. Report of a case.
Medical Annals District of Columbia 41(9):565-567, 1972.

4212
VINEBERG, S.E., AND E.P. WILLENS.
Observation and analysis of patient behavior in the rehabilitation hospital.
Archives Physical Medicine Rehabilitation 52:8-14, 1971.

4213
VINTILA, P.
Aspects of rehabilitation in 300 patients suffering myocardial infarct.
Atti della Società Italiana di Cardiologia 2:172-174, 1967.

4214
VIRU, A.A., P.K. KORGE, AND E.A. VIRU.
Interrelations between the adrenal glucocorticoid activity, the cardiovascular system, and the electrolyte metabolism during exhausting work.
Fiziologicheskii Zhurnal SSSR Imeni I.M. Sechenov 59(1):105-110, 1973.

4215
VISIOLI, O.
The diagnosis of coronary insufficiency, especially of the acute anginal form.
Ateneo Parmense Sezione 1 Acta Bio-Medica 41(1):5-59, 1970.

4216
VISSER, J.F.
The rehabilitation of patients with coronary sclerosis.
Nederlands Tijdschrift voor Geneeskunde 111:1923-1927, 1967.

4217
VLAICU, R., E. MACAVEI, AND I. PATIU.
Cross-sectional study of arterial pressure and serum lipids in coronary smokers and nonsmokers.
Medicina Internă 23(8):925-930, 1971.

4218
VLIERS, A.C.A.P., B. OESEBURG, K.R. VISSER, AND W.G. ZIJLSTRA.
Choice of detection site for the determination of cardiac output by thermal dilution: The injection thermistor catheter.
Cardiovascular Research 7 (1):133-138, 1973.

4219
VLIERS, A.C.A.P., K.R. VISSER, AND W.G. ZIJLSTRA.
Analysis of indicator distribution in the determination of cardiac output by thermal dilution.
Cardiovascular Research 7(1):125-132, 1973.

4220
VOEGTLIN, R., C. BRECHENMACHER, AND H. JEANMAIRE.
  Atrial arrhythmia due to virus infection.
  Journal Médical de Strasbourg 2(10):791-800, 1971.

4221
VOGEL, J.H., D. CORNISH, AND R.B. McFADDEN.
  Underestimation of ejection fraction with singleplane angiography in coronary artery disease: Role
  of biplane angiography.
  Chest 64: 217, 1973.

4222
VOGEL, J.H.K., Ed.
  Hypoxia, high altitude and the heart.
  Basel, Switzerland, S. Karger, 1970.

4223
VOGELSANG, A.
  Electrocardiogram and hard drugs.
  Lancet 2:324, 1973.

4224
VOGT, F.B., AND T. HALLEN.
  Electrocardiogram preprocessing unit.
  Aerospace Medicine 38:123-126, 1967.

4225
VOGT, J.J., M.T. MEYER SCHWERTZ, R. FOEHR, AND Г. GOLLE.
  Validation of a procedure for estimating the work load and the heat load from an analysis of
  continuous heart rate records.
  Travail Humain 35(1):131-142, 1972.

4226
VOHRA, J.K., J.T. DOWLING, AND G. SLOMAN.
  Idioventricular tachycardia in acute myocardial infarction.
  Medical Journal Australia 2:196-198, 1971.

4227
VOICULESCO, A., M. FREIFELD, AND I. BISTREANN.
  Aspects of heart dynamics and the electrocardiogram at rest and after effort in sillicosis.
  Poumon et le Coeur 24:229-237, 1968.

4228
VOLKOV, V.A., AND T.K. SEMENNIKOVA.
  Work capacity of patients having sustained myocardial infarction. (According to the data of long
  term observations and multichannel radioelectrocardiography).
  Terapevticheskii Arkhiv 43(2):29, 1971.

4229
VOLKOV, V.S.
  Adaptation of patients who have sustained myocardial infarction to physical exertion.
  Kardiologiya 11(7):75-81, 1971.

4230

VOLLMAR, F., H. GÜTHERT, M. BRANDT, ET AL.
Coronary sclerosis and its sequelae (statistical study on an unselected autopsy series). II. Myocardial infarction.
Zeitschrift für die Gesamte Innere Medizin und Ihre Grenzgebiete 26(14):451, 1971.

4231

VON DER GROEBEN, J.
Decision rules in electrocardiography and vectorcardiography.
Circulation 36:136-147, 1967.

4232

VON DER GROEBEN, J., D.D. FISHER, AND J.G. TOOLE.
Temporospatial frequency distribution of P, QRS, and T in normal man and woman.
American Heart Journal 75(4):487-509, 1968.

4233

VON DOSCICIN, V.L.
Therapy of cardiac arrhythmia with Verapamil.
Arzneimittel Forschung 20(9):1289-1290, 1970.

4234

VON EULER, U.S., C.A.GENZELL, L. LEVY, AND G. STRÖM.
Cortical and medullary adrenal activity in emotional stress.
Acta Endocrinologica 30:567, 1959.

4235

VON VOTEAL, B.E., L.G. LOZINSKIJ, V.A. GOLDBERG, M.G. VENEDIKTOVA, AND A. GRIBOVA.
The antiarrhythmic and coronary dilating properties of verapamil in patients with ischemic heart diseases.
Arzneimittel Forschung 20 (Suppl. 9A):1280-1284, 1970.

4236

VON ZIPFEL, J., J.D. MEYER-ERKELENZ, AND A. DIETZ.
Evaluation of the electrocardiogram during rest and exertion using various computer systems.
Verhandlungen der Deutschen Gesselschaft für Kreislaufforschung 37:445-449, 1971.

4237

VORBACH, H.
Rehabilitation following myocardial infarction
Medizinische Welt 24:1476-1482, 1968.

4238

VOSKANOV, M.A.
Effect of exercise therapy on the contractile function of the myocardium in patients with atherosclerosis of the coronary arteries. (Clinic-diagnostic study.)
Terapevticheskii Arkhiv 38(11):59-63, 1966.

4239

VOSLAROVA, Z., L. KUCEROVA, AND R. PAPEZOVA.
Changes of serum cholesterol and prebetalipoproteins in patients with ischaemic heart disease.
Sbornik Lekarsky 75:251, 1973.

4240
VOUKYDIS, P.C.
   The myocardium as a composite material: analysis.
   Bulletin Mathematical Biophysics 34(2):173-204, 1972.

4241
VOUKYDIS, P.C.
   Geometrical parameters of the individual myocardial fibers.
   Bulletin Mathematical Biophysics 34(2):205-211, 1972.

4242
VOUKYDIS, P.C.
   Application of the Gabor-Nelson theory in electrocardiography.
   Medical Biological Engineering 10:223-229, 1972.

4243
VUOPALA, U.
   Resumption of work after myocardial infarction in Northern Finland.
   Acta Medica Scandinavica (Suppl.)530:1, 1972.

4244
VYAZITSKY, P.O., AND A.I. SERGEEV.
   Condition of the cardiovascular system in acromegaly.
   Problemy Endokrinologii 18(4):31-34, 1972.

4245
VYDEN, J.K., AND E. CORDAY.
   The effect of cardiogenic shock on the superior mesenteric circulation.
   Modern Geriatrics 2(6):347-352, 1972.

4246
VYSOTSKAYA, V.D.
   Oxygen debt and physical performance capacity in persons with low arterial pressure.
   Sovetskaya Meditsina 35:48, 1972.

4247
WAGNER, G.S., C.R. ROE, L.E. LIMBIRD, ET AL.
   The importance of identification of the myocardial specific isoenzyme of creatine phosphokinase
   (MB form) in the diagnosis of acute myocardial infarction.
   Circulation 47(2):263-269, 1973.

4248
WAGNER, H.
   The effect of different walking distances on blood pressure and weight.
   Archiv für Physikalische Therapie 22(2):49-57, 1970.

4249
WAGNER, H.N., JR.
   Nuclear medicine in cardiovascular disease.
   Hospital Practice 7(9):108-116, 1972.

4250
WAGNER, J., J. KORSUKEWITZ, W. MEYER, ET AL.
   Carotid sinus stimulation.
   Deutsche Medizinische Wochenschrift 98:37, 1973.

4251
WAHLQVIST, M.L.
Substrate and hormone interrelationships in human myocardial metabolism.
Thesis, Uppsala University, Sweden, 1972.

4252
WAHLQVIST, M.L., L. KAIJSER, B.W. LASSERS, AND L.A. CARLSON.
Fatty acid as a determinant of myocardial substrate and oxygen metabolism in man at rest and during prolonged exercise.
Acta Medica Scandinavica 193(1-2):89-96, 1973.

4253
WAHLQVIST, M.L., L. KAIJSER, B.W. LASSERS, ET AL.
Glucocorticoid uptake and release by the human heart: Studies at rest, during prolonged exercise, and during nicotinic acid infusion.
Scandinavian Journal Clinical Laboratory Investigation 30(3):261-266, 1972.

4254
WAHREN, J. AND S. BYGDEMAN.
Onset of angina pectoris in relation to circulatory adaptation during arm and leg exercise.
Circulation 44(3):432-441, 1971.

4255
WAJDA, Z., W. KOZLOWSKI, J. GREZLIKOWSKI, D. LIPINSKA, ET AL.
Management of Morgan-Adams-Stokes syndrome using continuous epicardial and intraventricular pacing.
Polski Tygodnik Lekarski 24:5-7, 1969.

4256
WAKERLIN, G.E.
Reducing the risk factors of coronary heart disease.
Journal Rehabilitation 32:21, 1966.

4257
WAKLEY, E.J., AND M.J.S. LANGMAN.
Blood groups and plasma cholesterol esterification.
Cardiovascular Research 7:676-678, 1973.

4258
WAKLEY, E.J., M.J.S. LANGMAN, AND P.C. ELWOOD.
Blood group A sub-groups and serum cholesterol.
Cardiovascular Research 7:679-683, 1973.

4259
WALD, N., S. HOWARD, P.G. SMITH, AND K. KJELDSEN.
Association between atherosclerotic diseases and carboxyhaemoglobin levels in tobacco smokers.
British Medical Journal 1:761, 1973.

4260
WALKER, A.A., J.S. JANICKI, K.T. WEBER, R.O. RUSSELL JR., AND C.E. RACKLEY.
Equations for the calculation of mean ejection pressure.
Cardiovascular Research 7:567, 1973.

4261
WALLACE, A.
   Acute myocardial infarction.
   In: Julian, D.G. and M.F. Oliver, Eds., Acute myocardial infarction, p. 92.
   Edinburgh, Livingstone, 1968.

4262
WALLACE, A.G., AND R.A. ROSATI.
   Computers can change cardiology.
   Circulation 47(3):439-442, 1973.

4263
WALLOOPPILLAI, N.J., D.P. ATUKORALE, AND R. SURENDRAKUMAR.
   Coronary intensive care in Ceylon.
   Ceylon Medical Journal 17(2):63-67, 1972.

4264
WALSTON, A., II, AND M.E. KENDALL.
   Comparison of pulmonary wedge and left atrial pressure in man.
   American Heart Journal 86:159, 1973.

4265
WANG, K., F. GOBEL, D.F. GLEASON, AND J.E. EDWARDS.
   Complete heart block complicating bacterial endocarditis.
   Circulation 46(5):939-947, 1972.

4266
WANG, L., L. SCHLOFF, AND C.W. LILLEHEI.
   Hemodynamics at rest and supine exercise one year following mitral valve replacement by a
   Starr-Edwards prothesis.
   Circulation 34(4 Suppl. III):234, 1966.

4267
WANG, Y., R.J. MARSHALL, AND J.T. SHEPHERD.
   The effect of changes in posture and of graded exercise on stroke volume in man.
   Journal Clinical Investigation 39:1051, 1960.

4268
WANNENWETSCH, E.
   The success of rehabilitation with special consideration of unspecific pulmonary disease and
   heart-circulatory disease.
   Archiv für Physikalische Therapie 22(3):129-133, 1970.

4269
WARDEKAR, A., B. SON, C.D. GOSAYNIE, AND B. BERCU.
   Recurrent ventricular tachycardia successfully treated by excision of ventricular aneurysm.
   Chest 62(4):505-508, 1972.

4270
WARDLE, E.N.
   Long-term blood abnormalities in thrombosis.
   Lancet 2:442, 1973.

4271
WARDWELL, W.I.
A study of stress and coronary heart disease in an urban population.
Bulletin New York Academy Medicine 49:521-531, 1973.

4272
WARDWELL, W.I., AND C.B. BAHNSON.
Behavioral variables and myocardial infarction in Southeastern Connecticut heart study.
Journal Chronic Diseases 26(7):447-461, 1973.

4273
WAREMBOURG, H., M.E. BERTRAND, G. DUCLOUX, J.Y. KETELERS, AND A. CARRE.
Coronary output during rest and effort in coronary patients; correlations with coronary arteriography.
Archives des Maladies du Coeur et des Vaisseaux 65(1):105-115, 1972.

4274
WAREMBOURG, H., G. DUCLOUX, M. PAUCHANT, H. DELBECQUE, ET AL.
Ventricular-wall aneurysms following myocardial infarction. I. Indications for surgery and preoperative investigation.
Coeur et Médecine Interne 12:385, 1973.

4275
WAREMBOURG, H., J. LEKIEFFRE, G. FLAMENT, ET AL.
The importance of the vectorcardiogram for the diagnosis of left ventricular hypertrophy of the systolic type.
Archives des Maladies du Coeur et des Vaisseaux 65(9):1103-1112, 1972.

4276
WAREMBOURG, H., M. PAUCHANT, J. LEKIEFFRE, ET AL.
Predominating S waves in leads L1, L2, L3 in the course of chronic respiratory insufficiency.
Archives des Maladies du Coeur et des Vaisseaux 65(8):981-993, 1972.

4277
WARREN, J.E.
Myocardial infarction in an industrial population.
Archives Environmental Health 7:210-215, 1963.

4278
WARREN, W.D., J. SAURBEY, AND H.H. WANDALL.
Experimental study of oxygen differential therapy of ventricular fibrillation.
Surgery, Gynecology Obstetrics 117:677, 1963.

4279
WARSHAW, L.J.
Returning the cardiac to work.
Heart Bulletin 13:1, 1964.

4280
WARSHAW, L.J.
Employability of the patient with heart disease: how is it evaluated?
Journal Chronic Diseases 18:931-944, 1965.

4281
WARSHAW, L.J.
Rehabilitation after myocardial infarction.
Archives Environmental Health 10:109-112, 1965.

4282
WARSHAW, L.J.
Employability of cardiacs in industry.
Southern Medical Bulletin 54(3):31, 1966.

4283
WARSHAW, L.J.
Putting the patient with cardiac disease back to work.
Archives Environmental Health 12:651-654, 1966.

4284
WARSHAW, L.J.
The role of the industrial physician in rehabilitation of the cardiac.
Journal Occupational Medicine 8:514-515, 1966.

4285
WARSHAW, L.J.
Heart cases under workmen's compensation laws.
Journal Occupational Medicine 9:349-352, 1967.

4286
WARTAK, J.
ECG criteria for angina pectoris derived from resting Frank lead electrocardiograms.
Chest 58:42-48, 1970.

4287
WARTAK, J., J.A. MILLIKEN, AND J. KARCHMAR.
Computer program for pattern recognition of electrocardiograms.
Computers Biomedical Research 4:344-374, 1970.

4288
WASMUTH, C.E.
Law for the physician, pp. 15-30.
Philadelphia, Lea and Febiger, 1966.

4289
WASSERMAN, A.J., J.D. PROCTOR, F.J. ALLEN, AND V.E. KEMP, JR.
Human cardiovascular effects of alprenolol, a beta-adrenergic blocker: hemodynamic, anti-arrhythmic, and antianginal.
Journal Clinical Pharmacology 10:37-49, 1970.

4290
WASSERMAN, K.
Lactate and related acid base and blood gas changes during constant load and graded exercise.
Canadian Medical Association Journal 96:775-779, 1967.

4291
WASSERMAN, K., AND M.B. McILROY.
Detecting the threshold of anaerobic metabolism in cardiac patients during exercise.
American Journal Cardiology 14(6):844-852, 1964.

4292
WASSERMAN, K., A. NAIMARK, AND M.B. McILROY.
New method for continuous measurement of adequacy of cardiovascular response to exercise.
Circulation 24(4 Part 2):1066, 1961.

4293
WASSERMAN, K., B.J. WHIPP, S.N. KOYAL, AND W.L. BEAVER.
Anaerobic threshold and respiratory gas exchange during exercise.
Journal Applied Physiology 35:236-243, 1973.

4294
WASSERMIL, M., AND S. RODBARD.
Delayed return of QK interval to resting values after exercise in patients with heart disease.
Circulation 37-38 (Suppl. 6):202, 1968.

4295
WASSERMIL, M., AND M. TOOR.
Clinical and electrocardiographic observations of patients with ischemic heart disease during multistage submaximal exercise.
Cardiologia 53:158-174, 1968.

4296
WASSERMIL, M., AND M. TOOR.
Clinical and electrocardiographic responses to exercise in patients with coronary artery disease.
Israel Journal Medical Sciences 5(4):696-700, 1969.

4297
WASYLUK, J.
Effect of exercise on the electrocardiograms of patients after myocardial infarction.
Polski Tygodnik Lekarski 22(36):1364-1367, 1967.

4298
WATANABE, Y., K. NISHIJIMA, H. RICHMAN, AND E. SIMONSON.
Vectorcardiographic and electrocardiographic differentiation between cor pulmonale and anterior wall myocardial infarction.
American Heart Journal 84(3):302-309, 1972.

4299
WATERS, W.F., D.G. McDONALD, AND R.L. KORESKO.
Psychophysiological responses during analogue systematic desensitization and non-relaxation control procedures.
Behavioral Research Therapy 10:381-393, 1972.

4300
WATT, E.W., H.E. GAHAGEN, AND J. MENDEZ.
Serum lipids and body fat of young male college athletes.
Federation Proceedings 31(2):291, 1972.

4301
WAXMAN, M.B., AND A.G. WALLACE.
Electrophysiologic effects of bretylium tosylate on the heart.
Journal Pharmacology Experimental Therapeutics 183(2):264-274, 1972.

4302
WEAVER, N.K.
   Industry and the coronary worker.
   Journal Rehabilitation 32:77, 1966.

4303
WEAVER, N.K.
   Disability absenteeism of industrial workers with myocardial infarcts.
   American Heart Journal 62(4):457-461, 1961.

4304
WEAVER, N.K.
   Selective placement of the cardiac.
   Journal Occupational Medicine 8:516-517, 1966.

4305
WEBB, S.W., A.A.J. ADGEY, AND J.F. PANTRIDGE.
   Autonomic disturbance at onset of acute myocardial infarction.
   British Medical Journal 3:89-92, 1972.

4306
WEBER, D.J.
   Intravenous triamterene in the treatment of acute digitalis intoxication.
   Clinical Pharmacology Therapeutics 13(6):868-874, 1972.

4307
WEDGWOOD, J.
   Heart failure in old age.
   Postgraduate Medicine 52(4):179-183, 1972.

4308
WEE, A.S.T.
   Work after myocardial infarction. Effect on working capacity.
   Singapore Medical Journal 9(3):178-181, 1968.

4309
WEEDA, H.W.H.
   Arterial pressures during exercise in normals in patients with aortic coarctation and in patients
   with myocardial infarction.
   Malattie Cardiovascolari 10(1-2):265-273, 1969.

4310
WEEDA, H.W.H.
   Rehabilitation after myocardial infarction.
   Folia Medica Neerlandica 14:272-280, 1971.

4311
WEIL, J.V., E. BYRNE-QUINN, I.E. SODAL, J.S. KLINE, ET AL.
   Ventilatory control in normal man: Effects of acute exercise, chronic physical conditioning and
   chronic hypoxia.
   Chest 61 (Suppl.):45S-46S, 1972.

4312
WEILY, H.S., AND E. GENTON.
Pharmacokinetics of procainamide.
Archives Internal Medicine 130(3):366-369, 1972.

4313
WEINBLATT, E., ET AL.
Return to work and work status following first myocardial infarction.
American Journal Public Health 56:169-185, 1966.

4314
WEINBLATT, E., ET AL.
Prognosis of men after first myocardial infarction: Mortality and first recurrence in relation to selected parameters.
American Journal Public Health 58:1329-1347, 1968.

4315
WEINBLATT, E., S. SHAPIRO, AND C.W. FRANK.
Changes in personal characteristics of men over five years, following first diagnosis of coronary heart disease.
American Journal Public Health 61(4):831-842, 1971.

4316
WEINER, L., E.M. DWYER, JR., AND J.W. COX.
Left ventricular hemodynamics in exercise-induced angina pectoris.
Circulation 38:240-249, 1968.

4317
WEINMAN, J.
An appraisal of some noninvasive cardiovascular techniques.
Medical Biological Engineering 10:496-503, 1972.

4318
WEISS, N.S.
Cigarette smoking and arteriosclerosis obliterans: An epidemiologic approach.
American Journal Epidemiology 95(1):17-25, 1972.

4319
WEISS, R.A., AND P. KARPOVICH.
Energy cost of exercise for convalescents.
Archives Physical Medicine Rehabilitation 28:447, 1947.

4320
WEISS, S.M.
Psychological adjustment following open-heart surgery.
Journal Nervous Mental Disease 143(4):363-368, 1966.

4321
WEISSLER, A.M., L.C. HARRIS, AND G.D. WHITE.
Left ventricular ejection time index in man.
Journal Applied Physiology 18:919, 1963.

4322
WEISSLER, A.M., W.S. HARRIS, AND C.D. SCHOENFELD.
   Systolic time intervals in heart failure in man.
   Circulation 37:149-159, 1968.

4323
WEISSLER, A.M., P.G. PEELER, W. H. ROEHIL.
   Relationships between left ventricular ejection time, stroke volume, and heart rate in normal
   individuals and patients with cardiovascular disease.
   American Heart Journal 62:367, 1961.

4324
WELBORN, W.S.
   Effect of a new coronary vasodilator (NLT, Nilitil) for relief of angina pectoris.
   Proceedings Western Pharmacological Society 6:71, 1963.

4325
WELCH, H.G.
   Substrate utilization in muscle—Adaptations to physical effort.
   In: Naughton, J., H.K. Hellerstein, and I.C. Mohler, Eds. Exercise testing and exercise training in
   coronary heart disease, pp. 193-197. New York, Academic Press, 1973.

4326
WELCH, T.G., T.R. WHITE, R.P. LEWIS, P.I. ALTIERI, ET AL.
   Esophagopericardial fistula presenting as caridac tamponade.
   Chest 62(6):728-731, 1972.

4327
WELLENS, H.J., R.M. SCHUILENBURG, AND D. DURRER.
   Electrical stimulation of the heart in patients with ventricular tachycardia.
   Circulation 46:216-226, 1972.

4328
WELLENS, H.J.J., A. VERMEULEN, AND D. DURRER.
   Ventricular fibrillation occurring on arousal from sleep by auditory stimuli.
   Circulation 46(4):661-665, 1972.

4329
WELLER, P.
   Continuous treatment of the heart infarct using anticoagulants.
   Zeitschrift für Gesamte Innere Medizin und Ihre Grenzgebiete 23(7): 103-104, 1968.

4330
WELLS, C.L. AND E.R. BUSKIRK.
   Body temperatures during contralateral arm leg exercise.
   Medicine Science Sports 4(1):37-42, 1972.

4331
WELTI, J.J., P. BENAIM, AND D. FACQUET.
   Lasting recovery following electric shock treatment of a ventricular fibrillation with myocardial
   infarction.
   Presse Médicale 75(55):2845, 1967.

4332
WENDKOS, M.H.
    Electrocardiographic effects of marihuana.
    Journal American Medical Assocation 226:789, 1973.

4333
WENDKOS, M.H., AND K. WOLFF.
    Emotional correlates of angina pectoris.
    Journal American Geriatrics Society 16(8):845-858, 1968.

4334
WENDKOS, M.H., AND K. WOLFF.
    Emotional correlates of angina pectoris and their therapeutic implications.
    Israel Journal Medical Sciences 4(5):1126, 1968.

4335
WENDKOS, M.H., AND K. WOLFF.
    Emotional correlates of angina pectoris.
    Israel Journal Medical Sciences 5(4):723-726, 1969.

4336
WENGER, N.K.
    The use of exercise in the rehabilitation of patients after myocardial infarction.
    Journal South Carolina Medical Association 65(Suppl. 1):66-68, 1969.

4337
WENGER, N.K.
    Tables outlining cardiac conditioning program.
    Journal South Carolina Medical Association 65(Suppl. 1):102-104, 1969.

4338
WENGER, N.K.
    Physical conditioning after myocardial infarction. An early intervention program.
    Circulation 43-44(Suppl. 2):119, 1971.

4339
WENGER, N.K.
    Rehabilitation of the coronary patient.
    Delaware Medical Journal 44:104-106, 1972.

4340
WENGER, N.K.
    Early ambulation of patients after myocardial infarction.
    Cardiology 58(1):1-6, 1973.

4341
WENGER, N.K.
    Benefits of a rehabilitation program following myocardial infarction.
    Geriatrics 28:64, 1973.

4342
WENGER, N.K.
    The role of the physician in exercise testing and exercise training.
    In: Naughton, J., H.K. Hellerstein, and I.C. Mohler, Eds. Exercise testing and exercise training in coronary heart disease, pp. 395-401. New York, Academic Press, 1973.

4343
WENGER, N.K.
Early ambulation after myocardial infarction: Grady Memorial Hospital-Emory University School of Medicine.
In: Naughton, J., H.K. Hellerstein, and I.C. Mohler. Eds. Exercise testing and exercise training in coronary heart disease, pp. 324-328. New York, Academic Press, 1973.

4344
WENGER, N.K., C.A. GILBERT, AND W. SIEGEL.
Symposium: The use of physical activity in the rehabilitation of patients after myocardial infarction.
Southern Medical Journal 63:891-897, 1970.

4345
WENGER, N.K., C.A. GILBERT, AND M.Z. SKORAPA.
Cardiac conditioning after myocardial infarction. An early intervention program.
Cardiac Rehabilitation 2:17-22, 1971.

4346
WENGER, N.K., H.K. HELLERSTEIN, H. BLACKBURN, AND S.J. CASTRANOVA.
Uncomplicated myocardial infarction. Current physician practice in patient management.
Journal American Medical Association 224:511, 1973.

4347
WENGER, R.
Sociomedical problems of cardiology.
Wiener Klinische Wochenschrift 78:53-56, 1966.

4348
WENGER, R., ET AL.
On the analysis of electrocardiograms with deep S- spikes in the left thoracic leads.
Zeitschrift für Kreislaufforschung 55:98-109, 1966.

4349
WERKÖ, L.
Clinical value of physical conditioning in patients with manifest coronary heart disease. An introduction.
In: Larsen, O.A. and R.O. Malmborg, Eds. Coronary heart disease and physical fitness, Baltimore, University Park Press, 1971.

4350
WERTHEIMER, M., S. BLOOM, AND R.K. HUGHES.
Myocardial effects of pericardial tamponade.
Annals Thoracic Surgery 14(5):494-503, 1972.

4351
WERTLAKE, P.T., A.A. WILCOX, M.I. HALEY, AND J.E. PETERSON.
Relationship of mental and emotional stress to serum cholesterol levels.
Proceedings Society Experimental Biology Medicine 97:163, 1958.

4352
WESTERMANN, K.W.
Exertion electrocardiogram. Indications and results.
Deutsche Medizinishe Wochenschrift 94:439-441, 1969.

4353
WEXLER, B.C., AND J.T. JUDD.
   Hexosamine and beta-glucuronidase alterations during the acute onset and repair of isoproterenol induced myocardial infarction.
   Life Sciences 111(17):797-807, 1972.

4354
WHEATLEY, C.E., T.A. PRESTON, D.K. WEAVER, AND W.A. DEYOUNG.
   Complete heart block due to metastatic rhabdomyosarcoma.
   University Michigan Medical Center Journal 38(2):67-70, 1972.

4355
WHEELER, E.O., AND R.E. SCULLY.
   Complete heart block on electrocardiogram in 1916, with survival until 1972.
   New England Journal Medicine 288(6):308-315, 1973.

4356
WHEELER, R., AND J. CONWAY.
   The hemodynamic response to exercise in older subjects before and after propranolol.
   Clinical Research 17(2):270, 1969.

4357
WHIPP, B.J., AND K. WASSERMAN.
   Oxidative energy transfer during the nonsteady state phase of muscular work.
   Chest 61(2) (Suppl.):53S-56S, 1972.

4358
WHITE, P.D.
   The role of exercise in the aging.
   Journal American Medical Association 165:70, 1957.

4359
WHITE, P.D.
   The priority of rehabilitation in cardiovascular disease.
   Archives Physical Medicine Rehabilitation 45:592-596, 1964.

4360
WHITE, P.D.
   Place of exercise in cardiology.
   American Journal Cardiology 30(7):716, 1972.

4361
WHITE, R.I., JR.
   Technique and preliminary results of selective catheterization of patients with Blalock-Taussig shunts.
   Radiology 105(3):703-706, 1972.

4362
WHITEHOUSE, F.A.
   Some psycho-physiological factors in the evaluation of the work potential of the cardiac.
   Industrial Medicine Surgery 34:705-713, 1965.

4363
WHITEHOUSE, F.A.
   The cardiac work evaluation unit as a specialized team approach.
   Journal Rehabilitation 32:66, 1966.

4364
WHITEHOUSE, F.A.
   Psychologic factor in cardiac rehabilitation.
   New York State Journal Medicine 70:522-531, 1970.

4365
WHITSETT, T., AND J. NAUGHTON.
   Systolic time intervals in patients with ASHD.
   Clinical Research 16:438, 1968.

4366
WHITSETT, T., AND J. NAUGHTON.
   Systolic time intervals following exercise in healthy individuals and patients with atherosclerotic
   heart disease.
   Clinical Research 17(2):270, 1969.

4367
WHITSETT, T.L., AND J.P. NAUGHTON.
   The effect of exercise on systolic time intervals in sedentary and active individuals and rehabili-
   tated patients with heart disease.
   American Journal Cardiology 27:352-358, 1971.

4368
WIDOMSKA, C.T., AND S.H. MITURZYNSKA.
   One year observation of blood oxygenation and acid base equilibrium in patients with a history
   of myocardial infarction.
   Polski Tygodnik Lekarski 27:1432, 1972.

4369
WIDOMSKA, C.T., AND S.H. MITURZYNSKA.
   Blood oxygenation and acid base balance in shock during myocardial infarction.
   Polski Tygodnik Lekarski 27:1505, 1972.

4370
WIECKO, W.
   Sinus inhibition in paroxysmal atrial fibrillation.
   Polski Tygodnik Lekarski 27:1452, 1972.

4371
WIENER, F.
   Problems in rehabilitation and placement of the cardiac patient.
   Journal Occupational Medicine 8:471-476, 1966.

4372
WIENER, L., AND J.W. COX.
   Influence of stellate ganglion block on angina pectoris and the post-exercise electrocardiogram.
   American Journal Medical Sciences 252(3):289-195, 1966.

4373
WIENER, L., E.M. DWYER, JR., AND J.W. COX.
Left ventricular hemodynamics in exercise-induced angina pectoris.
Circulation 38(2):240, 1968.

4374
WIENER, L., E.M. DWYER, JR., AND J.W. COX.
Hemodynamic effects of nitroglycerin, propranolol, and their combination in coronary heart disease.
Circulation 39:623, 1969.

4375
WIENER, L., J.C. RIOS, AND R.A. MASSUMI.
Benign T wave inversion with elevated RS-T segment simulating myocardial injury.
American Heart Journal 67:684, 1964.

4376
WIGBOLDUS, A.H., J. URZUA, AND J.F. VILJOEN.
The "empty heart" phenomenon.
Journal Thoracic Cardiovascular Surgery 66:807, 1973.

4377
WIGLE, R.D., ET AL.
Return to work after myocardial infarction.
Canadian Medical Association Journal 104:210-212, 1971.

4378
WILBER, J.A., AND J.G. BARROW.
Hypertension-a community problem.
American Journal Medicine 52(5):653-663, 1972.

4379
WILDSMITH, J.A.W., W.G. DENNYSON, AND K.W. MYERS.
Results of resuscitation following cardiac arrest: a review from a major teaching hospital.
British Journal Anesthesia 44(7):716-720, 1972.

4380
WILENTZ, W.C.
Workmen's compensation problems: Casual relationship in cardiac deaths.
Journal Forensic Sciences 14:302-308, 1969.

4381
WILHELMSEN, L., G. GRIMBY, J. BJURE, B. EKSTROM-JODAL, M. AURELL, ET AL.
Physical activity, physical working capacity and its relation to coronary heart disease in men born in 1913.
Scandinavian Journal Clinical Laboratory Investigation Suppl. 24(110):111, 1969.

4382
WILHELMSEN, L., AND G. TIBBLIN.
Physical inactivity and risk of myocardial infarction in the men born in 1913 study.
In: Larsen, O.A. and R.O. Malmborg, Eds. Coronary heart diseases and physical fitness, Baltimore, University Park Press, pp. 251-255, 1971.

4383
WILHELMSEN, L., G. TIBBLIN, AND L. WERKÖ.
A primary preventive study in Gothenburg, Sweden.
Preventive Medicine 1:153-160, 1972.

4384
WILHELMSEN, L., H. WEDEL, AND G. TIBBLIN.
Multivariate analysis of risk factors for coronary heart disease.
Circulation 48:950, 1973.

4385
WILKERSON, J.E., AND E. EVONUK.
Changes in cardiac and skeletal muscle myosin ATPase activities after exercise.
Journal Applied Physiology 30:328, 1971.

4386
WILKIE, F., AND C. EISDORFER.
Intelligence and blood pressure in the aged.
Science 172:959-962, 1971.

4387
WILLEMS, D.
The question of coronary insufficiency signs at rest and with stress-ECG following alpha-acetyldigoxin.
Medizinische Welt 13:719-722, 1969.

4388
WILLEMS, D., AND H. KLEPZIG.
Significance of the nitrate test in an unclear work load-ECG.
Zeitschrift für Kreislaufforschung 59(4):304-314, 1970.

4389
WILLEMS, D., AND H. KLEPZIG.
The work-load electrocardiogram in bundle branch block and in the WPW syndrome in connection with the nitrate test.
Zeitschrift für Kreislaufforschung 59(4):315-322, 1970.

4390
WILLERSON, J.T., W.J. POWELL, JR., T.E. GUINEY, ET AL.
Improvement in myocardial function and coronary blood flow in ischemic myocardium after mannitol.
Journal Clinical Investigation 51:2989, 1972.

4391
WILLIAMS, G.D., AND G.S. CAMPBELL.
Long-term management of cardiac pacemakers with a systematic approach to malfunction: Report of 37 cases.
Surgery 66(4):644-654, 1969.

4392
WILLIAMS, H.J., C.W. JARVIS, W.A. NEAL, AND J.W. REYNOLDS.
Vascular thromboembolism complicating umbilical artery catheterization.
American Journal Roentgenology 116(3):475-486, 1972.

4393
WILLIAMS, J.C., M.C. DACE, I. KARACAN, R.L. WILLIAMS, ET AL.
  The risk of sleep in the cardiac patient.
  Clinical Medicine 17(1):64, 1969.

4394
WILMORE, J.H., R.N. GIRANDOLA, AND D.L. MOODY.
  Validity of skinfold and girth assessment for predicting alterations in body composition.
  Journal Applied Physiology 29:313-317, 1970.

4395
WILMORE, J.H., AND W.L. HASKELL.
  Use of the heart rate-energy expenditure relationship in the individualized prescription of exercise.
  American Journal Clinical Nutrition 24:1186-1192, 1971.

4396
WILMORE, J.H., J. ROYCE, R.N. GIRANDOLA, F.I. KATCH, AND V.L. KATCH.
  Physiological alterations resulting from a ten-week program of jogging.
  Medicine Science Sports 2:7-14, 1970.

4397
WILSON, E.M., A.J. RANIERI, JR., O.L. UPDIKE, AND J.F. DAMMANN, JR.
  An evaluation of thermal dilution for obtaining serial measurements of cardiac output.
  Medical Biological Engineering 10:179-191, 1972.

4398
WILSON, P.R., AND P.N. RUSSELL.
  Modification of psychophysical judgments as a method of reducing dissonance.
  Journal Personality Social Psychology 3:710-712, 1966.

4399
WILSON, R.S.E., T.H. MORRIS, AND J.R. REES.
  Cytomegalovirus myocarditis.
  British Heart Journal 34(8):865-868, 1972.

4400
WILTON-DAVIES, C.C.
  Computer-assisted monitoring of ECG's and heart sounds.
  Medical Biological Engineering 10:153-162, 1972.

4401
WINCOTT, E.A., AND F.I. CAIRD.
  Return to work after myocardial infarction.
  British Medical Journal 2:1302-1304, 1966.

4402
WINDISCHBAUER, G., AND H. SCHNETZ.
  Nil nocere! Iatrogenic hemopericardium with pericardial tamponade in acute benign nonspecific pericarditis.
  Münchener Medizinische Wochenschrift 114:2049, 1972.

4403
WINKLER, J.
Problems with employment of heart and circulatory patients in agriculture.
Zeitschrift für Aerztliche Fortbildung 59:826-827, 1965.

4404
WINNICK, J.P.
The prediction of maximum oxygen intake from recovery heart rates.
American Corrective Therapy Journal 26(1) 19-23, 1972.

4405
WINTER, D.A., P.M. RAUTAHARJU, AND H.K. WOLF.
Measurement and characteristics of overall noise content in exercise electrocardiograms.
American Heart Journal 74(3):324-331, 1967.

4406
WINTER, D.A., AND B.G. TRENHOLM.
Reliable triggering for exercise electrocardiograms.
IEEE Transactions Bio-Medical Engineering 16(1):75-79, 1969.

4407
WIRTH, K.E., AND K. SAWASDIMONGKOL.
On the effect of positive inotropic compounds on the contraction and relaxation of isolated heart preparations.
Basic Research Cardiology 68:256, 1973.

4408
WIRTZFELD, A.
Electrocardiographic observations in pacemaker-induced reciprocal ventricular beats.
Zeitschrift für Kreislaufforschung 61:891, 1972.

4409
WIRTZFELD, A., AND W. BAEDEKER.
Incidence of negative T-waves following pacemaker implantation.
Zeitschrift für Kreislaufforschung 61(9):828-841, 1972.

4410
WISE, J.R., JR.
Permanent pacing for symptomatic bradycardia.
Journal Maine Medical Association 63(12):269-272, 1972.

4411
WISEMAN, R.A.
Practolol. An analysis of clinical trials in cardiac dysrhythmias.
Acta Cardiologica 16:19-28, 1972.

4412
WISHNIE, H.A., T.P. HACKETT, AND N.H.CASSEM.
Psychological hazards of convalescence following myocardial infarction.
Journal American Medical Association 215(8):1292-1296, 1971.

4413
WITTICH, G.H.
Psychosomatic investigations on motion therapy in cardiovascular neuroses.
Verhandlungen der Deutschen Gesellschaft für Kreislaufforschung 32:154-158, 1966.

4414
WITTICH, G.H., AND E. ENKE-FERCHLAND.
Multidimensional integrated group therapy in psychosomatic rehabilitation.
Psychotherapy Psychosomatics 16(4-5):261-270, 1968.

4415
WIXSON, S.E.
Acute myocardial infarction computer applications.
Journal Association Advancement Medical Instrumentation 6(1):55-59, 1972.

4416
WOHLRAB, F., AND F. SCHEDEL.
The histochemical detection of changes in the enzyme activity of the human aorta wall and their relations to atherogenesis.
Deutsche Gesundheitswesen 27(31):1441-1450, 1972.

4417
WOIE, L., AND E.G. AKSNES.
A clinical evaluation of alpha-acetyldigoxin.
Nordisk Medicin 85(13) 404-408, 1971.

4418
WOJCICKI, J., AND R. CHRISTMAN.
Can lidocaine cause cardiac arrhythmia?
Wiadomosci Lekarskie 25(11):989-991, 1972.

4419
WOLF, H., P.J. MACINNIS, S. STOCK, ET AL.
Computer analysis of resting and exercise electrocardiograms.
Computers Biomedical Research 5:320, 1972.

4420
WOLF, H.K., P.J. MACINNIS, S. STOCK, ET AL.
Computer analysis of rest and exercise electrogardiograms.
Computers Biomedical Research 5(5):329-346, 1972.

4421
WOLF, H.K., P.J. MACINNIS, S. STOCK, ET AL.
The Dalhousie Program: A comprehensive analysis program for rest and exercise electro-cardiograms.
International Federation Information Processing Society TC-4 Working Conference, Hannover, West Germany, 1971. Amsterdam, The Netherlands. North Holland, 1972.

4422
WOLF, S.
Emotional stress and the heart.
Journal Rehabilitation 32:42, 1966.

4423
WOLF, S., M. BOGDONOFF, P.V. CARDON, JR., H.M. FOX, ET AL.
Psychological and sociological factors in cardiovascular disease.
Second National Conference Cardiovascular Diseases 1:235-246, 1964.

4424
WOLF, S., W.R. MCCABE, J. YAMAMOTO, C.A. ADSETT, AND W.W. SCHOTTSTAEDT.
Changes in serum lipids in relation to emotional stress during rigid control of diet and exercise.
Circulation 26:379, 1962.

4425
WOLF, S.G.
Cardiovascular reactions to symbolic stimuli.
Circulation 18:287, 1958.

4426
WOLF, S.G.
Stress and heart disease.
Modern Concepts Cardiovascular Disease 29:599, 1960.

4427
WOLFF, G.A., F. VEITH, AND B. LOWN.
A vulnerable period for ventricular tachycardia following myocardial infarction.
Cardiovascular Research 2:111, 1968.

4428
WOLFF, K.
Angina pectoris and emotional disturbances. Therapeutic implications.
Diseases Nervous System 30(6):401-404, 1969.

4429
WOLFSON, S., A.E. ACOSTA, L.I. ROSE, A.F. PARISI, AND K. ENGELMAN.
Effects of conditioning on plasma catecholamine levels during exercise in patients with coronary artery disease.
Clinical Research 19(4):714, 1971.

4430
WOLFSON, S., L.I. ROSE, J.E. BOUSSER, A.F. PARISI, ET AL.
Serum enzyme levels during exercise in patients with coronary heart disease: effects of training.
American Heart Journal 84:478-483, 1972.

4431
WOLLENBERGER, A., K. ONNEN, U. HINTERBERGER, ET AL.
Myocardial protein synthesis in acute myocardial hypoxia and ischemia.
Cardiology 56(1):48-64, 1971.

4432
WOLPERT, A., J.A. YARYURA-TOBIAS, AND L. KERTZNER.
Silent myocardial infarction in a chronic psychotic population.
Diseases Nervous System 32(4):280-283, 1971.

4433
WOLYVOVICS, M., A. BUTI, L.E. FOLLE, AND J. DIGHIERO.
Action of prenylamine lactate on angina pectoris. Simultaneous evaluation with double-blind test and ergometric bicycle.
Arquivos Brasileiros de Cardiologia 23(1):7-16, 1970.

4434
WONG, A.Y.K.
   A concentric layer model for estimating the energy expenditure of the left ventricle.
   Bulletin Mathematical Biophysics 32(4):581-598, 1970.

4435
WONG, A.Y.K., AND P.M. RAUTAHARJU.
   Relation of sarcomere lengths to filling pressures in normal and hypertrophied hearts.
   Bulletin Mathematical Biophysics 33(2):203-214, 1971.

4436
WONG, H.E., I.S. KASSER, AND R.A. BRUCE.
   Impaired maximal exercise performance with hypertensive cardiovascular disease.
   Circulation 39:633-638, 1969.

4437
WOOD, C.D., G.F. PERKINS, A.G. SMITH, AND J.M. REAUX.
   Response of the cardiovascular system in oxygen toxicity.
   Aerospace Medicine 43:162, 1972.

4438
WOODHILL, J.M., AND L. BERNSTEIN.
   Lowering serum cholesterol levels by dietary modification—a change in food habits, not a special
   diet.
   Medical Journal Australia 60-1:973, 1973.

4439
WOODS, J.W., AND W.B. BLYTHE.
   Management of malignant hypertension complicated by renal insufficiency.
   New England Journal Medicine 277(2):57-61, 1967.

4440
WOODWARK, G.M., AND M.R. GAUTHIER.
   Hospital education program following myocardial infarction.
   Canadian Medical Association Journal 106:665-667, 1972.

4441
WOOLEY, O.W., S.C. WOOLEY, AND R.B. DUNHAM.
   Can calories be perceived and do they affect hunger in obese and nonobese humans?
   Journal Comparative Physiology Psychology 80:250, 1972.

4442
WORMUTH, J., D. MATHEY, W. BLEIFELD, AND K.W. HEINRICH.
   Acidic-basic body content and disturbances of the heart rhythm in early myocardial infarction.
   Herz/Kreislauf 5:279, 1973.

4443
WOTMAN, S., J.T. BIGGER, JR., I.D. MANDEL, AND H.J. BARTELSTONE.
   Salivary electrolytes in the detection of digitalis toxicity.
   New England Journal Medicine 285:871, 1971.

4444
WRABEC, K., A. LUBIENIECKA, H. SZYDLIK, AND S. LUKASIK.
   Exercise therapy in the outpatient treatment of functional disturbances of cardiovascular type.
   Wiadomosci Lekarskie 25(8):649-654, 1972.

4445
WRABEC, K., AND L. PARADOWSKI.
Usefulness of electrocardiographic exercise tests: Master's two-step test and submaximal exercise test in the diagnosis of coronary failure.
Polski Tygodnik Lekarski 27:424-427, 1972.

4446
WRIGHT, K.E. JR., AND H. TOMODA.
Improved contractility with exercise in coronary artery disease.
Clinical Research 20(3):405, 1972.

4447
WRZESNIEWSKI, K.
Psychological problems of post-hospitalization rehabilitation of patients immediately after cardiac infarction.
Polski Tygodnik Lekarski 24(43):1663-1665, 1969.

4448
WRZESNIEWSKI, K.
Change of anxiety level in patients during sanatorium rehabilitation following myocardial infarction.
Polski Tygodnik Lekarski 26:996-998, 1971.

4449
WYNDER, E.L., AND P. HILL.
Blood lipids. How normal is normal?
Preventive Medicine 1:161-166, 1972.

4450
WYNDHAM, C.H.
Submaximal tests for estimating maximum oxygen intake.
Canadian Medical Association Journal 96:736-744, 1967.

4451
WYNDHAM, C.H.
The rehabilitation of patients with cardiovascular disease.
South African Medical Journal 41:987-991, 1967.

4452
WYNDHAM, C.H.
The problem of coronary heart disease with special reference to the influence of physical activity.
South African Medical Journal 43(23):720-723, 1969.

4453
WYNDHAM, C.H., AND G.K. SLUIS-GREMER.
The capacity for physical work of white miners in South Africa. III. The maximum oxygen intakes of normal miners and miners with cardiorespiratory diseases.
South African Medical Journal 43(4):3-8, 1969.

4454
WYNDHAM, C.H., N.B. STRYDOM, J.S. MARITZ, ET AL.
Maximum oxygen intake and maximum heart rate during strenuous work.
Journal Applied Physiology 14:927-936, 1959.

4455
WYNDHAM, C.H., N.B. STRYDOM, C.H. VAN GRAAN, A.J. VAN RENSBURG, ET AL.
Walk or jog for health. I. The energy costs of walking or running at different speeds.
South African Medical Journal 45:50-53, 1971.

4456
WYNDHAM, C.H., N.B. STRYDOM, C.H. VAN GRAAN, A.J. VAN RENSBURG, G.G. ROGERS, J.S. GREYSON, AND W.H. VAN DER WALT.
Walk or jog for health. II. Estimating the maximum aerobic capacity for exercise.
South African Medical Journal 45:53-57, 1971.

4457
WYNDHAM, C.H., W.H. VAN DER WALT, A.J. VAN RENSBURG, G.G. ROGERS, AND N.B. STRYDOM.
The influence of body weight on energy expenditure during walking on a road and on a treadmill.
Internationale Zeitschrift für Angewandte Physiologie einschliesslich Arbeitsphysiologie 29:285-292, 1971.

4458
WYNN, A.
Unwarranted emotional distress in men with ischaemic heart disease (IHD).
Medical Journal Australia 2:847-851, 1967.

4459
WYNN, A.
Rehabilitation of men with ischemic heart disease.
Israel Journal Medical Sciences 4(5):1127, 1968.

4460
WYNN, A.
Rehabilitation of men with ischemic heart disease.
Israel Journal Medical Sciences 5:791-793, 1969.

4461
YAMADA, K.
Which of ECG and VCG is superior in diagnosis?
Japanese Circulation Journal 31(11):1615-1652, 1968.

4462
YAMADA, K., M. OKAJIMA, K. HORI, ET AL.
Studies on the mechanism of ST-T alterations of electrocardiogram: with special reference to changes in unipolar surface electrogram and membrane potential during acutely induced myocardial ischemia.
Annual Report, Research Institute Environmental Medicine Nagoya University 19:41-50, 1972.

4463
YAMAKAWA, K., ET AL.
Considerations on the duration of bedrest after a myocardial infarct attack.
Japanese Journal Clinical Medicine 23:1775-1781, 1965.

4464
YAMAKAWA, K., K. KITAMURA, M. UESUGI, K. MINAMITANI, ET AL.
Exercise loading in rehabilitation of myocardial infarction cases.
Japanese Circulation Journal 29(11):1188, 1965.

4465
YAMAKAWA, K., K. KITAMURA, K. YAMAKURA, AND H. FURUYA.
Clinical evaluation of exercise tests using the radioelectrocardiograph.
Medical Electronics Biological Engineering 1:581, 1963.

4466
YAMANAKA, T., M. NAGATA, S. NOSOE, I. TAKAYAMA, ET AL.
Self fulfillment scale in neurosis and psychosomatic fear.
Journal Japanese Psychosomatic Society 12:330, 1972.

4467
YAMASAWA, I.
Serum enzyme patterns in acute ischemic heart disease with special reference to LDH isoenzymes
in intermediate types of ischemic heart disease, fresh myocardial infarction and cardiogenic shock.
Japanese Circulation Journal 37(5):509-531, 1973.

4468
YAMAZAKI, H., T. SANO, T. ODAKURA, K. TAKEUCHI, AND T. SHIMAMOTO.
Electrocardiographic and hematological changes by exercise test in coronary patients and pyridino-
lcarbamate pretreatment: A double-blind crossover trial.
American Heart Journal 79(5):640-647, 1970.

4469
YAMAZAKI, M., ET AL.
Two cases of angina pectoris complicated with ST rise by exercise.
Japanese Circulation Journal 35(6):717-718, 1971.

4470
YAMAZAKI, N.
Effects of heredity and environmental factors on development of myocardial infarction.
Japanese Circulation Journal 37(1):69, 1973.

4471
YANUSHKEVICHUS, Z.I., ET AL.
Use of consecutive statistical analysis for determining the hazard with respect to angina pectoris.
Kardiologiya 7(1):50-53, 1967.

4472
YARETZKY, A.
Indications for the use of cardiac pacemakers.
Family Physician 2(3):290-292, 1972.

4473
YASIN, S.
Measuring habitual leisure-time physical activity by recall record questionnaire.
In: Karvonen, M.J. and A.J. Barry, Eds. Physical activity and the heart, p. 372, Springfield, Ill.
Thomas, 1967.

4474
YASUI, S., M. YOKOI, N. OKAMOTO, Y. MIZUNO, ET AL.
Computer diagnosis of electrocardiograms by means of joint probability.
Israel Journal Medical Sciences 5(4):913-916, 1969.

4475
YATTEAU, R.F., AND E.S. ORGAIN.
Bedside diagnosis of postinfarction ventricular septal defect using the hydrogen-sensitive, platinum-tipped, wire electrode.
American Heart Journal 84(5):712-714, 1972.

4476
YEH, B.K., P. TAO, AND N. DE GUZMAN.
Mobitz type II AV block as manifestation of digitalis toxicity.
Journal Electrocardiology 5(1):74-77, 1972.

4477
YODFAT, Y.
The prevalence of cardiovascular disease in different ethnic and socioeconomic groups in Beit Shemesh, Israel.
Israel Journal Medical Sciences 8(10):1685-1694, 1972.

4478
YOKOI, M., Y. WATANABE, N. OKAMOTO, S. YASUI, AND Y. MIZUNO.
On-line computer diagnosis of arrhythmias on ECG by using small scale Digital Computer System.
Japanese Circulation Journal 33:129-138, 1969.

4479
YOKOI, M., S. YASUI, M. OKAJIMA, AND Y. MIZUNO.
Comparative studies on the diagnostic accuracy between the two diagnostic logic in electro-cardiographic interpretation.
Japanese Circulation Journal 33:51-58, 1969.

4480 YOSHIKAWA, T.
Rehabilitation of patients with psychosomatic deseases.
Journal Japanese Psychosomatic Society 12:352-353, 1972.

4481
YOSHIOKA, M., ET AL.
A study on apex cardiographic changes in a wave during exercise.
Japanese Circulation Journal 35(6):707, 1971.

4482
YOSHIMURA, S.
Problems in phonocardiographic diagnosis.
Japanese Circulation Journal 30:1560-1561, 1966.

4483
YU, P.N., C.A. IMBODEN, JR., S.M. FOX, III, AND T. KILLIP, III.
Coronary care unit. I and II.
Modern Concepts Cardiovascular Disease 34:23-30, 1965.

4484
YU, P.N., AND D.H. KRAMER.
    Management in the acute stage.
    Journal Rehabilitation 32:32, 1966.

4485
ZABAROVSKII, Y.Y.
    Hemodynamic characteristics in hypertensive patients during mental, emotional and physical stress.
    Latvijas psr Zinatnu Akademijas Vestis 13:104-114, 1973.

4486
ZADIONCHENKO, V.S.
    Long-term administration of Athromide to patients with coronary atherosclerosis.
    Kardiologiya 7(10):32-35, 1967.

4487
ZAITSEV, A.E.
    Cardiohemodynamics in patients with myocardial infarction during their rehabilitation by thera-
    peutic exercises.
    Kardiologiya 12(8):118-121, 1972.

4488
ZAITSEV, V.P.
    Certain problems of psychotherapy of patients with myocardial infarction.
    Kardiologiya 12:36-40, 1972.

4489
ZAMFIR, C., E. TURCU, B. MARINESCU, M. IONESCU, ET AL.
    Considerations on the rehabilitation of patients from the armed forces with ischemic cardiopathy.
    Medicina Interna 23(5):583-586, 1971.

4490
ZANDER, E.
    Deep psychological aspects of the hyperkinetic heart syndrome: Preliminary communication.
    Zeitschrift für Psychosomatische Medizin und Psychoanalyse 16:19, 1970.

4491
ZAPPALA, A.
    Influence of training and sex on the isolation and control of single motor units.
    American Journal Physical Medicine 49:348-361, 1970.

4492
ZÄZIWIL, E.S.
    Respiration as functional test of the heart.
    Schweizerische Medizinische Wochenschrift 100(4):193-196, 1970.

4493
ZBOROMIRSKII, V.V.
    Use of graded physical loads for early diagnosis of cardiac insufficiency in patients with aortic
    cardiac disease.
    Vrachebnoe Delo 1:56-59, 1971.

4494
ZEFT, H.J., S.D. PATTERSON, AND E.S. ORGAIN.
Propranolol in the long-term treatment of angina pectoris.
Annals Internal Medicine 70(5):1082, 1969.

4495
ZEINER-HENRIKSEN, T.
Cardiovascular disease symptoms in Norway: A study of prevalence and a mortality follow-up.
Journal Chronic Diseases 24(9):553-567, 1971.

4496
ZELIS, R., D.T. MASON, AND E. BRAUNWALD.
Control of skin and muscle circulation of the forearm during leg exercise in normal subjects and patients with congestive heart failure.
Clinical Research 15(4):453, 1967.

4497
ZELIS, R., D.T. MASON, AND E. BRAUNWALD.
Partition of blood flow to the cutaneous and muscular beds of the forearm at rest and during leg exercise in normal subjects and patients with heart failure.
Physiologist 10:357, 1967; Circulation Research 24:799-806, 1969.

4498
ZERA, E., AND A. ZBIEĆ.
Evaluation of rehabilitation after heart surgery.
Polski Tygodnik Lekarski 25:730-733, 1970.

4499
ZERDICK, J. AND H. MELLEROWICZ.
ST segment depression in the exercise electrocardiogram. Comparative ergometric electrocardiographic studies of the effect of the time factor on the ST segments in coronary insufficiency.
Zeitschrift für Kreislaufforschung 58:1128-1137, 1969.

4500
ZHDANENKO, V.G., M.S. LUKASHOVA, AND M.F. SHVETS.
State of contractile function of the cardiac muscle in persons under the age of 40 who have sustained myocardial infarction according to information from some instrumental methods of study.
Terapevticheskii Arkhiv 43(11):56-60, 1971.

4501
ZIEGELHOFFER, A., M. FEDELESOVA, AND K. SISKA.
The influence of exogenous ATP on cardiac metabolism in acute hypoxia.
Cardiology 56(1):136-142, 1971.

4502
ZILLI, A.
The rehabilitation of the sick affected by myocardial infarction.
Bollettino della Societá Italiana di Cardiologia 15(4):287-291, 1970.

4503
ZIMKIN, N.V., AND V.G. PAKHOTOV.
Variation of certain interrelated muscle activity parameters in stereotype movements.
Fiziologisheskii Zhurnal SSSR Imeni I.M. Sechenova 55:630-640, 1969.

4504

ZIMMER, H.G., C. TRENDELENBURG, AND E. GERLACH.
  Acceleration of adenine nucleotide synthesis de novo during development of cardiac hypertrophy.
  Journal Molecular Cellular Cardiology 4(3):279-282, 1972.

4505

ZIPES, D.P.
  The contribution of artificial pacemaking to understanding the pathogenesis of arrhythmias.
  American Journal Cardiology 28:211-222, 1971.

4506

ZIPES, D.P., AND C. FISCH.
  Supraventricular arrhythmias with abnormal QRS complex.
  Archives Internal Medicine 130(6):950-955, 1972.

4507

ZIPES, D.P., AND S.B. KNOEBEL.
  Rapid rate-dependent ventricular ectopy. Adverse responses to atropine-induced rate increase.
  Chest 62(3).255-258, 1972.

4508

ZIPFEL, J., J.D. MEYER-ERKELENZ, AND A. DIETZ.
  Evaluation of the electrocardiogram during rest and exertion using various computer systems.
  Verhandlungen der Deutschen Gesellschaft für Kreislaufforschung 37:445-449, 1971.

4509

ZOCHOWSKI, R.J., AND W. SERZYSKO.
  Earpiece dye dilution technique as a method for evaluation of haemodynamic changes during standardized effort test.
  Cor Vasa 13(1).50-63, 1971.

4510

ZOELCH, K.A.
  Prevention and rehabilitation of cardiovascular diseases.
  Fortschritte der Medizin 90:1213-1217, 1972.

4511

ZOHMAN, L.R.
  The expanding role of the rehabilitation counselor in returning the cardiac to work.
  Rehabilitation Record 12:1-5, 1971.

4512

ZOHMAN, L.R.
  Early ambulation of post-myocardial infarction patients: Montefiore Hospital.
  In: Naughton, J., H.K. Hellerstein, and I.C. Mohler, Eds. Exercise testing and exercise training in coronary heart disease, pp. 329-335, New York, Academic Press, 1973.

4513

ZOHMAN, L.R.
  Economic aspects of a stress testing and exercise training program.
  In:Naughton, J., H.K. Hellerstein, and I.C. Mohler, Eds. Exercise testing and exercise training in coronary heart disease, pp. 375-385, New York, Academic Press, 1973.

4514
ZOHMAN, L.R., AND J.S. TOBIS.
  The effect of exercise training of patients with angina pectoris.
  Archives Physical Medicine Rehabilitation 48:525-532, 1967.

4515
ZOHMAN, L.R., AND J.S. TOBIS.
  Cardiac Rehabilitation.
  New York, Grune and Stratton, 1970.

4516
ZONERAICH, O., AND S. ZONERAICH.
  Bigeminal rhythm, vectorcardiographic patterns in coronary artery disease.
  Journal Electrocardiology 5(3):265-271, 1972.

4517
ZUGIBE, F.T., T.L. CONLEY, P. BELL, JR., AND M. STANDISH.
  Enzyme decay curves in normal and infarcted myocardium.
  Archives Pathology 93(4):308-311, 1972.

4518
ZUKEL, W.J., R.H. LEWIS, P.E. ENTERLINE, R.C. PAINTER, ET AL.
  A short-term community study of the epidemiology of coronary heart disease. A preliminary report
  on the North Dakota study.
  American Journal Public Health 49:1630-1639, 1959.

4519
ZWIRN, P., E. SEBAOUN, A. FRANCESCHI, AND J. FONDARAI.
  Measurement of the systolic volume by external isotopic counting. Study on a model of curve
  gauging.
  Annales de Physique Biologique et Médicale 6(2):79-86, 1972.

4520
ZYZANSKI, S.J., AND C.D. JENKINS.
  Basic dimensions within the coronary-prone behavior pattern.
  Journal Chronic Diseases 22(12):781-795, 1970.

4521
ANONYMOUS.
  A four-pronged attack upon congestive heart failure.
  Patient Care 7:84, 1973.

4522
ANONYMOUS.
  An assessment of long-term anticoagulant administration after cardiac infarction. Second report of
  the working party on anticoagulant therapy in coronary thrombosis to the Medical Research
  Council.
  British Medical Journal 2:837-843, 1964.

4523
ANONYMOUS.
  Anticoagulant therapy. A clinical dilemma.
  Journal American Medical Association 187:27-40, 1964.

4524
ANONYMOUS.
   Anticoagulants in acute myocardial infarction.
   Journal American Medical Association 225(7):724, 1973.

4525
ANONYMOUS.
   Arrhythmias in acute myocardial infarction.
   Canadian Medical Association Journal 97(12):762-763, 1967.

4526
ANONYMOUS.
   Bibliography of short-term anticoagulant therapy in myocardial infarct. (1931-1964).
   Laval Médical 37:738-749, 1966.

4527
ANONYMOUS.
   Cardiac arrhythmias.
   Lancet 2:423, 1973.

4528
ANONYMOUS.
   Cardiac pacing in acute myocardial infarction.
   Journal Irish Medical Association 65(15):400, 1972.

4529
ANONYMOUS.
   Cardiac rehabilitation.
   Medical Journal Australia 2:946, 1973.

4530
ANONYMOUS.
   Cardiologic emergencies in the clinic and in practice.
   Herz/Kreislauf 5:308, 1973.

4531
ANONYMOUS.
   Clinical studies of myocardial infarction I. Hemodynamics in patients with acute myocardial
   infarction.
   Japanese Circulation Journal 37(9):1187-1188, 1973.

4532
ANONYMOUS.
   Closed panel conference. Present status of the management of congestive failure and advances in
   diuretic therapy.
   Journal New Drugs 1(4):160-191, 1961.

4533
ANONYMOUS.
   Coronary artery disease and rehabilitation.
   South African Medical Journal 40(7):130, 1966.

4534
ANONYMOUS.
   Coronary disease and competitiveness.
   British Medical Journal 1:1, 1969.

4535
ANONYMOUS.
   Danger of hypoglycaemia with use of propranolol.
   Medical Journal Australia 2:92, 1973.

4536
ANONYMOUS.
   Dialogue and therapeutic arguments with respect to the practical course of a treatment with digitalis.
   Revue du Practicien 23:3282, 1973.

4537
ANONYMOUS.
   Diet and coronary heart disease: A Council statement.
   Journal American Medical Association 222(13):1647, 1972.

4538
ANONYMOUS.
   Diet and coronary heart disease.
   American Journal Clinical Nutrition 26(1):53-54, 1973.

4539
ANONYMOUS.
   Early mobilization after uncomplicated myocardial infarction.
   Lancet 2:346, 1973.

4540
ANONYMOUS.
   Effect of diet on coronary heart disease mortality.
   Lancet 2:1266, 1973.

4541
ANONYMOUS.
   Enhancement of fibrinolytic activity.
   Lancet 2:716, 1973.

4542
ANONYMOUS.
   Exercise and coronary heart disease.
   Medical Letter Drugs Therapeutics 10:93-94, 1968.

4543
ANONYMOUS.
   Exercise and coronary patient.
   Medical Journal Australia 1:247, 1972.

4544
ANONYMOUS.
   Exercise and heart disease.
   Journal American Medical Association 200(2):173-174, 1967.

4545
ANONYMOUS.
Fibrinolytic activity, obesity, and coronary heart disease.
Journal American Medical Association 224(9):1288, 1973.

4546
ANONYMOUS.
Fitness, health, and motor behavior. Exercise and coronary heart disease.
Research News 22(5):3-10, 1971.

4547
ANONYMOUS.
Functional ergometric evaluation of patients with chronic myocardial infarction.
Minerva Cardiologica 21(11):759, 1973.

4548
ANONYMOUS.
Intercourse after myocardial infarction.
British Medical Journal 3:494, 1973.

4549
ANONYMOUS.
Ischemic heart disease—isotopes and epidemiology.
Medical Journal Australia 2(20):915-916, 1973.

4550
ANONYMOUS.
Long-term anticoagulant therapy after myocardial infarction. A study of 747 patients in 15 hospitals.
Journal American Medical Society 193:929-934, 1965.

4551
ANONYMOUS.
Metabolic changes of myocardial infarction.
Japanese Circulation Journal 37(9):1201-1202, 1973.

4552
ANONYMOUS.
Monitoring pacemaker in treatment of acute heart block.
British Medical Journal 4:784-785, 1972.

4553
ANONYMOUS.
Myocardial infarction in railway environment—medicoprofessional aspects concerning 100 cases.
Archives des Maladies Professionnelles 34(3):165, 1973.

4554
ANONYMOUS.
Prognostic importance of the electrocardiogram after myocardial infarction. Experience in the Coronary Drug Project.
Annals Internal Medicine 77(5):677-689, 1972.

4555
ANONYMOUS.
  Prognostic importance of premature beats following myocardial infarction. Experience in the
  Coronary Drug Project.
  Journal American Medical Association 223(10):1116-1124, 1973.

4556
ANONYMOUS.
  Prospect of computer diagnosis of cardiovascular disease. Informal meeting at the 6th international
  conference on Medical Electronics and Biological Engineering, Tokyo, 1965.
  Japanese Heart Journal 8:438-453, 1967.

4557
ANONYMOUS.
  Report of the inquiry on the training and resettlement of disabled persons.
  London, England. Her Majesty's Stationery Office, 1956.

4558
ANONYMOUS.
  Return to work after myocardial infarction.
  Scottish Medical Journal 12:325-326, 1967.

4559
ANONYMOUS.
  When should your coronary patients return to work?
  Patient Care 4:82-113, 1970.

4560
ANONYMOUS.
  The chief goal of computerized ECG evaluation is the ample relief of the overburdened doctor.
  Technische Gids voor Ziekenhuis en Instelling 41:503-517, 1972.

4561
ANONYMOUS.
  Tracings of changes of serum enzymes. Specially S-LDH-isoenzymes and abnormal electro-
  cardiogram on acute myocardial infarction.
  Japanese Circulation Journal 37(9):1187, 1973.

4562
ANONYMOUS.
  Treatment results and experiences in a coronary care unit.
  Opuscula Medica 16(7):227-233, 1971.

4563
ANONYMOUS.
  Walking through angina.
  British Medical Journal 2:904, 1966.

4564
ANONYMOUS.
  Working group on methodology of multifactor preventive trials in ischemic heart disease.
  Community Health 5:101, 1973.

4565
AMERICAN HEALTH FOUNDATION.
  Position statement on diet and coronary heart disease.
  Preventive Medicine 1:255-286, 1972.

4566
AMERICAN HEART ASSOCIATION.
  Ad Hoc Committee on Rehabilitation of the Young Cardiac, Council on Rheumatic Fever and
  Congenital Heart Disease, American Heart Association. Recreational activity and career choice
  recommendations for use by physicians, counseling physical education directors, vocational coun-
  selors, parents and young patients with heart disease.
  Circulation 43:459-464, 1971.

4567
AMERICAN HEART ASSOCIATION.
  Exercise testing and training of apparently healthy individuals. A handbook for physicians.
  New York, American Heart Association, Committee on Exercise, 1972.

4568
AMERICAN HEART ASSOCIATION.
  Explanation for proposed informed consent for exercise testing with attached forms for ap-
  parently healthy subjects and for people with heart disease.
  American Heart Association, Rehabilitation Committee. Memorandum CS 71524, June 1971.

4569
AMERICAN HEART ASSOCIATION.
  The heart future.
  In: Report of the Committee of Future Role. New York, American Heart Association, 1962.

4570
AMERICAN HEART ASSOCIATION.
  The National diet-heart study. Final report. American Heart Association Monograph No. 18.
  Circulation 37 (Suppl. 1):1-428, 1968.

4571
AMERICAN HEART ASSOCIATION.
  Work Evaluation Units. Newsletters.
  American Heart Association Vol. I, 1965.

4572
AMERICAN MEDICAL ASSOCIATION/AMERICAN ASSOCIATION FOR HEALTH, PHYSICAL ED-
  UCATION, AND RECREATION.
  Exercise and fitness.
  Journal American Medical Association 166(14):1744-1746, 1968.

4573
CHEST AND HEART ASSOCIATION, LONDON, ENGLAND.
  Preventive Techniques for the Modern Community. (Summaries of papers read at a two-day
  conference, March 2-3, 1971).

4574
COMMUNITY COUNCIL, HOUSTON, TEXAS.
  Report of the Rehabilitation Consultation Panel Project.
  Health Section, Community Council, Houston, Texas, March 1962.

4575
CORONARY DRUG PROJECT, RESEARCH GROUP.
  The Coronary Drug Project: Findings leading to discontinuation of the 2.5 mg/day estrogen
  group.
  Journal American Medical Association 226(6):652, 1973.

4576
FRENCH CARDIOLOGY SOCIETY.
  Advice of the French Cardiology Society with respect to return to work after a myocardial
  infarction.
  Presse Médicale 72(17):1034, 1964.

4577
INTER-SOCIETY COMMISSION FOR HEART DISEASE RESOURCES, ATHEROSCLEROSIS
  STUDY GROUP, AND EPIDEMIOLOGY STUDY GROUP.
  Primary prevention of the atherosclerotic diseases.
  Circulation 42:A55, 1970.

4578
METROPOLITAN LIFE INSURANCE CO. (U.S.A.)
  Detection and prognosis in coronary artery disease.
  Statistical Bulletin 49(6):2-4, 1968.

4579
METROPOLITAN LIFE INSURANCE CO. (U.S.A.)
  Prognosis in coronary heart disease among Metropolitan employees.
  Statistical Bulletin 50:6-8, 1969.

4580
METROPOLITAN LIFE INSURANCE CO. (U.S.A.)
  Regional variations in mortality from heart disease.
  Statistical Bulletin 53:3-6, 1972.

4581
NATIONAL DIET-HEART STUDY RESEARCH GROUP.
  The national diet—heart study final report.
  Circulation 37(Suppl.1):1, 1968.

4582
NATIONAL WORKSHOP ON EXERCISE.
  Proceedings National Workshop on exercise in the prevention, in the evaluation, and in the
  treatment of heart disease. (Myrtle Beach, South Carolina, 1969).
  Journal South Carolina Medical Association 65(Suppl. 1):1-105, 1969.
  Workshop Report I. Exercise and performance evaluation.
  Workshop Report II. Exercise and stress testing.
  Workshop Report III. Exercise programs for the prevention of heart disease.
  Workshop Report IV. Exercise and the treatment of heart disease.
  Workshop Report V. Exercise and rehabilitation..

4583
NEW YORK HEART ASSOCIATION.
  Criteria Committee of New York Heart Association. Diseases of the Heart and Blood Vessels:
  Nomenclature and Criteria for Diagnoses, 6th edition, pp. 112-113.
  Boston, Mass. Little Brown, 1953.

4584
PURDUE FARM CARDIAC PROJECT.
  Energy requirements for physical work.
  Agricultural Experiment Station, Research progress report No. 30. Lafayette, Indiana, 1961.

4585
SCANDINAVIAN COMMITTEE, ECG CLASSIFICATION.
  Scandinavian Committee on ECG Classification. "The Minnesota Code" for ECG classification.
  Adaptation to CR leads and modification of the code for ECG's recorded during and after
  exercise.
  Acta Medica Scandinavica (Suppl.)481:1-26, 1967.

4586
U.S. FEDERAL AVIATION AGENCY OFFICE.
  Problems in aeromedical certification. Cardiovascular response to exercise following myocardial
  infarction.
  Aviation Medicine 66(17):1-5, 1966.

4587
U.S. FEDERAL AVIATION AGENCY OFFICE.
  Clinical aviation medicine. A physical conditioning program for cardiac patients. A progress report.
  Aviation Medicine 66:5-9, 1966.

4588
U.S. DEPARTMENT OF HEALTH, EDUCATION, AND WELFARE. PUBLIC HEALTH SERVICE.
  The health consequences of smoking—a report of the Surgeon General, 1971.
  Washington, D.C., 1971.

4589
U.S. VETERANS ADMINISTRATION.
  Veterans Administration cooperative study group on antihypertensive agents. Effects of treatment
  on morbidity in hypertension. 2. Results in patients with diastolic blood pressure averaging 90
  through 114 mmHg.
  Journal American Medical Association 213:1143-1152, 1970.

4590
UNIVERSITY GROUP DIABETES PROGRAM.
  The University Group Diabetes Program—A study of the effects of hypoglycemic agents on
  vascular complications in patients with adult-onset diabetes.
  Diabetes 19(Suppl. 2):747, 1970.

4591
UNIVERSITY, STATE OF NEW YORK.
  Design for heart disease prevention programs.
  The University of the State of New York, State Education Department, and State of New York,
  Department of Health, Albany, N.Y., 1970.

4592
WORLD HEALTH ORGANIZATION.
  A programme for the physical rehabilitation of patients with acute myocardial infarction. Report
  of a Working Group: Freiburg im Breisgau, 1968.
  WHO Regional Office for Europe. Copenhagen, Denmark, 1968.

4593
WORLD HEALTH ORGANIZATION.
International work on cardiovascular diseases 1959-1969.
Geneva, Switzerland, 1969.

4594
WORLD HEALTH ORGANIZATION.
Psychological aspects of the rehabilitation of cardiovascular patients. Report on a working group,
Warsaw.
WHO Regional Office for Europe. Copenhagen, Denmark, 1969.

4595
WORLD HEALTH ORGANIZATION.
Rehabilitation of patients with cardiovascular diseases. Report on a Seminar, Noordwijk aan Zee,
2-7 October 1967.
WHO Regional Office for Europe. Copenhagen, Denmark, 1969. (Euro 0381)

4596
WORLD HEALTH ORGANIZATION.
Working group on methodology of multifactor preventive trials in ischaemic heart disease.
Community Health, 5:101, 1973.

4597
WORLD HEALTH ORGANIZATION.
Exercise tests in relation to cardiovascular function.
WHO Chronicle 22:386-389, 1968.

4598
WORLD HEALTH ORGANIZATION.
International action in cardiovascular diseases.
WHO Chronicle 23(9):395-404, 1969.

4599
WORLD HEALTH ORGANIZATION.
Ischaemic heart disease registers.
WHO Chronicle 24(1):11-13, 1970.

4600
WORLD HEALTH ORGANIZATION.
Society stress and disease.
WHO Chronicle 25(4):168-178, 1971.

4601
WORLD HEALTH ORGANIZATION.
Exercise tests in relation to cardiovascular function.
WHO Technical Report Series 388:5-28, 1968.

4602
WORLD HEALTH ORGANIZATION.
Rehabilitation of patients with cardiovascular disease.
WHO Technical Report Series 270, 1964.

Appendix[*]

4603
ABDULAEV, D.M., ET AL.
Dynamic study of the blood coagulation and anticoagulation system components in patients with myocardial infarct and chronic coronary insufficiency in relation to continuous and discontinuous anticoagulant treatment.
Azerbaidzhanskii Meditsinskii Zhurnal 1:3-14, 1964.

4604
ACREDSON, O., C. FÜRBERG, AND H. LINDERHOLM.
The effect of a ganglionic blocking agent (chlorisondamine) on electrocardiogram, physical work capacity and hemodynamics in patients with vasoregulatory asthenia.
Acta Medica Scandinavica (Suppl.)472:36-53, 1967.

4605
ADAMS, C.W.
Two-step tolerance test.
Journal American Medical Association 203:183, 1968; 204:178-179, 1968.

4606
ADAMS, C.W., D.B. EFFLER, A. KATTUS, ET AL.
Medical versus surgical therapy for ischemic heart disease.
Chest 58 (Suppl.1):293-314, 1970.

4607
ADAMS, C.W., AND R.G. KIGER.
Office evaluation of cardiac function by exercise.
Journal Tennessee Medical Association 62:209-217, 1969.

4608
AGNOLI, G.C., A. CARIANI, G. PINELLI, AND G.F. FERRETTI.
Anticoagulant therapy in myocardial infarct.
Cardiologia Pratica 13:804-811, 1962.

4609
ALDREDGE, J.L., AND A.J. WELCH.
Variations of heart rate during sleep as a function of the sleep cycle.
Electroencephalography Clinical Neurophysiology 35:193-198, 1973.

4610
ALIMURUNG, M.M.
Heart disease in the Philippines.
American Journal Cardiology 10:362, 1962.

4611
ANASTASSIADIS, C.T., AND J.E. SIVERTSON.
Myocardial infarction a few years experience in a Midwestern General Hospital.
Annals Internal Medicine 55:749-759, 1961.

* Citations in this section were considered useful after the main body of the *Guide to the Literature* was in press.

4612
ANDERSON, M.C., B. FURNASS, R. JENKINS, H. PANG, AND J. PENNINGTON.
Effects of three weeks' strenuous exercise on the cardiovascular fitness of young women.
Medical Journal Australia 2(21):966, 1973.

4613
ANDERSON, T.
Digitalis induced impotence.
Nordisk Medicin 75:334, 1966.

4614
ANDREWS, C.T., AND T.S. WILSON.
Vitamin C and thrombotic episodes.
Lancet 2:39, 1973.

4615
ARAVANIS, C., AND G. MICHAELIDES.
Cardiovascular diseases in Greece.
American Journal Cardiology 10:349, 1962.

4616
ASLAN, M.
Myocardial infarction. Analysis of 110 cases from diagnostic prognostic and therapeutic view-
points.
Western Medicine 2:342, 1961.

4617
AUSCHUTZ, F.
On the arteriosclerosis problem.
Wiener Medizinische Wochenschrift 114:115-118, 1964.

4618
AVOGARO, P., C. CAPRI, M. PAIS, AND G. CAZZOLATO.
Plasma and urine cortisol behavior and fat mobilization in man after coffee ingestion.
Israel Journal Medical Sciences 9(2):114, 1973.

4619
BAKER, J.D.
Lay diet clubs.
Obesity Bariatric Medicine 2(1):5, 1973.

4620
BANKS, R.E.
Myocardial infarction and normal coronary arteriogram–II.
American Journal Cardiology 32:126, 1973.

4621
BANNISTER, R., E. ASMUSSEN, K.W. DONALD, G. ROSE, ET AL.
Symposium on the meaning of physical fitness.
Proceedings Royal Society Medicine 62:1155-1191, 1969.

4622
BARBANO, G.
    On the control of anticoagulant therapy in myocardial infarct. Thrombo-elastography and Quick's time (consideration and comparison).
    Minerva Medica 55:612-618, 1964.

4623
BARNES, R., AND W.W. SCHOTTSTAEDT.
    The relation of emotional state to renal excretion of water and electrolytes in patients with congestive heart failure.
    American Journal Medicine 29:217, 1960.

4624
BARNETT, A.J., AND F.G. SILBERBERG.
    Long-term results of treatment of severe hypertension.
    Medical Journal Australia 2(21):960, 1973.

4625
BAROLDI, G.
    Significance of arterial obstructive lesions in early diagnosis of coronary heart disease.
    In: Halonen, P., and A. Loujiha, Eds. Early diagnosis of coronary heart disease. Proceedings, second Paavo Nurmi Symposium, Finland, 1971, pp. 49-66. Basel, S. Karger, 1973.

4626
BASHOUR, T., J. NAUGHTON, AND T. CHENG.
    Systolic time intervals in patients with artificial pacemakers.
    American Journal Cardiology 32:287-290, 1973.

4627
BASU, D.P.
    Anticoagulant therapy in cardiovascular diseases.
    Indian Practitioner 14:699-710, 1961.

4628
BEARD, E.F., AND C.A. OWEN.
    Cardiac arrhythmias during exercise testing in healthy men.
    Aerospace Medicine 44:286-289, 1973.

4629
BEAUMONT, J.L., G. ANGUERA, M.H. BUC, AND J. LÈNEGRE.
    Causes of myocardial infarct and treatment with anticoagulants.
    Naika 11:1203-1226, 1962.

4630
BECK, A.T.
    Sexuality and depression.
    Medical Aspects Human Sexuality 2:44-51, 1968.

4631
BEHR, G., AND P. BURTON.
    Heart-muscle magnesium.
    Laucet 2:450, 1973.

4632
BELBECK, L.W., AND J.B. CRITZ.
Effect of exercise on the plasma concentration of anorexigenic substance in man.
Proceedings Society Experimental Biology Medicine 142(1):19, 1973.

4633
BELOUSOV, S.S., M.E. GORKINA, AND M.A. MALAKHOVA.
Myocardial asynergy in ischemic heart disease and the influence of glyceryl trinitrate.
Kardiologiya 12:64-7, 1972.

4634
BENGTSSON, C.
Ischemic heart disease in women—material and methods.
Acta Medica Scandinavica (Suppl.)549:9-20, 1973.

4635
BENGTSSON, C.
Prevalence of ischemic heart disease in women in Goteborg, Sweden.
Acta Medica Scandinavica (Suppl.)549:21-26, 1973.

4636
BENGTSSON, C.
Incidence of myocardial infarction in women in Goteborg, Sweden.
Acta Medica Scandinavica (Suppl.)549:27-30, 1973.

4637
BENGTSSON, C., P. BJORNTORP, AND E. TIBBLIN.
Serum cholesterol and serum triglyceride levels in a population sample of women and in women
with ischemic heart disease.
Acta Medica Scandinavica (Suppl.)549:51-59, 1973.

4638
BENGTSSON, C., T. HALLSTRO, AND G. TIBBLIN.
Social factors, stress experience, and personality traits in women with ischemic heart disease,
compared to a population sample of women.
Acta Medica Scandinavica (Suppl.)549:82-92, 1973.

4639
BENGTSSON, C.
Physical activity in a population sample of women and in women with ischemic heart disease.
Acta Medica Scandinavica (Suppl.)549:93-96, 1973.

4640
BENGTSSON, C.
Prevalence of multiple risk factors for ischemic heart disease in women with and without known
ischemic heart disease.
Acta Medica Scandinavica (Suppl.)549:97-105, 1973.

4641
BENGTSSON, C., G. TIBBLIN, AND L. WILHELMS.
Risk factors for ischemic heart disease. Comparison between male and female population in
Goteborg, Sweden.
Acta Medica Scandinavica (Suppl.)549:106-113, 1973.

4642

BENOMAR, M., AND M. BERRADA.
Incidence and epidemiological features of myocardial infarction in young Maroccan adults.
Coeur et Médicine Interne 12:409, 1973.

4643

BERGSTROM, J., AND E. HULTMAN.
Muscle glycogen synthesis after exercise. An enhancing factor localized to the muscle cells in man.
Nature 210:309-310, 1966.

4644

BERKSON, D.M., S. STAMLER, AND W. JACKSON.
The precordial electrocardiogram during and after strenuous exercise.
American Journal Cardiology 18:43-51, 1966.

4645

BERKSON, D.M., J. STAMLER, H.A. LINDBERG, W.A. MILLER, E.L. STEVENS, ET AL.
Heart rate: an important risk factor for coronary mortality—Ten years experience of the Peoples Gas Co. Epidemiologic Study (1958-68).
In: Jones, R.J., Ed. Atherosclerosis, Second International Symposium, p. 382. New York, N.Y., Springer-Verlag, 1970.

4646

BERSHTEIN, S.A., AND O.V. BAZILYUK.
Changes in the hemodynamics and efferent sympathetic activity of some pressor cardiovascular reflexes in acute hypoxic hypoxia.
Fiziolohichnyi Zhurnal (Kiev) 18:769-78, 1972.

4647

BEVEGARD, S., A. HOLMGREN, AND B. JONSSON.
The effect of body position on the circulation at rest and during exercise with especial reference to the influence of stroke volume.
Acta Physiologica Scandinavica 49:279-298, 1960.

4648

BEVEGARD, B.S., A. HOLMGREN, AND B. JONSSON.
Circulatory studies in well-trained athletes at rest and during heavy exercise with special reference to stroke volume and the influence of body position.
Acta Physiologica Scandinavica 57:26-50, 1963.

4649

BHAN, A.K., AND J. SCHEUER.
Effects of physical conditioning on cardiac myosin.
Circulation 46 (Suppl. II):II-131, 1972.

4650

BIASE, G. DI, E. BONAVITA, I. SPAGNA, F. TABARRONI, AND F. FRANCESCONI.
New model study of residual heart power in cardiopathic patients in view of a rehabilitation program.
Giornale di Gerontologia 21:334, 1973.

4651
BIELAWSKI, J.
   Exercise electrocardiography.
   Journal Internal Medicine 15:10, 1972.

4652
BIERENBAUM, M.L., A.I. FLEISCHMAN, R.I. RAICHELSON, T. HAYTON, AND P.B. WATSON.
   Ten-year experience of modified-fat diets on younger men with coronary heart disease.
   Lancet 1:1404, 1973.

4653
BILLINGHURST, J.R.
   Coronary heart disease in Africa
   British Medical Journal 4:50, 1973.

4654
BIÖRCK, G.
   The biology of myocardial infarction.
   Circulation 37:1071-1085, 1968.

4655
BIORCK, G.
   Early diagnosis of coronary heart disease. What is it good for.
   In: Halonen, P. and A. Louhija, Eds. Early diagnosis of coronary heart disease, pp. 25-37. Basel,
   S. Karger, 1973.

4656
BIRKENHA, W.H.
   Early mobilization after umcomplicated myocardial infarction.
   Lancet 2:858-59, 1973.

4657
BISTENI, A., D. SODI-PALLARES, J. PONCE DE LEÓN, AND D. ARIZA.
   Polyparametric information of the electrocardiogram in injured tissue.
   In: Halonen, P. and A. Louhija, Eds. Early diagnosis of coronary heart disease, pp. 132-141.
   Basel, S. Karger, 1973.

4658
BJERNULF, A..
   Hemodynamic aspects of physical training after myocardial infarction.
   Acta Medica Scandinavica (Suppl.)548:1-50, 1973.

4659
BJORK, L.
   The value of different angiographic procedures in coronary heart disease.
   In: Halonen, P. and A. Loujiha, Eds. Early diagnosis of coronary heart disease, pp. 76-84. Basel,
   S. Karger, 1973.

4660
BJÖRNTORP, P., P. BERCHTOLD, G. GRIMBY, B. LINDHOLM, ET AL.
   Effects of physical training on glucose tolerance, plasma insulin, and lipids and on body
   composition in men after myocardial infarction.
   Acta Medica Scandinavica 192:439-43, 1972.

4661
BLACKBURN, H., H.L. TAYLOR, AND A. KEYS.
The electrocardiogram in prediction of five-year coronary heart disease incidence among men aged forty through fifty-nine.
Circulation 41 (Suppl. 1):1-154, 1970.

4662
BLACKET, R.B., B. LEELARTHAEPIN, A.J. PALMER, AND J.M. WOODHILL.
Coronary heart disease in young men a study of 70 patients with a critical review of etiological factors.
Australian, New Zealand Journal Medicine 3(1):39-62, 1973.

4663
BLACKMON, J.R., L.B. ROWELL, J.W. KENNEDY, ET AL.
Physiological significance of maximal oxygen intake in "pure" mitral stenosis.
Circulation 36:497-510, 1967.

4664
BLAKE, T.M.
Causes of myocardial infarct and treatment with anticoagulants.
Naika 11:1203-1226, 1962.

4665
BLAKE, T.M.
Anticoagulants for acute myocardial infarction. A discussion of the problem.
Geriatrics 18:291-295, 1963.

4666
BLAKE, T.M., E.R. ORR, AND J.W. SIMMONS.
Ineffectiveness of anticoagulants in myocardial infarction.
American Heart Journal 64:462-465, 1962.

4667
BLOOM, W.L.
Carbohydrates and water balance.
American Journal Clinical Nutrition 20:157-162, 1967.

4668
BLUMENFELD, A.
Heart attack: are you a candidate?
New York, Eriksson, 1965.

4669
BOGDONOFF, M.D., K.W. BACK, R.F. KLEIN, AND E.H. ESTES, JR.
The physiologic response to conformity pressure in man.
Annals Internal Medicine 57:389, 1962.

4670
BOGDONOFF, M.D., E.H. ESTES, JR., S.J. FRIEDBERG, AND R.F. KLEIN.
Fat mobilization in man.
Annals Internal Medicine 55:328, 1961.

4671
BONAMI, M., AND B. RIME.
Psychological approach to coronary disease, comparative analysis of the interviews with 20 patients suffering from myocardial infarcts.
Acta Psychiatrica Belgica 72:29-45, 1972.

4672
BONAMI, M., AND B. RIME.
An exploratory study of the precoronary personality by standardized analysis of thematic projective data.
Journal Psychosomatic Research 16:103-13, 1972.

4673
BONDE–PETERSEN, F., AND J. HENRIKSSON.
Effect of training with eccentric muscle contractions on skeletal muscle metabolities.
Acta Physiologica Scandinavica 88:564-70, 1973.

4674
BONJER, F.H.
Physical working capacity and energy expenditure.
In: Denolin, H., et al., Ed. Ergometry in cardiology. Boehringer, Mannheim, 1967.

4675
BONJER, F.H.
Relationship between working time, physical working capacity and allowable caloric expenditure.
Arbeitsmedizin, Sozialmedizin, Arbeitshygiene 22:66-93, 1968.

4676
BONNER, A.J., JR., H.N. SACKS, AND M.E. TAVEL.
Assessing the severity of aortic stenosis by phonocardiography and external carotid pulse recordings.
Circulation 48:247-252, 1973.

4677
BOOTSMA, B.K., A.J. HOELEN, J. STRACKEE, ET AL.
Analysis of R-R intervals in patients with atrial fibrillation at rest and during exercise.
Circulation 41:783-794, 1970.

4678
BORST, R.H., AND A. REICH.
The treatment of heart diseases: Pharmacology and clinical effects of Segontin (Prenylamin).
Herz Kreislauf 5:288, 1973.

4679
BORTZ, W.M., ET AL.
Fat, carbohydrate, salt and weight loss.
American Journal Clinical Nutrition 20:1104-1112, 1967.

4680
BORTZ, W.M., P. HOWAT, AND W.L. HOLMES.
Fat, carbohydrate, salt and weight loss: further studies.
American Journal Clinical Nutrition 21:1291-1301, 1968.

4681
BOUVRAIN, Y., C. MACREZ, I. KOMAROVER, AND M.C. COUTET.
Adaptation of cardiacs to work.
Archives des Maladies du Coeur et des Vaisseaux 57 (Suppl.):40-55, 1964.

4682
BOYLES, P.W.
Laboratory procedures and therapy in coronary thrombosis.
Journal American Medical Association 175:279-283, 1961.

4683
BRADLEY, R.
The "Heart Attack." Anticoagulants and the acute myocardial infarction.
Journal Kansas Medical Society 65:425-428, 1964.

4684
BRAUNWALD, E., J. ROSS JR., AND E.H. SONNENBLICK.
Mechanism of contraction of normal and failing heart.
Boston, Little Brown, 1968.

4685
BROD, J.
Influence of environmental factors on pathogenesis of hypertension.
Cardiologia 31:500, 1959.

4686
BROWN, D.F.
Blood lipids and lipoprotein atherogenesis.
American Journal Medicine 46:691, 1969.

4687
BROWN, D.F., AND J.T. DOYLE.
Pre-beta lipoproteinemia and serum triglycerides in health and in ischemic heart disease.
Circulation 33 (Suppl. 3):3, 1966.

4688
BROWN, J., G.J. BOURKE, G.F. GEARTY, ET AL.
Nutritional and epidemiological factors related to heart disease.
World Review Nutrition Dietetics 12:42, 1970.

4689
BROWN, K.W.G., AND R.L. MACMILLAN.
The effectiveness of the system of coronary care.
In: Meltzer, L.E. and J.D. Arend, Eds. Textbooks of coronary care pp. 52–57. Amsterdam, The Netherlands, Excerpta Medica, 1972.

4690
BRUCE, R.A., R. ELEADY-COLE, L.J. BENNETT, AND F. KUSUMI.
Divergent effects of antihypertensive therapy on cardiovascular responses and left ventricular function during upright exercise.
American Journal Cardiology 30(7):768, 1972.

4691
BRUCE, R.A., J.A. MAZARELLA, J.W. JORDAN, ET AL.
Quantitation of QRS and ST segment responses to exercise.
American Heart Journal 71:455-466, 1966.

4692
BRUENER, H., AND H. HOHLWECK.
A new method to record heart rate and respiratory rate inflight on cockpit crews.
Aerospace Medical Institute. Current Science Papers, pp. 21-33, Jan. 1973.

4693
BRUNNER, D., S. ALTMAN, N. MESHULAM, K. LOEBL, AND S. SCHWARTZ.
Low prevalence or absence of vascular disease in diabetic Yemenite Jews.
In: Shafrier, P. Impact of insulin on metabolic pathways. International symposium, Jerusalem,
Israel, Oct. 24-29, 1971, pp. 421-22. New York, Academic Press, 1972.

4694
BRYNTESON, P. AND W.E. SINNING.
The effects of training frequencies on the retention of cardiovascular fitness.
Medicine Science Sports 5(1):29, 1973.

4695
BURCH, G.E., AND A. ANSARI.
On prescribing the climate.
American Heart Journal 77:149, 1969.

4696
BURCH, G.E., AND T.D. GILES.
The burden of a hot and humid environment on the heart.
Modern Concepts Cardiovascular Disease 39:115-120, 1970.

4697
BURCH, G.E.A., ET AL.
A critique of aspects of methodological approaches to the role of the central nervous system in
cardiovascular disease.
Psychosomatic Medicine 26:432-453, 1964.

4698
BUSTAMANTE COSTA, U.
Rehabilitation of patients with cardiac diseases.
Third Latin-American meeting for social security. Quito, Ecuador, 1958.

4699
CAIN, H.D., ET AL.
Electrocardiographic monitoring of post-myocardial infarction activity.
Journal American Medical Association 178:946, 1961.

4700
CARDON, P.V., JR., AND R.S. GORDON, JR.
Rapid increase of plasma unesterified fatty acids in man during fear.
Journal Psychosomatic Research 4:5, 1959.

4701
CASH, J.D., AND D.G. WOODFIELD.
   Fibrinolytic response to moderate exercise in 50 healthy middle aged subjects.
   British Medical Journal 2:658, 1968.

4702
CASTLEDEN, C.M., AND P.V.COLE.
   Inhalation of tobacco smoke by pipe and cigar smokers.
   Lancet 2:21-22, 1973.

4703
CASTRO, C.M., AND L. DE SOLDATI.
   Results of anticoagulant treatment in 1000 patients.
   Prensa Medica Argentina 49:11012-11021, 1962.

4704
CATO, D.H.
   A technique for electrocardiography during exercise testing.
   Medical Journal Australia 2(21):971, 1973.

4705
CATTELL, R.B., AND H.W. EBER.
   The 16 personality factor questionnaire, 3rd edition.
   IPAT, Champaign, Ill.

4706
CHAPMAN, C., AND R. FRASER.
   Cardiovascular responses to exercise in patients with healed myocardial infarction.
   Circulation 9:347, 1954.

4707
CHAPMAN, C.B., J.H. FISHER, AND B.J. SPROULE.
   Behavior of stroke volume at rest and during exercise in human beings.
   Journal Clinical Investigation 39:1208, 1969.

4708
CHESTER, M.
   Current status of the use of anticoagulants in the treatment of myocardial infarct.
   Revista da Associacao Medica Brasileira 9:361-363, 1963.

4709
CHILDERS, R.W.
   Usefulness of extrasystole in cardiac diagnosis and prognosis.
   Medical Clinics North America 50:51–71, 1966.

4710
CHLOUVERAKIS, C.S.
   Controversies in medicine—Is obesity harmful?
   Obesity Bariatric Medicine 2:108, 194, 1973.

4711
CHURCH, C.F., AND H.N. CHURCH.
   Food values of portions commonly used. (11th edition)
   Philadelphia, J.B. Lippincott, 1970.

4712
CLEAVE, T.L., G.C. CAMPBELL, AND N.S. PAINTER.
Diabetes, coronary thrombosis, and the saccharine disease. (2nd edition)
Bristol, J. Wright, 1969.

4713
CLOAREC, M.
Myocardial infarction in the young adult less than 40 years old.
In: Laroche G. and L. Justin-Besancon, Eds. Les entretiens de Bichat Expansion Scientifique Francaise, pp. 155-156, Paris, 1970.

4714
CONSOLAZIO, C.F., R.E. JOHNSON, AND L.J. PECORA.
Physiological measurements of metabolic functions in man.
New York, Blakiston Division, McGraw—Hill, 1963.

4715
COOPER, J.B., AND A.W. HAHN.
Hybrid biological power cells for cardiac pacemakers. Materials evaluation.
IEEE Transactions Biomedical Engineering 20:336-345, 1973.

4716
COOPER, K.H.
Guidelines in the management of the exercising patient.
Journal American Medical Association 211:1663-1667, 1970.

4717
CORDAY, E., AND H.J.C. SWAN, EDS.
Myocardial infarction.
Baltimore, Williams and Wilkins, 1973.

4718
CRADDOCK, D.
Obesity and its management.
London, Livingston, 1969.

4719
CROPP, G.J., AND G.W. MANNING.
Electrocardiographic changes simulating myocardial ischemia and infarction associated with spontaneous intracranial hemorrhage.
Circulation 22:27-38, 1960.

4720
CROSTON, R.C., J.A. RUMMEL, AND F.J. KAY.
Computer model of cardiovascular control system responses to exercise.
Journal Dynamic Systems 95:301-307, 1973.

4721
DANFORD, H.G., D.A. DANFORD, J.E. MIELKE, AND L.F. PETERSON.
Echocardiographic evaluation of the hemodynamic effects of chronic aortic insufficiency with observations on left ventricular performance.
Circulation 48:253-262, 1973.

4722
DASHKEVICH, O.V.
Experimental analysis of conditions for onset of emotional stress.
Zhurnal Vysshei Nervnoi Deiatel'nosti 23:538-544, 1973.

4723
DAWBER, T.R., W.B. KANNEL, AND G.D. FRIEDMAN.
Vital capacity, physical activity and coronary heart disease.
In: Raab, W., Ed. Prevention of ischemic heart disease: Principles and practice, pp. 254.
Springfield, Ill. Thomas, 1966.

4724
DAYTON, S., AND M.L. PEARCE.
Prevention of coronary heart disease and other complications of atherosclerosis by modified diet.
American Journal Medicine 46:751, 1969.

4725
DEGRÉ, S., R. MESSIN, P. VANDERMOTEN, B. DEMARET, J.C. HAISSLY, P.H. SALHADIN, AND
H. DENOLIN.
Physiological-pathological aspects of muscular exercise in patients with myocardial infarction.
Acta Cardiologica 27:445-462, 1972.

4726
DENOLIN, H., L. KÖNIG, R. MESSIN, AND S. DEGRÉ.
Ergometry in cardiology.
Boehringer, Mannheim, 1967.

4727
DE NICOLA, P.
The laboratory diagnosis of coagulation defects.
Springfield, Ill. Thomas, 1955.

4728
DIMOND, E.G., AND P.F. TROTTA.
The advantages and disadvantages of using heparin as the other anticoagulant during the first 30
days after acute myocardial infarction.
Diseases Chest 40:214-216, 1961.

4729
DIMOND, G.E.
Assessment of functional recovery of men surviving first myocardial infarction.
American Heart Journal 65(6):832-838, 1963.

4730
DOBSON, M., A.E. TATTERSFIELD, M.W. ADLER, AND M.W. McNICOL.
Attitudes and long-term adjustment of patients surviving cardiac arrest.
British Medical Journal 3:207, 1971.

4731
DOICHINOV, A.
Anticoagulants in the treatment of myocardial infarct.
Suvremenna Meditsina 14:30-37, 1963.

4732
DOLL, R., AND A.B. HILL.
Mortality in relation to smoking: ten years' observations of British doctors.
British Medical Journal 1:1399, 1460, 1964.

4733
DRENICK, E.J., AND H.F. DENNIN.
Energy expenditure in fasting obese men.
Journal Laboratory Clinical Medicine 81(3):421, 1973.

4734
DUKE, M.
Bed rest in acute myocardial infarction. A study of physician practices.
American Heart Journal 82:486-491, 1971.

4735
DZEGELENOK, I.I., A.N. DOROSHENKO, AND A.G. SHIGIN.
A diagnostic program. Problems of predicting myocardial infarction on a digital computer.
In: Applied mathematics and cybernetics, pp. 254-258. Moscow, USSR. Izdatel'stvo Nauka, 1973.

4736
EGEBERG, O.
On the nature of the blood antihemophilic A factor (AHF = Factor VIII) increase associated with muscular exercise.
Scandinavian Journal Clinical Laboratory Investigation 15:202, 1963.

4737
EGGERS, P., K. VOGELBERG, AND E. ZYLMANN.
Clinical Study on 570 cases of myocardial infarct.
Münchener Medizinische Wochenschrift 104:2545-2548, 1962.

4738
EIDINOV, I.B.
On early anticoagulant therapy in acute thrombosis of coronary arteries of the heart.
Klinicheskaya Meditsina 39:115-122, 1961.

4739
ELLIOT, R.S., AND G. BRATT.
The paradox of myocardial ischemia and necrosis in young women with normal coronary arteriograms.
American Journal Cardiology 23:633, 1969.

4740
ENOS, W.F., R.H. HOLMES, J. BEYER.
Coronary disease among U.S. soldiers killed in action in Korea.
Journal American Medical Association 152:1090-1093, 1953.

4741
FAIVRE, G., J.M. GILGENKRANTZ, H. PETITIER, M. WEILLER, AND B. DODINOT.
Possibilities and limits of extrasystolic training in poisonings due to digitalis and quinidine.
Archives des Maladies du Coeur et des Vaisseaux 61:1373, 1968.

4742
FAUVRE, F.M., D.R. JOHN, AND L.E. WATKINS.
Cardiomyopathy secondary to pheochromocytoma.
California Medicine 117(4):58-60, 1972.

4743
FAZEKAS, J.F., ET AL.
Current therapeutic concepts of cerebral myocardial vascular disease.
Angiology 15:63-69, 1964.

4744
FEJFAR, Z.
Cardiovascular diseases become the greatest scourge of humanity.
Bulletin de la Société Internationale de Cardiologie 1:9, 1969.

4745
FITZGERALD, E.W., JR.
Anticoagulant control in acute myocardial infarction.
American Heart Journal 64:462-466, 1962.

4746
FLYNN, J.T., M.A.K. KENNEDY, AND S. WOLF.
Essential hypertension in one of identical twins: An experimental study of cardiovascular reactions in the Y twins.
Proceedings Association Research Nervous Mental Disease 29:954, 1950.

4747
FODOR, J.G., C.J. PFEIFFER, AND V.S. PAPEZIK.
Relationship of drinking water quality (hardness-softness) to cardiovascular mortality in Newfoundland.
Canadian Medical Association Journal 108:1369, 1973.

4748
FOULDS, G.A., AND K. HOPE.
Manual of the symptom sign inventory.
London, University of London Press, 1968.

4749
FRIEDBERG, C.K.
Should we abandon anticoagulant therapy in acute myocardial infarction?
Journal American Medical Association 180:307-328, 1962.

4750
FRIESINGER, G.C., I. LIKAR, R.O. BIERN, ET AL.
Vasoregulatory asthenia: a cause for false positive exercise electrocardiograms.
Circulation 32 (Suppl. II):90, 1965.

4751
FROMENT, C.
Anticoagulant therapy of cardiovascular diseases of ischemic origin.
Journal de Medécine et de Chirurgie Pratique 135:307-310, 1964.

4752
GALLIVAN, G.J., H. LEVINE, AND J. CANZONETTI.
Ischemic electrocardiographic changes after truncal vagotomy.
Journal American Medical Association 211:797-801, 1970.

4753
GAN, T.B.
Etiologic survey on selected cardiac patients in Djakarta.
Acta Cardiologica 16:147, 1961.

4754
GARRARD, C.L., JR., A.M. WEISSLER, AND H.T. DODGE.
The relationship of alterations in systolic time intervals to ejection fraction in patients with cardiac disease.
Circulation 42:455, 1970.

4755
GARRETT, H.L., J. MACBETH, AND G.V. MANN.
The reproducibility of a measurement of physical fitness.
Journal Chronic Diseases 23:559, 1971.

4756
GAUSE, R.L., AND B.G. BYNUM.
Ergometer Patent. Patent to (NASA) National Aeronautics and Space Administration, 10 July, 1973 (filed Nov. 29, 1971).

4757
GEIGER, H.J., AND N.A. SCOTCH.
The epidemiology of essential hypertension—A review with special attention to psychologic and sociocultural factors. I. Biologic mechanism and descriptive epidemiology. II. Psychologic and sociocultural factors in etiology.
Journal Chronic Diseases 16:1151-1182; 1183-1213, 1963.

4758
GERTEL, M., G.S. FOX, F.I. RABOW, AND D.H. GRAHAM.
The cardiovascular effects of pancuronium bromide during halothane anaesthesia.
Canadian Anaesthetists' Society Journal 19(6):599-606, 1972.

4759
GOLDBARG, A.N., J.R. MORAN, R.W. CHILDERS, ET AL.
Results and correlations of multistage exercise tests in a group of clinically normal business executives.
American Heart Journal 79:194-200, 1970.

4760
GOLDRICK, R.B., N. HAVENSTEIN, AND H.M. WHYTE.
Effects of caloric restriction and fenfluramine on weight loss and personality profiles of patients with long standing obesity.
Australian New Zealand Journal Medicine 3(2):131, 1973.

4761
GOLOVCHINER, I.E.
Invalidism in cardiovascular disease.
Zdravookhraveniya (SSSR) 9:22-26, 1963.

4762
GOMORI, P.
Some problems concerning the treatment of cardiac infarct with special reference to anticoagulant therapy.
Orvosi Hetilap 104:2310-2314, 1963.

4763
GORDON, E.S., ET AL.
A new concept in the treatment of obesity.
Journal American Medical Association 186(1):156-166, 1963.

4764
GORTVAI, G., ET AL.
Our experiences with lasting anticoagulant therapy.
Orvosi Hetilap 105:607-610, 1964.

4765
GOTTHEINER, V.
Long-range strenuous sports training for cardiac reconditioning and rehabilitation.
American Journal Cardiology 22:426, 1968.

4766
GOUFFAULT, J., J. VAN DEN DRIESCHE, J.C. PONY, P. COURGEON, AND R. THOMAS.
Conduction disturbances induced by piperazine. Clinical and experimental study.
Archives des Maladies du Coeur et des Vaisseaux 66:1289, 1973.

4767
GOULD, K.L., K. LIPSCOMB, G.W. HAMILTON, AND J.W. KENNEDY.
Left ventricular hypertrophy in coronary artery disease. A cardiomyopathy syndrome following myocardial infarction.
American Journal Medicine 55:595, 1973.

4768
GOULET, G., C. ALLARD, AND R. POIRIER.
Epidemiological study of a French Canadian population in a city. Factors associated with the coronary profile.
Coeur et Médecine Interne 7(2):257-262, 1968.

4769
GREEN, R.S., AND E.L. BORONSCHI.
Return to work of patients with angina pectoris and/or myocardial infarction.
Journal American Medical Association 172(8):783-789, 1960.

4770
GREENBAUM, D.
Heart-disease in South Vietnam.
Lancet 2:45, 1973.

4771
GREENLEAF, J.E., H.L. YOUNG, E.M. BERNAUER, R.H. AMBRUSTER, L.A. SAGAN, R. W. STALEY, L. JUHOS, W. VAN BEAUMONT, AND H. SANDLER.
Effects of isometric and isotonic exercise on body water compartments during 14 days bedrest.
Aerospace Medical Association. Preprints pp. 23-24. Las Vegas, Nevada, 1973.

4772
GROEN, J., B.K. TIJIONG, C.E. KAMMINGA, AND A.F. WILLEBRANDS.
Influence of nutrition, individuality and various forms of stress on serum cholesterol.
Voeding 13:556, 1952.

4773
GROEN, J.J., J.M. VAN DER VALK, N. TREURNIET, H. HEIJNINGEN, H. VAN KITS, G.J.S.
WILDE, AND H.E. PELSER.
Psychological factors in the causation of myocardial infarction.
Excerpta Medica. International congress series No. 182, 1968.

4774
GUMPERT, T.E.
Anticoagulant treatment in 104 male cases of acute myocardial infarction.
Lancet 1:399-400, 1962.

4775
GUSSENHOVEN, G.A.
The use of oral anticoagulants in coronary disease.
Nederlands Tijdschrift voor Geneeskunde 105:2260-2264, 1961.

4776
GUSSENHOVEN, G.A.
Role of anticoagulants in the treatment of myocardial infarct.
Belgisch Tijdschrift voor Geneeskunde 30:364-373, 1964.

4777
GUSTAFSON, J.E., G. WINOKUR, AND S. REICHLIN.
The effect of psychic-sexual stimulation on urinary and serum acid phosphatase and plasma
non-esterified fatty acids.
Psychosomatic Medicine 25:101, 1963.

4778
HAIMSOHN, J.S.
Myocardial infarction and normal coronary arteriogram-I.
American Journal Cardiology 32:125, 1973.

4779
HALPERIN, M., J. CORNFIELD, AND S.C. MITCHELL.
Effect of diet on coronary heart-disease mortality.
Lancet 2:438, 1973.

4780
HAMPTON, W.R.
Thrombolytic therapy and myocardial infarction.
Hartford Hospital Bulletin 17:66-73, 1962.

4781
HANDJANI, A.M., A EGHTEDARI, AND A. SHARIAT.
Acute myocardial infarction in Fars province, Iran: Characteristics based on an analysis of 200
cases.
Pahlavi Medical Journal 3(3):435-446, 1972.

4782
HANNAS, R.R.
   The case against using anticoagulants following acute myocardial infarction.
   Journal Oklahoma Medical Association 55:43-45, 1962.

4783
HANSEN, A.T.
   Does available evidence justify large-scale application of physical conditioning training in prevention and therapy of coronary heart disease?
   In: Larsen, O.A. and R.O. Malmborg, Eds. Coronary heart diseases and physical fitness, pp. 273-277, Baltimore, University Park Press, 1971.

4784
HARDEN, R.M.
   A method of intravenous administration of heparin in myocardial infarction.
   British Medical Journal 5365:1106-1107, 1963.

4785
HARTENAUER, G., R.L. DEWEES, AND E.M. KRIEGER.
   Acute myocardial infarction.
   Delaware Medical Journal 35:167-179, 1963.

4786
HELLERSTEIN, H.K., E.Z. HIRSCH, W. CUMLER, L. ALLEN, ET AL.
   Reconditioning of the coronary patient. A preliminary report.
   In: Likoff, W. and J.H. Moyer, Eds. Coronary Heart Disease, pp. 448-454.
   New York, Grune and Stratton, 1963.

4787
HERVEY, G.R.
   Regulation of energy balance.
   Nature 222:629, 1969.

4788
HILDEN, T., K. IVERSEN, F. RAOSCHON, AND M. SCHWARTZ.
   Anticoagulant therapy in acute myocardial infarction.
   Journal American Medical Association 183:903-904, 1963.

4789
HIMBERT, J., J. ROCHERMAURE, AND J. LENEGRE.
   Anatomical lesions in 100 cases with ventricular aneurysms following myocardial infarction.
   Archives des Maladies du Coeur et des Vaisseaux 59:1202, 1966.

4790
HINKLE, L.E., JR., S.T. CARVER, AND M. STEVENS.
   The frequency of asymptomatic disturbances of cardiac rhythm and conduction in Middle-aged men.
   American Journal Cardiology 24:629, 1969.

4791
HIRSCH, J., J.L. KNITTLE, AND L.B. SALANS.
   Cell lipid content and cell number in obese and nonobese tissue.
   Journal Clinical Investigation 45:1023, 1966.

4792
HOCHREIN, M., AND I. SCHLEICHER.
 Immediate therapeutic measures in myocardial infarct.
 Therapeutische Umschau 20:128-132, 1963.

4793
HOFFMAN, F.G.
 Effective subcutaneous heparin therapy in myocardial infarction.
 American Journal Medical Science 246:69-83, 1963.

4794
HOHNLOSER, E., AND H. BERGER.
 Critical observations on the therapy of heart infarct.
 Medizinische Wochenschrift 16:237-241, 1962.

4795
HOLMGREN, A.
 Vasoregulatory asthenia.
 In: Larson, O.A. and R.O. Malmborg Eds. Coronary Heart Disease and Physical Fitness, pp.
 34-37. Baltimore, University Park Press, 1971.

4796
HOUSTON, S., J.W. HODGE JR., D.D. OUSTERHOUT, AND F. LEONARD.
 The effect of α-cyanoacrylates on wound healing.
 Journal Biomedical Materials Research 3(2):281-289, 1969.

4797
HOWELL, R.W.
 Smoking and cholesterol.
 Lancet 2:446, 1973.

4798
HUEBER, E.F., AND H. NEUMANN.
 Clinical aspects and therapy of the atypical myocardial infarct.
 Wiener Klinische Wochenschrift 75:505-509, 1963.

4799
HUIDT, S., ET AL.
 On mortality in cardiac infarct. Five-year cases from a central hospital.
 Ugeskrift for Laeger 125:1787-1791, 1963.

4800
HUSSAMI, S.
 Anticoagulants and myocardial infarct.
 Revue Médicale du Moyen—Orient 18:482-484, 1961.

4801
IKEDA, M.
 Use of anticoagulant for cardiovascular diseases with special emphasis of the incidence of
 thromboembolism in Japan.
 Acta Gerontologica Japonica 38:1-16, 1961.

4802
IKKALA, E., G. MYLLYLÄ, AND H.S.S. SARAJAS.
Haemostatic changes associated with exercise.
Nature (London) 199:459, 1963.

4803
ILIESCU, C.C., AND L. ROMAN.
Coronary syndromes.
Bucharest, Romania. Editura Medicală, 1960.

4804
JAMES, T.N.
Pulse and impulse in the sinus node.
Henry Ford Hospital Medical Journal 15(4):275-299, 1967.

4805
JENSEN, W.N., AND L.S. LESSIN.
Membrane alterations associated with hemoglobinopathies.
Seminars in Hematology 7:409-426, 1970.

4806
JORDAN, H.A.
Weight regulation in man—Physiological and psychological factors.
Obesity Bariatric Medicine 2(2):42, 1973.

4807
KALLIONEAKI, J.L., AND H.A. SAORIVENA.
The A-B-O-Rh groups and myocardial infarction: association between the blood groups and the
patients' age, mortality rate in first month of illness and the requirement of anticoagulants.
Cardiologia (Basel) 41:109-112, 1962.

4808
KANNEL, G.T.
The Framingham Study, 20 years later: A case book of community studies.
Baltimore, Johns Hopkins Press, 1970.

4809
KANNEL, W.B., T.R. DAWBER, W.E. GLENNON, AND M.C. THORNE.
Preliminary report: The determinants and clinical significance of serum cholesterol.
Massachusetts Journal Medical Technology 4:11, 1962.

4810
KANNEL, W., T. DAWBER, A. KAGAN, N. REVOTSKIE, AND J. STOKES.
Factors of risk in the development of coronary heart disease—six year follow-up experience—the
Framingham study.
Annals Internal Medicine 55:33, 1961.

4811
KARVONEN, M.J., M. PEKKARINEN, P. METSÄLÄ, AND Y. RAUTANEN.
Diet and serum cholesterol of lumberjacks.
British Journal Nutrition 15:157, 1961.

4812
KATO, K., H. WATANABE, K. SUZUKI, A. OTA, ET AL.
Two cases with angina pectoris of variant form induced by an exercise stress test.
Japanese Circulation Journal 30(9):1276, 1966.

4813
KEEN, H.
Minimal diabetes and arterial disease: prevalence and the effect of treatment.
In: Camerini-Davalos, R.A., and H.S. Cole, Eds. Advances in metabolic disorders, (Suppl. 1) pp. 437. New York, Academic Press, 1970.

4814
KEYS, A.
The individual risk of coronary heart disease.
Annals New York Academy Science 134:1046-1056, 1966.

4815
KEYS, A.
Blood lipids in man—a brief review.
Journal American Dietetic Association 51:508, 1967.

4816
KEYS, A.
Prevention of coronary heart disease. Official recommendation from Scandinavia.
Circulation 38:227, 1968.

4817
KEYS, A., J.T. ANDERSON, AND F. GRANDE.
Prediction of serum cholesterol responses of man to changes in fats in diet.
Lancet 2:959, 1957.

4818
KEYS, A., N. KIMURA, A. KUSAKAWA, B. BRONTE-STEWART, N. LARSEN, AND M.H. KEYS.
Lessons from serum cholesterol studies in Hawaii, Japan and Los Angeles.
Annals Internal Medicine 48:83, 1958.

4819
KEYS, A., AND P.D. WHITE.
Cardiovascular epidemiology.
New York, Hoeber-Harper, 1956.

4820
KILAIDONIS, P., A. CONSTANTOPOULOS, AND C. ANDRIOTAKIS.
Application of anticoagulant therapy in 344 cases of myocardial infarction: statistical considerations and conclusions.
Praxis 50:507—511, 1961.

4821
KING, S.H., AND D.H. FUNKENSTEIN.
Religious practice and cardiovascular reactions during stress.
Journal Abnormal Psychology 55:135, 1957.

4822
KLAJMAN, A.
   Results of treatment of myocardial infarction without anticoagulants.
   Dapim Refuiim 22:307-311, 1963.

4823
KOBAYASHI, T., M. TAKEUCHI, T. KORO, AND A. TAWARD.
   Clinical application of telemeter electrocardiographic changes of cardiac diseases during routine exercise.
   Japanese Circulation Journal 27(12):896, 1963.

4824
KOMMERELL, B.
   The treatment of myocardial infarct with anticoagulants and streptokinase.
   Medizinische Klinik 58:928-933, 1963.

4825
KONISHI, F.
   Exercise equivalents of foods.
   Carbondale, Ill. Southern Illinois University Press, 1973.

4826
KROMAN, H., J. NODINE, S. BENDER, AND A. BREST.
   Lipids in normals and patients with coronary artery disease.
   American Journal Medical Sciences 248:571, 1964.

4827
KUO, P.T.
   Current metabolic-genetic interrelationship in human atherosclerosis.
   Annals Internal Medicine 68:449, 1968.

4828
KUSHELEVSKII, B.P.
   The therapeutic and preventive use of anticoagulants in cardiovascular diseases.
   Klinicheskaya Meditsina 41:16-20, 1963.

4829
LACHMAN, A.B., H.J. SEMLER, AND R.H. GUSTAFSON.
   Postural ST-T wave changes in the radioelectrocardiogram simulating myocardial ischemia.
   Circulation 31:557, 1965.

4830
LANARI, A., L. CHAIT, AND C. CAPURRO.
   Electrocardiographic effects of potassium. I. Perfusion through the coronary bed.
   American Heart Journal 67:357, 1964.

4831
LAPIERRE, A.
   Physical reeducation.
   Paris, France. Baillière, 1962.

4832
LASSER, N.L., AND S. KATZ.
   The occurrence of type II and type III hyperlipoproteinemia in a single kindred.
   Clinical Research 20:549, 1972.

4833
LEAK, D., AND A. GILCHREST.
Some considerations regarding the value of anticoagulants in acute myocardial infarction.
Scottish Medical Journal 7:512-515, 1962.

4834
LENÈGRE, J.
Clinical study and treatment of myocardial infarct.
Minerva Medica 54:2094, 1963.

4835
LENÈGRE, J., M. LEBLANC, AND J. BOUHEY.
Frequency and evolution of cardiovascular lesions at the working age.
Archives des Maladies du Coeur et des Vaisseaux 57(Suppl.):5-7, 1964.

4836
LEVITSKY, D.
Regulation of adiposity and the control of food intake. Presented at the First Annual Meeting of
the American Society of Clinical Nutrition and American Institute of Nutrition.
Cornell University, Aug. 14-17, 1973.

4837
LEVY, R.L.
A critique of certain measures presently employed in managing patients with cardiac infarction.
American Heart Journal 64:1-6, 1962.

4838
LIEBELT, R.A., S. ICHINOSE, AND N. NICHOLSON.
Regulatory influences of adipose tissue on food intake and body weight.
Annals New York Academy Science 131:559, 1965.

4839
LIEBERMAN, J.
Current appraisal of thrombolytic therapy. A critical review.
California Medicine 99:301-307, 1963.

4840
LINDEMAN, R., J. KYRIACOPOULOS, AND L. CONRAD.
Evaluation of a new single, oblique chest lead for the detection of electrocardiographic abnor-
malities.
American Heart Journal 64:24, 1962.

4841
LINDSAY. M.I., JR., ET AL.
Re-evaluation of therapy of acute myocardial infarction.
American Heart Journal 67:559-564, 1964.

4842
LOCKWOOD, D.R., J.E. LAMMERT, J.M. VOGEL, AND S.B. HULLEY.
Bone mineral loss during bedrest.
In: Frame, B., A.M. Parfitt, and H. Duncan, Eds. Proceedings, international symposium clinical
aspects Metabolic Bone Disease. Amsterdam, the Netherlands, Excerpta Medica, 1973.

4843
LOGAN, W.P.
    Mortality from coronary and myocardial disease in different social classes.
    Lancet 1:758, 1952.

4844
LOO, VAN D.E.
    Possibilities and limitations of combined fibrinolytic-anticoagulant therapy of myocardial infarction.
    Medizinische Klinik 58:1527-1529, 1963.

4845
LÖWIS of MENAR, P. VON, AND U.H. KLEMENS.
    Coincidence of abnormal carbohydrate tolerance and types of hyperlipoproteinaemia in patients with myocardial infarction.
    Arzneimittel-Forschung 22 (10a):1819-1823, 1972.

4846
LUFT, U.C.
    The effects of low concentrations of CO_2 on metabolic, respiratory and circulatory measurements during work and at rest. (Section A). The relationship between heart rate and metabolic rate. (Section B). Research report, contract NASA 9-7009, December 1971. Lovelace Foundation Medical Education Research, Albuquerque, New Mexico.

4847
MCCORMICK, W.J.
    Ascorbic acid as a chemotherapeutic agent.
    Archives Pediatrics 69(4):151-155, 1952.

4848
MCDONALD, G.L.
    Anticoagulants in myocardial infarction.
    Bulletin Postgraduate Committee Medicine, University of Sydney 19:226-230, 1963.

4849
MCNAMERA, J.J., M.A. MOLOT, J.E. STEMPLE, AND R.T. CATTING.
    Coronary disease in Vietnam casualties.
    Journal American Medical Association 216(7):1185-1187, 1971.

4850
MACIVER, J.
    Psychiatric aspects of cardiovascular diseases in industry.
    In: Warshaw, L.J., Ed. The heart in industry, pp. 317-345.
    New York, Hoeber, 1960.

4851
MARTINEZ-RIOS, A., B.C. BRUTO DA COSTA, K.A. CACENA-SELDNER, AND S.G. GENSINI.
    Normal electrocardiograms in the presence of severe coronary artery disease.
    American Journal Cardiology 25:320-324, 1970.

4852
MASAREI, J.R., M. SUMMERS, D.R. GURNOW, K.J. CULLEN, ET AL.
    Lipoprotein electrophoretic patterns, serum lipids and coronary heart disease.
    British Medical Journal 1:78, 1971.

4853
MASTER, A., F.M. WEISER, AND R. RABIN.
The emergency treatment of the complications of acute coronary artery occlusion.
Diseases Chest 42:457-473, 1962.

4854
MAY, L.M.
Comprehensive heparin therapy in coronary heart disease.
Texas State Journal Medicine 57:690-695, 1961.

4855
MELTZER, L., ET AL.
Prothrombin levels and fatality rates in acute myocardial infarction.
Journal American Medical Association 187:93-128, 1964.

4856
MENON, I.S., F.D. BURKE, P.A. SMITH, D.J. NEWELL, AND H.A. DEWAR.
A study of possible causes of increased fibrinolytic activity during exercise.
Thrombosis et Diathesis Haemorrhagica 21:287, 1969.

4857
MEZZASALMA, G., AND M. MORPURGO.
Rehabilitation of the cardiac patient.
Giornale di Gerontologia 11:4, 1963.

4858
MEZZASALMA, G., M. MORPURGO, A. PECILE, AND L. TESSARI.
On the behavior of lactic acid, pyruvic acid and lactic dehydrogenase in the blood of old people before and after muscular work.
Giornale di Gerontologia 7:216, 1969.

4859
MEZZASCLURE, G., C. SCARPAGGA, AND I. PICONE-CHIODO.
Clinico-statistical observations on myocardial infarction in a hospital population.
Ospedale Maggiore 49:258-259, 1961.

4860
MIASNIKOV, A.L.
The significance of disturbances of higher nervous activity in the pathogenesis of hypertensive disease. Proceedings, Prague Symposium, 1960. Pathogenesis of Hypertension, pp. 153.
London, Pergamon Press, 1962.

4861
MIHAIL, A., P. POPESCU, L. CHERASIM, AND X. PETRESCU.
Considerations on 50 cases of myocardial infarct.
Medicina Internă 14:687-691, 1962.

4862
MILLER, R.A.
How to live with a heart attack.
Radnor, Pa. Chilton, 1973.

4863

MIRONOVA, YU.P., G.V. GRACHEVA, AND V.P. MISHUROVA.
A study of serum creatine-kinase in evaluating the effect of cardioversion on the myocardium.
Kardiologiya 11:77, 1971.

4864

MOELLERING, R.C., JR., AND D.R. BASSETT.
Myocardial infarction in Hawaiian and Japanese males in Oahu; a review of 505 cases occurring between 1955 and 1964.
Journal Chronic Diseases 20:89, 1967.

4865

MONTOYE, H.G., P.W. WILLIS, G.E. HOWARD, AND J.B. KELLER.
Systolic pre-ejection period. Patients with heart disease compared to normal subjects.
Archives Environmental Health 21:425, 1970.

4866

MOSES, L., G.E. DANIELS, AND J.L. NICKERSON.
Psychogenic factors in essential hypertension.
Psychosomatic Medicine 18:471, 1956.

4867

MOUTIGLL, C.
Thrombosis, atherosclerosis and anticoagulants.
Journal Association Physicians India 11:257-267, 1963.

4868

MOULINIER, J.
The risks of anticoagulant treatment (necessity and difficulties of therapeutic control by the general practitioner).
Journal de Médecine de Bordeaux 138:1470-1474, 1961.

4869

NAGY, G., T. MIKE, AND S. BÉRO.
Myocardial infarction—a ten-year follow-up study in the Central State Hospital.
Orvosi Hetilap 102:788-793, 1961.

4870

NATOLI, A.
Therapy of myocardial infarction.
Progresso Medico (Napoli) 18:385-389, 1962.

4871

NORRIS, R.M.
Bundle-branch block and myocardial infarction.
Lancet 2:439, 1973.

4872

O'BRIEN, E.T., R.D. THORNES, M. WALDRON, AND M. O'GORMAN.
Physiology of fibrinolysis. 3. The effect of exercise on fibrinolysis in health and multiple sclerosis.
Irish Journal Medical Science 7:195, 1968.

4873
ORAM, S.
  Smoking and ischaemic heart disease.
  British Heart Journal 30:145, 1968.

4874
OSTRANDER, L.D., JR., B.J. NEFF, W.D. BLOCK, T. FRANCIS JR., AND F.H. EPSTEIN.
  Hyperglycemia and hypertriglyceridemia among persons with coronary heart disease.
  Annals Internal Medicine 67:34, 1967.

4875
OWREN, P.A.
  Critical study of tests for control of anticoagulant therapy.
  Thrombosis et Diathesis Haemorrhagica 7:294-306, 1962.

4876
OWREN, P.A.
  The results of anticoagulant therapy in Norway.
  Archives Internal Medicine 111:240-247, 1963.

4877
PAASKE, W.P., O. HENRIKSEN, P. SEJRSEN, AND S.L. NIELSEN.
  Should we stand all day?
  Lancet 2:444, 1973.

4878
PADMAVATI, S.
  A five-year survey of heart disease in Delhi.
  Indian Heart Journal 10:33, 1958.

4879
PADMAVATI, S.
  Epidemiology of cardiovascular disease in India, II. Ischemic heart disease.
  Circulation 25:711, 1962.

4880
PANTRIDGE, J.F., AND J.S. GEDDES.
  A mobile intensive care unit in the management of myocardial infarction.
  Lancet 2:271, 1967.

4881
PATTERSON, D., AND J. SLACK.
  Lipid abnormalities in male and female survivors of myocardial infarction and their first degree relatives.
  Lancet 1:393, 1972.

4882
PAYNE, R.W., M.B. EVESON, AND R.B. SLOANE.
  The relationship between blood cholesterol level and objective measures of personality.
  Journal Psychosomatic Research 7:23, 1963.

4883
PEGRUM G.D., K.M. HARRISON, S. SHAW, A. HASELTON, AND S. WOLFF.
Effect of prolonged exercise on platelet adhesiveness.
Nature (London) 213:301, 1967.

4884
PELL, S., AND C.A. D'ALONZO.
Acute myocardial infarction in a large industrial population: report of a 6 year study of 1,356 cases.
Journal American Medical Association 185:831, 1963.

4885
PENNINGTON, A.W.
The use of fat in a weight reducing diet.
Delaware State Medical Journal 23(4):79-86, 1951.

4886
PERLICK, E.Z.
Hazards of antithrombotic therapy.
Zeitschrift für Aerztliche Fortbildung 57:1242-1245, 1963.

4887
PERNOW, B., AND B. SALTIN.
Muscle metabolism during exercise.
New York, Plenum Press, 1971.

4888
PETERSEN, K.E.
Report on acute heart infarction treated without anticoagulants from
1945 to 1959.
Ugeskrift for Laeger 123:1131-1132, 1961.

4889
PEZOLD, F.A.
On the use of anticoagulant therapy in myocardial infarction.
Münchener Medizinische Wochenschrift 104:1549-1554, 1962.

4890
PIGOTT, V.M., D.H. SPODICK, E.H. RECTRA, AND A.H. KHAN.
Cardiocirculatory responses to exercise. Physiologic study by noninvasive techniques.
American Heart Journal 82:632, 1971.

4891
PILKINGTON, T.R.E., ET AL.
Diet and weight-reduction in the obese.
Lancet 1:856-858, 1960.

4892
PINCHERLE, G., AND H.B. WRIGHT.
Screening in the early diagnosis and prevention of cardiovascular diseases.
Journal College General Practitioners 12:380, 1967.

4893
PIVA, M., AND S. BONFANTI.
Clinical consideration on 95 cases of acute myocardial infarction with special reference to prognosis and therapy.
Minerva Medica 53:3695-3702, 1962.

4894
PLINER, P.L.
Effect of liquid and solid preloads on eating behavior of obese and normal persons.
Physiological Behavior 11(3):285, 1973.

4895
POOYA, M., J.C. RIOS, R. SARIN, AND R. MASSUMI.
Incidence and patterns of retrograde ventriculo-atrial conduction in man.
Circulation 39-40(Suppl. III):163, 1969.

4896
PORTO, J.
Social cardiology, our national and international plans.
Boletim do Centro de Cardiologia Médico-Social de Coimbra, (Portugal), 1961.

4897
PORTO, J.
Medico-social help for cardiac patients.
Boletim do Centro de Cardiologia Médico-Social de Coimbra, (Portugal), 1963.

4898
PORTO, J.
Cardiovascular diseases and their socio-economic reflections. Increasing need for help to cardiac patients.
Boletim do Centro de Cardiologia Médico-Social de Coimbra, (Portugal), 1964.

4899
PUDDU, V.
Cardiovascular diseases in Italy.
American Journal Cardiology 10(3):341-348, 1962.

4900
QUARFORDT, S.H., F. BOSTON, AND H. HILDERMAN.
Transfer of triglyceride between isolated human lipoproteins.
Biochimica Biophysica Acta 231:290, 1971.

4901
RABB, W.
Training, physical inactivity and the cardiac dynamic cycle.
Journal Sports Medicine Physical Fitness 6:38, 1966.

4902
RAHIMTOOLA, S.H., M.M. DIGILIO, A. EHSANI, H.S. LOEB, ET AL.
Changes in left ventricular performance from early after acute myocardial infarction to the convalescent phase.
Circulation 46:770-779, 1972.

4903
RATCLIFFE, H.L.
   Environmental factors and coronary disease.
   Circulation 27(4 Part 1):481, 1963.

4904
REMDE, W.
   The treatment of myocardial infarct with anticoagulants.
   Zeitschrift für Aerztliche Fortbildung 57:1237-1242, 1963.

4905
REMDE, W.
   The supervision of anticoagulant therapy.
   Zeitschrift für Aerztliche Fortbildung 57:1246-1249, 1963.

4906
RICHARDS, R.
   Anticoagulant therapy in acute myocardial infarction.
   Biochemical Clinics 1:137-148, 1963.

4907
RICHARDS, R., AND D.A. SCATON.
   Further observations on the value of anticoagulant therapy in the treatment of acute myocardial
   infarction.
   Scottish Medical Journal 6:559-564, 1961.

4908
RICHARDSON, J.F.
   Heart rate in middle-aged men.
   American Journal Clinical Nutrition 24:1476, 1971.

4909
RICHARDSON, J.F., AND G. PINCHERLE.
   Skinfold measurements of obesity in British businessmen.
   Journal Biosocial Studies 3:13, 1971.

4910
RIFKIND, B.
   Typing of hyperlipoproteinaemias.
   Atherosclerosis 11:545, 1970.

4911
RIFKIND, B.M., D. LAWSON, AND M. GALE.
   Diagnostic value of serum lipids and frequency of lipoprotein patterns in myocardial infarction.
   Journal Atherosclerosis Research 8:167, 1968.

4912
RIME, B., AND C. MERTENS.
   Incidence of psychologic and socio-cultural factors in the etiology of coronary disease.
   Annales Médicopsychologique 1:43-60, 1970.

4913
RIZZA, C.R.
   Effect of exercise on the level of antihaemophilic globulin in human blood.
   Journal Physiology 156:128, 1961.

4914
ROGER, G.R.
  Reflections on anticoagulant treatment.
  Clinique (Paris)56:553-580, 1961.

4915
ROSEN, J.L., AND G.L. BIBRING.
  Psychological reactions of hospitalized male patients to a heart attack.
  Psychosomatic Medicine 28:808-821, 1966.

4916
ROSEN, K.M., A. EHSANI, AND S.H. RAHIMTOOLA.
  Myocardial infarction complicated by conduction defect.
  Medical Clinics North America 57:155-166, 1973.

4917
ROSEN, K.M., R. HELLER, A. EHSANI, AND S.H. RAHIMTOOLA.
  Localization of site of traumatic heart block with HIS bundle reocrdings: Electrophysiologic
  observations regarding the nature of "split" H potentials.
  American Journal Cardiology 30:412-417, 1972.

4918
ROSENBERG, B.A.
  Acute myocardial infarction. I. Follow-up studies.
  New York State Journal Medicine 63:1791-1798, 1963.

4919
ROSENBLATT, D., AND E.A. SUCHMAN.
  Blue collar attitudes and information toward health and illness.
  In: Shostak, A.B. and W. Gomberg, Eds. Blue collar world, pp. 324-333.
  Englewood Cliffs, N.J. Prentice-Hall, 1964.

4920
ROSNER, S.W.
  Experience with exercise electrocardiography at a community hospital.
  In: Hoffman, B.F., Ed. Vectorcardiography 2. Amsterdam, North Holland Publishing Co., 1971.

4921
ROWE, M.J., M.A. DOLDER, B.J. KIRBY, AND M.F. OLIVER.
  Effect of a nicotinic acid analog on raised plasma-free fatty acids after acute myocardial
  infarction.
  Lancet 2:814-818, 1973.

4922
RUSHMER, R.F.
  Postural effects on the baselines of ventricular performance.
  Circulation 20:897, 1959.

4923
RUSSEK, H.I.
  Role of heredity, diet, and emotional stress in coronary heart disease.
  Journal American Medical Association 171:503, 1959.

4924
RUSSEK, H.I.
Present status of anticoagulant therapy in acute myocardial infarction.
Diseases Chest 43:541-543, 1963.

4925
RUSSEK, H.I.
Current myths and realities in anticoagulant therapy for coronary heart disease.
Medical Clinics North America 48:355-370, 1964.

4926
SAILER, S.
Myocardial infarction and arterial thromboses.
Wiener Medizinische Wochenschrift 113:93-95, 1963.

4927
SALA, G.
Clinical consideration on 300 cases of myocardial infarction.
Minerva Medica 54:3688-3692, 1963.

4928
SALANS, L.B., S.W. CUSHMAN, AND R.E. WEISMANN.
Studies of human adipose tissue: Adipose cell size and number in nonobese and obese patients.
Journal Clinical Investigation 52:929, 1973.

4929
SCHMITT, R.C.
Demographic statistics of Hawaii, 1778-1965.
Honolulu, University of Hawaii Press, 1968.

4930
SCHOR, S.J., K.A. ELSON, K.O. ELSON, AND J.P. DUNN.
An evaluation of the periodic health examination: A study of factors discriminating between survival and death for coronary artery disease.
Annals Internal Medicine 61:1006, 1964.

4931
SCHREIBER, R., A. NOVOTNY, V. DVORAK, AND J. CHYBA.
Thrombo-embolic disease. Thrombo-embolic complications of myocardial infarction.
Casopis Lekaru Ceskych 102:125-130, 1963.

4932
SEAMAN, A.J.
An overview of anticoagulant therapy for coronary artery disease.
American Journal Medicine 33:717-730, 1962.

4933
SHANOFF, H.M., J.A. LITTLE, AND A. CSIMA.
Studies of male survivors of myocardial infarction. XII. Relation of serum lipids and lipoproteins to survival over a ten-year period.
Canadian Medical Association Journal 103:927, 1970.

4934
SHAPIRO, A.P.
   Psychophysical mechanism in hypertensive vascular disease.
   Annals Internal Medicine 53:64, 1960.

4935
SHELDON, W.H., AND R. BALL.
   Physical characteristics of the Y twins and their relation to hypertension.
   Proceedings Association Research Nervous Mental Diseases 29:962, 1950.

4936
SIEKERT, R.G.
   Cardiac dysrhythmia and transient cerebral ischaemic attacks.
   Lancet 2:444, 1973.

4937
SIEVERS, J.
   Myocardial infarction. Clinical features and outcome in three thousand thirty-six cases.
   Acta Medica Scandinavica 175(Suppl.):406, 1964.

4938
SIGLER, L.H.
   Abnormalities in the electrocardiogram induced by emotional strain. Possible mechanisms and
   implications.
   American Journal Cardiology 8:807, 1961.

4939
SIGLER, L.H.
   Long survival following myocardial infarction. Report on 255 patients living ten years or longer
   after the first attack.
   American Journal Cardiology 9(4):547-557, 1962.

4940
SLACK, J., AND N.C. NEVIN.
   Hereditary aspects of hyperlipidemic states.
   In: Casdorph, H.R., Ed. Treatment of the hyperlipidemic states, pp. 121.
   Springfield, Ill. Thomas, 1971.

4941
SOKOLOW, M.
   Personality and predisposition to essential hypertension.
   In: Pathogenesis of essential hypertension. Proceedings, Prague Symposium, May 22-29, 1960.
   Oxford, Pergamon Press, 1962.

4942
SOULIER, J.-P., AND T. MOUDALAKI.
   Sudden death in a recent heart infarction.
   Nederlands Tijdschrift voor Geneeskunde 106:2228-2232, 1962.

4943
SPAIN, D.M., D.J. NATHAN, AND M. GELLIS.
   Weight, body type and the prevalence of coronary atherosclerotic heart disease in males.
   American Journal Medical Sciences 245:63, 1963.

4944
SPODICK, D.H., AND V.M. QUARRY-PIGOTT.
  Effects of posture on exercise performance. Measurement of systolic time intervals.
  Circulation 48:74, 1973.

4945
STERNE, J.
  The treatment of myocardial infarction during the first two days.
  Clinique (Paris):57:547-550, 1962.

4946
STEVENSON, I., C.H. DUNCAN, AND H.S. RIPLEY.
  Changes in the electrocardiogram with variations in the emotional state.
  Geriatrics 6.164, 1951.

4947
STORSTEIN, L.
  Physical activity and myocardial infarction.
  Nordisk Medicin 65:9, 1961.

4948
STRÖMGREN, L.S.
  Anticoagulant treatment of acute myocardial infarction. The importance of adequate dosage for
  the course of the disease.
  Acta Medica Scandinavica 175:473-481, 1964.

4949
SWAN, H.J.C., W. GANZ, J. FORRESTER, ET AL.
  Catherization of the heart in man with use of a flow-directed balloon-tipped catheter.
  New England Journal Medicine 283:447-451, 1971.

4950
TAGGART, P., D. GIBBONS, AND W. SOMERVILLE.
  Some effects of motor-car driving on the normal and abnormal heart.
  British Medical Journal 4:130, 1969.

4951
TAYLOR, H.
  Coronary heart disease in physically active and sedentary populations.
  Journal Sports Medicine Physical Fitness 2:73, 1962.

4952
TAYLOR, S.H., J. ANDERSON, AND A. KEYS.
  Physical activity serum cholesterol and other lipids in man.
  Proceedings, Society Experimental Biology Medicine 95:383, 1957.

4953
TAYLOR, S.H., K.W. DONALD, AND J.M. BISHOP.
  Circulatory studies in hypertensive patients at rest and during exercise.
  Clinical Science 16:351-376, 1957.

4954
THOMAS, C.B.
   The precursors of hypertension.
   Medical Clinics North America 45:259, 1961.

4955
THOMAS, T., C. CALHOUN, C.O.T. BALL, R.S. ANDERSON, AND G.R. MENEELY.
   Acute myocardial infarction in 90 Negro patients. Clinical manifestations and immediate mortality.
   American Journal Cardiology 8:178, 1961.

4956
THOMPSON, G.R., AND A.M. GOTTO, JR.
   Ileal bypass in the treatment of hyperlipoproteinaemia.
   Lancet 2:35, 1973.

4957
THORPE, G.L.
   Treating overweight patients.
   Journal American Medical Association 165(11):1361-1365, 1957.

4958
TROMBOLD, J.C., R.C. MOELLERING, JR., AND A. KAGAN.
   Epidemiological aspects of coronary heart disease and cerebrovascular disease. The Honolulu Heart
   Program.
   Hawaii Medical Journal 25:231, 1966.

4959
UDANI, P.M., ET AL.
   Carbohydrates deprivation syndrome.
   Indian Pediatrics 9:311-322, 1972.

4960
UEDA, H.
   Cardiovascular diseases in Japan.
   American Journal Cardiology 10:371, 1962.

4961
UNGERLEIDER, H., AND E. HIGGINS.
   Prognosis of cardiovascular disease: An insurance appraisal.
   American Journal Cardiology 13(5):576-584, 1964.

4962
URSCHEL, H.C., M.A. RAZZUK, R.E. WOOD, AND D.L. PAULSON.
   Factors influencing patency of aortocoronary artery saphenous vein grafts.
   Surgery 72(6):1048-1063, 1972.

4963
VAINBAUM, Y.S.
   Scheme of motor regimen for patients with ischemic heart disease.
   Voprosy Kurortologii Fizioterapii Lechebnoy Fizicheskoy Kultury 36(6):549, 1971.

4964
VAKIL, R.J.
   Cardiovascular diseases in India.
   American Journal Cardiology 10:380, 1962.

4965
VAN BEAUMONT, W., H.L. YOUNG, AND J.E. GREENLEAF.
Influence of isometric and isotonic exercise during bedrest on changes in plasma volume, plasma protein concentration and content during $+G_2$ acceleration.
Aerospace Medical Association. Preprints pp. 19-20. Las Vegas, Nevada, 1973.

4966
VARNAUSKAS, E.
Studies in hypertensive cardiovascular disease with special reference to cardiac function.
Scandinavian Journal Clinical Laboratory Investigation 7 (Suppl. 17):1-117, 1955.

4967
VENNING, E.H., I. DYRENFORTH, AND J.C. BECK.
Effect of anxiety upon aldosterone excretion in man.
Journal Clinical Endocrinology 17:1005, 1957.

4968
VEREL, D.
Anticoagulants: another view.
British Medical Journal pp. 5417, 1964.

4969
WAHLBERG, F., AND B. THOMASSON.
Glucose tolerance in ischaemic cardiovascular disease.
In: Dickens, F., P.J. Randle, and W.J. Whelan, Eds. Carbohydrate metabolism and its disorders, p. 185. New York, Academic Press, 1968.

4970
WEINSTEIN, A.
Anticoagulation . . . how long?
Journal Tennessee Medical Association 54:59-60, 1961.

4971
WEISSLER, A.M., W.S. HARRIS, AND C.D. SCHOENFELD.
Bedside technics for the evaluation of ventricular function in man.
American Journal Cardiology 23:577, 1969.

4972
WELCH, C., W.L. PROUDFIT, F.M. SONO, JR., AND E.K.SHIREY.
Cinecoronary angiography in young men.
Circulation 42(4):647-652, 1970.

4973
WELTI, J.J.
Anticoagulant treatment.
Cahiers du Collège de Médecine des Hospitaux de Paris 5:49-55, 1964.

4974
WENDKOS, H.W.
Unstable T-waves in persons without organic heart disease.
American Heart Journal 28:549-567, 1944.

4975
WERKÖ, L., AND H. LAGERLOF.
Studies on circulation in man: cardiac output and blood pressure in right auricle, right ventricle and pulmonary artery in patients with hypertensive cardiovascular disease.
Acta Medica Scandinavica 133:427-436, 1949.

4976
WEXLER, J.
The controversial anticoagulants.
Maryland State Medical Journal 11:110-111, 1962.

4977
WHITE, P.D.
Heart disease. (4th edition)
New York, Macmillan, 1951.

4978
WILDE, G.J.S., AND H.E. PELSER.
Acute myocardial infarction.
Haarlem, the Netherlands, Bohn, 1965.

4979
WILLIAMS, B., AND P.D. WHITE.
Rehabilitation of the cardiac patient.
American Journal Cardiology 7(3):317-319, 1961.

4980
WILSON, W., G.B. LEE, AND K. AMPLATZ.
Biplane selective coronary arteriography via percutaneous transfemoral approach.
American Journal Roentgenology, Radium Therapy, Nuclear Medicine 100:332-340, 1967.

4981
WILSON, W.S., S.B. HULLEY, M.I. BURROWS, AND M.Z. NICHAMAN.
Serial lipid and lipoprotein responses to the American Heart Association fat-controlled diet.
American Journal Medicine 51:491, 1971.

4982
WINTERS, W.G., D.M. LEAMAN, AND R.A. ANDERSON.
The effect of exercise on intrinsic myocardial performance.
Circulation 48:50, 1973.

4983
WOLF, S., P.V. CARDON, JR., E.M. SHEPARD, AND H.G. WOLFF.
Life stress and essential hypertension. A study of circulatory adjustments in man.
Baltimore, Williams and Wilkins, 1955.

4984
WRIGHT, I.S.
A bear by the tail? The discontinuance of anticoagulant therapy.
Diseases Chest 40:454-456, 1961.

4985
WRIGHT, I.S.
Evaluation ofanticoagulant therapy for myocardial infarction.
Lancet 2:654-656, 1962.

4986
WRIGHT, I.S., ET AL.
   Evaluation of anticoagulant therapy for myocardial infarction.
   American Heart Journal 66:842-846, 1963.

4987
WRIGHT, I.S.
   Anticoagulant therapy a matter of discrimination.
   Journal Egyptian Medical Association 46:327-342, 1963.

4988
XENAKES, E., D. DOUVAS, AND PH. KOSTEAS.
   Statistical study of the anticoagulant management of myocardial infarct.
   Hellenike Iatrike 31:266-273, 1962.

4989
YAMANAKA, M.
   Studies on the methods of control and of administration of drugs for anticoagulant therapy.
   Japanese Circulation Journal 27:136-141, 1963.

4990
YOUNG, O.M., ET AL.
   Effect on body composition and other parameters in obese young men of carbohydrate level of
   reduction diet.
   American Journal Clinical Nutrition 24:290-296, 1971.

4991
YOUNG, W., R.L. HOTOVEC, AND A.G. ROMERO.
   Tea and atherosclerosis.
   Nature 216:1015, 1967.

4992
ZUIDEMA, P.J.
   Angina pectoris and coronary thrombosis in Djakarta, 1947-51.
   Documenta de Medicina Geographica et Tropica 4:378, 1952.

4993
ANONYMOUS
   ECG monitors: safety, interference, test program.
   Spri Rad 6:1, 1971.

4994
ANONYMOUS
   Helping the heart patient go back to work.
   Industrial Medicine Surgery 41:16, 1972.

4995
ANONYMOUS
   Prevention of C.H.D. The fats in the fire.
   Journal American Medical Association 215:1813, 1971.

4996
ANONYMOUS
  Psychological hazards of convalescence after myocardial infarction.
  Lancet 1:1055, 1071.

4997
ANONYMOUS
  Sodium heparin vs. sodium warfarin in acute myocardial infarction. Conclusions based on study of
  798 cases at 13 hospitals.
  Journal American Medical Association 189:555-562, 1964.

4998
AMERICAN COLLEGE OF CARDIOLOGY.
  Cardiac and other organ transplantation in the setting of transplant science as a national effort.
  Fifth Bethesda Conference of the American College of Cardiology.
  American Journal Cardiology 22:896-912, 1968.

4999
AMERICAN HEART ASSOCIATION.
  Mass field trials of the diet-heart question. Their significance, timeliness, feasibility, and applica-
  bility. American Heart Association Monograph No. 28.
  New York, American Heart Association, 1969.

5000
CIBA, INTERNATIONAL SYMPOSIUM
  Essential hypertension—an international symposium.
  Berne, June 7-10, 1960. Berlin, Springer-verlag, 1960.

5001
COUNCIL ON REHABILITATION, INTERNATIONAL SOCIETY OF CARDIOLOGY.
  Myocardial infarction. How to prevent. How to rehabilitate.
  Bruxelles, Belgium. International Society Cardiology, 1973.

5002
PRAGUE SYMPOSIUM
  The pathogenesis of essential hypertension.
  Proceedings Prague Symposium, May 22-29, 1960.
  Oxford, Pergamon Press, 1962.

5003
TIMBERLINE CONFERENCE
  Timberline Conference on the psychophysiological aspects of cardiovascular diasease.
  Timberline Lodge, Portland, Oregon.
  Psychosomatic Medicine Supplement, July-August 1964.

5004
U.S. NATIONAL HEALTH SURVEY
  Heart conditions and high blood pressure.
  Health Statistics, Series B, No. 13. Washington, D.C.
  U.S. Department Health, Education, Welfare, 1960.

5005
WORLD HEALTH ORGANIZATION
  The prodromal symptoms of myocardial infarction and sudden death. Report on a working group.
  Regional Office for Europe, Copenhagen. (EURO 8204-3).

Author Index

Balke, B. 0186, 0187, 0188, 0189, 2861, 2862, 2863, 2901, 2902, 2903, 2904, 2924, 3038, 4113
Ball, C.O.T. 4955
Ball, K. 0190, 4126
Ball, K.P. 0191
Ball, R. 4935
Balogh, Z. 0192, 4000
Baltaxe, H.A. 2319
Balter, M.B. 2676
Bandera, L. 0312, 1295, 1296
Banerjea, J.C. 0193
Banerjee, A. 1292
Banks, R.E. 4620
Bannister, R. 4621
Bantea. C. 0194
Banzhaf, E. 3117
Bao, O. 3534
Baptista, G. 2861
Barachet, M. 3160
Baragan, J. 3126
Baranov, V.A. 0195, 0196
Barats, S.S. 0197
Barbano, G. 4622
Barbeau, A. 0730
Barber, J.M. 0395
Barbosa, F.J. 3493
Barbosa, J. 0198
Barbotin, M. 0705
Barckow, D. 0199
Barczewski, W. 2106
Bardet, J. 0994, 2638
Barin, P. 3355
Barlow, J.B. 2193, 3167, 3168
Barmeyer, J. 3402
Barnard, C.N. 3617
Barnard, R.J. 0200, 0201, 4069
Barnes, R. 4623
Barnes, R.J. 0202
Barness, L.A. 1018
Barnett, A.J. 4624
Barnett, G.O. 0203, 1406, 2460
Barold, S. 0499
Baroldi, G. 4625
Baron, P. 0429
Barr, I. 2426, 3840
Barritault, L. 2648
Barrow, J.G. 4378
Barry, A.J. 0204, 0205, 0754, 1902, 3769
Barry, H.J. 0206
Barry, W.H. 0207
Bartel, A.G. 0208, 0561
Bartels, C.T. 2269
Bartels, H. 0501, 3604
Bartels, R.L. 1083
Bartelstone, H.J. 0209, 4443
Barth, P. 0210
Bartoli, E. 0920
Bartoszewski, J. 0857

Barwolf, A. 3372
Barylak, J. 0141, 0144, 2120, 3443
Bashour, T. 0599, 0600, 4626
Bassett, D.R. 0211, 4864
Bassler, T.J. 0212
Bastiaans, J. 0213
Basu, D.P. 4627
Basu, S.K. 0214
Basu, T.K. 0177
Batchlor, C. 1474, 2015
Bateman, M. 1528, 1529, 1530, 1836
Bates, B.B. 1837
Batsevich, A.A. 0215
Battock, D.J. 0216, 0217
Baubinene, A.V. 0218
Bauer, B. 2079
Bauer, R.D. 3081
Baum, O.V. 0219
Bauman, D.J. 0220
Baumann, P.C. 0221, 2354
Baumgarten, C. 3257
Baumgartl, P. 2055
Bay, G. 0375
Bazilyuk, O.V. 4646
Beard, E.F. 0222, 3047, 4628
Beauffigeau, A. 0429
Beaumont, J.-L. 4629
Beaver, W.L. 4293
Beck, A.T. 4630
Beck, D. 0223, 0224
Beck, J.C. 4967
Beck, R.H. 0225, 0226
Beck, R.J. 3036
Beck, W. 0227, 0228, 3617
Becker, A.E. 0229
Becker, M.C. 0230
Becker, M.J. 0229
Becklake, M.R. 2037
Beckman, C.B. 0840
Beckurth, J.R. 0231
Bédard, P. 1969
Bedford, E. 0232
Bednarzewski, J. 0233
Bedrak, E. 0234
Bedynek, J.L. 3059
Beer, G. 0234
Beering, S.C. 3370
Befeler, B. 0235
Beg, M.A. 3970
Begg, T.B. 3304
Behar, S. 1892
Behar, V.S. 0208
Behr, G. 4631
Beiser, G.D. 0236, 0237, 0965, 0966, 0968, 0971, 1346, 1347, 1348, 3275, 3395
Beland, A.J. 0358
Belaya, N.A. 0042
Belbeck, L.W. 4632
Belknap, E.L. 1635, 3376

Brooks, W.W. 0314
Broustet, J.P. 0416, 0428, 0429
Broustet, P. 0290, 0416
Browe, J.H. 0430
Brown, A.E. 1173
Brown, D.F. 0419, 0431, 0889, 4686, 4687
Brown, D.J. 2578
Brown, H. 0270
Brown, H.B. 0432, 0433
Brown, J. 4688
Brown, K. 3799
Brown, K.W.G. 0434, 0831, 4689
Brown, L.B. 0435
Brown, R.G. 0436
Brown, R.I.F. 1420
Brown, R.W. 0437
Brown, W.K. 3348
Brown, W.V. 2335
Browne, I.W. 0438
Brox, D. 2637
Brozek, J. 0439, 0440, 1979
Bruce, A. 0456
Bruce, E.R. 2349
Bruce, R.A. 0441, 0442, 0443, 0444, 0445,
    0446, 0447, 0448, 0449, 0450, 0451, 0452,
    0453, 0454, 0455, 0457, 0611, 0820, 0821,
    0823, 0853, 1291, 1707, 1708, 1709, 1710,
    1711, 1908, 1909, 1919, 2477, 2481, 2817,
    2847, 4068, 4436, 4690, 4691
Bruce, T.A. 0458, 0463, 4042
Bruch, J. 0187
Bruener, H. 4692
Bruhn, J. 2917
Bruhn, J.G. 0028, 0459, 0460, 0461, 0462,
    0463, 0464, 0465, 2906, 2907, 2908, 2909,
    3343
Brummer, P. 0466
Brundage, B.H. 0467
Brunner, D. 0468, 0469, 0470, 0471, 0472,
    0473, 0474, 0475, 0476, 0477, 2701, 4693
Bruno, L. 0312, 1296
Bruno, M.S. 3997
Brunzell, J.D. 0478
Brusca, A. 0083
Bruschke, A.V.G. 0135, 0479
Brusis, O.A. 0480
Bruto Da Costa, B.C. 4851
Bryant, L.R. 0758
Brynteson, P. 4694
Bubel, M.S. 2651
Buc, M.H. 4629
Buchbinder, N.A. 0481
Bucher, J. 4141
Bucher, R. 3295
Buchheit, H. 2157
Büchner, C. 0361
Buckberg, G.D. 0201, 0690
Buckley, M.J. 0914
Bucklin, R. 0482

Buczynski, E. 3904
Budingen, F. 0483
Budwai, P.S. 1441
Buell, P. 0415, 0484
Buley, L.E. 0485
Buncher, C.R. 1324
Bunde, C.A. 0486, 1434
Bunnell, I.L. 2192
Buoncristiani, U. 0696
Burch, G.E. 0487, 0488, 0489, 0490, 0491,
    0492, 0493, 0494, 0495, 0496, 3137, 4695,
    4696
Burch, G.E.A. 4697
Burchell, H.B. 1586, 2546
Burchett, G. 0226
Burdeshaw, J.A. 3698
Burford, C.L. 0663
Burgalassi, S. 0497
Burgess, J.H. 1042
Burggraf, G.W. 0498, 1041
Burgos Cornejo, J. 3110
Burian, W. 2150
Burkart, F. 0499, 2860, 3295
Burke, C.E. 0222
Burke, F. 2686
Burke, F.D. 4856
Burkhardt, H. 0500
Burlando, A. 1608
Burlando, A.G. 1619, 1620
Burlando, A.J. 0524
Burns, N. 3751
Burrell, F. 0716
Burrmann, H. 0501, 3604
Burrows, M.I. 4981
Burry, H.C. 0502
Burstein, A.G. 0757
Burton, A.C. 0503
Burton, H. 1054
Burton, P. 4631
Burvill, M.J. 4079
Buskirk, E. 4012, 4021
Buskirk, E.R. 0504, 0505, 0506, 0507, 1859,
    1860
Buslenko, N.S. 0508
Busnengo, E. 0509, 0510, 0511
Bustamante Costa, U. 4698
Buston, W.M. 2785
Buti, A. 4433
Butkus, A. 3054
Butler, J.C. 2091
Butler, V.P., Jr. 0512, 3793
Butterfield, W.J.H. 2997
Buttram, W.R., Jr. 0513
Buxman, J. 0514
Buyukozturk, K. 0515
Buzina, R. 0516
Buzoianu, V. 1431, 1432
Buzzi, A. 0517
Byers, S.O. 3387

Byers, W.S. 1366
Bygdeman, S. 4254
Bynum, B.G. 4756
Byrne-Quinn, E. 4311

Cabrol, A. 3339
Cacace, L. 3966
Cacena-Seldner, K.A. 4851
Caceres, C.A. 0854, 1676, 2270
Cachovan, M. 3159
Cady, L.D. 0534, 0535, 1262, 1280
Cady, L.D., Jr. 0518, 0519
Caesar, K. 1802
Caffrey, B. 0520, 0521, 0522
Cahen, P. 0523
Cain, H.D. 0524, 0525, 4699
Caird, F.I. 4401
Calabrò, R. 3547
Calatayud, J.B. 0854, 1676
Calay, G. 0081
Caldwell, A.B. 0300, 0302, 0303
Caldwell, J.R. 0526, 0527
Caldwell, T.B. 2671
Calesnick, B. 0528
Calhoun, C. 4955
Califano, J.E. 0529
Calise, S.J. 0226
Call, R.W. 0530, 0531
Callaghan, J.C. 2258
Calleja, H.B. 0532
Calva, E. 2265
Calvin, J.R. 0533
Calvy, G.L. 0534, 0535
Campbell, D.A. 0536
Campbell, E.J.M. 1656
Campbell, G.C. 4712
Campbell, G.S. 4391
Campbell, L. 3457
Campbell, W.B. 4059
Campeau, L. 0390
Campion, B.C. 0074, 0075
Candiolo, G. 0537
Canivet, J. 3082
Canizares, C. 0538
Canizares, F. 0538
Cannata, D. 3532
Cantone, A. 0539
Cantwell, J.D. 0540, 0541, 0542, 1051
Canzoneri, J., III 4160
Canzonetti, J. 4752
Caplan, R.D. 1143
Capone, R.J. 2410
Caponnetto, S. 2576
Capp, M.P. 2569
Capri, C. 4618
Capurro, C. 4830
Caputi, A.P. 2562

Caquet, R. 0543
Carabatos, C. 2951
Caracta, A.R. 1842, 1843
Carbajal, B. 0517
Cardillo, T.E. 0544
Cardon, P.V., Jr. 4423, 4700, 4983
Cardus, D. 0545, 0546, 0547, 0548, 4158
Cariani, A. 4608
Caris, T.N. 2248
Carlton, R.A. 1383
Carli, A. 2763
Carli, C.D. 0729
Carlson, L.A. 0386, 0549, 0550, 2227, 4252
Carlson, R.G. 0551, 2320
Carlson, W.S. 3431
Carmo, E.J.S., Jr. 0379
Carnes, G.C. 0552
Carp, C. 3862
Carrasco, H. 3440
Carre, A. 4273
Carre, R. 3126
Carretero, O.A. 0526
Carriere, S. 3844
Carroll, A. 3388
Carroll, D.G. 0553
Carroll, W.M. 1661
Carruthers, M. 3819, 3986
Carruthers, M.O. 0554
Carson, P. 0555
Carson, V. 2927
Carter, R.E., Jr. 3851
Caruso, D. 4082
Carver, S.T. 4790
Casaccia, M. 1301
Casar, F.P. 0556
Casari, A. 0362
Case, R.B. 3070, 3071
Cash, J.D. 0557, 0558, 0768, 4701
Cassel, J. 0559, 0561
Cassel, J.C. 0560, 1884, 2047
Cassem, N.H. 0562, 0563, 1459, 1460, 1461,
    4412
Cassens, R.G. 3274
Cassidy, J. 0127, 0128
Castellanos, A. 0564
Castellanos, A., Jr. 0565, 2275, 2276
Castelli, W.P. 1874, 1875, 1879
Castillo, A. 4114
Castillo, C.A. 3426, 3427
Castillo, C.S. 0564
Castle, L.W. 0566
Castleden, C.M. 4702
Caston, J. 0567
Castranova, S.J. 4346
Castro, C.M. 4703
Casucci, G. 4091
Catalano, V. 3155
Cataldi, S. 2562
Cataliotti, C. 1026

Chung, K.J. ,1385
Chuquimia, R. 3246
Church, C.F. 4711
Church, H.N. 4711
Chyba, J. 4931
CIBA, International Symposium 5000
Cibulski, A.A. 0636
Cihak, J. 0637
Clancy, D.L. 2998
Clancy, R.L. 0638
Clark, R.J. 0639
Clark, V.A. 0588
Clarke, A.M. 0640
Claudon, D.G. 0229
Clausen, J.P. 0641, 0642, 0643, 0644, 0645,
    0646, 4099
Cleave, T.L. 4712
Clejan, S. 0162
Clemente, R. 2550
Clemmons, R.S. 3627
Cleveland, G.L. 1797
Cleveland, S.E. 0647
Cline, M.E. 1640
Cline, R.E. 0648
Clinton Miller, M. III 3343
Cloarec, M. 4713
Clode, M. 1656
Cluver, E.H. 1823
Clyman, B. 0530
Clyman, C. 0531
Cobb, L.A. 0444, 0649
Cobb, S. 0527, 1905
Cobbin, L.B. 1358
Coblence, B. 3126
Cobo, L. 0650
Cochrane, R. 0651
Cody, D.V. 2472
Coffin, L.H. 0535
Cogan, O.J. 2490
Coghlan, N. 2838
Cohen, B.S. 1388
Cohen, E. 0652
Cohen, H. 0653
Cohen, H.C. 0654
Cohen, H.D. 3680
Cohen, H.E. 2680
Cohen, J. 3578
Cohen, L.S. 0408, 0655, 0235, 3733, 4025
Cohen, O. 2708
Cohen, R.J. 0655
Cohen, S. 0992
Cohen, S.I. 3895
Cohn, J.N. 1986
Cohn, K. 3967
Cohn, K.E. 1043, 1340, 3254
Cohn, L.H. 0656
Cohn, P.F. 0657, 0658, 0659, 0660
Cokkinos, D.V. 2247
Colao, G. 0661

Colbert, J.N. 0662
Cole, P.V. 4702
Coleman, A.E. 0663
Coleman, A.J. 0664, 0665, 0666, 0885
Coleman, H.N. III 1443
Colemont, A. 2274
Coles, D. 0286
Coles, D.M. 1389
Colin, W. 0667
Collier, C.R. 3657
Collignon, P. 0668
Collins, F.B. 0669
Collins, J.G. 1054
Collins, W.S. 2978
Colón, A.A. 0344, 1219, 1220
Coltart, D.J. 0670
Colton, C.K. 0671
Columbaro, R.L. 3009
Community Council, Houston, Texas 4574
Conley, T.L. 4517
Connell, M.D. 0672
Conner, W.T. 1521
Conners, R.B. 3303
Connolly, J.E. 0673
Connor, S.L. 0677
Connor, W.E. 0675, 0676, 0677
Conolly, M.E. 0674, 1251
Conrad, H. 0678
Conrad, L. 4840
Conrad, L.L. 0679
Conradi, E. 0680
Conradsson, T. 0681
Conradsson, T.B. 3489
Conroy, D.V. 3696, 3698
Consolazio, C.F. 4714
Constantinides, E.D. 0682
Constantopoulos, A. 4820
Conte, J. 3515
Conti, C.R. 0683
Conway, J. 1851, 1852, 4356
Coodley, E.L. 0684
Cook, K.J. 0685
Cook, L.P. 0686
Cooley, D.A. 1252, 4102
Cooper, G. 1443
Cooper, J. 2268
Cooper, J.B. 4715
Cooper, J.K. 1098, 3889
Cooper, K.H. 0687, 0688, 0689, 3370, 4716
Cooper, L. 0567
Cooper, M. 0445, 2173, 2174
Cooper, N. 0690
Cooper, R. 0691
Cope, G.D. 0692
Cope, J.A. 0358
Copeland, G.D. 0427, 0693
Copeman, J.W. 0530
Corbin, M. 1137, 1392
Corcoran, A.C. 0694

Corday, E. 0695, 1099, 3440, 4245, 4717
Corea, L. 0696
Cornfield, J. 0697, 1474, 4779
Cornil, A. 0281
Cornish, D. 4221
Cornoni, J.C. 0561, 1884
Coronary Drug Project, Research Group 4575
Corredor Morales, A. 3110
Corsini, G. 1117
Cortes-Alicea, M. 1219
Cortis, B. 2446
Corya, B.R. 2491
Cosby, R.S. 0698, 0699
Coscarelli, L. 0247
Cosin Aguilar, J. 3007
Costas, R., Jr. 0344, 1219, 1220
Coste, A. 4106
Costeas, F. 0700
Costill, D.L. 0701
Costiloe, J.P. 3606, 3607
Cotes, J.E. 0702, 0703
Cotoi, S. 1231
Cottier, P. 0704
Coudert, J. 2781
Coulshed, N. 0983, 0984, 0985
Coulson, A.H. 0588, 3277
Council on Rehabilitation, International
    Society of Cardiology 5001
Courgeon, P. 4766
Coutet, M.C. 4681
Coutts, K.D. 2528
Couturier, Y. 0705, 2063
Covalt, D.A. 1265, 1266, 1269
Covarrubias, E. 2781
Covell, J. 3356
Covell, J.W. 0706, 0707, 3829
Covic, M. 3638
Cox, J.L. 0708
Cox, J.R. 0709
Cox, J.R., Jr. 0710
Cox, J.W. 0919, 4316, 4372, 4373, 4374
Cox, J.W., Jr. 0427
Craddock, D. 4718
Craig, C.P. 0711
Craige, E. 1075, 3336, 3891
Cramer, D.B. 1318
Cramer, G. 2534
Crampton, R.S. 0712, 0713
Crane, M.G. 1760
Cranefield, P.F. 1682, 1683
Crawford, D.W. 3190
Crawford, M.D. 0714, 2795
Creditor, M.C. 0715
Cress, R.H. 0716
Creteanu, G. 0717
Crews, J. 0718
Crews, T.L. 0146
Criley, J.M. 2339
Crislip, R.L. 0421

Cristal, N. 0719
Cristodoresco, R. 0720
Critz, J.B. 0721, 4632
Crockett, L.K. 0722
Cronin, R.F.P. 0323, 0723
Croog, S.H. 0724, 0725, 0726, 0727
Cropp, G.J. 4719
Crosbie, S.M. 0915
Cross, D.F. 0728
Croston, R.C. 4720
Crown, S. 1721
Croxson, M.S. 2972
Cruickshank, J.C. 0764
Crumpton, C.W. 3426
Cruz-Vidal, M. 1219
Csima, A. 4933
Cucchini, F. 0729
Cuche, J.L. 0730
Cucurachi, L. 0731
Cuddy, T.E. 0153, 2853
Cuilliere, M. 0607
Cull, J.G. 0732
Cullen, K.J. 4852
Cullhed, I. 0099, 0100, 0733, 0734, 0799,
    0800, 1664, 1729
Cumler, W. 4786
Cumming, G.R. 0735, 0736, 0737, 0738,
    0739, 3928
Cundey, P.E., Jr. 0146
Cunningham, D.A. 0721
Cunningham, D.J.C. 0740
Cunningham, R.J. 2697
Cunninghame Green, R.A. 3802
Cuomo, A. 2879
Curd, J.G. 3794
Cureton, T. 1690, 2758
Cureton, T.K. 3769
Currens, J.H. 0741
Curry, G.C. 2390, 2402
Curzi, G. 3648
Cushman, S.W. 4928
Custovic, F. 3131
Cutcher, B. 2082, 2084
Cutforth, E. 2841
Cybulska, B. 0296
Czaplicki, S. 0051, 0742, 0743
Czitober, H. 3292
Czopf, J. 4000
Czula, R. 1912

Dace, M.C. 4393
Dack, S. 2613, 2615
Dadd, M.J. 0744
Dagenais, G.R. 0360, 0745, 0746
Dahl, L.K. 0747
Dahlbäck, O. 0748
Dahllöf, A-G. 1691

Dahn, I. 0748
Daily, B.N.J. 0749
Daily, P.O. 0207
Dalderup, L.M. 0750
Dall, J.L.C. 0751
D'Alonzo, C.A. 3112, 3113, 4884
Dalton, B. 0752
Daly, E. 0753
Daly, J.W. 0204, 0754
Damato, A.N. 0280, 0755, 1208, 1843, 2392, 2393, 3095
Damir, A.M. 0756
Dammann, J.F., Jr. 4397
Damon, A. 3175
Dan, A.J. 0757
Danford, D.A. 4721
Danford, H.G. 4721
Daniel, T.M. 0708
Daniels, G.E. 4866
Danielson, G.K. 0758, 1139
Danielson, R.A. 2478
Danilov, IU, E. 0759
Danilova, K.M. 3810
Danilow, J.J. 0760
Danilowicz, D.A. 0761
Dannemann, H. 0762, 2434
Danzig, R. 3964
Daoud, F.S. 0763
D'Arbela, P.G. 4117
Darbonne, A. 0992
Darby, S. 0764
D'Arcy, V. 0765
Darling, R.C. 0766
Darmady, J.M. 0767
Darsinos, J. 2823
Das, P.C. 0768
Dasgupta, S. 2833
Dashkevich, O.V. 4722
Da Silva, W.N. 0769, 0770
Datato, A.N. 3798
Datey, K.K. 0771
Datlow, D.W. 2596
Datnow, B. 3679
Datsenko, I.I. 0772
Dauber, T.R. 1880
Daugherty, E.A. 1073
David, N.A. 3192
David, P. 3265
Davidson, L.A.G. 0436
Davies, C.T.M. 0773, 0774, 0775
Davies, D.S. 0674
Davies, H. 1236, 4059
Davies, M. 0776
Davies, M.H. 0777
Davies Jones, G.A.B. 0709
Davila, R. 3504
Davydova, A.A. 0778
Dawber, T. 4810
Dawber, T.R. 0780, 1876, 2557, 4723, 4809

Dawidowicz, A. 0779
Dawson, A.A. 0781
Dawson, J.E. 0541
Day, H.W. 0782
Day, W.C. 3109, 3442
Dayrit, C. 0001
Dayton, S. 4724
De Ambroggi, L. 3411
De Angelis, L. 0783
Dear, W.E. 0222
Deasy, L.C. 0784
De Bakey, M.E. 0785
De Benedictis, N. 0084
DeBisschop, G. 2814
DeBra, D.W. 2756
Debroczi, T. 1712
DeBusk, R.F. 0786, 3857
Decker, D.D. 0787
Decortis, A. 2279
De Coster, A. 0788
De Geest, H. 3145
Degré, S. 0788, 4169, 4725, 4726
De Guia, R. 1376
Deherdt, P. 0818
Deitz, R.D. 1126
De Jongh, D. 0527
De Keyser, J.W. 3177
Dekker, A. 0722
Dekova, A.M. 1001
De La Chapelle, C.E. 0789, 0790
Delahaye, A. 0791
Delahaye, J.P. 1744
De La Iglesia, F.A. 0792
Delamare, J. 1081
De Lang, P.A. 0850
Delaye, J. 1352
Delbecque, H. 4274
Delbue, C. 0793
Delcourt, R. 2109
Deleixhe, A. 0794
De Leon, C. 0538
Delgado, S. 0795
De Lippenholtz, L.P. 2938
Delius, L. 0796, 0797, 0798, 0801
Delius, W. 0799, 0800
Deliyiannis, S. 0240, 0241
Deller, S. 2344
Delman, A.J. 0802
Deloche, A. 4185
Del Rio, C. 2247
Demaney, M.A. 0803
Demaret, B. 4725
DeMartino, A. 1377
Dembo, A.G. 0804
Demedts, M. 0805
Demeester, M. 2109, 2110
De Mello, W.C. 0806
De Micheli, A. 0807, 2665
Denborough, M.A. 0808, 2419

De Neve, M. 0809
Dengler, H.J. 0810
De Nicola, P. 4727
Denier Von Den Gon, J.J. 0372
Denis, B. 0166
Denison, D.M. 0811
Dennin, H.F. 4733
Dennis, L.H. 0655
Dennyson, W.G. 4379
Denolin, H. 0069, 0788, 2214, 4169, 4726
De Palma, R.G. 0812, 3371
Depasquale, N.P. 3997
De Paula, P. 3236
Depouill, J. 0523
De Quattro, V. 0813
Derevici, I. 0814
Derman, U. 0279
Dervillée, E. 0815
Deryagina, G.P. 0816
Desanctis, R.W. 0817, 1738, 2148
Desche Labarthe, S. 0543
Deschryer, C. 0818
De Silva, G.U. 2994
Desser, K.B. 0251, 0257, 0259, 0261
Detry, J.M.R. 0819, 0820, 0821, 0822, 0823,
  3423, 3424
Deuschle, K.W. 0825
Deutsch, E. 0824
Deutscher, S. 0826
Devera, L.B. 0695
De Vernejoul, P. 2647, 2648
Devine, C.E. 0827
De Vita, V.T. 2595, 2596
DeVito, J.J. 1397
DeVreker, R. 4203
Dewar, H.A. 0828, 2686, 4856
Dewees, R.L. 4785
DeWeese, J.A. 0829, 2813
De Wijn, J.F. 0830
Deyer, K. 1241
DeYoung, W.A. 4354
Dhalla, N.S. 4081
Dhawan, B.N. 1445
Dhurandhar, R.W. 0831, 0832, 0833
Diaco, N.V. 0200
Diard, F. 0834
Diaz, F.V. 0835
Di Blasi, I. 3502
Dibner, R.D. 1213
Dick, D.E. 0284
Dick, T.B.S. 3922
Dicovsky, C. 0836
Diehl, H.J. 0837, 3832
Diekmeier, L. 0838
Dienstl, F. 0839
Dietz, A. 4236, 4508
Dietzman, R.H. 0840
Dighiero, J. 1063, 4433
Digilio, M.M. 4902

Di Giorgi, S. 0329, 0841, 3067, 3068, 3069,
  3072, 3073
Dijkema, F.K. 0842
Dikshit, K. 3201, 3202
Di Leo, M. 0908
Di Lieto, M. 1376
Dill, D.B. 0843
Di Luzio, V. 3648
Di Michele, A. 3114
Dimitriu, C.G. 0844
Dimnik, R. 0845
Dimond, E.G. 0252, 0253, 0254, 0255, 0260,
  1307, 4728
Dimond, G.E. 0846, 0847, 4729
Dinsmore, R.E. 3198
Di Nunzio, H. 2245
Dionisio, S.D. 0848
Di Paolo, E. 0849
Di Prampero, P.E. 2556
Dirken, J.M. 3278, 3565
Dirnagl, K. 3611
Dissmann, T. 2759
Distelbrink, C.A. 0850
Dixon, W. 0589
Djiane, P. 0851, 3666
Dlin, B.M. 0852
Doan, A.E. 0853, 1622
Doane, B.L. 3219, 3220, 3221
Dobosiewicz, K. 2979
Dobrow, R.J. 0854
Dobrowolski, L.A. 0855, 0856
Dobrzanski, T. 0867
Dobson, M. 0867, 4730
Dock, D.S. 3333
Dock, W. 0858, 0859
Dodek, A. 0860
Dodge, H.T. 4754
Dodinot, B. 0861, 3134, 3135, 4741
Doenecke, P. 0862
Dohba, N. 0863
Dohrenwend, B.P. 0864
Doichinov, A. 4731
Doig, A. 4030
Dolabchian, Z.L. 0865
Dolan, P. 3866
Doll, R. 4732
Dollery, C.T. 0674, 0866, 2085
Dombeck, D.H. 2095
Domenichini, G. 2650
Dominian, J. 0867
Donald, K.W. 0105, 2243, 4621, 4953
Donaldson, A. 3779
Donat, K. 0868
Donath, H. 2984
Donegan, M.E. 2695
Doney, H. 1932, 1933
Dongier, M. 0869
Donofrio, G. 1381
Donoso, E. 2614

Edelman, M. 0608
Edelstein, S.G. 1395
Ederer, F. 0926
Edgett, J.W. 2698
Edgill, M. 2476
Edhag, O. 0927, 0147
Edmunds, L.H. 1040
Edwards, J.E. 0229, 3855, 4265
Edwards, R.H.T. 0928
Effert, S. 1049
Effler, D.B. 4606
Efskind, L. 1190, 3764
Egeberg, O. 0929, 4736
Eggers, P. 4737
Eghtedari, A. 4781
Egmond, W.G. 0135
Ehn, L. 3488
Ehrenkranz, M. 1274
Ehrenstein, W. 2186
Ehrlich, L. 2424
Ehsani, A. 3245, 3372, 3373, 4902, 4916, 4917
Eich, R.H. 3801
Eichhorn, R.L. 0930
Eidinov, I.B. 4738
Eie, H. 3926
Einstein, R. 1358
Eisdorfer, C. 4386
Eisenberg, H. 0931
Eisenreich, R. 0932
Ekblom, B. 0355, 0933, 0934, 0935, 1543
Ekelund, L-G. 0936
Ekstrom-Jodal, B. 3754, 4381
Elber, E. 3146
Eleady-Cole, R. 4690
Elena, R. 1063
Elestad, M.H. 1962
Eliakim, M. 0240, 0241, 0937, 0938
Eliot, R.S. 0939, 0940
Eliseo, V. 0941
El-Keiy, A.M. 3834
Elkeles, R.S. 0942
El-Khatib, M.R. 2234
Ellestad, M.H. 0358, 0943, 1886, 2548
Elliot, R.S. 4739
Elliott, S. 0107
Elliott, W.C. 1645, 2059, 2060, 2490
Ellis, J.G. 0255
Ellison, R.C. 2741, 2742
Ellner, O. 3555
Elmfeldt, D. 0944, 2118, 3535, 3536, 4188
El-Rakhawy, M.T. 0035
El-Sherif, N. 0945, 0946
Elson, K.A. 4930
Elson, K.O. 4930
Elwood, P.C. 4258
Elzinga, G. 0842
Emara, A. 1562

Emerson, P.A. 1506
Emmrich, J. 3402
Enderle, J. 0947
Enesco, I. 0948
Engel, G.L. 0949
Engelhardt, K. 0950
Engell, H.C. 3735
Engelman, K. 3193, 4429
Enger, S.C. 0951
English, T.A.H. 0952
Engstedt, L. 0386, 0953
Enke-Ferchland, E. 4414
Enos, W.F. 4740
Enrico, J.F. 3130
Enterline, P.E. 4518
Entman, M.L. 2569, 3628
Epois, A. 0954
Epstein, E.J. 0983, 0984, 0985
Epstein, F.H. 0613, 0955, 0956, 0957, 0958, 0959, 0960, 0961, 0962, 0963, 1812, 3043, 3044, 3878, 4874
Epstein, S.E. 0236, 0237, 0412, 0655, 0964, 0965, 0966, 0967, 0968, 0969, 0970, 0971, 1319, 1320, 1344, 1345, 1346, 1347, 1348, 1965, 2998, 3275, 3276, 3395
Erbstoesser, H. 0972
Erfurt, J.C. 1516
Erickson, L. 0973
Ericsson, B. 0975
Ericsson, M. ,0974
Erikssen, J. 0976
Ertem, G. 0601, 4191
Escher, J.W. 0802
Eshchar, Y. 0895
Eshkol, D. 2331, 4210
Eskwith, I.S. 0977
Espino Vela, J. 2370
Esrig, B. 2216
Estandia, A. 1189
Esterly, J.R. 3029
Estes, E.H., Jr. 3357, 4669, 4670
Esu, M.P. 0605, 2398, 2399
Ettinger, P.O. 0036, 0978
Evang, K. 0979
Evans, D.W. 3239
Evans, J.G. 3214
Evans, J.M. 1355, 1367, 1368
Evans, J.R. 1760
Evans, R.B. 0980
Evans, R.W. 2698
Evans, W. 0981
Eventov, A.Z. 0042
Eveson, M.B. 4882
Evonuk, E. 4385
Ewing, D.J. 0982
Ewing, K. 1442
Ewy, G.A. 3316, 3319
Exner, I. 1697

Friedberg, G.K. 4749
Friedberg, H.D. 1165
Friedberg, S.J. 4670
Friedemann, M. 2860
Friedman, E.H. 1166, 1167, 1168, 1169,
  1170, 1610, 1611, 1612, 1613, 1614, 1619,
  1620
Friedman, G.D. 1171, 1876, 2038, 2039, 4723
Friedman, H.S. 3370
Friedman, L. 0719
Friedman, L.D. 1172
Friedman, M. 0383, 1173, 1174, 1175, 1176,
  1177, 1178, 3385, 3386, 3387, 3388, 3389,
  3390, 3391, 3392
Friedman, R. 0948, 2615
Friedman, S. 0671
Friedman, W.F. 3356
Friedrich, G. 1179
Friesen, W.J. 1180
Friesinger, G.C. 0745, 1074, 1181, 1866,
  3410, 4750
Frisius, H. 0199
Fritz, P.J. 1182
Froberg, J. 4036
Froelicher, V.F. 1183, 1184
Froer, K.-L. 2278
Froggatt, P. 1784
Frohlich, E.D. 1185
Froment, A. 1186
Froment, C. 4751
Froment, R. 1186, 1187, 1744
Frost, H. 1188
Froufe, D.J. 1189
Froufe, J. 2857
Fröysaker, T. 1190, 3764
Fry, D.L. 0203
Frye, R.L. 1403, 1404, 1859, 1860, 2466,
  3987
Fuccella, L.M. 1191
Fuenning, S.I. 3369
Fujimori, Y. 3949
Fujimura, S. 3077
Fujinami, T. 1192
Fujino, M. 2134
Fujita, Y. 1193, 1194
Fukuda, S. 1935
Fulton, M. 0105
Fumagalli, C. 0087, 0289
Funatsu, T. 1765
Fung, Y-C 1195
Funke, H.D. 1196
Funkenstein, D.H. 4821
Fürberg, C. 1197, 1198, 4604
Furbetta, D. 1199
Furman, K.I. 0234
Furman, R.H. 1200
Furnass, B. 4612
Furnival, C.M. 3803
Furukawa, I. 2008

Furuya, H. 1201, 4465
Futenma, A. 3551
Fuyuno, Y. 2954
Fyfe, T. 0915

Gabe, I.T. 0412
Gable, A.J. 3335
Gabor, G. 1202
Gabriel, H.P. 0761
Gach, J. 0081
Gadermann, E. 1203
Gadzhiev, S.A. 1204
Gaffney, T.E. 1858
Gahagen, H.E. 4300
Galazka, A. 1205
Galbiati, C. 3411
Galbraith, A. 1206
Galbraith, H.J.B. 1521
Gale, G.E. 2193
Gale, M. 4911
Galea, E.G. 1207
Galizzi, J., Jr. 3508
Gallagher, H.S. 3566
Gallagher, J.J. 1208, 1843
Gallagher, P.J. 1209
Gallen, W.J. 1959
Galli, F. 3502
Gallivan, G.J. 4752
Gallo, B. 2790
Galluzzi, N.J. 3798
Galyean, J.R., III 0342
Gambetta, M. 0348, 2398, 2387
Gamboa, R. 1210
Gan, T.B. 4753
Ganassi, M. 1211
Gander, M. 3485
Gandjour, A. 1212
Ganelina, I.E. 1213, 1214, 1215, 1216
Gangola, R. 2864
Ganten, D. 1217
Ganten, U. 1217
Ganz, W. 1218, 4949
Ganzoni, N. 2669
Gaos, C. 4048
Garashov, B.N. 4134
Garcia, E. 0222
Garcia Alfageme, A. 3504
Garcia-Palmieri, M.R. 0344, 1219, 1220
Garcia Pont, P.H. 3252
Gardikas, K. 3887
Gardner, G.W. 0200
Gardner, M.J. 2796, 2799
Gardner, M.M. 1061
Garello, L. 1221
Garfinkel, H.J. 1222
Garfinkel, L. 1501
Garland, I.W. 2508

Garrard, C.L., Jr. 4754
Garrett, H.L. 1223, 2544, 3691, 4755
Garrison, G.E. 1224, 2479, 2480
Garrity, T.F. 1225, 1226, 1227
Gartlan, J.L., Jr. 0251, 0261
Gascho, J.A. 0713
Gaspary, F. 1228
Gatchel, R.J. 4112
Gattheiner, V. 1229
Gatz, R.N. 2407
Gau, G.T. 1230
Gaudy, M. 3667
Gault, J.H. 3409
Gault, J.R. 0412
Gaus, E. 2076
Gause, R.L. 4756
Gausi, C. 2770
Gauthier, M.R. 4440
Gavrilescu, S. 1231, 1232, 1233
Gay, M.L. 4067
Gazes, P.C. 1234, 1235
Gazetopoulos, N. 1236
Gearty, G.F. 4688
Geary, F.J. 1237
Geddes, J.S. 0025, 1238, 4880
Geddes, L.A. 1239, 1240, 4160
Geffen, L.B. 3458
Geiger, H.J. 4757
Geill, T. 1509
Geisler, G.F. 2198
Geismar, P. 1241
Geiss, W.P. 4095
Geissler, W. 1242
Geivers, H. 1243
Geizerova, H. 1244
Gelband, H. 2852, 3374
Gelernter, H.L. 1245
Gelfand, D. 1246, 1247
Gelfand, E.T. 4022
Geller, A.J. 2616, 2617
Gellis, M. 4943
Genda, A. 1248
Gensini, G.G. 0329, 1249
Gensini, S.G. 4851
Gent, G. 2245
Genton, E. 4312
Gentry, W.D. 1250
Gentsch, T.O. 2394
Genzell, C.A. 4234
Geoghegan, M. 1733
George, C.F. 1251
Gerami, S. 1252
Gerard, R. 3956
Gerasimenko, Yu.A. 1253, 1254
Gerber, M.A. 0265
Gerbrandt, M.J. 0787
Gerlach, E. 4504
Gero, S. 1255
Gersh, B.J. 1256

Gershberg, A.L. 1257, 1258
Gershen, R.J. 1107
Gershengorn, K. 1464
Gertel, M. 4758
Gertler, M.M. 0519, 0534, 0535, 1259, 1260,
    1261, 1262, 1263, 1264, 1265, 1266, 1267,
    1268, 1269, 1270, 1271, 1272, 1273, 1274,
    1275, 1276, 1277, 1278, 1279, 1280, 1281,
    1282, 1283, 1284, 1285, 1286, 1287, 2261,
    2262, 3166, 3514
Gertz, E.W. 3828
Geser, H. 1288
Gettes, L.S. 0763, 1289, 1290, 3954
Gey, G. 0445, 1291
Ghahrama, A. 0366
Gherasim, L. 4861
Ghose, J.C. 1292
Ghuys, E. 3177
Gialafos, J. 1523
Giallo, P. Del 1293
Gianelly, R.E. 1294
Giani, P. 0312, 1064, 1065, 1295, 1296
Giannini, S.D. 1297
Giard, P. 1298
Giardina, E-G.V. 1299, 3937
Gibbons, D. 4950
Gibby, R.G., Jr. 1300
Gibby, R.G., Sr. 1300
Gibelli, A. 1301
Gibson, R.V. 1005
Gibson, T.C. 1302
Giddings, J.A. 0698, 0699
Giegler, I. 1303, 1430
Giese, W.K. 1304, 1305
Gifford, R.W., Jr. 1306
Gigliogi, L. 0289
Giknis, F.L. 1307
Gilatowska, B. 4080
Gilberstadt, H. 1311
Gilbert, C.A. 4344, 4345
Gilbert, L. 3080
Gilbert, R. 0165, 1308, 1309, 1310
Gilchrest, A. 4833
Giles, T. 0496
Giles, T.D. 4696
Gilgenkrantz, J.M. 3181, 4741
Gillies, D.D. 1312
Gillmann, H. 1313
Gilman, L.B. 3237
Gilmore, J.P. 0638, 2724
Gilmour, D.P. 2496
Gilmour, K.E. 4145
Gilson, J.S. 1314
Gima, A.S. 3051
Ginefra, P. 3493
Ginn, W.M. 1315
Ginnouch, J. 0104
Gioffre, M. 2808
Girandola, R.N. 4394, 4396

Girotti, A.L. 2656
Gisolfi, C.V. 1316
Gittleman, B. 1047
Giudicelli, J.F. 0365
Giuliani, E.R. 2467, 3984, 3987
Giusti, C. 3544
Gjol, N. 1317
Gladova, M.A. 3170
Glagov, S. 1318, 2351
Glancy, D.L. 0968, 1319, 1320, 1321
Glaskin, A. 3723
Glazunov, I.S. 1322
Gleason, D.F. 4265
Glennon, W.E. 1876, 4809
Glick, G. 0654, 3827
Gloster, J. 1528, 1529, 1530, 1836
Glueck, C.J. 1323, 1324
Glushneva, Z.Ya. 2115
Gobel, F. 1574, 4265
Gobel, F.L. 2027
Goble, A.J. 0437, 0808, 2419
Goch, J.H. 1325, 1326
Goddard, R.F. 1327
Godfrey, C., III 1621
Godic, V. 3934
Godman, M.J. 2243
Goenen, M. 1328
Goerke, L.S. 0589
Gofstein, R.M. 0430
Golas, R.M. 2779
Gold, H. 0695
Gold, H.K. 1329
Gold, W.M. 1330
Goldbarg, A. 1619, 1620
Goldbarg, A.N. 1331, 1332, 1333, 1334, 4759
Goldberg, C. 0653
Goldberg, H. 2877, 2878
Goldberg, L.I. 1335, 1714
Goldberg, R.T. 1336
Goldberg, S.J. 1337
Goldberg, V.A. 4235
Goldberger, E. 1172
Goldbloom, R.B. 1018
Goldbourt, U. 2664
Goldman, M.J. 1338
Goldreyer, B.N. 0307, 1339
Goldrick, R.B. 4760
Goldschlager, N. 1340
Goldschmidt, O.F. 2098
Goldsmith, R. 1341
Goldstein, J. 3521
Goldstein, J.L. 1342, 1343, 1582
Goldstein, R.E. 0968, 0971, 1344, 1345,
    1346, 1347, 1348, 3275, 3395
Goldstein, S. 1349, 1400, 1401
Goletz, E. 2054
Golle, F. 4225
Golle, R. 2709
Gollnick, P.D. 1350

Golovchiner, I.E. 4761
Golubev, I.S. 1351
Gomori, P. 4762
Gomprecht, R.F. 1370, 1371, 1372, 1373,
    1374
Goncalves, J. 0903
Gonin, A. 1352
Gonzalez-Lavin, L. 1353
Gooch, A.S. 1354, 1355, 1356, 2595, 2596,
    2882, 3758
Goodale, R. 3324
Goode, R.C. 1357
Goodluck, P.L. 3674
Goodman, A.H. 1358
Goodwin, J.F. 0928, 1984
Goodyer, A.V.N. 2646
Goossens, A. 2110
Gordon, E.E. 1359
Gordon, E.S. 3038, 4763
Gordon, G.M. 0802
Gordon, R.S., Jr. 4700
Gordon, T. 1360, 1361, 1362, 1874, 1878,
    1879
Gorkina, M.E. 4633
Gorlich, H.D. 1363
Gorlin, R. 0064, 0657, 0658, 0659, 0660,
    1072, 1364, 1365, 1502, 1645, 2143, 2322,
    2704, 2818, 3065
Gorman, P. 2722
Gorman, P.A. 0854, 1109, 1366, 1367, 1368
Gormsen, J. 2233
Gortvai, G. 4764
Gosaynie, C.D. 4269
Gossain, V. 0038
Gossrau, R. 3584
Goswami, M. 1374, 1375
Goswami, M.K. 1370
Goto, N. 1369
Gotsman, M.S. 0106, 2340, 2341
Gott, V.L. 2740
Gottheiner, V. 4765
Gotto, A.M., Jr. 4956
Gottsch, L.G. 1281
Gotzoyannis, S. 2124
Gouffault, J. 4766
Gould, K.L. 4767
Gould, L. 1370, 1371, 1372, 1373, 1374,
    1375, 1376, 1377
Goulet, C. 4768
Gozo, E.G., Jr. 0654
Grabin, S. 0049
Grace, W.J. 1378, 1379, 1380, 1381, 1382,
    2736
Gracheva, G.V. 4863
Graettinger, J.S. 1383
Graff, H. 1384
Grafnetter, D. 1244
Graham, C. 0786
Graham, D.H. 4758

Guzman, S.V. 1452, 1453
Gvozdova, L.G. 1454, 2115
Gyntelberg, F. 1455
Gyulai, F. 1456

Haas, W. 2207
Haasis, R. 1457, 1802
Haber, E. 0238, 3793, 3794, 3795, 3796
Haber, L.D. 1458
Hackel, D.B. 2569
Hackett, T.P. 0310, 0438, 0563, 1459, 14(
    1461, 3012, 4412
Hadden, D.R. 1462
Haeger, K. 0975
Haenni, B. 0374, 1463
Haferkamp, O. 3554
Hafkenschiel, J.H. 1073
Haft, J. 2538
Haft, J.I. 1464, 3895
Haft, J.L. 1465
Hagan, J. 1466, 1467
Hagemeij. F. 4193
Hagenfeldt, L. 1468, 1469
Hagens, J.H. 2246
Haghfelt, T. 1470
Hagino, K. 0167, 0168
Hahn, A. 1471
Hahn, A.W. 4715
Hahn, C. 0581, 0989
Hahn, P. 0624, 1472, 1473
Haider, R. 1366, 1983, 1984, 2910
Haimsohn, J.S. 4778
Haissly, J.C. 4725
Haisty, W.K., Jr. 1474
Hakkila, J. 1475, 1476
Halberstam, M.J. 1477, 1478, 1479
Haley, M.I. 4351
Halhuber, M.J. 1480, 1481, 1482, 1483, 1484,
    1485, 3611, 3918
Halim, S. 2759
Halkin, H. 1486
Hall, C.A. 1345
Hall, K.V. 1190, 2957, 3764
Hall, P. 0355
Hall, R.J. 1487
Hall, Y. 3879
Hallén, A. 0099, 0100, 0101, 0102
Hallen, T. 4224
Hallermann, F.J. 2466, 3513
Hallman, G.L. 1252
Halloran, K.H. 1489, 1490
Hallstro, T. 4638
Halonen, P. 1488
Halperin, M. 4779
Halpern, A. 3672
Halpern, J.W. 1491
Halpern, M. 3120

Ham, G.C. 1492
Hamby, R.I. 1442, 1493
Hamer, J. 1494, 1495, 1496, 3694, 3712,
    3713
Hames, C.G. 0561, 1884, 2479, 2480, 3011,
    3757, 3767
Hamet, A. 3144
Hamilton, G.W. 4767
Hamilton, H.B. 1914
Hamilton, M. 1521
Hammarsten, J.F. 0568
Hammer, J. 1497
Hammermeister, K.E. 4059
Hammersen, F. 1498
Hammersten, J.F. 3123
Hammett, V.B.O. 1499
Hammond, E. 1500
Hammond, E.C. 1501
Hampson, L.G. 1042
Hampton, J.R. 1502
Hampton, W.R. 4780
Hamwi, G.J. 4132
Han, J. 1503, 1504, 1505, 2256
Hancock, E.W. 1043, 2001
Handjani, A.M. 4781
Handley, A.J. 1506
Haney, T. 1250
Hannas, R.R. 4782
Hanrath, P. 0345, 1507
Hansen, A.T. 4783
Hansen, H.W. 1508
Hansen, P. 1509
Hansen, P.F. 1510
Hanson, J.S. 1477, 1511, 1512, 1513, 1514,
    1749, 2329, 3983
Hanssen, L.W. 0479
Hansson, L. 0273
Hanzlik, J. 1515, 4080
Hara, M. 2858
Harada, K. 1248
Harbauer, G. 0862
Harbold, N.B., Jr. 2467, 3984
Harburg, E. 1516
Hardarson, T. 1724
Harden, R.M. 4784
Harding, P.R. 0124
Hardway, R.M., III 2644
Hardy, R.E. 0732
Hardyck, D.C. 1517
Harken, D.E. 1518
Harkness, J.P. 1054
Harland, W.A. 1519
Harper, C.R. 3783
Harpur, J.E. 1520, 1521
Harris, A. 1522, 1523, 1524
Harris, A.W. 1525
Harris, C.N. 0125, 1526, 1886
Harris, D. 0506
Harris, L.C. 4321

Harris, P. 1527, 1528, 1529, 1530, 1836, 3644
Harris, R. 1531, 1532, 1533, 1534
Harris, W.E. 0421
Harris, W.S. 1535, 1536, 2660, 3196, 3197, 4322, 4971
Harrison, C.E. 1443
Harrison, D.C. 0047, 0207, 0786, 1294, 1537, 1970
Harrison, G.M. 2930
Harrison, K.M. 4883
Harrison, R.G. 0035
Harrison, S.G.C. 1538
Harrison, T.R. 1539
Harrison, W.K. 1315
Harrison, W.K., Jr. 3996
Hart, J.T. 1540
Härtel, G. 1541
Hartenauer, G. 4785
Hartley, L.H. 1542, 1543, 1544, 1995, 3109, 3512
Hartung, C. 0108
Hartung, G.H. 1545
Hartwell, A.S. 1395
Harumi, K. 1546, 2844, 2845
Harvald, B. 1547
Harvard, C.W.H. 1548, 1549
Harvey, R.M. 1017, 1550
Hasan, M. 0181
Haselton, A. 4883
Hashiba, K. 1551
Hashida, E. 1552, 1553, 1554
Hashimoto, Y. 2842
Hasik, J. 1555
Haskell, W.L. 0916, 1101, 1102, 1103, 1104, 1105, 1106, 1110, 1556, 1557, 1558, 1559, 1560, 1919, 4014, 4395
Haspel, L.U. 1561
Hassanein, M. 1562
Hatch, F.T. 1206
Hatcher, C.R., Jr. 1563
Hatle, L. 3351
Hatt, P.Y. 1546, 1846
Hattingberg, I., Von 1565, 1566, 1567, 1568, 1569, 1570
Hau, T.F. 1571
Haveliwala, H.K. 4118
Havenstein, N. 4760
Haviar, V. 1572, 1573
Hawker, R. 0286
Hawkins, H. 1574
Hawkins, H.M. 0940
Hay, D.R. 1575, 1576
Hayakawa, H. 2539, 2540, 2541
Hayase, S. 1577
Hayat, J.C. 2763
Hayner, N.S. 3044
Hayt, D. 2538
Hayton, T. 0304, 1048, 4652
Haywood, J. 1579

Haywood, L.J. 1578
Hazan, S.J. 1580
Hazeki, T. 1581
Hazzard, W.R. 0478, 1342, 1343, 1582
Heady, J.A. 2797, 2798
Healy, M.K. 3147
Heath, M.J. 1583
Heberer, G. 1584
Heck, H. 3140
Heck, K. 2207
Hedvall, G. 1585
Hefner, L.L. 2744
Hegge, F.N. 1586
Hegyeli, A.F. 2285, 2289
Hehl, F.J. 2982
Hehrlein, F.W. 1587
Heidrich, H. 0199
Heidrich, R. 1588
Heijningen, H. 4773
Heikkilä, J. 1967
Hein, C. 1589
Heine, B. 1590
Heine, H. 1591
Heine, M. 0747
Heinle, R.A. 1592
Heinonen, O.P. 1593, 1809
Heinrich, K.W. 1507, 4442
Heinz, N. 1594
Heinzelmann, F. 0916, 1595, 1596
Heisig, B. 3257
Heisterkamp, C.A. 2644
Helander, E. 1415
Helbig, W. 2458
Helfant, R. 0755
Helfant, R.H. 1072, 3581
Hellberg, K. 0316
Helle, I. 0375
Hellems, H.K. 3791
Heller, E.M. 1597, 1598, 1599, 1600
Heller, L.J. 1601
Heller, R. 4917
Heller, S.S. 1122
Hellerstein, H.K. 0688, 1084, 1167, 1168, 1169, 1170, 1247, 1602, 1603, 1604, 1605, 1606, 1607, 1608, 1609, 1610, 1611, 1612, 1613, 1614, 1615, 1616, 1617, 1618, 1619, 1620, 1621, 1622, 1671, 1919, 2911, 3240, 4123, 4124. 4346, 4786
Hellmuth, G.A. 1623, 1624, 1625, 1626, 1627, 1628, 1629, 1630, 1631, 1632, 1633, 1634, 1635, 1811
Hellmuth, P.J. 1633
Hellstrom, R. 1636
Helmer, O.M. 0998
Helmsworth, J. 0271
Heltman, J. 1637, 1638
Hemenway, W.G. 0182
Henderson, H.S. 3616
Henderson, J.A. 1622

Holmkjaer, P.M. 1789
Holsinger, J.W. 0940
Holt, D.E. 1307
Holt, J.H. 3696, 3697
Holtz, H. 1697
Holzer, J. 1698, 1699
Holzman, D. 0922
Holzmann, M. 1700
Honeyman, M.S. 1701
Hong, S.K. 2774
Honick, G.L. 0679
Hood, O.C. 1971
Hood, W.B., Jr. 0238, 2143, 2425, 2431, 4018
Hood, W.P., Jr. 1702, 1075, 3352
Hoon, R.S. 3759
Hope, K. 4748
Hopewell, W.S. 1703
Hopkins, B.E. 0692, 4019
Hoppes, W.L. 1618
Horan, L.G. 1055, 1704
Horgan, J.H. 1705
Hori, K. 4462
Hori, M. 3949
Horibe, T. 1668
Horman, M.J. 3842
Horn, H.E. 0882, 0883
Horn, H.R. 0658
Horna, C. 3448
Hornbaker, J.H., Jr. 1706
Hornsten, T.R. 0449, 0450, 1617, 1618, 1619,
    1620, 1621, 1707, 1708, 1709, 1710, 1711,
    2817
Horvath, I. 2633
Horvath, M. 1712
Horvath, S.M. 1713
Horwitz, D. 1335, 1714
Horwitz, L.D. 2303, 2402, 3100
Horwitz, N.H. 0685
Horzela, T. 0899
Hosmer, D. 0453
Hosono, K. 1715, 3006, 3548
Hotovec, R.L. 4991
Hotta, S. 3990
Hottenrott, C. 0690
Houk, P. 4181
House, J. 3507
Houston, J.D. 3733
Houston, S. 4796
Howard, D. 1716
Howard, E.J. 1717
Howard, G.E. 4865
Howard, J. 1718
Howard, J.C., Jr. 1719
Howard, M.R. 3694
Howard, S. 4259
Howat, P. 4680
Howe, G.L. 4045
Howell, M.L. 1720
Howell, R.W. 1721, 4797

Hoy, J. 0185
Hoyt, W.F. 1722
Hrubec, Z. 1723
Hsi, B.P. 1169
Hubay, C.A. 0812
Huber, O. 2030, 2031
Hubner, P.J.B. 1724
Huddell, B. 0852
Hudson, W.A. 3644
Hueber, E.F. 4798
Huebschmann, H. 1725, 1726
Huep, W.W. 1727
Huet, C. 2975
Hugenhol, P.G. 4193
Hugenholtz, P.G. 2741, 3346
Hughes, F.C. 1728
Hughes, R.K. 4350
Huhti, E. 3994, 3995
Huidt, S. 4799
Hule, V. 1639
Hull, R. 1729
Hullemann, K.D. 1473
Hulley, S.B. 4842, 4981
Hullin, R.P. 3882
Hultgren, H.N. 3991
Hultman, E. 1730, 1731, 1732, 4643
Humblet, L. 0668
Hume, R. 1733
Humphrey, D.C. 1306
Humphreys, M.H. 0920
Humphries, J.O. 1706
Hunt, D. 3476, 3477
Huntington, C.S. 1734
Hunyor, S.N. 1389
Hupka, K. 1735
Hurjui, V. 0717
Hurst, J.W. 2985, 3592
Hurst, W.D. 3347
Hurwitz, R.A. 1337
Hurych, J. 1904
Hurzeler, P.A. 1736
Husaini, M. 3488
Hussain, A.T. 3776
Hussami, S. 4800
Hutchinson, J.C. 1040
Hüttemann, U. 3625
Hutter, A.M. 1737
Hutter, A.M., Jr. 0817, 1738, 2148
Hutton, I. 1739
Hyatt, K.H. 1740
Hyland, J.W. 3897

Iakovlev, N.N. 2281
Iannetti, M. 2576
Iano, T. 2332
Iarussi, D. 2790
Iatridis, S.G. 1741

Iatsenko, K.S. 1982
Ibrahim, M. 1744, 4093
Ibrahim, M.A. 1742, 1743
Ichinoe, S. 4838
Ichinose, H. 3138
Ichinose, S. 3989
Ida, M. 1745
Igarashi, M. 1668
Ignatieva, I.F. 0873
Iguchi, K. 2844
Iida, M. 1587
Iimura, O. 1746
Iino, S. 2948, 2949
Ikai, M. 2179
Ikeda, M. 4801
Ikeda, Y. 2068, 2070, 2071
Ikkala, E. 1747, 1748, 4802
Ikkos, D. 1749
Ikram, H. 2959
Iliescu, C.C. 4803
Ilmurzynska, K. 1750
Ilyushina, I.P. 0111
Imboden, C.A., Jr. 4483
Imhof, P. 1191
Imparato, A.M. 1751
Improta, M. 2879
Imura, N. 1752
Inama, K. 1753
Inamori, K. 0167
Ingram, C.G. 2502
Ingram, G.I.C. 1754
Ingvaldsen, P. 2022, 2023
Inoue, T. 1552, 1553, 1554
Insull, B. 2363
Inter-Society Commission for Heart Disease
    Resources, Atherosclerosis Study Group,
    and Epidemiology Study Group 4577
Ionescu, M. 4489
Ionescu, S. 1432
Ionescu, V. 1755
Irisawa, A. 1757
Irisawa, H. 1756, 1757
Irvine, R.O.H. 1758
Isaacs, J.H. 1759
Isawa, Y. 3005
Isbell, M.W. 0125
Isenberg, E.L. 3123
Iseri, L.T. 1760, 1885
Ishida, S. 0104
Ishii, Y. 1761
Ishikawa, H. 1762, 2072
Ishikawa, K. 1763
Ishikawa, T. 3945
Ishiko, T. 1764
Ishimi, Z. 1248
Ishise, S. 1765
Isobe, J.H. 4145
Isom, O.W. 1766
Israel, S. 1767, 1768

Itakura, S. 0863
Itano, M. 3966
Itasaka, Y. 1769
Ithuralde, M.M. 1490
Ito, H. 1577
Ito, M. 2955
Ito, T. 2114, 3551
Ito, Y. 2068, 2069
Iuster, Z. 2024
Ivancic, R. 3131
Ivanitskaya, I.N. 3188, 3975
Iversen, F. ,1241
Iversen, K. 0625, 4788
Iwatsuka, T. 3990
Iyengar, C.K.S. 1770
Iyengar, S.R.K. 1770
Izmalkova, N.M. 3762

Jachuck, S.J. 1771
Jackson, D. 2559
Jackson, D.H. 1772
Jackson, F.W. 1773
Jackson, J.C. 1641
Jackson, J.R. 2585
Jackson, L.K. 3407
Jackson, W. 4644
Jackson, W.E. 2631
Jacob, D. 0126
Jacobs, C.F. 1774
Jacobs, D. 1775
Jacobs, J.J. 2493
Jacobs, W. 1035
Jacobsen, J.G. 2461
Jacobson, J.H., II 3281
Jacobson, L. 2463
Jacobson, L.B. 1776
Jacono, A. 2790
Jaeger, M. 1777
Jaffe, H.L. 2613, 2618
Jagannadhan, T.G. 3250
Jageneau, A. 3562
Jahn, E. 1591
Jahn, H. 2983
Jain, P.C. 3867
Jakob, R. 1179
Jakobs, C. 0194
Jakubik, A. 1778, 1779
James, D.C. 0309
James, T.N. 1780, 1781, 1782, 1783, 1784,
    1785, 4145, 4146, 4804
Janeway, R. 3179
Janicka, K. 2449
Janicki, J.S. 4260
Jankovics, A. 3820
Jankowski, L.W. 1786
Jantsch, H. 1787
Janushkevichius, Z.I. 1788

Kamagaki, M. 3967
Kamath, S.A. 3674
Kamenker, S.M. 1869, 3719
Kamminga, C.E. 4772
Kamon, E. 1870
Kampmeier, R.H. 1871
Kamyar, R. 2114
Kanehisa, T. 1936
Kanie, T. 2003
Kannel, G.T. 4808
Kannel, W. 4810
Kannel, W.B. 0887, 1360, 1361, 1362, 1872,
    1873, 1874, 1875, 1876, 1877, 1878, 1879,
    1880, 1881, 1882, 2557, 4723, 4809
Kantrowitz, A.R. 1883
Kanyerezi, R.B. 4117
Kaplan, B.H. 0561, 1884
Kaplan, B.M. 0654
Kaplan, M.A. 0119, 0126, 1526, 1885, 1886
Kaplan, S. 0271
Kaplan, S.M. 1887
Kaplinsky, E. 1486
Karacan, I. 4393
Karamycshev, F.I. 1888
Karassi, A. 0844
Kärävä, R. 3222
Karchmar, J. 4287
Karczewska, Z. 3415
Karczewski, T. 2224
Kardash, V.A. 1889
Kariv, I. 1890, 1891, 1892, 1949, 1950, 1951,
    1952, 1953, 1954, 1955, 1956
Karlefors, T. 0627
Karliner, J.S. 1699, 1893, 2355
Karlöf, I. 2257
Karlsson, J. 0987
Karnafel, W. 1894
Karnegis, J.N. 1895
Karnell, J. 0953
Karobath, H. 4141
Karpati, P. 1896
Karpenko, L.I. 1213
Karpman, V.L. 1897
Karpovich, P. 4319
Karpovich, P.V. 1898
Karppanen, H. 1899
Karstens, R. 1900, 2076
Karvonen, M.J. 1901, 1902, 3217, 3223, 3224,
    4128, 4129, 4811
Kasahara, Y. 1903
Kasahara, Y.L. 0167
Kasalicky, J. 1904
Kasatani, T. 0167
Kasch, F.W. 0393
Kaserman, D.R. 0530, 0531
Kasl, S.V. 1905
Kaspar, A. 2976
Kasparian, H. 2775, 2872, 2976, 3321
Kasprzykowski, V. 2961

Kassebaum, D.G. 0860, 1906, 1907
Kasser, I.S. 1908, 1909, 2847, 4436
Kasser, S. 0456
Kassirskii, G.I. 4116
Kastansky, I. 0986
Kastenschmidt, L.L. 3274
Kastor, J.A. 1910, 1911
Kasuga, Y. 3548
Katayama, T. 1551
Katch, F.I. 1912, 2463, 4396
Katch, V.L. 4396
Kathcli, C.R. 4146
Katila, M. 1154, 1155, 1156, 1913
Kato, H. 1914, 3333, 4067
Kato, K. 1915, 2130, 2131, 4812
Katsilabros, L. 1916
Katsilabros, N.L. 1916
Katsumaro, Y. 1201
Katsura, S. 0444
Kattus, A. 4606
Kattus, A.A. 0200, 0201, 1058, 1917, 1918,
    1919, 1920, 1921, 1922, 2509, 2510, 2511,
    2512, 2513, 3800
Katz, A.M. 1923
Katz, L.N. 1924, 1925, 1926
Katz, M.R. 2877, 2878
Katz, S. 4832
Katzschmann, R. 1927
Kaufman, A. 0417
Kaufman, J.M. 1928
Kaufman, W.S. 1084
Kavanagh, T. 1929, 1930, 1931, 1932, 1933
Kawai, C. 1934
Kawai, N. 4135
Kawamura, H. 2788
Kawano, T. 1935, 1936
Kawasaki, S. 1765
Kay, F.J. 4720
Kazemi, H. 0044
Kazik, M. 1937
Kazuo, K. 1201
Kazutoshi, M. 1201
Keatinge, W.R. 0373
Kedra, M. 1938, 1939, 1940
Keegan, D.A.J. 0025
Keelan, P. 1941
Keen, H. 4813
Keeney, C.E. 1942
Keifer, H. 0361
Keihara, C. 1745
Keiper, C. 3751
Keith, R.A. 1943, 1944
Keller, J.B. 4865
Keller, L. 1255
Kellermann, J.J. 0895, 1890, 1891, 1945,
    1946, 1947, 1948, 1949, 1950, 1951, 1952,
    1953, 1954, 1955, 1956
Kellershohn, C. 2647
Kellett, R.J. 1521

Kelliher, G.J. 1957
Kelly, A.E. 1249
Kelly, E.H. 0302
Kelly, E.R. 0410
Kelly, J.J. 3487
Kelly, J.J., Jr. 3254
Kelly, R.J. 1815, 2196, 2197
Kelman, G.R. 1052
Kelman, H.R. 1958
Kelser, G.A. 0600, 2304
Kelser, G.A., Jr. 0599
Kelso, G.F. 1959
Keltner, A. 2568
Kemp, G.L. 0943, 1960, 1961, 1962
Kemp, H.G. 1072, 2818
Kemp, V.E., Jr. 4289
Kendall, M.E. 4264
Kendrick, Z. 3178
Kenedi, P. 1963
Kennedy, J.W. 0341, 2091, 4663, 4767
Kennedy, M.A.K. 4746
Kennedy, O.G. 1964
Kennedy, R.J. 1380
Kenner, H.M. 3899
Kent, K.M. 1965
Kentala, E. 1966, 1967
Kentala, E.S. 1476
Kenzler, W. 1968
Keon, W.J. 1969
Kepic, S. 3098
Kerber, R.E. 1970
Kerdiles, Y. 2406
Kerkhof, A.C. 0336
Kermarec, J. 3124, 3125
Kertzner, L. 4432
Keshishian, J.M. 1971
Kesteloot, H. 3145
Ketelers, J.Y. 4273
Keul, J. 1648
Keyes, J.W. 1972
Keyling, W. 1697
Keys, A. 0334, 0335, 0337, 0439, 0516, 0973,
    1973, 1974, 1975, 1976, 1977, 1978, 1979,
    4013, 4015, 4661, 4814, 4815, 4816, 4817,
    4818, 4819, 4952
Kezdi, P. 1980, 2107
Khaja, F. 1981, 3531
Khalfen, E.Sh. 1982
Khan, A.H. 1983, 1984, 5890
Khan, M.Z. 3970
Khanna, P.K. 1985, 3759
Kharitonova, V.V. 2302
Khatri, I.M. 1986
Khattri, H.N. 1441
Khoi, N. 3186
Khomenok, V.P. 1987
Khoo, K.L. 1988
Kida, H. 1989
Kidd, L. 3673

Kidera, G.J. 2142, 3783, 3784
Kidson, M.A. 1990, 1991
Kief, H. 1992
Kieny, R. 1993
Kiger, R.G. 4607
Kiil, F. 0012
Kilaidonis, P. 4820
Kilbom, A. 1543, 1994, 1995, 3512
Kilcoyne, M.M. 1996, 1997
Killip, T. 1998, 1999, 2803
Killip, T., III 4483
Kilpatrick, D.G. 2000, 3773
Kim, G.E. 1751
Kimball, R. 2001
Kimbiris, D. 2238
Kimera, Z. 2002
Kimura, E. 2003, 2004, 2005
Kimura, K. 2876
Kimura, N. 0104, 2006, 2007, 2008, 2009,
    2010
Kincaid, D.T. 2011, 2012
Kinch, S.H. 0419, 0888, 0889
King, D.J. 2013
King, J. 1392
King, L.T. 2014
King, R. 1666
King, S.H. 4821
Kingaby, G.L. 0811
Kingsley, B. 0515
Kini, P.M. 1763, 2015
Kinlein, M.L. 2016
Kinlen, L.J. 2017
Kinoshita, M. 1670
Kirby, B.J. 4921
Kircheiner, B. 2018
Kirchmair, H. 1485
Kirchoff, H.W. 2019
Kireev, P.M. 2020
Kirk, C.J.C. 0347
Kirkeby, K. 2021, 2022, 2023, 2956
Kirsten, E. 2024
Kiseleva, Z.M. 0112
Kishii, T. 2068
Kishikawa, M. 1192
Kishimoto, M. 2025
Kishon, Y. 1805
Kiss, E. 2026
Kitamura, K. 2027, 4464, 4465
Kitchell, J.R. 2681, 2682
Kitchin, A. 0775
Kitchin, A.H. 2028
Kitchiner, D. 2340
Kits Van Heijiningen, H. 2029
Kiveloff, B. 2030, 2031
Kivowitz, C. 2032
Kjeldsen, K. 4259
Kjellberg, S.R. 2033
Kjellmer, I. 1585
Kjelsberg, M. 3879

Kosinski, J. 3445
Kosminski, S. 2121
Kosowsky, B. 2428
Kosowsky, B.D. 2122, 2393
Kössling, F. 2057
Kossling, F.K. 2123
Kosteas, Ph. 4988
Kostis, J.B. 0245, 2124
Kothari, L.K. 2125
Kotov, A.P. 2126
Kottke, F.J. 2127, 2128
Kowal, S.J. 2129
Koyal, S.N. 4293
Koyama, S. 2130, 2131
Koyanagi, T. 2132
Koziara, Z. 1939
Kozlowski, S. 2100, 2101, 2102
Kozlowski, W. 4255
Kozlova, Z.P. 2133
Kozuka, T. 2134
Kozul, V. 2135
Kozyreva, S.A. 0294, 0295
Krachenbuhl, J.R. 2136
Kraevsky, Y.M. 1215
Kramer, A.A. 0042, 0050, 3434
Kramer, D.H. 1985, 4484
Kramer, J.C. 2137
Kramer, K.D. 2138
Kramer, P. 2139
Kramer, S.G. 0669
Kramm, H. 1484, 2140
Kranz, P.D. 1464, 1465
Krasemann, E.O. 0363, 2141
Krasnikov, V.E. 3853
Krasno, L.R. 2142
Krasnow, N. 1365, 2143, 2322
Kraszewska, Z. 0141, 3443
Kraus, H. 2144, 2145
Kraus, W.L. 0184
Krause, E.G. 2146
Krause, H. 2079
Krausman, D.T. 2147
Krauss, B. 2208
Krauss, K.R. 2148
Krauthamer, M.J. 1129
Kravitz, A.R. 2149
Krayenbuhl, H.P. 2150, 2668
Krebs, H. 1817, 2151
Kreisler, B. 1892
Kreitmann, P. 0871
Kremer, G. 2057
Krenn, J. 1787
Kretschmer, W. 2152
Kreulen, T.H. 0658
Kreuzer, H. 2153
Kreuzer, P. 0663
Krieger, E.M. 4785
Krikler, D.M. 2154, 3863, 3864
Krishchian, E.M. 0865

Kristal, J.J. 2327
Kristinsson, A. 0928
Kroes, F. 2405
Kroll, M.S. 2489
Kroman, H. 4826
Krotkiewski, M. 2155
Krotz, J. 1451
Krovetz, L.J. 1397, 2579
Kruchinina, N.A. 2156
Krueger, D.E. 3052
Krug, A. 2157, 4041
Krüger, K. 2158
Kruger, R.P. 2159
Krukovskaya, Z.V. 0041
Krutovskaya, O.V. 2160
Krylov, A.A. 2161
Krzywanek, H.J. 3238
Kubicek, F. 2028, 2162, 2163
Kubicek, W.G. 2127
Kubler, W. 2164
Kubo, S. 3499
Kuborskii, A.P. 2932
Kucerova, L. 4239
Kuch, J. 2239, 2240
Kuchel, O. 0730
Kuchin, N.N. 2165
Kudchodkar, B.J. 3809
Kudo, H. 1652
Kuhn, E. 2166, 4153
Kuhn, F.M. 2167
Kuhn, P. 2168, 2169
Kuhn, R. 1759
Kuida, H. 0073
Kukes, V.G. 3762
Kukolevsky, G.M. 1897
Kukushkin, N.I. 2170
Kula, J.J. 0931
Kulak, L.L. 2171
Kulbertus, H. 0668
Kulbertus, H.E. 2172
Kulharni, R.K. 2286
Kuller, L. 2173, 2174, 2175
Kumagai, T. 2643
Kumakura, S. 2189
Kumar, S. 2448
Kumar, V. 0038
Kumekin, U.P. 0873
Kunio, Y. 1201
Kunwar, K.B. 0181
Kunze, D. 2176
Kuo, P.T. 2177, 4827
Kuplic, J.B. 2178
Kupper, L.L. 2047
Kuramochi, M. 2843, 4027
Kuramoto, K. 2179, 4028
Kurland, G.S. 3157
Kuroda, Y. 2179
Kurucz, R.L. 2180
Kusa, O. 2181

Manelis, G. 0471, 0472, 0473
Mangelsdorf, E. 3847
Mangili, F. 2555
Mangiola, S. 2543
Manheimer, D.I. 2676
Mani, M.M. 2464
Maniscalco, A. 1381
Mann, A. 1952, 1954
Mann, G.V. 1223, 2544, 2545, 3691, 4755
Mann, R.H. 2546
Manninen, V. 1541
Manning, G.W. 4719
Manning, J. 1385
Mansour, K. 1563
Mant, A.K. 2547
Manvi, K.N. 2548
Maranhao, V. 2877, 2878
Marchand, P. 2990
Marche, J. 1728
Marchet, H. 3236
Marchionni, R. 2550
Marcus, H. 2032
Marcus, H.S. 1218
Marder, L. 3627
Marec-Seidel, V. 2549
Maretic, Z. 2551
Margaria, R. 2552, 2553, 2554, 2555, 2556
Margolis, J.R. 1879, 2557
Margolis, N. 1608
Marik, S. 1608, 1619, 1620
Marinescu, B. 4489
Maritz, J.S. 4454
Mark, A.L. 3531
Mark, H. 2558
Mark, R.J. 2559
Markiewicz, M. 2239, 2560
Markowski, S. 1637, 1638
Marks, A.D. 2561
Marks, H.H. 3325, 3326, 3327
Marmo, E. 2562
Marmorston, J. 0980
Maroko, P.R. 2563, 2564
Maron, B.J. 2565, 2579
Marriott, H.J.L. 2566, 2567, 3965
Marshall, R. J. 4267
Marshall, T.K. 1784
Marshall, W.L. 2568
Marsili, P. 4190
Martin, A.M., Jr. 2569
Martin, C.M. 2470, 2570, 2571
Martin, H.L. 2572, 2573, 2574
Martin, J.F. 2325
Martin, R.H. 3921
Martinez, A. 0538
Martinez, J. 0593
Martinez-Rios, A. 4851
Martini, G. 2575
Martini, U. 2576
Martin-Noel, P. 0166

Martins Correia, J.F. 3806
Martynov, I.F. 2577
Martz, B.L. 0997, 0998
Martz, R. 2578
Marx, E. 3286
Masangkay, M.P. 3613
Masarei, J.R. 4852
Mascaretti, L. 2777
Mascher, G. 1386
Masica, D.N. 2579
Masironi, R. 0069, 2214
Maslova, K.K. 2580
Mason, B. 2581
Mason, D.T. 0412, 2410, 2582, 2583, 2584,
    2804, 3409, 3505, 4496, 4497
Mason, J.K. 2585
Mason, R.E. 0745, 1181, 2586, 2587, 2588,
    2589
Massari, C. 2556
Massey, B.H. 2743
Massey, F.J., Jr. 0384, 0590
Massie, J. 2590
Massie, J.F. 2591
Massing, G.K. 0884
Massoni, G. 2592
Massumi, R. 4895
Massumi, R.A. 2593, 2594, 2595, 2596, 2597,
    3186, 3316, 3317, 3318, 3319, 3320, 4004,
    4375
Master, A. 4853
Master, A. M. 2598, 2599, 2600, 2601, 2602,
    2603, 2604, 2605, 2606, 2607, 2608, 2609,
    2610, 2611, 2612, 2613, 2614, 2615, 2616,
    2617, 2618, 2619, 2620, 2621, 2622, 2623,
    2624, 2625, 2626, 2627, 2628, 2629, 2630
Mastropaolo, J.A. 2631
Mastroyannis, H. 0700
Matarazzo, R.G. 2632
Matarese, S. 2790
Mate, K. 2633
Mateef, D. 2634
Matell, G. 0953
Mateshvili, G.G. 2635
Mather, H.G. 2636
Mathew, T.H. 3335
Mathews, D.K. 1083, 1084, 2180
Mathey, D. 4442
Mathieu, P. 3134, 3135
Mathisen, H.S. 2637
Mathivat, A. 2638
Mathur, A. 0376
Mathur, P.P. 2639
Matic, T. 3176
Matlof, H.J. 0047
Matloff, J.M. 3077, 3200
Matson, J.L. 3897
Matsubara, H. 2640
Matsuda, T. 2641, 2642
Matsumoto, M. 2643

Matsumoto, S. 1989
Matsumoto, T. 2644
Matsuo, S. 0259, 1551, 2645
Matsushita, S. 4028
Matsuura, T. 2646
Mattage, R. 0849
Matteo, J.Di. 2647, 2648
Mattes, L.M. 3862
Mattie, E.C. 1024
Mattingly, T.W. 0173, 2649
Mattioli, G. 2650
Mattioli, L.F. 1330
Matusova, A.P. 2651
Matzdorff, F. 2652, 2653, 2654
Maugh, T.H., II 2655
Maurat, J.P. 2136
Mauser, R. 0839
Mautner, B. 2656
Mavrogeorgis, E. 2124
Maxwell, G.M. 3427
May, L.M. 4854
Mayer, B. 3738
Mayer, J. 2483, 2657, 2658, 3656
Maynard, A.T. 2514
Mayo, M. 0698, 0699
Mayou, R. 2659
Mayron, B. 2660
Mayron, B.R. 3196, 3197
Mazarella, J.A. 4691
Mazeno, M. 3515
Mazzoni, A. 3883
Meade, J.H., Jr. 1078, 1079
Meade, T.W. 2661, 3678
Mecl, A. 2662
Medalie, J.H. 1863, 2663, 2664
Medrano, G.A. 0807, 2665
Meerkamm, F. 2666
Meerson, F.Z. 2667
Meesmann, W. 3596
Mehmel, H.C. 2668
Meier, F. 2669
Meier, M.A. 3600
Meier, R. 3757
Meier, W. 2150
Meier-Liehl, T. 3517
Meigs, J.W. 2670, 2671
Meijler, F.L. 0372, 4172
Meijne, N.G. 2384
Meinders, A.E. 0576
Meinecke, B. 3405
Melamed, S.B. 2672
Melendez, L. 1495
Mel'grano, F. 0434
Melicow, M.M. 2673
Melik-Akhnazorov, A.S. 1869
Melin, J. 1541
Melkonian, E. 3680
Mellerowicz, H. 2674, 2675, 4499
Mellinger, G.D. 2676

Mellink, H.M. 2384
Mellon, L.J. 2677
Meloche, R. 3215
Meltzer, L. 4855
Meltzer, L.E. 2678, 2679, 2680, 2681, 2682
Melzer, L. 1832
Memetov, K.A. 3719
Ménard, J. 2683
Menashe, V.D. 0423
Mendel, D. 3263
Mendelson, S.H. 1799
Mendez, J. 0506, 4300
Mendez, L. 2684
Meneely, G.R. 4955
Menotti, A. 2687, 2688, 2689, 3262, 3452
Mensen, H. 2690
Mercer, C.J. 2972, 2973, 2974
Merceron, R. 2691
Merker, C. 3374
Merkulova, E.Yu. 2932
Merli, M. 2692
Mermet, B. 0871
Merriman, J.E. 2693, 2694, 2695, 2696
Mershon, J.C. 2697, 2698
Merskey, C. 0891
Mertens, C. 2699, 2700, 3645, 3646, 3647, 4912
Mertens-Strythagen, J. 3619
Merx, W. 0345, 1507
Meshulam, N. 0470, 0474, 0475, 0476, 0477,
    2701, 4693
Messenbourg, B.A.P. 2702
Messer, J.V. 0183, 0314, 1365, 2703, 2704
Messin, R. 0788, 4169, 4725, 4726
Messinger, H.B. 2267
Messmer, B.J. 1252
Metcalfe, J. 4136
Metelitsa, V.I. 0050, 2705, 2706
Metivier, J. 2707
Metropolitan Life Insurance Co. (U.S.A.)
    4578, 4579, 4580
Metsala, P. 4811
Metz, K.F. 1870
Meulemans, G. 2700
Meuwissen, O.J.A.T. 2708
Meyer, A.-E. 2709
Meyer, J. 2710
Meyer, J.F. 3348
Meyer, W. 4250
Meyer-Erkelenz, J.D. 4236, 4508
Meyer Schwertz, M.T. 4225
Meythaler, M. 2207
Mezey, K.C. 2711
Mezzasalma, G. 4857, 4858
Mezzasclure, G. 4859
Mgeladze, N.V. 2712
Miall, W.E. 1053
Miasnikov, A.P. 4860
Mibukura, Y. 2004
Miccoli, A. 0297

Moran, J.R. 4759
Morand, P. 0424, 3266
Moravec, J. 1564
Morbelli, E. 2777
Morch, J.E. 2525
Mordkoff, A.M. 2778, 2779
Moreira, A.C. 2780
Moret, P. 2781
Moreyra, E. 2782, 2827
Morgan, E.J. 0635
Morgan, H.G. 2508
Morgan, W.P. 2783
Morgans, C.M. 2784, 2785
Mori, F. 2007
Mori, H. 2786, 2787, 2788
Mori, K. 1765, 2789
Mori, S. 0087, 0289
Mori, Y. 1551
Moriarty, R. 3545
Morishima, A. 2070
Morledge, J.H. 0444
Morlley, D.M. 0430
Moro, C.O. 2790
Morpurgo, M. 1301, 4857, 4858
Morra, C.A. 2791
Morris, E. 2792
Morris, G. 3587
Morris, J.J., Jr. 2497, 2498
Morris, J.N. 2793, 2794, 2795, 2796, 2797,
    2798, 2799, 3678
Morris, J.T. 2800
Morris, T.H. 4399
Morris, W.H.M. 2801, 2802
Morrison, J. 2803
Morrison, R.B.I. 3214
Morrison, S.L. 0105
Morrow, A.G. 2804, 3826
Morrow, D.H. 2407
Morse, D. 3758
Morse, R.L. 2805
Mortarino, G. 0312, 1295, 2196
Mortier, G. 0809
Morton, E.V.B. 2806
Morton, S.D. 2959, 2960
Morwood, J. 2807
Mosbech, J. 1241
Moscatello, B. 2808, 3533
Moschos, C.B. 2809, 2810
Moses, C. 2811
Moses, L. 4866
Moshkov, Y.N. 2812
Mosinger, M. 2814, 2815
Moss, A.J. 0829, 1349, 1399, 1400, 1401,
    2813
Mossard, J.M. 2816
Mosslacher, H. 3772
Most, A.S. 0660, 1072, 2817, 2818, 2819
Mota, E. 2820
Motles, E. 3354

Motomiya, T. 2304, 2856
Motte, G. 0391, 2412
Mottonen, M. 2821
Motulsky, A.G. 1342, 1343, 1582
Mouallem, H. 0242
Moudalaki, T. 4942
Moulinier, J. 4868
Moulopoulos, S.D. 2822, 2823
Moutigll, C. 4867
Mowe, G. 2824, 2825
Mower, M.M. 2740
Moxley, R.T. 0916, 2826
Moyano, A. 2827
Moyer, J.H. 2828, 3655
Moyes, D.G. 0885
Moynahan, E.J. 3172
Mozel, A.I. 4116
Mruk, K. 0615
Muckerheide, M. 1136
Mueller, H. 1867
Mueller, M. 2829
Muenster, J.J. 1383
Mufson, M.A. 0534
Muhlberg, H. 2830, 2831
Muir, J.R. 2832
Mukerjee, A.B. 2833
Mukharlyamov, N.M. 3719
Mukherjee, A.K. 3500
Mukherjee, S.K. 2834
Mukhorin, B.P. 2108
Mulcahy, R. 1021, 1022, 2835, 2836, 2837,
    2838
Mulch, J. 1587
Mulder, D.G. 0690
Mulholland, H.C. 0025
Muller, C. 0976
Muller, E.A. 2839, 2840
Muller, J.N. 1958
Muller, R. 1031
Muller, O. 2957
Muller, O.F. 0242, 0243, 2044, 0246
Muller, R. 2376
Muller-Wiefel, H. 4041
Mullins, C.B. 0923, 2402, 3100
Mundth, E.D. 1440
Mundy, G.R. 2841
Munro, H.N. 2388
Munro, J.F. 3888
Murai, K. 1670
Muraki, H. 2842
Murao, S. 2845
Murata, K. 2843
Muratore, E. 3552
Murayama, M. 2844, 2845
Murota, K. 0167
Murov, M.A. 3692
Murphy, E.A. 4047
Murphy, G.W. 2846
Murray, A. 0456

Murray, J.A. 3686
Murray, J.J. 1521
Murray, M.J. 2847, 2848
Murthy, V.K. 1578
Muti. R. 2849
Myburgh, D.P. 2851
Myerburg, R.J. 2852
Myers, K.W. 4379
Myllylä, G. 1747, 1748, 4802
Mylon, E. 4051
Mymin, D. 2559, 2853, 4105
Myojyo, S. 0863
Myrsten, A.-L. 2854
Myrtek, M. 0988
Mysliwiec, M. 2855

Nachnani, G. 2304
Nachnani, G.H. 2856
Nadal-Ginard, B. 2857
Nadas, A.D. 0039
Nadas, A.S. 3738
Nadzhimitdinov, L.T. 3170
Nagasaka, T. 2858
Nagata, M. 4466
Nagatomo, A. 1989
Nagayama, T. 2786
Nagel, M.R. 2859
Nager, F. 2860
Nagle, F. 2861, 2902, 2903, 2921
Nagle, F.J. 2862, 2863
Nagle, R. 2864, 2865
Nagle, R.E. 2866
Nagy, G. 4869
Nahun, L.H. 2867, 2868
Naimark, A. 2869, 4292
Nair, K.G. 2870
Nairn, J.R. 2502
Najafi, H. 2871
Najmi, M. 0892, 2872
Nakagawa, K. 2842
Nakakura, S. 2008
Nakamura, T. 2873
Nakamura, Y. 0863, 3548
Nakano, J. 2874
Nakano, O. 0167
Nakao, K. 1670
Nakayama, M. 2875
Nakayama, R. 2876
Nakayama, T. 1248
Nakayama, Y. 2009, 2010
Nakhjavan, F.K. 2877, 2878
Nakhoul, J. 2391
Nanda, N. 1385
Nanda, N.C. 0583, 0771
Napier, J.A. 3287
Napolitano, D. 2879
Nardelli, A. 3451, 3452

Narula, O.S. 2880
Narusawa, T. 2948, 2949
Nash, C.B. 0913
Nash, F.A. 2881
Natali, G. 4190
Natarajan, G. 2882
Nathan, D.J. 4943
Nathan, M.J. 2883
National Diet-Heart Study Research
    Group 4581
National Workshop on Exercise 4582
Natoli, A. 4870
Naughton, J. 0187, 0188, 0568, 0757, 1919,
    2228, 2229, 2722, 2884, 2885, 2886, 2887,
    2888, 2889, 2890, 2891, 2892, 2893, 2894,
    2895, 2896, 2897, 2898, 2899, 2900, 2901,
    2902, 2903, 2904, 2905, 2906, 2907, 2908,
    2909, 2910, 2911, 2912, 2913, 2914, 2915,
    2916, 2917, 2918, 2919, 2920, 2921, 2922,
    2923, 2924, 2925, 2926, 2929, 3088, 3089,
    3671, 4365, 4366, 4626
Naughton, J.P. 0184, 1108, 1109, 1110, 2462,
    2660, 2862, 2863, 2966, 3196, 3197, 4367
Navashina, E.G. 2020
Nawada, Y. 2954
Nayler, W.G. 2927, 2928
Naylor, W.S. 1980
Nazario, E. 1219, 1220
Neal, C. 2929
Neal, H. 1073
Neal, W.A. 4392
Neblett, C.R. 2930
Nebolon, J. 0128
Nechaev, S.I. 0756
Nedde, W. 1514
Nedde, W.H. 1511
Nedeljkovic, S. 2931
Nedostupov, S.P. 2932
Neel, J.L. 3268
Neff, B.J. 4874
Neff, R.K. 1809, 2718
Neil, E. 1650
Neill, W.A. 2322, 2703
Neilson, J.M. 2028
Neilson, J.M.M. 0775
Neimann, J.L. 0861
Nelemans, F.A. 2708
Nelson, A.M. 2933
Nelson, J. 2286
Nelson, W.H. 0124
Nelson, W.R. 1684
Nemenova, Yu.M. 2115
Nemes, V. 2633
Nemiroff, M. 0916
Neophyto, M. 0555
Nerdrum, H.J. 2934
Nerem, R.M. 2935
Neri, L.C. 0078
Nestel, P.J. 0808, 2419

Palma, A. 3055
Palmer, A.J. 4659, 4662
Palmer, J. 3056
Palmer, K.N. 0781
Palmero, H.A. 0260
Pandit, V. 1932, 1933
Pandolf, K.B. 1870
Pang, H. 4612
Pani, K.C. 2644
Panse, V.N. 3674
Pantridge, J.F. 0025, 1238, 3057, 3058, 4305, 4880
Panzram, G. 3117
Papadopoulos, N.M. 3059
Papageorge's, N.P. 0127
Pape, J. 3060
Papezik, V.S. 4747
Papezova, R. 4239
Papp, J.G. 3976
Papp, O.A. 3061
Paradowski, L. 4445
Paramonova, E.G. 2115, 3026, 3063, 3064
Parisi, A.F. 4429, 4430
Parker, D. 4042
Parker, D.P. 1526, 1886
Parker, G.W. 3065
Parker, J.O. 0498, 0841, 1550, 1981, 3066, 3067, 3068, 3069, 3070, 3071, 3072, 3073, 3531
Parks, J.W. 2798
Parley, K. 3074
Parlin, R.W. 4013, 4015
Parmley, L.F., Jr. 1919
Parmley, W.W. 2032, 3075, 3076, 3077, 3200, 3201, 3202, 4083
Parratt, J.R. 2773, 3078
Parsonnet, V. 3079, 3080, 3419
Partanen, T. 1647
Partlová, E. 2088
Pasch, T. 3081
Passa, P. 3082
Passmore, R. 0774, 3085
Passoni, F. 0021
Passowicz, L. 3083, 3084
Pasternac, A. 1072, 2742
Pastorini, C. 2576
Patel, D.J. 1406
Pathak, C.L. 3086
Patiu, I. 4217
Paton, B.C. 1814
Patrushev, V.I. 3087
Patterne, D. 1219
Patterson, D. 4881
Patterson, J. 2922, 2923
Patterson, J.A. 3036, 3088, 3089
Patterson, S.D. 4494
Pattison, D.C. 2799
Patton, R.D. 0755
Pauchant, M. 4274, 4276

Paul, L.T. 3090
Paul, O. 1111, 2250, 3091, 3092, 3093, 3094
Paulay, K.L. 3095
Paulev, P.E. 3096
Paulin, S. 3543
Paulson, D.L. 4962
Paunescou-Podeanu, A. 3097
Pavelchuk, L.K. 0041
Pavlik, L. 3098
Pavlov, V.M. 2672
Pavlovic, J. 1497
Payne, G.H. 0916
Payne, P.R. 3099
Payne, R.M. 3100
Payne, R.W. 4882
Pazzanese, D. 3101
Pchelintsev, V.P. 3102
Peal, S. 3103
Pearce, M.L. 0003, 0004, 1058
Pearman, H.E. 3191
Pearson, H.E.S. 3104
Pearson, J.S. 3105
Pearson, N.G. 2636
Pechar, G. 1912
Pechar, G.S. 2463
Pechar, J. 4153
Pecile, A. 4858
Pecora, L.J. 4714
Pedersen, A. 3106
Pedersen, O.F. 3108
Pedersen-Bjergaard, O. 2018, 3107
Pedraza, N.M. 3109
Pedrote Guinea, J.A. 3110
Peeler, P.G. 4323
Peffer, C.J. 0890
Pegrum, G.D. 4883
Pekkarinen, M. 4128, 4129, 4811
Pelides, L.J. 3111
Pell, S. 3112, 3113, 4884
Pellegrini, A. 2692
Pellegrino, L. 3114
Pelligra, R. 3679
Pelser, H.E. 3115, 4978
Penaloza, D. 3448
Penberton, J. 2503
Penido, J.R.F. 1395
Penney, J.P.M. 3116
Pennington, A.W. 4885
Pennington, J. 4612
Pense, G. 3117
Pentecost, B.L. 0267, 0268, 0764, 3118
Pepine, C.J. 0169, 0248, 3119
Pereira-Miguel, J.M. 3120
Pereira-Miguel, M.J. 3120
Perez, C.F. 3121
Perez, F.F. 3122
Perez, L.H. 0593
Perkins, G.F. 4437
Perlick, E.Z. 4886

Rabow, F.I. 4758
Rackley, C.E. 0884, 3311, 3352, 3476, 3477, 3478, 3479, 4260
Radford, M.D. 3239
Radhakrishnamurthy, B. 3866
Radi, M. 1787
Radke, H.M. 3323
Radke, J.D. 3240
Raffle, P.A.B. 2797, 2798
Raffo, M. 3241
Raftery, E.B. 1804, 1806
Rahe, R. 4037
Rahe, R.H. 0306, 2365, 2366, 3242, 3243, 3244, 4038, 4039
Rahimtoola, S.H. 3245, 3246, 3372, 3373, 4095, 4902, 4916, 4917
Raichelson, R.E. 0304, 4652
Raine, J. 3247
Raines, A. 2328
Raines, J.K. 0766
Raizner, A.E. 3248
Raj, D.V. 3249
Rajagopalan, R.S. 3250
Ralston, H.J. 3251
Raman, K. 0762
Rambousek, R. 1980
Ramchand, S. 1770
Ramirez, E.A. 3252
Ramirez, O. 3655
Ramos, O.L. 3253
Rampulla, C. 1301
Ramsay, F. 3011
Ramsey, F. 3757
Ranchhod, R. 2961
Rand, M.A. 2778
Rand, N.M. 3724
Ranganathan, N. 0024
Ranieri, A.J., Jr. 4397
Rankin, J. 3038
Rao, B.S. 3254
Rao, S. 4005, 4006
Raoschen, F. 4788
Rapaport, E. 3255
Rapoport, M.Y. 3256
Raskin, P. 2386
Rasmuson, T. 0026, 0098
Rasmussen, P.A. 1510
Raspa, E.G. 3049
Rass, E. 2055
Rastan, D. 3257
Rastan, H. 3257
Ratcliffe, H.L. 4903
Rater, D. 3258
Rath, G.J. 1964
Ratnoff, O.D. 0029
Rausch De Traubenberg, N. 3259
Rautaharju, P. 0336
Rautaharju, P.M. 3260, 3261, 3262, 4405, 4435

Rautanen, Y. 4811
Rawlins, M.D. 3263
Rayman, R.B. 3264
Raynaud, J. 3265
Raynaud, P. 3265, 3267, 3268, 3669
Raynaud, R. 3266, 3267, 3268, 3269
Razzuk, M.A. 4962
Rea, W.J. 0923
Read, K.L.Q. 2636
Reaume, R. 2632
Reaux, J.M. 4437
Rechnitzer, P.A. 0721, 3270, 3271, 3272, 3273
Recine, G. 3547
Rectra, E.H. 4890
Reddy, C.V.R. 1370, 1371, 1732
Reddy, K.V. 3249
Reddy, M.V.V. 3274
Redfors, A. 3022
Redwood, D.R. 0986, 0970, 1345, 1347, 1348, 1965, 3275, 3276, 3395
Reeder, L.G. 3277, 3278, 3565
Rees, J.R. 4399
Rees, W.D. 3279
Reeves, T.J. 1078, 1539, 1839, 2309, 2310, 3280, 3696, 3697, 3699, 3700, 4048
Reeves, T.I. 1077
Regensburger, D. 3257
Reginster-Haneuse, G. 0794
Reich, A. 4678
Reich, T. 3281
Reichel, F. 0002
Reichert, P. 0320, 0321, 3282
Reichle, F.A. 3283
Reichlin, S. 4777
Reid, D.D. 3284, 3285
Reid, D.S. 3111
Reid, E.A.S. 0723
Reid, J.V.O. 2499
Reid, M.S. 2211
Reidmeister, J.C. 3286
Reiff, G.G. 3287
Reindell, H. 0361, 2098, 3288, 3400, 4011, 3402, 3405
Reinhold, D. 3289, 3290, 3291
Reinhold, U. 3291
Reis, R.L. 0968
Reiser, M.F. 0184, 2268
Reiterer, W. 3292
Religa, H. 3981
Relke, W. 2056
Remde, W. 4904, 4905
Remington, R.D. 3287, 3293
Remion, M. 2236
Remmlinger, H. 3294
Reneman, R.S. 4168
Renggli, L. 3925
Renker, U. 3296
Renyi Vamos, F., Jr. 3815

Sarin, R.K. 4004
Sarker, K. 1292
Saroff, A.L. 3937
Sasamoto, H. 3548
Saslaw, M.S. 3549
Saslow, G. 3550
Sassa, H. 3551
Sassi, G. 2554
Sassu, P. 0605, 2398, 2399
Satake, T. 2858
Sato, K. 2134
Satta, G. 0082
Sauer, H.I. 2944
Saulnier, J.P. 0861
Saurbey, J. 4278
Savagnone, E. 3552
Savela, J. 1160
Sawasdimongkol, K. 4407
Säwe, U. 0276, 3034, 3553
Scandinavian Committee, ECG Classification 4585
Scarpagga, C. 4859
Scaton, D.A. 4907
Schaal, S.F. 3946
Schachenmayr, W. 3554
Schacke, G. 3555
Schacter, J. 0916
Schaefer, F. 1810
Schaefer, J. 4041
Schaefer, R.A. 1985
Schaff, G. 0902
Schaffer, A.I. 3579
Schalch, D.S. 1401
Schaller, K. 3556
Schamroth, L. 3446, 3557, 3558, 3559, 3560
Schane, W.P. 3561
Schaper, W. 1243, 3562
Schar, M. 3563, 3564, 3565
Schattenberg, T.T. 1139
Schatz, J. 3321
Schatz, J.W. 3566
Schaudig, A. 3567
Schauer, J. 2357
Schauf, G.E. 3568
Schecter, N. 3569
Schedel, F. 4416
Scheffel, H. 2593
Scheib, E.T. 3545
Scheier, I.H. 3570
Scheiffarth, F. 3571
Scheinman, M. 3572
Scheinman, M.M. 0006, 3573, 3574
Schekelle, R.B. 2250
Scheler, F. 2139
Schellborn, W. 1868
Scherf, D. 3575, 3576, 3577, 3578, 3579, 3580
Scherlag, B.J. 3581
Scherstén, T. 0326, 1691

Scheuer, J. 3582, 4649
Schick, K. 3583
Schiebler, T.H. 3584
Schiefer, H. 3585
Schiffman, J. 1220
Schildberg, F.W. 1584
Schiller, E. 3586, 3587
Schilling, D. 2209
Schilling, W. 3588
Schimmler, W. 3589
Schirmer, W. 3590
Schjonsby, H.P. 3591
Schlaak, M. 1810
Schlager, M. 3399
Schlant, R. 1034
Schlant, R.C. 1035, 2985, 3592
Schlarb, K. 3593
Schleicher, I. 1678, 4792
Schlesinger, P. 3594
Schlesinger, Z. 3595
Schleusing, G. 2357, 2830, 2831
Schley, G. 3596
Schloff, L. 4266
Schluger, J. 3597
Schlussel, H. 3598
Schmidt, A. 2654
Schmidt, A.M. 0073
Schmidt, C. 1212
Schmidt, F.L. 3599
Schmidt, G.B. 3600
Schmidt, H. 1591
Schmidt, K. 2654
Schmidt, K.H. 3163
Schmidt, R. 1697
Schmitt, R.C. 4929
Schmitthenner, J.E. 1073
Schmutzler, H. 2675, 3601, 3602
Schnaper, H. 0922
Schneider, B. 3603
Schneider, H. 0501, 3604
Schneider, K.W. 3605
Schneider, R.A. 3606, 3607
Schnellbacher, K. 3406, 3608
Schnetz, H. 4402
Schoenfeld, C.B. 4196
Schoenfeld, C.D. 1536, 4322, 4971
Schoenfeld, M.R. 1172
Schollmeyer, P. 3609, 3610
Schöner, S. 2752
Schopl, S.R.M. 3611
Schopman, F.J. 0057
Schor, S.J. 4930
Schork, M.A. 1516, 3293
Schott, A. 3580
Schottstaedt, W.W. 4424, 4623
Schouten, J. 3612
Schowengerdt, C.G. 3613
Schrama, P.G.M. 3278
Schramm, G. 1584

Silvester, L.J. 1813
Silvij, S. 3740
Simborg, D.W. 3741
Sime, W.E. 3742
Simmons, J.W. 4666
Simmons, R. 3743
Simmons, R.L. 3842
Simmons, W.S. 1182
Simon, A.B. 3744
Simon, A.L. 3745
Simon, R. 1281
Simonov, V.I. 0876
Simons, C. 2080
Simonson, E. 0973, 1979, 3004, 3431, 3746, 3747, 3748, 3749, 3750, 3751, 3752, 3753, 4298
Simonsson, B.G. 3754
Simoons, M.L. 0135
Simpson, F.O. 0827, 3755, 3756
Simpson, M. 3011
Simpson, M.T. 3757
Simpson, T. 0555
Sinclair, G. 2735
Singer, E. 3758
Singh, B.K. 0600
Singh, I. 3759
Singh, J. 3760
Singh, M.D. 0260, 1307
Singh, S.P. 0925
Sinha, B.C. 4109
Sinha, S.N. 2853
Sinning, W.E. 3761, 4694
Sinnott, J.C. 0723
Siska, K. 4501
Sivertson, J.E. 4611
Sivkov, I.I. 3762
Sjoerdsma, A. 1335
Sjögren, A. 0147, 1468, 3763
Sjögren, A.-L. 1156
Sjostrand, T. 2033
Skachova, J. 0637
Skagseth, E. 1190, 3764
Skavronsky, V.I. 3765
Skelton, C.L. 3830
Skinner, J. 0506, 1690, 3404
Skinner, J.S. 1112, 1113, 1114, 3766, 3767, 3768, 3769
Skjaeggestad, O. 3770
Skoluda, D. 2057
Skoogh, B.E. 3754
Skorapa, M.Z. 4345
Skouby, A.P. 0625
Skoufas, P. 2412
Skrien, T. 2590
Slack, J. 3771, 4881, 4940
Slama, R. 2413
Slany, J. 3772
Slater, A. 0245, 3773
Slavin, D. 2275

Sleight, P. 0740, 3774
Slidziewski, K. 0141, 3443, 3444
Sloan, A.W. 2488
Sloan, J.M. 3775
Sloane, R.B. 4882
Slobodin, V.B. 2358
Slodki, S.J. 3776
Sloman, G. 2760, 3335, 3777, 3778, 3779, 3780, 3781, 4226
Sloman, J.G. 4151
Slone, D. 1809
Sluis-Gremer, G.K. 4453
Smessart, A.A. 2736
Smets, P. 3177
Smid, J. 1497
Smith, A.G. 4437
Smith, A.L., Jr. 3782
Smith, A.L., Sr. 3782
Smith, B. 2866
Smith, C. 2929
Smith, C.I. 1716
Smith, D. 2760
Smith, E.R. 1965
Smith, G. 2767
Smith, G.H. 3785
Smith, H.J. 3786
Smith, H.W. 0693
Smith, J.E. 3783, 3784
Smith, L.E. 3787
Smith, P.A. 4856
Smith, P.G. 4259
Smith, R. 3788
Smith, R.E. 2471
Smith, R.F. 3789, 3790, 3791
Smith, T.W. 0238, 3652, 3792, 3793, 3794, 3795, 3796
Smith, W.K., Jr. 3797
Smith, W.L. 1815, 2196, 2197
Smith, W.M. 1550, 3798
Smithen, C. 3840
Smithen, C.S. 3799
Smokler, P.E. 3800
Smulyan, H. 3801
Smyllie, H.C. 3802
Smyth, N.P.D. 1971
Sneppe, R. 2236
Snoeckx, L. 3562
Snow, H.M. 3803
Snow, P.J.D. 3804
So, C.S. 3805
Soares Da Costa, J. 3806
Soares, Da Costa, T. 3806
Sobel, A. 3498
Sobel, B.E. 2043, 2564
Soboleva, V.A. 0041
Sobolova, V. 3807
Sobrino, R. 1219
Sodal, I.E. 4311
Söderholm, B. 3808

Sodermar, T. 0974
Sodhi, H.S. 3809
Sodi Pallares, D. 0807, 2665, 4657
Soffer, D. 0719
Sohn, Y.J. 2328
Sokolov, B.P. 3810
Sokolov, V.V. 3813
Sokolow, M. 4941
Solanki, S.V. 3811
Soldati, L.De. 4703
Solden, A. 2772
Soloff, L.A. 1126, 1127, 1128, 3812
Solomonova, L.N. 3813
Solti, F. 3814, 3815
Somani, P. 2189
Somer, H. 2104
Somer, T. 1159
Somerville, J. 3817
Somerville, W. 3818, 3819, 3986, 4950
Sommelet, P. 3134, 3135
Sommer, A. 3816
Sommer, L. 0366
Sommer, L.S. 0368
Somogyi, G. 3820
Somogyi, J.C. 3821
Son, B. 4269
Sones, F.M. 3054
Sones, F.M., Jr. 3822
Song, H. 3823
Sonka, J. 0999
Sonnenberg, S. 3906
Sonnenblick, E.H. 0411, 3075, 3076, 3824,
    3825, 3826, 3827, 3828, 3829, 3830, 3860,
    4144, 4684
Sono, F.M., Jr. 4972
Sood, N.K. 4117
Soots, G. 0906
Sopina, N.V. 3831
Sorauf, T. 1811
Sordahl, L.A. 3628
Sorge, F. 0837, 3631, 3832
Sorlie, P. 1882
Sörnäs, R. 2376
Sorokin, M. 3833
Sorokina, E.I. 3853
Sorour, A.H. 3834
Sosa, E. 3148
Sosa, J.A. 0323, 0723
Sotirakis, L. 0700
Soukupová, K. 3835
Soule, A.B. 1477
Soulier, J.-P. 4942
Sousa, P.A. 3836
Southwick, E.G. 2571
Sowton, E. 0185, 0499, 3799, 3837, 3838,
    3839, 3840, 3863, 3864
Sowton, G.E. 1495, 1496
Spach, M.S. 2569
Spagna, I. 4650

Spain, D.M. 3841, 4943
Spalding, D. 3149
Spangler, R.D. 2378, 3842
Spann, J.F. 3076
Spann, J.F., Jr. 3481
Sparkman, D.R. 0278, 2316, 3843
Sparks, H.V. 384
Spear, A. 3845
Spears, W.R. 1740
Specht, D.F. 3846, 3847
Spector, H.T. 1336
Spelman, M.S. 3848
Spencer, F. 1276, 1277, 1278
Spencer, F.C. 1766
Spencer, M.E. 3849
Spencer, W.A. 0413, 3850, 3851, 4158, 4160
Speranskii, G.N. 3852
Speransky, N.I. 3853
Spiegel, M. 2353, 3854
Spiekerman, R.E. 3855
Spinelli, S.P. 0770
Spitzer, H. 3856
Spivack, A.P. 0786, 3857
Spodick, D.H. 3146, 3858, 4890, 4944
Spoerri, Th. 3859
Spoerry, A. 2545
Spotniz, H.M. 3860
Sprague, H.B. 3861
Sprangler, R.D. 1814
Spring, G.K. 0029
Springer, E.B. 3894
Spritzer, R.C. 3862
Sproule, B.J. 2745, 4707
Spurrell, R.A.J. 3863, 3864
Spycher-Braendli, C.B. 3865
Srimal, R.C. 1445
Srinivasan, S.R. 3866
Srivastava, B.N. 3867
Srivastava, M.C. 3759
Staehelin, B. 3868
Staffeldt, E.S. 3108
Stahl, C. 3649
Staller, B. 0892
Stallmann, F.W. 0890, 3153, 3154
Stamatelopoulos, S.F. 3730
Stamler, J. 2631, 3869, 3870, 3871, 3872,
    3873, 3874, 3875, 3876, 3877, 3878, 3879,
    3880, 3881, 4645
Stamler, R. 3881
Stamler, S. 4644
Stampfer, M. 0236, 0237, 0965, 0966, 0971,
    1345
Stanaway, R.G. 3882
Stancari, V.di 3883
Standaert, F.G. 2328
Standish, M. 4517
Stanek, V. 1904
Stanford, W. 0648
Stankowska, K. 2449

Tarlinto, M. 1312
Tashiro, H. 2010
Taskar, P.K. 4001
Taskinen, P. 3223, 3224
Tatinian, N.G. 0865
Tatsumi, S. 4002
Tattersfield, A.E. 4003, 4730
Taubert, K. 3685
Tausch, H. 1697
Tavel, M.E. 4676
Tavernier, J. 0834
Tavormina, V. 2849
Tawakkol, A. 2597, 3320, 4004
Tawara, I. 1762, 2072
Taward, A. 4823
Taylor, A.W. 4005, 4006
Taylor, D.J.E. 2960, 4007
Taylor, H. 4951, 4952
Taylor, H.L. 0334, 0335, 0336, 0337, 0338,
  . 0507, 0973, 3431, 4008, 4009, 4010, 4012,
  4013, 4014, 4015, 4016, 4021, 4661
Taylor, H.S. 1919
Taylor, J.L. 4017
Taylor, J.O. 4018
Taylor, L. 1979
Taylor, R.R. 0692, 3076, 4019
Taylor, S.H. 2516, 3689, 4953
Taylor, W. J. 1397, 4021
Taylow, M.P. 3802
Teasdale, S.J. 0832
Tector, A.J. 4022
Teichholz, L.E. 0658
Teichmann, W. 4023
Teixeria, A.R.L. 0079
Tejerina, R.M. 4024
Temkin, L.P. 4025
Templer, D.I. 4026
Terasawa, F. 2843, 4027, 4028
Terjung, R.T. 4029
Terry, G. 4030
Tessari, L. 4858
Tessler, M.P. 0564
Teuns, J.P. 4031
Teyssandier, M.J. 4032
Thadani, U. 0619
Thanabalsundram, R.S. 4033
Thayer, R. 4006
Theorell, T. 2373, 4034, 4035, 4036, 4037,
  4038, 4039, 4040
Thiede, A. 4041
Thiel, H.G. 4042
Thirwell, M.P. 4043
Thockloth, R.Mc. 4044
Thom, A.R. 4045
Thomas, C. 3515, 4046
Thomas, C.B. 4047, 4954
Thomas, D.P. 2149
Thomas, H.D. 4048
Thomas, H.E., Jr. 0780

Thomas, H.V. 4049
Thomas, L.L.M. 3183
Thomas, M. 3111, 1805, 4050
Thomas, M.L. 0080
Thomas, P.C. 3047
Thomas, R. 4766
Thomas, R.M. 4051
Thomas, T. 4955
Thomasson, B. 4969
Thomopoulos, D. 3887
Thompson, A.J. 1184
Thompson, D.F.J. 4052
Thompson, D.J. 0611, 3133
Thompson, G.R. 4956
Thompson, H.K., Jr. 3744
Thompson, J.I. 4053
Thompson, M. 0722, 4054
Thompson, M.E. 4211
Thompson, P.L. 4055
Thompson, R.H. 1859, 1860
Thompson, W.B. 1734
Thompson, W.M., Jr. 4056
Thonig, S. 3631
Thorn, G.W. 2425
Thorne, J.L. 0073
Thorne, M.C. 4809
Thornes, R.D. 4872
Thornton, J.V. 4058
Thorpe, G.L. 4957
Thorpe, P. 4057
Thorsen, T. 0375
Thulesius, O. 3808
Thumala, A. 4059
Thurman, A.E. 0463
Thurn, P. 2385
Thys, J.P. 0281
Tibbell, B. 4063
Tibblin, E. 4637
Tibblin, G. 0944, 1244, 2118, 4060, 4061,
  4062, 4382, 4383, 4384, 4188, 4638, 4641
Tiedemann, T. 1868
Tiedt, N. 4064
Tijiong, B.K. 4772
Tikoff, G. 0073
Tiliagos, M.R. 4065
Tillman, K. 4066
Tillman, P. 2074
Tillotson, J. 1914
Tillotson, J.L. 4067
Timberline Conference 5003
Timio, M. 0696
Timmis, H.H. 0636
Ting, N. 4068
Tinti, P. 0087
Tipton, C.M. 4069
Tisher, C.C. 3616
Titus, J.L. 4070
Tiwari, N.M. 4071
Tjoe, S.L. 4072

Westling, H. 0627, 0628, 0748
Westura, E.E. 3842
Wexler, B.C. 4353
Wexler, J. 4976
Wheatley, C.E. 4354
Wheeler, E.F. 3099
Wheeler, E.O. 4355
Wheeler, R. 4356
Wherry, R.J., Jr. 3790
Whipp, B.J. 4293, 4357
Whipple, I.T. 3742, 3876
White, G.D. 4321
White, P.D. 0741, 1262, 1280, 1281, 3182,
    4358, 4359, 4360, 4819, 4977, 4979
White, R.I., Jr. 4361
White, T. 0628
White, T.R. 4326
Whitehorn, W.V. 1601
Whitehouse, F.A. 4362, 4363, 4364
Whiteman, H.W. 1307
Whiter, H.H. 1262, 1274, 1279, 1280, 1282,
    1283, 1284, 1285, 1286, 1287, 2262
Whitfield, A.G.W. 0436
Whiting, R. 2122, 2428
Whiting, R.B. 3198
Whitlock, L.S. 1853
Whitney, L.H. 1666
Whitsett, T. 2909, 4365, 4366
Whitsett, T.L. 4367
Whyte, H.M. 4760
Wibler, J.A. 4378
Wick, R.L. 2171, 3669
Widimsky, J. 1904
Widomska, C.T. 4368, 4369
Wiecko, W. 4370
Wiener, F. 4371
Wiener, L. 0919, 3119, 3566, 4372, 4373,
    4374
Wieszmann, B. 2074
Wigboldus, A.H. 4376
Wiggins, C.W. 0679
Wigle, E.D. 0024
Wigle, R.D. 4377
Wilburne, M. 1759
Wilcken, D.E.L. 0744, 2459
Wilcox, A.A. 4351
Wilde, G.J.S. 4978
Wildenthal, K. 2746
Wildsmith, J.A.W. 4379
Wilentz, W.C. 4380
Wiley, J.E. 2758
Wilhelms, L. 3535, 4641
Wilhelmsen, L. 2118, 3536, 3537, 3538, 4061,
    4189, 4381, 4382, 4383, 4384
Wilhelmsson, C. 4188
Wilhelmsson, C.E. 4189
Wilkerson, J.E. 4385
Wilkie, F. 4386
Will, H. 2146

Willebrands, A.F. 4772
Willems, D. 4387, 4388, 4389
Willems, J.L. 2015
Willens, E.P. 4212
Willerson, J.T. 4390
Williams, B. 4979
Williams, B.T. 2743
Williams, D.O. 2866
Williams, H.J. 4392
Williams, J. 3369
Williams, J.C. 4393
Williams, J.F. 3624
Williams, J.F., Jr. 3827
Williams, J.H. 0695
Williams, R.L. 4393
Williamson, D.H. 1817
Willis, P.W. 4865
Willis, R.E. 2478
Wilmore, J.H. 4394, 4395, 4396
Wilson, D.E. 0671
Wilson, E.M. 4397
Wilson, P.R. 4398
Wilson, R.S.E. 4399
Wilson, T.S. 4614
Wilson, W. 2255, 4980
Wilson, W.S. 4981
Wilton-Davies, C.C. 4400
Winckler, G. 0338
Wincott, E.A. 4401
Windischbauer, G. 4402
Winfield, M.E. 2512, 2513
Wing, H. 2249
Winkler, J. 4403
Winkler, O. 1608
Winkler, W.Th. 3859
Winnick, J.P. 4404
Winokur, G. 4777
Winston, M. 0621
Winston, M.M. 3218
Winter, D.A. 2853, 4105, 4405, 4406
Winter, R. 2074
Winternitz, M.C. 4051
Winters, W.G. 4982
Winters, W.L. 1127, 1128
Wintner, I. 1956
Wirth, K. 0810
Wirth, K.E. 4407
Wirtzfeld, A. 4408, 4409
Wirz, P. 2668, 3485
Wise, J.R., Jr. 4410
Wiseman, R.A. 4411
Wishnie, H.A. 4412
Wissler, R.W. 2351
Wit, A.L. 0280
Wittich, G.H. 4413, 4414
Wixson, S.E. 4415
Wohlgemuth, B. 4064
Wohlgemuth, P. 4064
Wohlrab, F. 4416

Yi, C. 3823
Yipintsoi, T. 2466
Yodfat, Y. 4477
Yokoi, M. 4478, 4479
Yokoi, N. 4474
Yorifuji, S. 4084
Yoshida, K. 2005
Yoshida, M. 1248
Yoshikawa, T. 4480
Yoshimura, S. 4482
Yoshioka, M. 1551, 4481
Yoshitada, Y. 1201
Youmans, E.L. 3849
Young, D.R. 3679
Young, D.T. 3352
Young, H.L. 4965, 4771
Young, J.L. 0942
Young, M.W. 1493
Young, O.M. 4990
Young, W. 4991
Yu, P.N. 0829, 2846, 4483, 4484
Yuhasz, M.S. 0721, 3271, 3273
Yurchak, P.M. 1911, 2143

Zabarovskii, Y.Y. 4485
Zadionchenko, V.S. 4486
Zaferman, D.M. 1982
Zagami, A. 0247
Zahir, M. 1376, 1377
Zaitsev, A.E. 4487
Zaitsev, V.P. 3720, 3721, 4488
Zajtchuck, R. 1353
Zaladinova, N.B. 2160
Zamalloa, O. 2247
Zamfir, C. 4489
Zander, E. 4490
Zappala, A. 4491
Zaragoza, A.J. 2259
Zaret, B.L. 2040
Zatelli, R. 2522
Zatokovenko, V.F. 1020
Zäziwil, E.S. 4492
Zbieć, A. 4498
Zbinden, E. 1288
Zboromirskii, V.V. 4493
Zborowska-Sluis, D.T. 2037
Zechner, A. 0689

Zeft, H.J. 4494
Zeigler, R.K. 0548
Zeiner-Henriksen, T. 4495
Zelenka, V. 3807
Zelis, R. 2410, 3505, 4496, 4497
Zera, E. 4498
Zerdick, J. 4499
Zerykier, F. 0477
Zetterquist, S. 0927, 2403
Zhdanenko, V.G. 4500
Zhdanova, S.M. 0050
Zhukovsky, V.D. 3982
Zhuravleva, A.I. 2812
Ziad Sinno, M. 3246
Ziegelhoffer, A. 4501
Ziegler, W.G. 0882, 0883
Zieske, H. 2332
Zijlstra, W.G. 4218, 4219
Zilli, A. 4502
Zimkin, N.V. 4503
Zimmer, H.G. 4504
Zimmerman, A.K. 1676
Zimmerman, H.A. 0803, 3031
Ziolkowski, L. 2102
Zipes, D.P. 2044, 4504, 4506, 4507
Zipfel, J. 4508
Zisman, F.I. 1446
Zlady, G.M. 1724
Zochowski, R.J. 0141, 3443, 4509
Zoelch, K.A. 4510
Zohman, B.L. 3474
Zohman, L.R. 1736, 1919, 4075, 4076, 4077,
    4511, 4512, 4513, 4514, 4515
Zöllner, N. 2096
Zoneraich, O. 4516
Zoneraich, S. 4516
Zsoter, T.T. 4043
Zubarev, R.P. 2531
Zuchowska, J. 0608
Zucker, I.R. 3080, 3419
Zugibe, F.T. 4517
Zuidema, P.J. 4992
Zukel, W.J. 1723, 4518
Zwirn, P. 4519
Zykin, N.N. 2932
Zylmann, E. 4737
Zyzanski, S. 3011
Zyzanski, S.J. 1795, 1796, 1796, 4520

Subject Index

Carbon dioxide 1490, 2253, 4846
Carbon disulphide 1647
Carbon monoxide (intoxication) 0072, 0772
Carboxyhaemoglobin levels 4259
Cardiac 2961, 4385
Cardiac activities 2069, 2116
Cardiac adaptations 3582
Cardiac adjustment 3455
Cardiac adrenergic preponderance 3236
Cardiac arrest 0182, 0268, 0367, 0453, 0493,
    0897, 1386, 2258, 2968, 3003, 3219, 4379
Cardiac arrythmias 2189, 2275, 2308, 2422,
    4527
Cardiac capacity & control 0444, 1354, 1467,
    2190, 2278, 2408
Cardiac care, pre-hospital 2339
Cardiac catheterization 0039, 0194, 0229,
    0423, 0599, 1507
Cardiac deaths 1827, 1828, 1830, 1864, 4380
Cardiac decompensation 3753
Cardiac defects, acquired 2208
Cardiac disease 0224, 0271, 0293, 0487, 0864,
    2208, 2213, 2323, 3007, 3089, 4283
Cardiac dysrhythmia 4936
Cardiac function 0412, 0863, 1117, 1149,
    1156, 1193, 1194, 1308, 1309, 1365, 1431,
    1444, 1618, 1622, 2208, 2412, 2927, 3096,
    3204, 4607
Cardiac electric field 3716
Cardiac employment (employees) 1627, 1628,
    3737, 3790, 4124
Cardiac evaluation 3970
Cardiac glucosides 2946
Cardiac glycoside 1182, 2139, 2930
Cardiac hypertrophy 2870
Cardiac insufficiency 2278
Cardiac massage 0991, 1643
Cardiac muscle 3076, 3205
Cardiac myosin 4649
Cardiac output 0158, 0188, 0256, 0312, 0445,
    0644, 0645, 0900, 0927, 0934, 0994, 1043,
    1127, 1128, 1185, 1512, 1543, 1585, 2196,
    2197, 2413, 2450, 2451, 4397, 4975
Cardiac pacemakers (See also Pacemakers)
    0438, 0598, 0601, 0700, 1389, 1399, 1463,
    1587, 2291, 4392, 4528
Cardiac pain 2401
Cardiac patient 2237, 2263, 2443, 2791, 2868,
    2892, 2895, 2900, 2907, 2908, 2914, 2918,
    2920, 2947, 2999, 3009, 3049, 3127, 4282,
    4283, 4284, 4291, 4304, 4362, 4371, 4393,
    4753, 4897
Cardiac rhythm 1068, 1354, 1383, 1412, 2450,
    4790
Cardiac rehabilitation 2792, 3166, 3221, 4364,
    4371, 4529
Cardiac rupture 1317, 1497, 3110

Cardiac shape 2159
Cardiac size 2159
Cardiac stroke volume (See Heart stroke
    volume)
Cardiac supervisors 1628
Cardiac surgery 0753, 0761, 0829, 0852, 0904,
    0914, 0947, 1122, 1139, 1190, 1242, 1311,
    1336, 1337, 1580, 1642, 2246, 2883
Cardiac tamponade 3226, 4326
Cardiac transportation 4107
Cardiac troubles, functional 3256, 3263
Cardiac valvular disease 2153
Cardiac volume 3422, 4148
Cardiac work 1626, 1629,1630, 1811, 1954,
    3418, 3698, 4363
Cardiacs 1624, 4274, 4282, 4283
Cardialgic neurosis 2313
Cardiocirculatory adaptation 2781, 4890
Cardiogenic shock 0030, 0081, 0368, 0569,
    0840, 0914, 1698, 1699, 2095, 2368, 2459,
    2559, 2879, 3006, 3349, 3995, 4245, 4467
Cardiography 3797
Cardiohemodynamics 4487
Cardiokinetic drug 3360
Cardiological instrumental methods 3494
Cardiologic emergencies 4530
Cardiology 0232, 0869, 0887, 0938, 1847,
    2006, 2013, 3858, 4262, 4347, 4360, 4898
Cardiomegaly 0860
Cardiomyopathy 0003, 0052, 0492, 0860,
    0928, 1055, 2870, 2995, 3019, 3172, 3493,
    4001, 4742
Cardiopathic patient 3453
Cardiopathy 0293
Cardiopulmonary system 1766, 2357, 2886,
    3037, 3220, 4094
Cardiorespiratory 0992, 1011, 1014, 1073,
    1301, 1513, 1528, 1619, 2888, 2913
Cardiosclerosis 3030
Cardiotachometer 2435
Cardiotoxic 1867
Cardiovascular adaptation 2282, 3141, 3215,
    4029
Cardiovascular clinics 3297
Cardiovascular conditioning 0878
Cardiovascular control system 4720
Cardiovascular death 1774, 1841
Cardiovascular diagnosis 1722, 1777, 4015
Cardiovascular disease 1752, 1857, 1878, 1887,
    2007, 2041, 2230, 2253, 2440, 2944, 3044,
    3137, 3158, 3174, 3180, 3210, 3230, 3231,
    3277, 3294, 3306, 3381, 3491, 3552, 3598,
    3634, 3659, 3880, 3975, 4014, 4200, 4207,
    4423, 4436, 4451, 4477, 4495, 4510, 4593,
    4615, 4697, 4744, 4761, 4879, 4892, 4898,
    4899, 4960, 4961, 4964, 4966, 5003
Cardiovascular disorders 1755, 1972

0414, 0430, 0431, 0432, 0433, 0534, 0549,
0595, 0620, 0675, 0731, 0747, 0793, 0830,
0915, 0926, 0931, 0977, 1018, 1047, 1048,
1130, 1144, 1200, 1206, 1357, 1454, 1509,
1878, 1901, 1914, 2007, 2115, 2155, 2221,
2273, 2299, 2318, 2530, 2536, 2933, 3010,
3021, 3046, 3061, 3062, 3063, 3064, 3087,
3218, 3253, 3345, 3435, 3474, 3598, 3677,
3821, 3888, 3969, 4051, 4997, 4123, 4424,
4438, 4537, 4540, 4570, 4581, 4619, 4652,
4891, 4923
Digital computer 2344, 2460, 3657, 3715,
3845, 4478, 4735
Digitalis 0010, 0237, 0592, 0717, 1067, 1126,
1160, 1272, 1319, 1376, 1393, 1716, 1792,
1820, 1859, 1860, 1906, 1934, 2015, 2094,
2215, 2424, 2426, 2540, 2583, 3000, 3315,
3795, 3796, 3911, 4536, 4613, 4741
Digitalis intoxication 0209, 0238, 0512, 0751,
1027, 1029, 1165, 1371, 1820, 1910, 1911,
2272, 2882, 3157, 3374, 3820, 3966, 3987,
4306, 4443, 4476
Digitalis poisoning 0147, 0692
Digoxin 0447, 0512, 0810, 0910, 1180, 1541,
1860, 2024, 2098, 2472, 3694, 3794
Diisopyramide phosphate 2639
Dipyridamole 1159, 1171
Diphenidol 2540
Diphenylhylantoin 3923
Diphosphoglycerate 3686
Disability 2126, 2659, 3586, 3634, 4303, 4557
Disadvantaged 0662
Discordant pairs 2364
Discharged patient 1958
Disease, chronic 3457, 3496, 3643
Disease, incidence 3364
Disease, detection 3487
Disease, modern 2158
Disease severity 2060
Discussion 2573
Disopyramide 3114
Dissonance, reduce 4378
Distal run-off 4086
Distance runners 3983
Distress 3279
Distribution 3247
Diuretics 0167, 0977, 2085, 3685, 4532
District Hospital (Brzozow) 2210
Diurnal variation 3395
Diverticulum 4102
Dizziness 2697
Dock electromagnetic ballistocardiograph 3313
Dopamine 0081, 0730, 1698, 1699, 1714,
3377, 3458, 3648
Doppler ultrasonic flowmeter 0251, 2124
Dosage 1792, 3599, 3852
Double atriogram 3531
Double-blind trial 1941, 3252, 3500, 3798,
4057, 4433, 4469

Double atrial heterotopic rhythm 3532
Doxycyline 3913
Dreaming 2978
Dressler syndrome 1637
Droperidol 2438
Drugs, 0284, 0634, 0675, 0781, 0793, 1153,
1293, 1306, 1364, 1464, 1502, 2031, 2202,
2221, 2676, 2756, 2946, 2986, 3277, 3816,
4223
Drug action 3375
Drug addiction 0543
Drug management 1972
Drug therapy 3465
Drug treatment 1819, 2166, 3893
Ductus artheriosus 2440
Dye densitometer 1789
Dye-dilution method 1512, 2006, 4509
Dynamic changes 4097
Dynamic electrocardiography 2178
Dynamic handgrip (DYN) 4025
Dynamic programming method 1982
Dysrhythmia 0074, 0075, 0387, 1771, 2236,
3799

ECG interpretation 3917, 4479
ECG peculiarities 3661, 4176
ECG seminary 2206
ECG synthesis 4138
Echocardiography 0003, 0004, 0583, 0744,
1058, 1075, 1385, 1814, 2045, 3892, 3967
Economic aspects 3221, 3590, 4513
Ectopic beat 1980, 3965, 4189
Edema 1031, 1498, 1555
Edrophonium 0541, 3157
Education 1130, 1666, 3884, 4440
Effectiveness, process 3180, 3445, 3488, 3640,
3681, 4010, 4203
Effects, cardiac conditions 3272, 3273, 3281,
3291, 3293, 3372, 3374, 3406, 3498, 3517,
3531, 3533, 3596, 3608, 3639, 3648, 3660,
3685, 3690, 3711, 3712, 3732, 3743, 3750,
3768, 3769, 3779, 3801, 3804, 3819, 3827,
3831, 3834, 3840, 3852, 3895, 3897, 3911,
3927, 3945, 3954, 3983, 4087, 4124, 4151,
4182, 4245, 4499
Effort syndrome 0896
Effort test 1777, 3241, 4509
Ehlers Danlos syndrome 2524
Eisenmenger syndrome 3419
Ejection fraction 3352, 4221
Ejection pressure 4260
Ejection time 4321, 4323
Electric shock treatment 0720, 4331
Electrical heart position 0364
Electrical instability 2428
Electrical pacing 0281, 0862, 3485
Electrical reversion 2422
Electrical stability 1965
Electrical stimulation 2150, 3644

Heart tissue 3619
Heart treatment 2167
Heart valve prosthesis 2331
Heart volume 0100, 1062, 1149, 2033, 2367
Heart wounds 2108
Hematocrit 4061
Hematology 4468
Hemiblock 0362, 1963, 4191
Hemiplegia 1211
Hemodialysis 2955, 2966, 2998, 3025
Hemodilution 0656
Hemodynamic alterations 3519, 3975, 4509
Hemodynamic effects 1818, 2131, 2238, 2252,
    2441, 2996, 3202, 3424, 3540, 3624, 3785,
    3988, 4181, 4289, 4374, 4721
Hemodynamic events 2193, 2398
Hemodynamic response 1680, 1819, 1852,
    1915, 1986, 2014, 2329, 2399, 3068, 3254,
    3539, 3673, 3711, 3713, 3801, 4136, 4356
Hemodynamic sequelae 3518
Hemodynamic status 3724
Hemodynamic studies 0073, 0153, 0185, 0236,
    0237, 0255, 0274, 0297, 0345, 0368, 0406,
    0423, 0498, 0499, 0605, 0627, 0628, 0669,
    0733, 0736, 0739, 0748, 0822, 0841, 0914,
    0919, 0927, 0954, 0978, 1017, 1034, 1035,
    1041, 1063, 1072, 1079, 1146, 1154, 1231,
    1233, 1340, 1376, 1377, 1403, 1404, 1493,
    1536, 1581, 2534, 2595, 2989, 3067, 3427,
    3476, 3503, 4059, 4531
Hemodynamics 1727, 1739, 1765, 1788, 1819,
    1885, 2027, 2130, 2164, 2352, 2442, 2458,
    2872, 2878, 2889, 2997, 3069, 3070, 3072,
    3186, 3377, 3423, 3434, 3476, 3477, 3483,
    3513, 3541, 3542, 3543, 3719, 3730, 3763,
    3902, 3993, 4003, 4050, 4116, 4193, 4266,
    4316, 4485, 4604, 4646, 4658
Hemodynamics, rest 2257, 4266
Hemoglobin 0014, 2033, 3158, 3344, 3686,
    3945
Hemoglobinopathies 2306, 4805
Hemolytic anemias 2307
Hemorrhage 3331, 3354
Hemorrhagic diathesis 3981
Hemostasis-inducing compounds 2286
Hemostatic agents 2284, 4802
Hemostatics approach 1748
Heparin 0386, 0808, 1506, 1618, 2715, 4784,
    4793, 4854
Heparin-induced lipolysis 1618
Hepatic cirrhosis 0768
Hepatic diseases 0768, 1071
Heredity 1260, 1516, 2364, 2366, 2376, 3138,
    3164, 3474, 4470, 4923
Hexobendine 2562
Hexonium electrophoresis 2932
Hexosamine 4353
High blood pressure 3910
HIP study 3683, 3684

HIS bundle 0599, 0755, 1208, 1700, 2518,
    4106, 4155
HIS bundle, ECG 3581, 3799, 3863, 3944
Histochemistry 2123, 3584, 4416
Histoenzymatic 3810
Histopathology 3412, 3413
Hoarseness 0487
Hoehenried 2140, 3918
Holland 3939
Home care 1411, 2636, 3928
Homemaker 1039
Homeostatic factor 3514
Homeostasis 3033
Hormones 0538, 1401, 4251
Hospital (Hospitalization) 0140, 0144, 0868,
    0880, 1132, 1179, 1367, 1520, 1521, 1658,
    1738, 2025, 2120, 2416, 2429, 2636, 2732,
    3421, 3433, 3444, 3534, 3607, 4003, 4018,
    4212, 4440
Hunger 4441
HV intervals 3373
Hycanthone 3508
Hydralazine 3798
Hydrochlorothiazide 3437
Hydrogen 4475
Hydrogen sulfide baths 2318
Hydroxycorticoids 0420, 0619
6-Hydroxydopamine 1445
[4-2-Hydroxy-3-isopropylaminopropoxy)]
    acetanilide 0172, 3713
Hydroxylase, beta- 3458
Hypercapnia 0740
Hypercholesterolemia 0331, 0340, 2273, 3809
Hyperexcitation syndrome 2721
Hyperglycemia 0087, 0348, 0771, 2216, 3044,
    4874
Hyperglyceridemia 2177
Hyperhemolysis 1026
Hyperkalemia 0182, 2389
Hyperkinetic 0169, 2376, 4490
Hyperlipaemia 0539, 3120, 3387
Hyperlipidemia 0812, 1013, 1323, 1342, 1343,
    1582, 1861, 2260, 3924, 4940
Hyperlipoproteinemia 0085, 0162, 0343, 0837,
    0970, 1134, 1324, 2220, 2221, 2333, 3505,
    3631, 3771, 3922, 4832, 4910, 4956
Hyperproteinemia 1988, 2335
Hypertension 0045, 0050, 0054, 0167, 0231,
    0273, 0340, 0378, 0393, 0397, 0526, 0527,
    0590, 0616, 0626, 0678, 0694, 0704, 0715,
    0747, 0777, 0781, 0813, 0866, 0982, 0998,
    1003, 1023, 1024, 1025, 1063, 1140, 1141,
    1185, 1186, 1253, 1282, 1288, 1306, 1424,
    1441, 1480, 1494, 1511, 1517, 1540, 1590,
    1680, 1718, 1818, 1819, 2202, 2222, 2291,
    2329, 2441, 2462, 2479, 2483, 2530, 2580,
    2581, 2683, 2756, 2759, 2828, 2932, 3087,
    3091, 3149, 3164, 3215, 3545, 4589, 4624,
    4685, 4746, 4757, 4866, 4934, 4935, 4941,

Patient monitoring 2338, 2344
Patient training 0042, 0274, 0275
Patient transportation 4019
Pediatrician 2199
Pennsylvania 2462
Pentaerythritol tetranitrate 2142
Pentanitrol 1510
Perception 3545
Performance 0205, 0216, 0217, 0354, 0378,
0505, 1450, 1513, 1764, 3146
Perforation 3226
Perfusion state 0368
Perhexiline maleate 0346, 0486, 1434
Pericardial effusion 2593
Pericardial infusion 3320
Pericardial tamponade 4350, 4402
Pericarditis 0106, 0722, 1005, 2341, 3241,
4402
Pericardium 2975
Peripheral arterial disease 3304, 3631
Peripheral arterial insufficiency 4063
Peripheral atherosclerosis 3371
Peripheral circulation 3743
Peripheral resistance 2399
Peripheral vascular disease 3832
Peripheral vascular occlusions 2080
Personal adjustment 0930
Personal characteristics 0930, 2420, 2908,
3040, 3149, 4315
Personal factors 4206, 4315
Personality 0061, 0062, 0133, 0143, 0369,
0439, 0521, 0522, 0622, 0647, 0776, 0894,
0988, 1125, 1166, 1215, 1311, 1517, 1613,
1614, 1721, 1742, 1778, 1943, 1990, 1991,
2152, 2778, 3238, 3329, 3380, 3703, 3882,
4066, 4198, 4201, 4705
Personality conflict 4170
pH 1490, 1758
Pharmacodynamic effect 3533
Pharmacokinetics 3652, 4312
Pharmacological agents 0113, 0114, 0528,
1332, 2377, 2711
Pharmaco-physical treatment 2152
Pharmacotherapy 3621
Phenprocoumon 0808
Phentermine 3888
Phentolamine 1983, 3995
Phenytoin 0249, 0925, 4151
Phillipines 4610
Philosophy 3462
Phonocardiogram 0054, 0127, 0128, 0215,
0787, 0907, 0908, 1204, 1561, 2124, 2447,
2875, 3122, 3715, 3978, 4135, 4482
Phosphates 2061
Phosphatides 2176
Phospholipid 1182, 2317
Phosphorated compound 1020
Phosphorous, inorganic 2789
Physiatrist 1359

Physical ability 3402
Physical activity 0187, 0206, 0226, 0468,
0472, 0506, 0507, 0538, 0561, 0687, 0779,
0830, 0874, 0979, 0990, 1087, 1090, 1094,
1101, 1105, 1108, 1109, 1110, 1111, 1112,
1113, 1114, 1118, 1144, 1220, 1261, 1341,
1557, 1558, 1596, 1686, 1829, 1862, 1872,
1882, 1902, 1976, 2233, 2281, 2888, 2906,
2907, 2912, 2918, 2920, 2926, 2953, 3050,
3177, 3189, 3235, 3287, 3293, 3363, 3538,
3635, 3717, 3757, 3767, 3841, 3876, 4008,
4009, 4012, 4016, 4128, 4381, 4344, 4452,
4473, 4639, 4723, 4947
Physical capacity 2100, 3403
Physical characteristics 3674
Physical conditioning 0205, 0618, 0641, 1223,
1604, 1606, 1608, 1619, 1620, 1947, 1951,
2903, 3240, 3509, 3510, 3743, 4338, 4349
Physical conditioning, chronic 4311
Physical education 3849, 3920
Physical effort 2325, 3102, 3434, 4325
Physical endurance 3928
Physical exercise 0132, 0195, 0279, 0409,
0474, 0475, 0602, 0653, 0911, 1096, 1155,
1159, 1581, 1741, 1869, 2097, 2101, 2185,
2338, 2386, 3236, 3406, 3562, 3852, 3975,
4186
Physical exercise, lack 3236
Physical exertion 0110, 0111, 0145, 0166,
0312, 0329, 0377, 0378, 0539, 0603, 0606,
0804, 1264, 1834, 3002, 3030, 3035, 3719,
4214, 4229
Physical fitness 0068, 0186, 0189, 0306, 0392,
0502, 0688, 0689, 0735, 1044, 1061, 1147,
1158, 1170, 1449, 1455, 1499, 1688, 1720,
1925, 1966, 2019, 2077, 2166, 2223, 2921,
2950, 3038, 3337, 3398, 3442, 3537, 3691,
3693, 3807, 3849, 3876, 3928, 4066, 4069,
4140, 4621, 4755
Physical follow-up treatment 0282
Physical illness 3191, 4205, 4206
Physical inactivity 1120, 1183, 4382
Physical loading 0308, 1802, 4493
Physical performance 1327, 1332, 2213, 2279,
2887, 2914, 2981, 4246
Physical reconditioning 1857, 2083, 4166
Physical rehabilitation 1966, 3445, 3912, 4167
Physical strain 1671, 3404, 3585, 4116, 4485
Physical stress 2207, 2218
Physical therapy 1964, 3289
Physical training 0204, 0274, 0275, 0326,
0642, 0644, 0645, 0646, 0667, 0809, 0818,
0820, 0823, 0875, 0933, 0935, 0975, 1007,
1145, 1146, 1148, 1149, 1151, 1152, 1154,
1156, 1157, 1316, 1414, 1448, 1511, 1514,
1543, 1552, 1696, 1801, 1818, 1913, 1956,
1967, 1994, 1995, 2018, 2113, 2212, 2455,
2784, 2886, 2908, 3107, 3183, 3222, 3276,
3340, 3400, 3403, 3423, 3512, 3535, 3536,

Pressor effect 2202
Pressure flow dynamics 2863
Pressure lability 2271
Pressure volume relations 3356
Presystolic gallop 1373
Prevention 0019, 2544, 2684, 2690, 2705,
    2754, 2793, 2881, 2893, 2939, 3228, 3234,
    3284, 3536, 3555, 3643, 3719, 3872, 3876,
    3923, 4052, 4121, 4134, 4510, 4573, 4591
Primary preventive study 1901, 4383
Prinodolol 0130
Prinzmetal's angina 0021, 0833, 1352, 3806,
    4185
Procaine amide 1299, 4312
Procaine blockade 2133
Procedure 3341, 4225
Processing unit 4224
Professional cardiopaths 3259
Professional liability 2190
Professional people 1979, 3295, 3469
Progeny, infarct parents 1803
Prognosis 0175, 0888, 1009, 1010, 1119, 1129,
    1238, 1258, 1460, 1467, 1561, 1715, 1723,
    1903, 2013, 2025, 2169, 2418, 2969, 3027,
    3133, 3198, 3217, 3473, 3683, 3724, 3848,
    3960, 4193, 4314, 4555, 4709
Program course 4171
Prolonged work test 3679
Pronethaloe 0319
Propranidid 3160
Prophylaxis 2205, 2692, 2993, 3118
Propranolol (Inderal) 0064, 0096, 0115, 0130,
    0216, 0217, 0273, 0280, 0437, 0666, 0670,
    0736, 0739, 0746, 0876, 0919, 0928, 1019,
    1030, 1160, 1289, 1290, 1294, 1333, 1345,
    1453, 1479, 1495, 1496, 1522, 1577, 1664,
    1724, 1728, 1941, 2276, 2353, 2874, 2943,
    3156, 3372, 3406, 3472, 3597, 3722, 3804,
    3897, 3911, 4043, 4083, 4374, 4494, 4535,
    4536
Prosthesis, implantation 3170
Protein, concentrated 3940
Prothrombin 4855
Psychiatric, factors 1642, 1779, 2292, 3760,
    4850
Psychiatry 0029, 0402, 0563, 0682, 0814,
    0857, 0897, 1580, 1642, 3193, 3552, 3621,
    3907
Psychic changes, problems 3720
Psychic factors 1848, 2187, 3720, 4161, 4773,
    4915
Psychic stress 1649
Psychoanalysis 0213
Psycho-bioclinical relationships 3647
Psychobiological factors 1424, 1720, 4412
Psychodynamic 0224, 0272, 1473, 1571, 1835,
    1900, 2029, 2080
Psychogalvanic reflex 4197
Psychological adaptation 0013, 0570, 0572,
    0573, 0726, 0852, 1006, 1461, 1515, 1642

Psychological adjustment 1642, 3665, 4320
Psychological aspects 1667, 1924, 3449, 3456,
    3491, 3569, 3658, 3723, 4046, 4490
Psychological factors 0066, 0370, 0389, 0520,
    0567, 0570, 0571, 0572, 0573, 0724, 0726,
    0838, 0852, 0867, 0904, 1006, 1021, 1022,
    1038, 1061, 1171, 1420, 1459, 1461, 1499,
    1515, 1570, 1632, 1642, 1649, 1667, 1793,
    1794, 2268, 2982, 3123, 3721, 3738, 3971,
    4040, 4320, 4364, 4423
Psychologic impact 2244
Psychological patterns 1743
Psychological problems 0039, 0206, 0293,
    0496, 0556, 0761, 0798, 0949, 1363, 1539,
    1569, 1588, 3103, 3121, 4078, 4447
Psychological stress 2089
Psychological studies 2250, 3105, 3115, 3187
Psychology 0059, 0139, 0144, 0459, 0662,
    0759, 0801, 0896, 1677, 1701, 2100, 3312,
    4912
Psychometry 3702
Psychopharmacological 1405, 2167
Psycho-physiological factors 3520, 3550, 3909,
    4362
Psycho-physiological judgments 4398
Psychophysiological responses 4299
Psychophysiology 0988, 1175, 3680
Psychosexual 0179
Psychosocial factors 0465, 0950, 1143, 1170,
    1288, 1391, 1399, 1400, 1401, 1423, 1595,
    2365, 3243, 3674, 3848, 4034, 4035, 4037,
    4038
Psychosocial stress 3916
Psychosomatic factors 0168, 0223, 0287, 0624,
    0651, 0796, 0869, 1472, 1492, 1590, 1668,
    1745, 1762, 1864, 1887, 1935, 2072, 3005,
    3136, 3329, 3714, 3868, 3909, 3956, 4150,
    4413, 4466, 4480
Psychosomatic medicine 1847
Psychosomatic rehabilitation 4414
Psychotherapy 0028, 0798, 1968, 2076, 3621,
    3622, 3859, 3884, 4488
Psychosis (Prevention) 2246
Psychotic population 4432
Psychotropic factors 1719, 1867, 2166, 3277
Public Health Dept. 3101
Public speaking 3986
Puerto Rico 0344, 1219
Pulmonary artery 3245
Pulmonary autograft 3817
Pulmonary cancer 4190
Pulmonary cardiopathy 3588
Pulmonary circulation 3625
Pulmonary disease 3037, 4268
Pulmonary edema 0860
Pulmonary hypertension 1840
Pulmonary perfusion 0044
Pulmonary pressure 0788, 3065
Pulmonary problems 0214, 0860, 1309, 2441,
    2443

Pulmonary stenosis 0736, 0739
Pulmonary vascular bed 1807
Pulmonary wedge 4264
Pulse 0005, 1205, 1243, 2447, 2876, 3099
Pulse contour method 0046
Pulse frequency 1802
Pulse pressure height 3664
Pulse rate 2033, 2087
Pulse stimulation 3950
Pulse volume recorder 0766
Pulsus alternans 3077
Purkinje cell 2264
Purkinje fiber 3374
Pyridinol carbonate 4468
Pyruvates 1528, 1529, 2265, 3300

Q-A2 interval 1456, 2875
Q-second sound interval 4095
Q-section 3 3583
Q-II interval 3776
QK interval 4294
QQF theory 3568
QRS, loop 1967, 3004, 3863, 4232, 4506
QT interval 0510, 0511, 1126, 1427, 3138
Q-T ratio 1960, 3353
QX/QT ratio 3353
Qualitative composition 2115
Quantitative analysis 2015, 3716, 3790
Quantitative diagnosis 2045, 4163
Quantitative effects 3240
Quantitative radionuclide angiocardiography
     1837
Questionnaire 0769, 1171, 3287
Quinidine 0720, 0807, 0913, 0976, 1394, 4083

RF conditioning 1955
RR-interval 0372, 1474, 1578
RS-T segment 0604, 4375
R-V interval 1299, 1554
Race 2944
Race factor 0397, 1718, 3841, 3879, 4477
Radicular pain syndrome 2896
Radioactive chromium 2161
Radiocardiography 3492, 3526
Radioelectrocardiogram 0141, 0240, 0241,
     0242, 0243, 0244, 0246, 0606, 0742, 0743,
     1188, 1201, 2113, 3443, 4228, 4465
Radioelectrocardiograph 2949
Radiography 3139
Radiography, automated 2159
Radioimmunoassay 3458, 3652, 3792, 3793,
     4175
Radiology 0834, 1729
Radiology chest findings 3543
Radio-telemetry 2067, 3555
Railroad 4013, 4016
Railways and myocardial infarction 3128, 4553
Rate-dependent factors 3711, 4507
Rating scale 3587

Rauwolfia serpentina 3798
Reactive behavior 4031
Readaptation 0424, 4166, 4199
Rebound phenomenon 4164
Recall record questionnaire 4473
Reciprocal ventricular beats, 4408
Recirculation 1693
Recognition 3315
Reconditioning 3237
Recording speed 3146
Recovery 2225, 2958, 3177, 4331, 4729
Recreational activities 2102, 3690, 4054
Rectum 3003
Recurrence rate 3271
Red blood cell membrane 2305
Redox potential 2265
Re-employment 3737
Reflexogenic areas 1650
Refractory angina pectoris 1928
Refractory cardiac edema 3668
Refractory heart failure 3655, 4030
Refractory periods 1842
Regional differences 3881
Regional health administration 1935
Rehabilitated patients 1948, 4367
Rehabilitation 0017, 0019, 0040, 0041, 0049,
     0070, 0082, 0084, 0093, 0136, 0137, 0138,
     0139, 0140, 0141, 0144, 0163, 0193, 0212,
     0214, 0230, 0283, 0315, 0322, 0363, 0369,
     0371, 0404, 0413, 0416, 0428, 0429, 0476,
     0477, 0480, 0514, 0540, 0553, 0661, 0682,
     0753, 0759, 0783, 0786, 0797, 0798, 0801,
     0835, 0868, 0878, 0996, 1009, 1010, 1011,
     1012, 1038, 1050, 1059, 1203, 1213, 1214,
     1242, 1247, 1257, 1273, 1331, 1336, 1391,
     1408, 1421, 1422, 1473, 1475, 1480, 1481,
     1482, 1483, 1484, 1515, 1531, 1533, 1534,
     1567, 1568, 1569, 1570, 1572, 1575, 1597,
     1607, 1617, 1659, 1667, 1735, 2188, 2200,
     2230, 2263, 2421, 2437, 2454, 2814, 2824,
     2850, 2865, 2909, 2915, 2979, 3032, 3049,
     3055, 3165, 3170, 3210, 4268, 4367, 4529,
     4533, 4566, 4574, 4592, 4595, 4602, 4857,
     4979
Rehabilitation counselor 4511
Rehabilitation facilities 0759, 0760, 1253,
     1254, 1484, 3611, 3961, 4212
Rehabilitation potential 2082, 3850
Rehabilitation problems 3721, 4371
Rehabilitation programs 0524, 0732, 1229,
     1253, 1254, 1388, 1556, 4073, 4075, 4341,
     4656
Rehabilitation success 4268
Religion 0726, 4026
Religious identity 2201
Renal arteriovenous fistula 0080
Renal circulation 1131
Renal diseases 3879, 4439
Renal elimination 2139

Technical advances 2121
Technique 3303, 3320, 3593
Tecumseh study 0962, 0963, 1812, 3043
Telecardiology, simultaneous multiload 2229
Telemetry 0084, 1489, 1736, 1855, 2002, 2081, 2338, 3773
Temperature 0701, 0843, 0967, 0971, 1203, 1316, 3003, 3053, 4330
Temporal relationships 3071
Temporospatial frequency 4232
Tension 0584, 2399, 3074
Terbutaline 1728
Terminal artery disease 2057
Test 0001, 0043, 0661, 1044, 4017, 4047, 4079, 4120, 4180, 4450, 4492
Test behavior 4173, 4174
Tetrahydronaphthalene 1013
Tetralogy of Fallot 0423, 1330
Thailand 3999
Thalassotherapy 0760
Theophylline ethylenediamine 2808
Theory 2121
Therapeutic exercise 3520, 3660, 4487
Therapeutic implications 2141, 2149, 2989, 3228, 4334, 4792
Therapeutic study 3763
Therapeutic suppression 3228
Therapeutic training 3290
Therapy 0224, 0324, 0375, 0393, 0399, 0597, 1009, 1010, 1463, 1547, 1602, 1603, 2205, 2406, 2941, 3105, 3425, 3431, 3440, 3470, 3538, 3598, 3681, 3756, 3793, 3798, 3831, 3907, 3963, 3995, 4202, 4233, 4238, 4444
Thermal balance 1083
Thermal responses 4021
Thermal stress 3430
Thermistor catheter 4218
Thermodilution 0421, 1585, 4218, 4219, 4397
Thiopentone 0664
Third heart sound 2086
TcH2O 3253
Thoracic impedance 1240
Thoracotomy 2975
Threshold determination 3726
Thrombangitis obliterans 4063
Thromboembolism 0400, 0403, 4931
Thrombogenesis 2304, 2856
Thrombolysis 4203
Thrombolytic therapy 4839
Thrombophlebitis 2967
Thromboresistant polymers 2287
Thrombosis 0229, 1506, 1509, 1674, 2810, 2997, 4270, 4614, 4867
Thrombotic cerebrovascular disease 3514
Thyroiditis 1593
Thyrotoxicosis 2461
Thyroxine 1519
Tilt table testing 3348
Timberline conference 3550

Time factor 3974, 4037, 4499
Time intervals 2208, 2597, 3191
Time parameter 3865
Tiprenolol, DL- 3346
Tissue adhesives 2286
Tobacco (See also Smoking) 0126, 0617, 1374, 2038, 3467, 3469, 4259
Tolamidol 0124
Tolbutamine 3048
Tolerance 3158
Tomo-echography 2136
Tonus reactivity 4137
Topography 3836
"Total" surface waveform 2112
Toxic 1820
Trace elements 3486
Tracings 3146
Trained subjects 2144, 2186, 3398, 3399, 3511, 3687, 3708, 3807, 3907, 3927, 4006, 4112, 4140, 4491
Training 3171, 3178
Training effects 3330, 3429, 4099, 4183, 4430
Training levels 3940
Training regime 3706
Tranquilizer 3277, 3470, 3640
Transesophageal atrial pacing 2770
Transfer conditions 2044
Transmembrane potential 2079, 3203, 3374
Transmural electrocardiograph 3574
Transpeptidase activity 0104
Transplantation (organ) 4998
Transthoracic direct current shock 1383
Transvenous electrode catheter 3997
Trasicor 0876, 1191, 3156
Treadmill test 0067, 0117, 0122, 0127, 0236, 0318, 0648, 0943, 0973, 0974, 1050, 1073, 1137, 1184, 1193, 1194, 1356, 1886, 1918, 1960, 1961, 2060, 2078, 2349, 2382, 2861, 3089, 3330, 3348, 3742, 3800, 4457
Treatment 3250, 3309, 3379, 3435, 3461, 3643, 3753, 3784, 3813, 3815, 3831, 3837, 3887, 3953, 3957, 3980, 3981, 4030, 4053, 4094, 4097, 4115, 4117, 4269, 4369
Treatment by excision 4269
Triad 3671
Triangular test 2398
Tricuspid insufficiency 3122
Tricuspid regurgitation 3318
Tricuspid valve 1865
Trifascicular 0298, 3319, 3890
Trigger mechanism 3228
Triggering 4406
Triglycerides 0090, 0419, 0478, 0550, 3054, 3819, 4900
Trypsin 3887
Tuberculous myocarditis 2105
Twins 2364, 2365, 2366
Two-step tolerance test 4605

Vocational counseling 1466, 2815, 2962, 3210, 3259
Vocational health 1629
Vocational medicine 1630
Voice analysis test 1173
Volumetric calibration 2286
Vulnerability 3229, 4187, 4427

Walking 0060, 0373, 1494, 1786, 3032, 3179, 3251, 4115, 4248, 4455, 4456, 4457
War veterans 1857
Warm up, simulated 2919
Water 0146, 0701, 0714, 0811, 1841
Water-electrolyte regulation mechanism 3499
Wave amplitude 2716
Wave transmission 3845
Waveform analysis 3260
Waveform identification 3303
Waveform information 2111, 2112
Waveform patterns 3262, 3846, 3847, 4481
Weight 1870, 2783, 3305, 4248
Weightlessness 0936
Weight loss 1834
Wenckeback AV block 2880
Western Collaborative Group Study 1795, 3384, 3391, 3392
Whites 2291, 3137
Wisconsin 1623
Without cardiac failure 2096, 3409
Without heart block 3837
Wives (wife) 2023
Wolff-Parkinson-White syndrome 2394, 2800, 3820, 3181, 3346, 3560, 3783, 3944, 4176
Women 2463, 2484, 2581
Work 0095, 0101, 0129, 0148, 0154, 0158, 0159, 0189, 0197, 0317, 0369, 0388, 0406, 0415, 0472, 0473, 0511, 0571, 0574, 0609, 0610, 0616, 0941, 0987, 1003, 1037, 1045, 1062, 1116, 1199, 1417, 1569, 1621, 1623, 1635, 1832, 1862, 1927, 2033, 2454, 3053, 3127, 3169, 3376, 3743, 3768, 3898, 4005, 4126, 4133, 4134, 4214, 4283, 4308, 4454

Work assessment 0095, 0096, 0100, 0101, 0156, 0639, 1036, 2314
Work capacity (See Physical work capacity) 2825, 3141
Work classification unit 1629, 1630
Work environment 2326, 3051
Work, ergometric 2675
Work evaluation units 1626, 2084
Work physiology 2053
Work potential 4362
Work status 3669, 4313
Work stressor tests 3672
Work tolerance 1316, 3769
Work, type 0154, 0189, 0197, 0369, 0473
Working age 1966
Workload 0895, 1198, 1542, 2439, 4225, 4388
Workload ECG 4388, 4389
Workmen's compensation 0278, 0401, 1623, 1624, 1627, 1633, 1634, 1635, 4058, 4285, 4380
Workshop 1808
WPW syndrome 4389
Wrestler 1833

X-ray 0972, 1477, 1657, 3306
Xenon[133]   0607, 0643, 0899, 1693, 3734

Yemenites 0470
Yoga 1015, 2125, 3480, 4118
Young adults 3125, 3131
Young people 1900, 2080, 3267, 3417, 3474, 3510, 3589, 3661, 3752, 3808, 3910, 3926, 3930

Zinc 0614
Zonal myocardial ischemia 1645

List of Publications Cited

Abstracts Soviet Medicine
Academia Peruana de Cirugia
Academy Medicine New Jersey Bulletin
Acta Anatomica (Basel)
Acta Anesthesiologica (Padova)
Acta Biologica et Medica Germanica
Acta Cardiologica
Acta Cardiologica (Suppl.)
Acta Clinica Belgica
Acta Dermato-Venereologica
Acta Diabetologica Latina
Acta Endocrinologica
Acta Endocrinologica Scandinavica
Acta Gerontologica Japonica
Acta Haematologica Japonica
Acta Medica Academiae Scientiarum Hungaricae
Acta Medica Philippina
Acta Medica Scandinavica
Acta Medica Scandinavica (Suppl.)
Acta Neurologica
Acta Neurologica et Psychiatrica Belgica
Acta Orthopaedica Scandinavica (Suppl.)
Acta Paediatrica Scandinavica
Acta Paediatrica Scandinavica (Suppl.)
Acta Physiologica Scandinavica
Acta Physiologica Scandinavica (Suppl.)
Acta Psychiatrica Belgica
Acta Societatis Medicorum Upsaliensis
Acta Universitatis Uppsala
Activitas Nervosa Superior
Aerospace Medicine
Akademiia Nauk Armianskoi SSR, Doklady
Akita Central Hospital Medical Journal
Alabama Journal Medical Science
American Academy Occupational Medicine
American Association Industrial Nurses Journal
American Corrective Therapy Journal
American Family Physician
American Heart Association Monograph
American Heart Journal
American Journal Cardiology
American Journal Clinical Nutrition
American Journal Clinical Pathology
American Journal Diseases Children
American Journal Epidemiology
American Journal Medical Electronics
American Journal Medical Sciences
American Journal Medicine
American Journal Nursing
American Journal Obstetrics Gynecology
American Journal Occupational Therapy
American Journal Pathology
American Journal Physical Medicine
American Journal Physiology
American Journal Psychiatry
American Journal Public Health
American Journal Roentgenology, Radium Therapy, Nuclear Medicine
American Journal Surgery
American Psychologist
American Review Respiratory Diseases
American Surgeon
Anaesthesia
Anesthesist
Anais Paulistas de Medicina e Cirurgia
Anales de la Facultad de Medicina, Universidad Nacional Mayor de San Marcos de Lima
Anatomischer Anzeiger
Anestesia e Rianimazione
Anesthésie Analgésie Réanimation
Angiologica
Angiology
Anglo-German Medical Review
Annales Academiae Scientiarum Fennicae Series A V, Medica
Annales de Biologie Clinique
Annales de Cardiologie et d'Angéiologie (Paris)
Annales de Chirurgie
Annales de Médecine Interne
Annales Médicopsychologique
Annales de Physique Biologique et Médicale
Annali della Sanita Pubblica
Annals Clinical Laboratory Science
Annals Clinical Research
Annals Internal Medicine
Annals New York Academy Sciences
Annals Surgery
Annals Thoracic Surgery
Annual Report, Research Institute Environmental Medicine Nagoya University
Annual Review Medicine
Annual Review Physiology
Applied Therapeutics
Arbeitsmedizin, Sozialmedizin, Arbeitshygiene
Arbeitsphysiologie
Archiv für Kreislaufforschung
Archiv für Physikalische Therapie Balneologie und Klimatologie
Archive für Klinische Medizin
Archives Environmental Health
Archives General Psychiatry

Archives Internal Medicine
Archives Internationales de Pharmacodynamie et de Therapie
Archives des Maladies du Coeur
Archives des Maladies du Coeur et des Vaisseaux
Archives des Maladies Professionelles de Médecine du Travail et de Sécurité Sociale
Archives Otolaryngology
Archives Pathology
Archives Pediatrics
Archives Physical Medicine Rehabilitation
Archives des Sciences Physiologiques
Archives Surgery
Archives Union Médicale Balkanique
Archivio E. Maragliano di Patologiae Clinica
Archivio per le Scienze Mediche
Archivos de la Fundacion Roux-Ocefa
Archivos del Instituto de Cardiologia de Mexico
Archiwum Medycyny Sadowej i Kryminologii
Arizona Medicine
Arkhiv Patologii
Arquivos Brasileiros de Cardiologia
Arzneimittel-Forschung
Arztliche Forschung
Asian Journal Medicine
Ateneo Parmense
Ateneo Parmense Sezione 1 Acta Bio-Medica
Atherosclerosis
Atti della Società Italiana di Cardiologia
Australasian Annals Medicine
Australasian Radiology
Australian New Zealand Journal Medicine
Australian New Zealand Journal Psychiatry
Aviation Medicine
Azerbaidzhanskii Meditsinskii Zhurnal

Balneologia Polska
Basic Research Cardiology
Behavioral Research Therapy
Behavioral Science
Belgisch Tijdschrift voor Geneeskunde
Bibliotheca Cardiologica
Biochemical Clinics
Biochimica Biophysica Acta
Biologiya Meditisina
Biomedical Sciences Instrumentation
Biomedizinische Technik
Biophysics
Blut
Boletim do Centro de Cardiologia Médico-Social de Coimbra
Boletim da Sociedade Portuguesa de Cardiologia
Boletin de la Asociacion Medica de Puerto Rico
Bollettino della Società Italiana di Cardiologia
Bordeaux Médical

Bratislavske Lekarske Listy
British Heart Journal
British Journal Anesthesia
British Journal Anaesthesiology
British Journal Haematology
British Journal Industrial Medicine
British Journal Medical Psychology
British Journal Nutrition
British Journal Pharmacology
British Journal Pharmacy Chemotherapy
British Journal Preventive Social Medicine
British Journal Psychiatry
British Journal Social Clinical Psychology
British Medical Journal
Bruxelles Médical
Bulletin Academy Medicine New Jersey
Bulletin Mathematical Biophysics
Bulletin New York Academy Medicine
Bulletin de Physio-Pathology Respiratoire
Bulletin Polish Medical Science History
Bulletin Postgraduate Committee Medicine, University of Sydney
Bulletin der Schweizerischen Akademie der Medizinischen Wissenschaften
Bulletin de la Société Internationale de Cardiologie
Bulletin de la Société Internationale de Chirurgie
Bulletin de la Société Médicale d'Afrique Noire de Langue Francaise
Byulleten Eksperimental'noi Biologii i Meditsiny

Cahiers d'Anesthésiologie
Cahiers du Collège de Médecine des Hôspitaux de Paris
Cahiers de Kinesitherapie
Calcified Tissue Research
California's Health
California Medicine
Canadian Anaesthetists' Society Journal
Canadian Journal Physiological Pharmacology
Canadian Journal Physiology Pharmacology
Canadian Journal Public Health
Canadian Journal Surgery
Canadian Medical Association Journal
Canadian Medical Journal
Cardiac Rehabilitation
Cardiologia
Cardiologia Pratica
Cardiology
Cardiology Digest
Cardiovascular Clinics
Cardiovascular Research
Cardiovascular Research Center Bulletin
Casopis Lekaru Ceckych
Ceskoslovenske Zdravotnictvi
Ceylon Medical Journal
Chemistry

Chest
Chimie Therapeutique
Chirurg
Chirurgie Pratique
Circulation
Circulation Research
Cleveland Clinic Quarterly
Clinica Terapeutica
Clinical Chemistry
Clinical Medicine
Clinical Nutrition
Clinical Orthopaedics
Clinical Pharmacology Therapeutics
Clinical Research
Clinical Science
Clinician
Clinique
Coeur et Médecine Interne
Coimbra (Universidade) Medecinal
Community Health
Comparative Biochemistry and Physiology A:
    Comparative Physiology
Comprehensive Psychiatry
Comptes Rendus Société Biologique
Computers Biomedical Research
Connecticut Medical Journal
Consultant
Cor et Vasa
Corse Méditerranée Médicale
Cuore e Circolazione
Current Therapeutic Research Clinical Experi-
    mental

Danish Medical Bulletin
Dapim Refuiim
Das Offentliche Gesundheitswesen
Delaware Medical Journal
Deutsche Archiv für Klinische Medizin
Deutsche Gesundheitswesen
Deutsche Medizinische Wochenschrift
Dia Medico
Diabetes
Diagnostica
Diagnostik
Disease-a-Month
Diseases Chest
Diseases Nervous System
Dissertation Abstracts
Dissertation Abstracts, International Section B
    Science and Engineering
Documenta de Medicina Geographica et
    Tropica
Doklady Akademii Nauk SSSR
Drug Intelligence Clinical Pharmacy
Duodecim

Eksperimentnal'naya Khirurgia i Anestezi-
    ologiya
Electroencephalography Clinical Neurophysi-
    ology
Emergency Medicine
Erfahrungsheilkunde
Ergonomics
Europa Medicophysica
European Journal Clinical Pharmacology
European Journal Pharmacology
European Surgical Research
Evolution Médicale
Excerpta Medica
Experimental Medicine Surgery

Federation Proceedings
Finska Lakaresallskapets Handliger
Fiziologia Normală Patologică
Fiziologicheskii Zhurnal SSSR
Fiziologisheskii Zhurnal SSSR Imeni I.M.
    Sechenova
Fiziolohichnyi Zhurnal
Folia Angiologica
Folia Cardiologica (Milano)
Folia Clinica Internacional (Barcelona)
Folia Medica
Folia Medica Neerlandica
Folia Morphologica
Försvarsmedicin
Fortschritte auf dem Gebiete der Roentgen-
    strahlen und der Nuklearmedizin
Fortschritte der Medizin

Gaslini
Gazette Médicale de France
Gazzetta Internazionale de Medicina Chirugia
Gazzetta Italiana di Cardiologia
Geneeskundige Gids
Geriatrics
Gerontologia Clinica
Gerontologist
Gigiena i Sanitariya
Gigiena Truda Professional'nye Zabolevaniya
Giornale di Batteriologia, Virologia ed Immuno-
    logia
Giornale di Gerontologia
Giornale di Igiene e Medicina Preventiva
Giornale Italiano di Cardiologia
Giornale di Psichiatria e di Neuropatologia
Group for the Advancement of Psychiatry,
    Symposium
Grudnaia Khirurgia
Gruzica i Choroby Pluc

Haematologica
Harefuah Journal Israel Medical Association
Hartford Hospital Bulletin
Hawaii Medical Journal
Health Service Reports
Heart Bulletin
Heart Lung
Heilberufe
Hellenic Armed Forces Medical Review
Hellenike Iatrike
Helvetica Medica Acta
Henry Ford Hospital Medical Journal
Herz Kreislauf
Higiena i Zdraveopazvane
Hippokrates
Hisotchemie
Hospital Community Psychiatry
Hospital Practice

IEEE Transactions Bio-Medical Engineering
Indian Heart Journal
Indian Journal Medical Science
Indian Medical Forum
Indian Medical Journal
Indian Pediatrics
Indian Practitioner
Industrial Medicine Surgery
Institute Electrical Electronics Engineers,
    Transactions Biomedical Engineering BME
Instrumentation
Internal Medicine Digest
International Journal Biometeorology
International Journal Clinical Experimental
    Hypnosis
International Journal Epidemiology
International Journal Group Psychotherapy
International Journal Psychiatry
International Journal Psycho-Analysis
Internationale Zeitschrift für Angewandte
    Physiologie
Internationale Zeitschrift für Angewandte
    Physiologie einschliesslich Arbeits-
    physiologie
Internationales Archiv für Arbeitsmedizin
Internist
Irish Journal Medical Science
Israel Journal Medical Sciences

Japanese Circulation Journal
Japanese Heart Journal
Japanese Journal Anesthesiology
Japanese Journal Clinical Medicine
Japanese Journal Medicine
Johns Hopkins Medical Journal
Journal Abnormal Psychology

Journal American College Health Association
Journal American Dietetic Association
Journal American Geriatric Society
Journal American Medical Association
Journal American Medical Women's Association
Journal American Osteopathic Association
Journal Applied Physiology
Journal Arkansas Medical Society
Journal Association Advancement Medical In-
    strumentation
Journal Association Physicians India
Journal Atherosclerosis Research
Journal Biomedical Materials Research
Journal Biosocial Science
Journal Biosocial Studies
Journal Bone Joint Surgery
Journal Brasileiro de Doencas Toracicas
Journal Cardiovascular Surgery
Journal Chronic Diseases
Journal Clinical Endocrinology
Journal Clinical Investigation
Journal Clinical Laboratory Investigation
Journal Clinical Pathology
Journal Clinical Pharmacology
Journal Clinical Psychology
Journal College General Practitioners
Journal Comparative Physiology Psychology
Journal Consulting Clinical Psychology
Journal Dynamic Systems
Journal Egyptian Medical Association
Journal Electrocardiology
Journal Experimental Medicine
Journal Forensic Sciences
Journal Gerontology
Journal Health Human Behavior
Journal Health Social Behavior
Journal Human Sexuality
Journal Indian Medical Association
Journal Internal Medicine
Journal Iowa Medical Society
Journal Irish College Physicians Surgeons
Journal Irish Medical Association
Journal Japanese Psychomatic Society
Journal Japanese Society Internal Medicine
Journal Kansas Medical Society
Journal Laboratory Clinical Medicine
Journal Louisiana State Medical Society
Journal Maine Medical Association
Journal de Médecine de Bordeaux
Journal Medical Association Alabama
Journal Medical Association Georgia
Journal Medical Association Thailand
Journal Medical Society New Jersey
Journal Médical de Strasbourg
Journal Medical Surgery
Journal Medicine
Journal Molecular Cellular Cardiology
Journal Mount Sinai Hospital
Journal National Cancer Institute

Journal Nervous Mental Disease
Journal New Drugs
Journal Nuclear Medicine
Journal Nutrition
Journal Oklahoma State Medical Association
Journal Oral Medicine
Journal Osaka City Medical Center
Journal Pediatrics
Journal Personality Social Psychology
Journal Pharmacology Experimental Therapeutics
Journal Pharmacology Experimental Therapy
Journal Pharmacy Pharmacology
Journal Philippine Federation Private Medical Practitioners
Journal Philippine Medical Association
Journal Physiologie
Journal Physiology (London)
Journal Psychosomatic Research
Journal de Radiologie et d'Electrologie
Journal Rehabilitation
Journal Respiratory Disease
Journal Royal College Physicians
Journal School Health
Journal des Sciences Médicales de Lille
Journal South Carolina Medical Association
Journal Sport Medicine
Journal Sports Medicine Physical Fitness
Journal Steroid Biochemistry
Journal Surgical Research
Journal Tennessee Medical Association
Journal Thoracic Cardiovascular Surgery
Journal Thoracic Surgery
Journal Tokyo Medical College

Kardiologia Polska
Kardiologiya
Kazanskii Meditsinkii Zhurnal
Klinische Medizin
Klinische Wochenschrift
Klinicheskaya Meditsina
Korean Journal Internal Medicine

Laboratory Investigation
Lancet
Landarzt
Langenbecks Archiv für Chirurgie
Latvijas psr Zinatnu Akademijas Vestis
Laval Médical
Lekarska Veda v Zahranici
Life Sciences
Life Sciences, Part II, Biochemistry, General and Molecular Biology
Lijecnicki Vjesnik
Lyon Médical

Magyar Belorvosi Archivum
Malattie Cardiovascolari
Manitoba Medical Review
Maroc Médical
Maryland State Medical Journal
Massachusetts Journal Medical Technology
Materia Medica Polona
Mayo Clinic Proceedings
Médecine Tropicale
Medica Mundi
Medical Annuals District of Columbia
Medical Aspects Human Sexuality
Medical Biological Engineering
Medical Clinics North America
Medical Digest
Medical Economics
Medical Electronics Biological Engineering
Medical Journal Australia
Medical Letter Drugs Therapeutics
Medical Record Annals
Medical Research Engineering
Medical Times
Medical Trial Technique Quarterly
Medical Tribune
Médicale du Canada
Medicina (Rijeka)
Medicina Clinica
Medicina Española
Medicina Interna
Medicina dello Sport
Medicine
Medicine Science Sports
Medicine Sport
Medicinski Glasnik
Medikon
Medizin und Ernährung
Medizin und Sport
Medizinische Klinik
Medizinische Monatsschrift
Medizinische Technik
Medizinische Welt
Medizinische Wochenschrift
Metabolism
Metamedica
Methods Information Medicine
Microvascular Research
Milbank Memorial Fund Quarterly
Military Medicine
Minerva Anestesiologica
Minerva Cardioangiologica
Minerva Cardiologica
Minerva Medica
Minnesota Medicine
Modern Concepts Cardiovascular Diseases
Modern Geriatrics
Modern Medicine
Modern Treatment
Monatsschrift für Kinderheilkunde
Mount Sinai Journal Medicine
Münchener Medizinische Wochenschrift

Nagoya Journal Medical Science
Nagoya Journal Medicine
Naika
National Conference Cardiovascular Diseases
Nature
Naturwissenschaften
Nederlands Milk Dairy Journal
Nederlands Tijdschrift voor Geneeskunde
Neurology
New England Journal Medicine
New York State Journal Medicine
New Zealand Medical Journal
Nippon Acta Radiologica
Nippon University Medical Journal
Nordisk Medicin
Northwest Medicine
Nosokomejaka Chronika
Nouvelle Presse Médicale
Novosti Meditsinskogo Priborostroeniia
Nuclear Medizin
Nursing Research
Nursing Times

Obesity Bariatric Medicine
Öffentliche Gesundheitswesen
Ohio State Medical Journal
Opuscula Medica
Orvosi Hetilap
Ospedale Maggiore

Pahlavi Medical Journal
Patient Care
Patologia Polska
Pediatric Clinics North America
Pediatrics
Pennsylvania Medicine
Perceptual Motor Skills
Pflügers Archiv (European Journal Physiology)
Pharmacologia Clinica
Physical Fitness Research Digest
Physical Therapy
Physiological Behavior
Physiological Reviews
Physiologist
Physiotherapy
Policlinico: Sezione Pratica
Polish Medical Journal
Polski Przeglad Chirurgizny
Polski Tygodnik Lekarski
Polskie Archiwum Medycyny Wewnetrznej
Postgraduate Medical Journal
Postgraduate Medicine
Poumon et le Coeur
Pracovni Lekarstvi
Practitioner

Praxis
Praxis der Psychotherapie
Prensa Médica Argentina
Presse Médicale
Prevent
Preventive Medicine
Problemy Endokrinologii
Proceedings Association Research Nervous Mental Disease
Proceedings International Congress Gerontology
Proceedings Medical Section American Life Convention
Proceedings of the National Meeting Biophysics Biotechnology, Finland
Proceedings New England Cardiovascular Society
Proceedings Nutrition Society
Proceedings Royal Society London, B.
Proceedings Royal Society Medicine
Proceedings Society Experimental Biology Medicine
Proceedings Western Pharmacological Society
Progress Cardiology
Progress Cardiovascular Diseases
Progress Report Medicophysical Institute TNO
Progresso Medico
Protectio Vitae
Przeglad Epidemiologiczny
Przeglad Lekarski
Psychiatric Communications
Psychiatrie, Neurologie und Medizinische Psychologie
Psychiatry Digest
Psychiatry Medicine
Psychological Medicine
Psychological Reports
Psychopharmacologia
Psychosomatic Medicine
Psychosomatics
Psychotherapy Psychosomatics
Public Health Reports

Quarterly Journal Medicine
Quarterly Journal Studies on Alcohol

Radiation Data Reports
Radiologica Medica
Radiology
Rassegna Geriatria
Rassegna Internazionale di Clinica e Terapia
Rassegna di Medicina Sperimentale
Recenti Progressi in Medicina
Rehabilitacia
Rehabilitation

Rehabilitation Literature
Rehabilitation Record
Research Communications Chemical Pathology
  Pharmacology
Research News
Research Quarterly
Research Quarterly American Association for
  Health, Physical Education, Recreation
Revista Argentina de Cardiologia
Revista de la Asociacion Médica Argentina
Revista Brasileira Cardiovascular
Revista Clinica Expañola
Revista da Associacao Medica Brasileira
Revista del Colegio Medico de Guatemala
Revista Espanola de Cardiologia
Revista Medica de Chile
Revista Medica de Cordoba
Revista Medico-Chirurgicală a Societatii de
  Medici și Naturaliști din Iași
Revista de Sanidad e Higiene Pública
Revista da Sociedade Brasileira de Medicina
  Tropical
Revue Epidémiologie Médecine Sociale Santé
  Publique
Revue Lyonnaise Médicale
Revue Médicale de Dijon
Revue de Médecine Psychosomatique (Paris)
Revue de Médecine de Tours
Revue Médicale de Liège
Revue Médicale du Moyen-Orient
Revue Médicale Suisse Romande
Revue de Neuropsychiatrie Infantile
Revue du Praticien
Revue de Réadaptation
Revue Roumaine de Médecine Interne
Revue Roumaine de Physiologie
Rheumatologia Balneologia Allergologia
Rheumatology and Physical Medicine
Rhode Island Medical Journal
Riforma Medica
Rivista degli Infortoni e delle Malattie Profes-
  sionali
Rivista Istituto Vaccinogeno Consorzi Provincia
  Antituberculosi, Milano
Rivista di Medicina Aeronautica e Spaziale

Sangre
Sbornik Lekarsky
Sbornik Vědeckých Praci Lékařské Fakulty
  Karlovy Universitas
Scandinavian Archives Physiology
Scandinavian Journal Clinical Laboratory In-
  vestigation
Scandinavian Journal Clinical Laboratory In-
  vestigation (Suppl.)
Scandinavian Journal Rehabilitation Medicine
Scandinavian Journal Thoracic Cardiovascular
  Surgery

Schweizerische Medizinische Wochenschrift
Schweizerische Zeitschrift für Sportmedizin
Science
Scottish Medical Journal
Second National Conference Cardiovascular
  Diseases
Semaine des Hôpitaux de Paris
Seminars in Hematology
Sexual Behavior
Sexulogy
Singapore Medical Journal
Social Medicinsk Tidskrift
Social Science Medicine
Sociology Science Medicine
South African Medical Journal
Southern Medical Bulletin
Southern Medical Journal
Sovetskaya Meditsina
Spri Rad
Srpski Arhiv za Celokupno Lekarstvo
Statistical Bulletin
Stroke
Studii și Cercetări de Fiziologie
Sudebno-Meditsinskaia Ekspertiza
Surgery
Surgery Gynecology Obstetrics
Suvremenna Meditsina

Technische Gids voor Ziekenhuis en Instelling
Terapevticheskii Arkhiv
Texas Medicine
Texas State Journal Medicine
Therapeutische Umschau
Therapie
Therapie der Gegenwart
Therapiewoche
Thorax
Thoraxchirurgie
Thoraxchirurgie Vaskuläre Chirurgie
Thrombosis et Diathesis Haemorrhagica
Tidsskrift for den Norske Laegeforening
Tijdschrift voor Aangepaste Werkvoorziening
Tijdschrift voor Geneeskunde
Tidjdschrift voor Sociale Geneeskunde
Tohoku
El Torax
Transactions American Society Artificial In-
  ternal Organs
Transactions Association Life Insurance Medi-
  cal Directors of America
Transactions New York Academy Sciences
Transactions Royal Society Tropical Medicine
  Hygiene
Transactions Society Occupational Medicine
Travail Humain
Triangle
Tropical Geographical Medicine
Trudy Vornezhskogo Meditsinskogo Instituta

Ugeskrift for Laeger
Union Médicale du Canada
University Michigan Medical Center Journal
Upsala Journal Medical Sciences

Vascular Diseases
Vascular Surgery
Verhandlungen der Deutschen Gessellshaft für
    Innere Medizin
Verhandlungen der Deutschen Gesellschaftt für
    Kreislaufforschung
Vestnik Akademii Meditsinskikh Nauk SSSR
Vestnik Khirurgii Imenii Grekova
Viaţa Medicală
Virginia Medical Monthly
Vnitrni Lekarstir
Voeding
Voprosy Kurortologii Fiziotherapii i Lechebnoi
    Fizicheskoy Kul'tury
Voprosy Pitaniya
Voprosy Reumatisma
Vrachebnoe Delo

West Virginia Medical Journal
Western Medicine
Wiadomosci Lekarskie
Wiener Klinische Wochenschrift
Wisconsin Medical Journal
World Health Organization Chronicle
World Health Organization Technical Report
    Series
World Review Nutrition Dietetics

Yale Journal Biological Medicine

Zdravookhranenie Belorusskii
Zdravookhranenie Kazakhstana
Zeitschrift für Aerztliche Fortbildung (Jena)
Zeitschrift für Allgemeine Medizin der Landarzt
Zeitschrift für Alternsforschung
Zeitschrift für Angewandte Bäder- und Klima-
    heilkunde
Zeitschrift für Erkrankungen der Atmungs-
    organe
Zeitschrift für Experimentelle und Angewandte
    Psychologie
Zeitschrift für Gesamte Experimentalle Medizin
Zeitschrift für die Gesamte Hygiene
Zeitschrift für die Gesamte Hygiene und Ihre
    Grenzgebiete
Zeitschrift für Gesamte Innere Medizin
Zeitschrift für die Gesamte Innere Medizin und
    Ihre Grenzgebiete
Zeitschrift für Innere Medizin
Zeitschrift für Kardiologie
Zeitschrift für Kreislaufforschung
Zeitschrift für Physikalische Medizin
Zeitschrift für Physiotherapie
Zeitschrift für Praktische Anaesthesie und
    Wiederbelebung
Zeitschrift für Praeventiv Medizin
Zeitschrift für Psychosomatische Medizin und
    Psychoanalyse
Zhurnal Eksperimental'noi i Teoreticheskoi
    Fizikii
Zhurnal Vysshei Nervnoi Deiatel'nosti

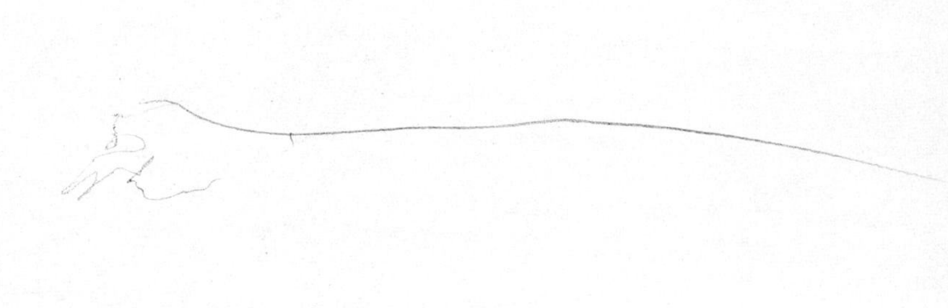